PDxMD

Differential Diagnosis
with Clinical Benchmarks

PDxMD Differential Diagnosis is dedicated by the staff of PDxMD to Fiona Foley and the entire Editorial Faculty for their leadership in the development of new and innovative ways of organizing information in support of quality patient care.

PDxMD

Differential Diagnosis

with Clinical Benchmarks

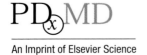

An Imprint of Elsevier Science

Philadelphia ■ St Louis ■ London ■ Sydney ■ New York ■ Toronto

PDxMD
An imprint of Elsevier Science

Publisher:	Steven Merahn, MD
Project Managers:	Caroline Barnett, Lucy Hamilton, Zak Knowles
Programmer:	Narinder Chandi
Production:	Aoibhe O'Shea – GMS UK, Alan Palfreyman – PTU
Designer:	Jayne Jones
Layout:	The Designers Collective Limited

Printed in China by RDC Group

PDxMD
Elsevier Science
The Curtis Center
625 Walnut Street,
Philadelphia, PA 19106

The
Publisher's
policy is to use
**paper manufactured
from sustainable forests**

ISBN 1-932141-00-6

Introduction

What is PDxMD?

PDxMD is a new, evidence-based primary care clinical information system designed to support your judgment with practical clinical information. The content is continuously updated by expert contributors with the latest on evaluation, diagnosis, management, outcomes and prevention – all designed for use at the point and time of care.

First and foremost, PDxMD is an electronic resource. This book gives you access to just a fraction of the content available on-line. At www.pdxmd.com, you will find:

- Over 330 signs and symptoms and more than 1180 conditions set out in a unique matrix system that enables you to search for information according to your patient's chief complaint
- Information on more than 450 medical conditions and more than 750 drugs and other therapies, organized in condition-specific 'MediFiles'
- Patient information sheets on 300 topics for you to customize and hand to your patient during consultation

About this book

PDxMD Differential Diagnosis with Clinical Benchmarks is a print version of the electronic Differential Diagnosis tools (DDxFiles) found on PDxMD. This book is divided into two parts:

Part One: Differential Diagnosis is a series of more than 330 tables, organized in alphabetical order by Chief Complaint. Each table provides lists of potential diagnoses sorted by age and relative prevalence.

Part Two is an alphabetical listing of more than 1180 Clinical Benchmarks – twelve clinical findings and features associated with specific diagnoses:

- Onset
- Male:Female Ratio
- Ethnic prevalence
- Character of symptomatology
- Location of signs and symptoms
- Patterns of signs and symptoms
- Precipitating Factors
- Relieving Factors
- Clinical Course
- Co-Morbidities
- Procedure Results
- Test Findings

These Clinical Benchmarks provide comprehensive diagnostic decision support, including rapid comparison between potential diagnoses. This approach allows for individual patient differences by focusing on the physician's thought process as central to appropriate diagnosis.

Introduction

How to use this book
The two parts of this book can be used individually or together.

To use Part One: Differential Diagnosis
Chief Complaints are listed in alphabetical order. Find the table associated with your patient's chief complaint. Look under the appropriate age range column to review the list of possible diagnoses. Select one or more that may be applicable based on your current assessment of the patient.

The diagnoses are listed in order of relative, not absolute, prevalence, based on general review of epidemiologic and other health statistics data. If there are multiple complaints, select a 'lead complaint' and compare between the relevant Clinical Benchmarks to help shape your diagnostic decision.

To use Part Two: Clinical Benchmarks
Clinical Benchmarks are listed by diagnosis in alphabetical order. Based on your clinical judgment or your use of the tables in Part One, find the Clinical Benchmarks for the diagnoses under consideration and compare and contrast them to the patient. As necessary, compare Clinical Benchmarks between diagnoses to help further define the patient's profile. Clinical Benchmarks can facilitate your thinking regarding the evaluation and workup necessary to confirm your patient's condition or status.

If you require additional information on the diagnostic evaluation or management of a specific medical condition, see the relevant volume from the PDxMD Medical Conditions Series or the electronic version of PDxMD (www.pdxmd.com).

How are DDxFiles created?
PDxMD is created using a special process of Collaborative Authoring. This process allows medical information to be reviewed and synthesized from multiple sources – including but not limited to peer-reviewed articles, evidence databases, guidelines and position papers – and by multiple individuals, organized around and integrated into a standard 'template' that matches the needs of primary care physicians in practice.

The templates used here are the Differential Diagnosis tables arranged by chief complaint, age, and relative prevalence found in Part One, and the twelve-point Clinical Benchmarks found in Part Two.

The Differential Diagnosis tables were prepared by a team of physicians led by Editorial Advisory Board member David Fairchild. The individual diagnostic pathways that comprise the Clinical Benchmarks sections were written by specialist physicians. Dr Fairchild worked closely with the team throughout to ensure that the information is accurate and properly organized. Online DDxFiles are constantly reviewed and updated: the material presented here represents a snapshot in time of the electronic Differential Diagnosis tool.

A complete list of Editorial Faculty and staff of PDxMD is provided below. All Editorial Faculty, and specifically the Editorial Advisory Board members, participate in PDxMD as individuals and not as representatives of, or on behalf of, their affiliated institutions or associations and any indication of their affiliation with a specific institution or association should not be taken as an endorsement of PDxMD or any participation of their institution or association with PDxMD.

Introduction

Continuous Product Improvement

PDxMD is committed to continuous quality improvement and welcomes any comments, suggestions and feedback from the professional community. Please send any ideas or considerations regarding this volume or any other volume in the PDxMD series via e-mail to feedback.pdxmd@elsevier.com or to PDxMD, Elsevier Science, The Curtis Center, 625 Walnut Street, Philadelphia, PA 19106.

Acknowledgments

PDxMD would like to thank the following for their kind permission to reproduce images:

Gary White, Associate Clinical Professor, Department of Dermatology, University of California, San Diego, CA
Acne rosacea (p402), Acne vulgaris (p402), Alopecia areata (p411), Atopic dermatitis (p423), Basal cell carcinoma (p431), Behçet's disease (p432), Bullous pemphigoid (p438), Cellulitis (p444), Contact dermatitis (p459), Corns (p460), Drug reaction (pp471, 473), Dupuytren's contracture (p474), Erythema multiforme (p482), Erythema nodosum (p483), Folliculitis (p493), Furunculosis (p495), Herpes simplex (p512, P, L), Herpes zoster (p513), Hidradenitis suppurativa (p513), Impetigo (p523), Ingrown nail (p525), Lichen planus (p536), Lichen sclerosis (p536), Melanoma (p546), Onychomycosis (p565), Paronychia (p572), Photodermatitis (p579), Pityriasis rosea (p580), Pityriasis versicolor (p580), Psoriasis (p593), Ringworm (p606), Scabies (p609), Seborrheic dermatitis (p611), Seborrheic keratosis (p612), Squamous cell carcinoma (p620), Stasis dermatitis (p621), Stevens-Johnson syndrome (p621), Sunburn (p624), Systemic lupus erythematosus (p625), Vitiligo (p645).

Myron Yanoff, Professor & Chair, Department of Ophthalmology, MCP Hahnemann University, Philadelphia, PA
Bacterial conjunctivitis (p428), Cataract (p442), Corneal abrasion (p459), Episcleritis (p481), Glaucoma (p500), Herpes simplex (p512, C), Hordeolum (p515), Retinoblastoma (p602), Sarcoidosis (p608), Scleritis (p610), Uveitis (p640), Viral conjunctivitis (p643).

Basil Zitelli, Professor of Pediatrics, University of Pittsburgh School of Medicine, Children's Hospital of Pittsburgh, Pittsburgh PA
Child abuse (p448), Down syndrome (p471), Teething (p626).

Editorial Faculty and Staff

Executive Committee

Editorial Faculty and Staff

Editorial Board

Editorial Faculty and Staff

Editorial Faculty and Staff

Editorial Faculty and Staff

Differential Diagnosis Contributors

David G Fairchild, MD, MPH
Primary Care, Signs & Symptoms
Brigham and Women's Hospital
Boston, MA

James Bastian, MD
Pediatrics
Brigham & Women's Hospital
Wellesley, MA

Gordon Baustian, MD
Family Medicine
Director of Medical Education and
Residency
Cedar Rapids Medical Education
Foundation
Cedar Rapids, IA

Neil Bhattacharyya, MD, FACS
Otology, Laryngology
Assistant Professor of Otology and
Laryngology
Brigham and Women's Hospital
Boston, MA

Nabil Chehade, MD
Urology
Urology Department
Kaiser Permanente Medical Center
Parma, OH

Mary E Colpoys, MD
Pediatrics
Alewife Brook Community Pediatrics
Arlington, MA

Joshua M Cooper, MD
Cardiology
Fellow in Cardiovascular Medicine
Brigham and Women's Hospital
Boston, MA

Phillip W Cushman, MD
Psychiatry
Clinical Assistant Professor of Psychiatry
University of Florida College of Medicine
Gainesville, FL

Fred F Ferri, MD, FACP
Family Medicine
Clinical Professor
Brown University of Medicine, Chief
Division of Internal Medicine
Fatima Hospital, St Joseph's Health
Services
Providence, RI

David S Geller, MD, FAAP
Pediatrics
Patriot Pediatrics
Bedford, MA

Shalini Goyal, MD
General Medicine
Instructor of Medicine, Harvard Medical
School
Associate Physician, Department of
General Medicine
Brigham and Women's Hospital
Boston, MA

James A Greenberg, MD
Obstetrics, Gynecology
Vice Chairman
Department of Obstetrics/Gynecology
Brigham and Women's/Faulkner Hospitals
Boston, MA

Galen Henderson, MD
Pulmonology
Pulmonary and Critical Care Medicine
Brigham and Women's Hospital
Boston, MA

Francine Hennessey, MD
Pediatrics, Adolescent Medicine
Patriot Pediatrics
Bedford, MA

Russell C Jones, MD, MPH
Family Medicine
Dartmouth Medical School
New London, NH

Editorial Faculty and Staff

Editorial Faculty and Staff

John Stamatoyannopoulos
Molecular Oncology
Dana Farber Cancer Institute
Boston, MA

Lisa L Strate, MD, MPH
Gastroenterology
Instructor in Medicine
Harvard Medical School
Division of Gastroenterology
Brigham and Women's Hospital
Boston, MA

Jonathan Strongin, MD, PhD
Pulmonology
Medical Director of Respiratory Care
Cambridge Health Alliance
Cambridge, MA

Barry Tils, MD
Emergency Medicine
Department of Emergency Medicine
Newton-Wellesley Hospital
Newton, MA

Sigal Yawetz, MD
Infectious Diseases
Division of Infectious Diseases
Brigham & Women's Hospital
Boston, MA

Staff

Management Team
Fiona Foley, Steven Merahn, MD,
Daniel Pollock, Zak Knowles,
Howard Croft, Tanya Thomas, Lucy
Hamilton, Julie Volck, Bill Bruggemeyer,
Andrea Ford

Editorial Team
Anne Dyson, Sadaf Hashmi, Debbie
Goring, Louise Morrison, Ellen Haigh,
Robert Whittle, Claire Champion, Caroline
Barnett, Laurie Smith, Li Wan, Paul
Mayhew, Carmen Jones, Fi Ward

Technical Team
Martin Miller, Narinder Chandi, Roy
Patterson, Aaron McGrath, John Wylie,
Sarah Craze, Cameron Sangster

We would also like to acknowledge the
extraordinary contributions of the
following individuals to the
conceptualization and realization of
PDxMD over the initial years of its growth
and development:

Tim Hailstone, Jonathan Black,
Alison Whitehouse, Jayne Harris, Angela
Baggi, Sharon Bambaji, Sam Bedser,
Layla van den Bergh, Stuart Boffey,
Siobhan Egan, Helen Elder,
Mark Mitchenall, Chris Moodie, Tony
Pollard, Simon Seljeflot, Liz Southey, Tim
Stentiford, Matthew Whyte

Part One

Differential Diagnosis

- Chief Complaints are listed in alphabetical order.

- Find the table associated with your patient's Chief Complaint.

- Look under the appropriate age range column to review the list of possible diagnoses.

- Select one or more that may be applicable based on your current assessment of the patient.

The diagnoses are listed in order of relative, not absolute, prevalence, based on general review of epidemiologic and other health statistics data.

If there are multiple complaints, select a 'lead complaint' and compare between the relevant Clinical Benchmarks to help shape your diagnostic decision.

Emergency Rule Out conditions shown in red. Entries in blue are for information only
Conditions are listed in approximate order of prevalence for this age range

Abdominal bloating

Baby (0-1 yr)	Child (1-12 yr)	Adolescent (12-18 yr)	Adult (18-45 yr)	Middle Age Adult (45-65 yr)	Senior Adult (65+ yr)
Aerophage	Aerophage	Aerophage	Aerophage	Aerophage	Aerophage
Intestinal obstruction	Nonabsorbable carbohydrate	Intestinal obstruction	Intestinal obstruction	Intestinal obstruction	Intestinal obstruction
Nonabsorbable carbohydrate	Carcinoid syndrome	Fatty food intolerance	Irritable bowel syndrome	Irritable bowel syndrome	Gastroenteritis
Gastroenteritis	Intestinal obstruction	Gastroenteritis	Gastroenteritis	Gastroenteritis	Nonabsorbable carbohydrate
Celiac disease	Gastroenteritis	Chronic fatigue syndrome	Chronic fatigue syndrome	Chronic fatigue syndrome	Celiac disease
Giardiasis	Celiac disease	Nonabsorbable carbohydrate	Celiac disease	Carcinoid syndrome	Fatty food intolerance
Carcinoid syndrome	Fatty food intolerance	Celiac disease	Fatty food intolerance	Fatty food intolerance	Carcinoid syndrome
Lactose intolerance	Giardiasis	Irritable bowel syndrome	Carcinoid syndrome	Nonabsorbable carbohydrate	Irritable bowel syndrome
Gastric dilation	Irritable bowel syndrome	Carcinoid syndrome	Nonabsorbable carbohydrate	Celiac disease	Lactose intolerance
Imperforate anus	Gastric dilation	Giardiasis	Lactose intolerance	Lactose intolerance	Giardiasis
		Lactose intolerance	Giardiasis	Giardiasis	Chronic fatigue syndrome
		Gastric dilation			

Baby (0-1 yr)	Child (1-12 yr)	Adolescent (12-18 yr)	Adult (18-45 yr)	Middle Age Adult (45-65 yr)	Senior Adult (65+ yr)
Neuroblastoma	Constipation	Constipation	Hepatomegaly	Hepatomegaly	Hepatomegaly
Germ cell ovarian cancer	Encopresis	Pregnancy	Fecal mass	Fecal mass	Abdominal aortic aneurysm
Sex cord/stromal ovarian cancer	Intussusception	Trauma	Splenomegaly	Diverticular disease	Colon cancer
Carcinoid syndrome	Germ cell ovarian cancer	Sex cord/stromal ovarian cancer	Crohn's disease	Epithelial cell ovarian cancer	Pancreatic cancer
Hepatoma	Trauma	Hodgkin's disease	Ulcerative colitis	Splenomegaly	Epithelial cell ovarian cancer
Epithelial cell ovarian cancer	Sex cord/stromal ovarian cancer	Carcinoid syndrome	Pancreatic pseudocyst	Germ cell ovarian cancer	Germ cell ovarian cancer
Pyloric stenosis	Hepatoma	Hepatoma	Hepatoma	Hepatoma	Hepatoma
Nephroblastoma (Wilms' tumor)	Carcinoid syndrome	Germ cell ovarian cancer	Carcinoid syndrome	Sex cord/stromal ovarian cancer	Sex cord/stromal ovarian cancer
	Neuroblastoma	Epithelial cell ovarian cancer	Sex cord/stromal ovarian cancer	Carcinoid syndrome	Fecal mass
	Nephroblastoma (Wilms' tumor)	Crohn's disease	Germ cell ovarian cancer	Colon cancer	Carcinoid syndrome
	Epithelial cell ovarian cancer	Ulcerative colitis	Epithelial cell ovarian cancer	Pancreatic cancer	Gastric cancer
	Crohn's disease	Acute leukemia	Diverticular disease	Gastric cancer	Metastatic cancer
	Ulcerative colitis	Non-Hodgkin's lymphoma	Abdominal aortic aneurysm	Metastatic cancer	Metastatic neoplasm of the liver
	Volvulus	Encopresis	Colon cancer	Metastatic neoplasm of the liver	Diverticular disease
	Acute leukemia		Pancreatic cancer	Pancreatic pseudocyst	Splenomegaly
			Gastric cancer	Abdominal aortic aneurysm	Pancreatic pseudocyst
			Metastatic neoplasm of the liver	Crohn's disease	Crohn's disease
			Metastatic cancer	Ulcerative colitis	Ulcerative colitis

Emergency Rule Out conditions shown in red. Entries in blue are for information only

Conditions are listed in approximate order of prevalence for this age range

Abdominal pain, chronic/recurrent

Emergency Rule Out conditions shown in red. Entries in blue are for information only
Conditions are listed in approximate order of prevalence for this age range

Baby (0-1 yr)	Child (1-12 yr)	Adolescent (12-18 yr)	Adult (18-45 yr)	Middle Age Adult (45-65 yr)	Senior Adult (65-yr)
Urinary tract infection	Urinary tract infection	Urinary tract infection	Dysmenorrhea	Irritable bowel syndrome	Irritable bowel syndrome
Intestinal obstruction	Constipation	Constipation	Irritable bowel syndrome	Peptic ulcer	Peptic ulcer
Intussusception	Psychosomatic	Hepatoma	Peptic ulcer	Acute pancreatitis	Acute pancreatitis
Hypercalcemia	Irritable bowel syndrome	Dysmenorrhea	Hypercalcemia	Cholecystitis	Cholecystitis
Carcinoid syndrome	Henoch-Schönlein purpura	Irritable bowel syndrome	Hepatoma	Hypercalcemia	Hypercalcemia
Henoch-Schönlein purpura	Abdominal migraine	Henoch-Schönlein purpura	Henoch-Schönlein purpura	Poliomyelitis	Henoch-Schönlein purpura
Hepatoma	Hypercalcemia	Abdominal migraine	Endometriosis	Henoch-Schönlein purpura	Poliomyelitis
Poliomyelitis	Depression	Psychosomatic	Cholecystitis	Hepatoma	Hepatoma
Volvulus	Hepatoma	Hypercalcemia	Crohn's disease	Carcinoid syndrome	Ischemic bowel disease
Typhoid fever	Intussusception	Typhoid fever	Poliomyelitis	Crohn's disease	Ulcerative colitis
Posterior urethral valves	Carcinoid syndrome	Poliomyelitis	Ulcerative colitis	Ulcerative colitis	Carcinoid syndrome
Constipation	Typhoid fever	Depression	Acute pancreatitis	Typhoid fever	Crohn's disease
Chronic fatigue syndrome	Poliomyelitis	Carcinoid syndrome	Ruptured/ hemorrhagic ovarian cyst	Ischemic bowel disease	Adrenal insufficiency
	Peptic ulcer	Peptic ulcer	Carcinoid syndrome	Adrenal insufficiency	Typhoid fever
	Acute pancreatitis	Acute pancreatitis	Typhoid fever	Pancreatic cancer	Pancreatic cancer
	Renal calculi	Renal calculi	Ovarian torsion	Epithelial cell ovarian cancer	Gastric cancer
	Crohn's disease	Crohn's disease	Intestinal obstruction	Gastric cancer	Epithelial cell ovarian cancer
	Ulcerative colitis	Ulcerative colitis	Adrenal insufficiency	Intestinal obstruction	Intestinal obstruction
	Sexual abuse	Sexual abuse	Pancreatic cancer	Porphyria	Porphyria
	Chronic lead poisoning	Chronic lead poisoning	Epithelial cell ovarian cancer	Chronic fatigue syndrome	Chronic fatigue syndrome
	Esophagitis	Esophagitis	Porphyria		
	Sickle cell anemia	Sickle cell anemia			
	Chronic fatigue syndrome	Chronic fatigue syndrome			

4

Baby (0-1 yr)	Child (1-12 yr)	Adolescent (12-18 yr)	Adult (18-45 yr)	Middle Age Adult (45-65 yr)	Senior Adult (65+yr)
			Ischemic bowel disease Gastric cancer Chronic fatigue syndrome		

Abdominal pain, generalized/periumbilical

Emergency Rule Out conditions shown in red. Entries in blue are for information only
Conditions are listed in approximate order of prevalence for this age range

Baby (0-1 yr)	Child (1-12 yr)	Adolescent (12-18 yr)	Adult (18-45 yr)	Middle Age Adult (45-65 yr)	Senior Adult (65+ yr)
Gastroenteritis	Gastroenteritis	Gastroenteritis	Gastroenteritis	Constipation	Constipation
Constipation	Constipation	Constipation	Constipation	Gastroenteritis	Urinary tract infection
Urinary tract infection	Encopresis	Encopresis	Intestinal parasites	Urinary tract infection	Gastroenteritis
Chlamydia pneumoniae	Irritable bowel syndrome	Testicular torsion	Testicular torsion	Acute pancreatitis	Abdominal abscess
Intestinal parasites	Urinary tract infection	Rocky Mountain spotted fever	Rocky Mountain spotted fever	Irritable bowel syndrome	Intestinal obstruction
Lactose intolerance	Psychosomatic	Irritable bowel syndrome	Irritable bowel syndrome	Intestinal obstruction	Rocky Mountain spotted fever
Diabetes mellitus in children	Testicular torsion	Allergic reactions and anaphylaxis	Acute appendicitis	Acute appendicitis	Intestinal parasites
Campylobacter infection	Rocky Mountain spotted fever	Urinary tract infection	Intestinal obstruction	Renal calculi	Acute iron toxicity
Behçet's syndrome	Addison's disease	Chlamydia pneumoniae	Addison's disease	Rocky Mountain spotted fever	Irritable bowel syndrome
Rocky Mountain spotted fever	Intestinal parasites	Psychosomatic	Campylobacter infection	Allergic reactions and anaphylaxis	Addison's disease
Testicular torsion	Lactose intolerance	Intestinal parasites	Behçet's syndrome	Acute iron toxicity	Allergic reactions and anaphylaxis
Acute iron toxicity	Acute iron toxicity	Acute iron toxicity	Acute iron toxicity	Testicular torsion	Chlamydia pneumoniae
Allergic reactions and anaphylaxis	Diabetes mellitus in children	Addison's disease	Allergic reactions and anaphylaxis	Peritonitis	Acute pancreatitis
Abdominal abscess	Allergic reactions and anaphylaxis	Behçet's syndrome	Chlamydia pneumoniae	Chlamydia pneumoniae	Campylobacter infection
Intussusception	Chlamydia pneumoniae	Campylobacter infection	Acute pancreatitis	Addison's disease	Abdominal aortic aneurysm
Intestinal obstruction	Diabetic ketoacidosis	Lactose intolerance	Abdominal abscess	Behçet's syndrome	Behçet's syndrome
Necrotizing enterocolitis	Meckel's diverticulum	Diabetic ketoacidosis	Urinary tract infection	Campylobacter infection	Abdominal aortic dissection
Pseudomembranous colitis	Sickle cell anemia	Meckel's diverticulum	Abdominal aortic dissection	Ischemic bowel disease	Ischemic bowel disease
	Campylobacter infection	Sickle cell anemia	Peritonitis	Intestinal parasites	Acute appendicitis
	Behçet's syndrome	Peritonitis	Chronic renal failure	Abdominal abscess	Peritonitis
	Intestinal obstruction	Intestinal obstruction	Ischemic bowel disease	Abdominal aortic dissection	Chronic renal failure

Baby (0-1 yr)	Child (1-12 yr)	Adolescent (12-18 yr)	Adult (18-45 yr)	Middle Age Adult (45-65 yr)	Senior Adult (65+ yr)
	Peptic ulcer	Peptic ulcer	Meckel's diverticulum	Abdominal aortic aneurysm	Porphyria
	Chronic lead poisoning	Abdominal abscess	Porphyria	Chronic renal failure	Meckel's diverticulum
	Peritonitis	Cholecystitis	Abdominal aortic aneurysm	Porphyria	Renal calculi
	Abdominal abscess	Pseudomembranous colitis	Pseudomembranous colitis	Meckel's diverticulum	Pseudomembranous colitis
	Intussusception			Mesenteric adenitis	Testicular torsion
	Volvulus			Puerperal infection (endometritis)	
	Cholecystitis			Pseudomembranous colitis	
	Pseudomembranous colitis				

Abdominal pain, generalized/periumbilical (continued)

Emergency Rule Out conditions shown in red. Entries in blue are for information only
Conditions are listed in approximate order of prevalence for this age range

Baby (0-1 yr)	Child (1-12 yr)	Adolescent (12-18 yr)	Adult (18-45 yr)	Middle Age Adult (45-65 yr)	Senior Adult (65+yr)
Colic	Constipation	Constipation	Constipation	Constipation	Constipation
Constipation	Colic	Irritable bowel syndrome	Irritable bowel syndrome	Diverticular disease	Diverticular disease
Volvulus	Irritable bowel syndrome	Colic	Crohn's disease	Irritable bowel syndrome	Irritable bowel syndrome
Cystitis	Cystitis	Muscular strain	Ulcerative colitis	Muscular strain	Muscular strain
Bladder trauma	Bladder trauma	Abdominal hernias	Cystitis	Crohn's disease	Colon cancer
Imperforate anus	Muscular strain	Cystitis	Pelvic inflammatory disease	Bladder trauma	Cystitis
Abdominal abscess	Abdominal hernias	Crohn's disease	Bladder trauma	Cystitis	Abdominal abscess
	Crohn's disease	Ulcerative colitis	Muscular strain	Ulcerative colitis	Bladder trauma
	Ulcerative colitis	Bladder trauma	Abdominal hernias	Abdominal hernias	Abdominal hernias
	Abdominal abscess	Pelvic inflammatory disease	Diverticular disease	Pelvic inflammatory disease	Crohn's disease
	Volvulus	Abdominal abscess	Abdominal abscess	Abdominal abscess	Ulcerative colitis
	Intussusception	Inguinal hernia	Colon cancer	Colon cancer	Volvulus
		Endometriosis	Volvulus	Volvulus	Herpes zoster, shingles
		Ovarian torsion	Inguinal hernia	Herpes zoster, shingles	Intussusception
			Herpes zoster, shingles	Inguinal hernia	
			Ovarian torsion	Intussusception	

8

Baby (0-1 yr)	Child (1-12 yr)	Adolescent (12-18 yr)	Adult (18-45 yr)	Middle Age Adult (45-65 yr)	Senior Adult (65 yr)
Colic	Colic	Colic	Acute pancreatitis	Acute pancreatitis	Acute pancreatitis
Bacterial pneumonia	Viral pneumonia	Viral pneumonia	Pyelonephritis	Splenomegaly	Splenomegaly
Subdiaphragmatic abscess	Bacterial pneumonia	Bacterial pneumonia	Splenomegaly	Pyelonephritis	Pyelonephritis
Abdominal abscess	Mycoplasmal pneumonia	Mycoplasmal pneumonia	Bacterial pneumonia	Bacterial pneumonia	Bacterial pneumonia
Pleural effusion	Pyelonephritis	Pyelonephritis	Viral pneumonia	Viral pneumonia	Viral pneumonia
Splenomegaly	Pleurisy	Pleurisy	Mycoplasmal pneumonia	Mycoplasmal pneumonia	Mycoplasmal pneumonia
	Pleural effusion	Pleural effusion	Splenic infarct	Pleurisy	Herpes zoster, shingles
	Subdiaphragmatic abscess	Endometriosis	Endometriosis	Pericarditis	Pleurisy
	Acute pancreatitis	Ovarian torsion	Ovarian torsion	Endometriosis	Pleural effusion
	Abdominal abscess	Acute pancreatitis	Pleurisy	Ovarian torsion	Myocardial infarction
	Splenomegaly	Subdiaphragmatic abscess	Pleural effusion	Myocardial infarction	Pericarditis
	Pericarditis	Splenomegaly	Myocardial infarction	Pleural effusion	Aspiration pneumonia
		Herpes zoster, shingles	Herpes zoster, shingles	Abdominal abscess	Abdominal abscess
		Abdominal abscess	Subdiaphragmatic abscess	Herpes zoster, shingles	Splenic infarct
		Myocardial infarction	Pericarditis	Subdiaphragmatic abscess	Subdiaphragmatic abscess
		Pericarditis	Abdominal abscess	Aspiration pneumonia	
			Aspiration pneumonia	Splenic infarct	

Emergency Rule Out conditions shown in red. Entries in blue are for information only
Conditions are listed in approximate order of prevalence for this age range

Abdominal pain, left upper quadrant

Emergency Rule Out conditions shown in red. Entries in blue are for information only
Conditions are listed in approximate order of prevalence for this age range

A — Abdominal pain, right lower quadrant

Baby (0-1 yr)	Child (1-12 yr)	Adolescent (12-18 yr)	Adult (18-45 yr)	Middle Age Adult (45-65 yr)	Senior Adult (65+yr)
Colic	Acute appendicitis	Acute appendicitis	Acute appendicitis	Acute appendicitis	Colon cancer
Cystitis	Colic	Colic	Ruptured/ hemorrhagic ovarian cyst	Crohn's disease	Acute appendicitis
Budd-Chiari syndrome	Muscular strain	Muscular strain	Crohn's disease	Ulcerative colitis	Epithelial cell ovarian cancer
Bladder trauma	Ruptured/ hemorrhagic ovarian cyst	Functional benign ovarian tumor	Cystitis	Colon cancer	Germ cell ovarian cancer
Chronic lead poisoning	Cystitis	Cystitis	Ulcerative colitis	Muscular strain	Sex cord/stromal ovarian cancer
	Budd-Chiari syndrome	Budd-Chiari syndrome	Pelvic inflammatory disease	Cystitis	Cystitis
	Bladder trauma	Pelvic inflammatory disease	Prostatitis	Budd-Chiari syndrome	Budd-Chiari syndrome
	Functional benign ovarian tumor	Bladder trauma	Muscular strain	Epithelial cell ovarian cancer	Functional benign ovarian tumor
	Crohn's disease	Prostatitis	Budd-Chiari syndrome	Germ cell ovarian cancer	Diverticular disease
	Ulcerative colitis	Ruptured/ hemorrhagic ovarian cyst	Diverticular disease	Sex cord/stromal ovarian cancer	Crohn's disease
	Abdominal abscess	Ectopic pregnancy	Colon cancer	Bladder trauma	Ulcerative colitis
	Chronic lead poisoning	Crohn's disease	Bladder trauma	Functional benign ovarian tumor	Bladder trauma
	Meckel's diverticulum	Ulcerative colitis	Epithelial cell ovarian cancer	Diverticular disease	Muscular strain
	Intussusception	Abdominal abscess	Germ cell ovarian cancer	Prostatitis	Prostatitis
	Insect and spider bites and stings	Chronic lead poisoning	Sex cord/stromal ovarian cancer	Ischemic bowel disease	Herpes zoster, shingles
		Meckel's diverticulum	Functional benign ovarian tumor	Herpes zoster, shingles	Abdominal abscess
		Intussusception	Ectopic pregnancy	Abdominal abscess	Pelvic inflammatory disease
		Renal calculi	Abdominal abscess	Pelvic inflammatory disease	Ischemic bowel disease
		Insect and spider bites and stings	Ischemic bowel disease	Chronic lead poisoning	Chronic lead poisoning
				Intussusception	Intussusception

List continues on next page

Baby (0-1 yr)	Child (1-12 yr)	Adolescent (12-18 yr)	Adult (18-45 yr)	Middle Age Adult (45-65 yr)	Senior Adult (65+ yr)
			Herpes zoster, shingles Chronic lead poisoning Intussusception Renal calculi Insect and spider bites and stings	Renal calculi Insect and spider bites and stings	Renal calculi Insect and spider bites and stings

Abdominal pain, right lower quadrant (continued)

Emergency Rule Out conditions shown in red. Entries in blue are for information only
Conditions are listed in approximate order of prevalence for this age range

Abdominal pain, right upper quadrant/epigastrium

Baby (0-1 yr)	Child (1-12 yr)	Adolescent (12-18 yr)	Adult (18-45 yr)	Middle Age Adult (45-65 yr)	Senior Adult (65+ yr)
Gastritis	Gastritis	Gastritis	Cholecystitis	Cholecystitis	Cholecystitis
Viral hepatitis	Viral hepatitis	Viral hepatitis	Gastritis	Biliary tract disease	Biliary tract disease
Pyelonephritis	Irritable bowel syndrome	Irritable bowel syndrome	Peptic ulcer	Gastritis	Gastritis
Biliary tract disease	Pyelonephritis	Biliary tract disease	Acute pancreatitis	Viral hepatitis	Viral hepatitis
Acute pancreatitis	Bacterial pneumonia	Pyelonephritis	Viral hepatitis	Peptic ulcer	Peptic ulcer
Bacterial pneumonia	Viral pneumonia	Bacterial pneumonia	Alcoholic hepatitis	Acute pancreatitis	Acute pancreatitis
Cardiac tamponade	Mycoplasmal pneumonia	Viral pneumonia	Pyelonephritis	Pyelonephritis	Pyelonephritis
Pleural effusion	Pleurisy	Mycoplasmal pneumonia	Biliary tract disease	Irritable bowel syndrome	Irritable bowel syndrome
Pleurisy	Cardiac tamponade	Cardiac tamponade	Abdominal hernias	Alcoholic hepatitis	Alcoholic hepatitis
Peptic ulcer	Pleural effusion	Amebic dysentery	Acute appendicitis	Myocardial infarction	Myocardial infarction
Subdiaphragmatic abscess	Biliary tract disease	Pancreatic cancer	Irritable bowel syndrome	Pancreatic cancer	Pancreatic cancer
Pyogenic liver abscess	Acute pancreatitis	Pleurisy	Cardiac tamponade	Cardiac tamponade	Cardiac tamponade
Pericarditis	Peptic ulcer	Pleural effusion	Fitz-Hugh-Curtis syndrome (ascending PID)	Acute appendicitis	Acute appendicitis
	Cholecystitis	Fitz-Hugh-Curtis syndrome (ascending PID)	Myocardial infarction	Pericarditis	Pericarditis
	Subdiaphragmatic abscess	Acute pancreatitis	Amebic dysentery	Cardiac tamponade	Bacterial pneumonia
	Pyogenic liver abscess	Peptic ulcer	Bacterial pneumonia	Amebic dysentery	Pleurisy
	Pericarditis	Cholecystitis	Pancreatic cancer	Bacterial pneumonia	Viral pneumonia
	Insect and spider bites and stings	Subdiaphragmatic abscess	Pyogenic liver abscess	Pleurisy	Mycoplasmal pneumonia
		Pyogenic liver abscess	Subdiaphragmatic abscess	Viral pneumonia	Abdominal hernias
		Pericarditis	Pericarditis	Mycoplasmal pneumonia	Herpes zoster, shingles
		Insect and spider bites and stings	Bacterial pneumonia	Abdominal hernias	Pleural effusion
			Viral pneumonia	Herpes zoster, shingles	Aspiration pneumonia
			Mycoplasmal pneumonia	Pleural effusion	Pyogenic liver abscess
				Aspiration pneumonia	

A

Baby (0-1 yr)	Child (1-12 yr)	Adolescent (12-18 yr)	Adult (18-45 yr)	Middle Age Adult (45-65 yr)	Senior Adult (65+ yr)
			Pleurisy Pleural effusion Herpes zoster, shingles Aspiration pneumonia Gastric cancer Insect and spider bites and stings	Pyogenic liver abscess Subdiaphragmatic abscess Gastric cancer Fitz-Hugh-Curtis syndrome (ascending PID) Insect and spider bites and stings	Subdiaphragmatic abscess Gastric cancer Fitz-Hugh-Curtis syndrome (ascending PID) Insect and spider bites and stings

Abdominal pain, right upper quadrant/epigastrium (continued)

13

Emergency Rule Out conditions shown in blue are for information only
Conditions are listed in approximate order of prevalence for this age range

Abdominal rigidity

Baby (0-1 yr)	Child (1-12 yr)	Adolescent (12-18 yr)	Adult (18-45 yr)	Middle Age Adult (45-65 yr)	Senior Adult (65+yr)
Necrotizing enterocolitis	Acute appendicitis	Acute appendicitis	Acute appendicitis	Acute appendicitis	Acute appendicitis
Insect and spider bites and stings	Peritonitis	Ruptured/ hemorrhagic ovarian cyst	Ectopic pregnancy	Acute pancreatitis	Acute pancreatitis
Tetanus	Tetanus	Tetanus	Ruptured/ hemorrhagic ovarian cyst	Intestinal perforation	Intestinal perforation
Peritonitis	Insect and spider bites and stings	Ectopic pregnancy	Insect and spider bites and stings	Diverticular disease	Insect and spider bites and stings
	Ruptured/ hemorrhagic ovarian cyst	Insect and spider bites and stings	Acute pancreatitis	Cholecystitis	Peritonitis
	Crohn's disease	Pelvic inflammatory disease	Intestinal perforation	Insect and spider bites and stings	Tetanus
	Ulcerative colitis	Peritonitis	Tetanus	Tetanus	Diverticular disease
		Crohn's disease	Diverticular disease	Peritonitis	Peptic ulcer
		Ulcerative colitis	Cholecystitis	Crohn's disease	Cholecystitis
			Crohn's disease	Ulcerative colitis	Crohn's disease
			Ulcerative colitis	Peptic ulcer	Ulcerative colitis
			Peptic ulcer	Ectopic pregnancy	
			Pelvic inflammatory disease	Ruptured/ hemorrhagic ovarian cyst	
			Peritonitis	Pelvic inflammatory disease	

Baby (0-1 yr)	Child (1-12 yr)	Adolescent (12-18 yr)	Adult (18-45 yr)	Middle Age Adult (45-65 yr)	Senior Adult (65+ yr)
Fracture	Fracture	Fracture	Callus	Callus	Callus
Callus	Callus	Callus	Fracture	Osteoarthritis	Osteoarthritis
Enchondroma	Enchondroma	Enchondroma	Paget's disease	Fracture	Fracture
Osteoma	Osteoma	Exostosis (osteochondroma)	Metastatic cancer	Paget's disease	Paget's disease
Osteosarcoma	Osteosarcoma	Osteoma	Acromegaly (pituitary gigantism)	Metastatic cancer	Metastatic cancer
Periosteal fibrosarcoma	Periosteal fibrosarcoma	Osteosarcoma	Multiple myeloma	Acromegaly (pituitary gigantism)	Acromegaly (pituitary gigantism)
Exostosis (osteochondroma)	Exostosis (osteochondroma)	Periosteal fibrosarcoma	Periosteal fibrosarcoma	Multiple myeloma	Multiple myeloma
		Metastatic cancer	Exostosis (osteochondroma)	Periosteal fibrosarcoma	Periosteal fibrosarcoma
			Enchondroma	Exostosis (osteochondroma)	Exostosis (osteochondroma)
			Osteoma	Enchondroma	Enchondroma
			Osteosarcoma	Osteoma	Osteoma
				Osteosarcoma	Osteosarcoma

Emergency Rule Out conditions shown in red. Entries in blue are for information only
Conditions are listed in approximate order of prevalence for this age range

15

Emergency Rule Out conditions shown in red. Entries in blue are for information only
Conditions are listed in approximate order of prevalence for this age range

Baby (0-1 yr)	Child (1-12 yr)	Adolescent (12-18 yr)	Adult (18-45 yr)	Middle Age Adult (45-65 yr)	Senior Adult (65+yr)
Drug withdrawal	Drug reaction	Drug reaction	Diabetic hypoglycemia	Diabetic hypoglycemia	Diabetic hypoglycemia
Non-diabetic hypoglycemia	Non-diabetic hypoglycemia	Drug withdrawal	Anxiety	Anxiety	Drug withdrawal
Thrombotic thrombocytopenic purpura	Post-traumatic stress disorder	Post-traumatic stress disorder	Drug withdrawal	Drug withdrawal	Anxiety
Drug reaction	Thrombotic thrombocytopenic purpura	Depression	Manic depression	Thrombotic thrombocytopenic purpura	Manic depression
	Manic depression	Manic depression	Delirium	Manic depression	Delirium
	Delirium	Thrombotic thrombocytopenic purpura	Thrombotic thrombocytopenic purpura	Delirium	Thrombotic thrombocytopenic purpura
	Diabetic hypoglycemia	Delirium	Hyperthyroidism	Myocardial infarction	Myocardial infarction
	Drug withdrawal	Non-diabetic hypoglycemia	Myocardial infarction	Hyperthyroidism	Hyperthyroidism
	Diabetes mellitus in children	Diabetic hypoglycemia	Depression	Depression	Depression
	Hyperthyroidism	Hyperthyroidism	Post-traumatic stress disorder	Post-traumatic stress disorder	Post-traumatic stress disorder
		Diabetes mellitus in children			

Baby (0-1 yr)	Child (1-12 yr)	Adolescent (12-18 yr)	Adult (18-45 yr)	Middle Age Adult (45-65 yr)	Senior Adult (65+ yr)
Not relevant to this age group	Parietal lobe lesion	Parietal lobe lesion Dementia	Ischemic stroke Brain tumor Head injury	Ischemic stroke Brain tumor Head injury	Ischemic stroke Brain tumor Head injury

Emergency Rule Out conditions shown in red. Entries in blue are for information only
Conditions are listed in approximate order of prevalence for this age range

17

Emergency Rule Out conditions shown in red. Entries in blue are for information only
Conditions are listed in approximate order of prevalence for this age range

Baby (0-1 yr)	Child (1-12 yr)	Adolescent (12-18 yr)	Adult (18-45 yr)	Middle Age Adult (45-65 yr)	Senior Adult (65+yr)
Seborrheic dermatitis	Ringworm	Ringworm	Male pattern baldness	Male pattern baldness	Male pattern baldness
Ringworm	Trauma	Trauma	Ringworm	Alopecia areata	Ringworm
Nutritional deficiencies	Burns	Psoriasis	Alopecia areata	Ringworm	Pityriasis versicolor
Psoriasis	Seborrheic dermatitis	Seborrheic dermatitis	Pityriasis versicolor	Pityriasis versicolor	Alopecia areata
Child abuse	Child abuse	Drug reaction	Seborrheic dermatitis	Seborrheic dermatitis	Seborrheic dermatitis
Reflex sympathetic dystrophy	Nutritional deficiencies	Anorexia nervosa	Postpartum hair loss	Postpartum hair loss	Hypothyroidism
Trauma	Reflex sympathetic dystrophy	Reflex sympathetic dystrophy	Hypothyroidism	Hypothyroidism	Systemic lupus erythematosus
Burns	Drug reaction	Child abuse	Systemic lupus erythematosus	Systemic lupus erythematosus	Syphilis
Drug reaction	Alopecia areata	Nutritional deficiencies	Psoriasis	Psoriasis	Basal cell carcinoma
Hypothyroidism	Iron deficiency anemia	Alopecia areata	Lichen planus	Discoid lupus erythematosus	Trichotillomania
Alopecia areata	Trichotillomania	Burns	Reflex sympathetic dystrophy	Reflex sympathetic dystrophy	Reflex sympathetic dystrophy
Ectodermal dysplasia	Hypothyroidism	Hypothyroidism	Discoid lupus erythematosus	Syphilis	Squamous cell carcinoma
Hypopituitarism	Psoriasis	Iron deficiency anemia	Syphilis	Trichotillomania	Hypopituitarism
	Hypopituitarism	Trichotillomania	Trichotillomania	Squamous cell carcinoma	Discoid lupus erythematosus
		Hypopituitarism	Squamous cell carcinoma	Hypopituitarism	Psoriasis
			Hypopituitarism	Lichen planus	Amyloidosis
			Burns	Burns	Burns
			Nutritional deficiencies	Nutritional deficiencies	Nutritional deficiencies
			Scleroderma	Basal cell carcinoma	Lichen planus
			Basal cell carcinoma	Scleroderma	Scleroderma
			Amyloidosis		Iron deficiency anemia

18

Baby (0-1 yr)	Child (1-12 yr)	Adolescent (12-18 yr)	Adult (18-45 yr)	Middle Age Adult (45-65 yr)	Senior Adult (65+yr)
			Iron deficiency anemia AIDS	Amyloidosis Iron deficiency anemia AIDS	

Amenorrhea, secondary

Emergency Rule Out conditions shown in red. Entries in blue are for information only
Conditions are listed in approximate order of prevalence for this age range

Baby (0-1 yr)	Child (1-12 yr)	Adolescent (12-18 yr)	Adult (18-45 yr)	Middle Age Adult (45-65 yr)	Senior Adult (65+yr)
Not relevant to this age group	Not relevant to this age group	Pregnancy	Pregnancy	Menopause	Not relevant to this age group
		Oral contraception	Oral contraception	Pregnancy	
		Ectopic pregnancy	Stress	Oral contraception	
		Stress	Ectopic pregnancy	Stress	
		Hypothyroidism	Hypothyroidism	Drug reaction	
		Polycystic ovarian disease	Menopause	Hypothyroidism	
		Drug reaction	Low body mass index	Low body mass index	
		Anorexia nervosa	Ruptured/ hemorrhagic ovarian cyst	Polycystic ovarian disease	
		Low body mass index	Drug reaction	Functional benign ovarian tumor	
		Ruptured/ hemorrhagic ovarian cyst	Polycystic ovarian disease	Epithelial cell ovarian cancer	
		Functional benign ovarian tumor	Anorexia nervosa	Germ cell ovarian cancer	
		Endometrial scarring	Pituitary eosinophilic adenoma (prolactinoma)	Sex cord/stromal ovarian cancer	
		Thyroiditis	Hypopituitarism	Ruptured/ hemorrhagic ovarian cyst	
		Pituitary eosinophilic adenoma (prolactinoma)	Secondary amenorrhea (hypothalmic dysfunction)	Endometrial scarring	
		Hypopituitarism	Secondary amenorrhea (premature ovarian failure)	Pituitary eosinophilic adenoma (prolactinoma)	
		Mullerian dysgenesis	Functional benign ovarian tumor	Anorexia nervosa	
		Non-functioning chromophobe pituitary adenoma	Endometrial scarring	Hypopituitarism	
		Plague			

Baby (0-1 yr)	Child (1-12 yr)	Adolescent (12-18 yr)	Adult (18-45 yr)	Middle Age Adult (45-65 yr)	Senior Adult (65+ yr)
			Non-functioning chromophobe pituitary adenoma Epithelial cell ovarian cancer Germ cell ovarian cancer Sex cord/stromal ovarian cancer Mullerian dysgenesis Plague	Secondary amenorrhea (hypothalmic dysfunction) Secondary amenorrhea (premature ovarian failure) Non-functioning chromophobe pituitary adenoma Mullerian dysgenesis Plague	

Amenorrhea, secondary (continued)

Emergency Rule Out conditions shown in red. Entries in blue are for information only
Conditions are listed in approximate order of prevalence for this age range

Baby (0-1 yr)	Child (1-12 yr)	Adolescent (12-18 yr)	Adult (18-45 yr)	Middle Age Adult (45-65 yr)	Senior Adult (65+yr)
Not relevant to this age group	Post-concussive syndrome	Post-concussive syndrome	Postictal/ postseizure phase	Psychosomatic	Alzheimer's disease
	Trauma	Trauma	Temporal lobe epilepsy	Postictal/ postseizure phase	Drug reaction
	Postictal/ postseizure phase	Psychosomatic	Post-concussive syndrome	Drug reaction	Postictal/ postseizure phase
	Psychosomatic	Migraine headache	Trauma	Post-concussive syndrome	Wernicke's encephalopathy
	Brain injury	Brain injury	Brain injury	Transient ischemic attack	Transient ischemic attack
	Migraine headache	Transient ischemic attack	Transient ischemic attack	Brain injury	Brain injury
	Temporal lobe epilepsy	Drug reaction	Psychosomatic	Trauma	Psychosomatic
	Encephalitis	Postictal/ postseizure phase	Wernicke's encephalopathy	Alzheimer's disease	Migraine headache
	Drug reaction	Temporal lobe epilepsy	Migraine headache	Temporal lobe epilepsy	Post-concussive syndrome
	Transient ischemic attack	Encephalitis	Encephalitis	Wernicke's encephalopathy	Trauma
			Drug reaction	Migraine headache	Temporal lobe epilepsy
			Alzheimer's disease	Encephalitis	Encephalitis

Baby (0-1 yr)	Child (1-12 yr)	Adolescent (12-18 yr)	Adult (18-45 yr)	Middle Age Adult (45-65 yr)	Senior Adult (65-yr)
Iron deficiency anemia	Iron deficiency anemia	Iron deficiency anemia	Anemia due to acute blood loss	Colon cancer	Colon cancer
Sickle cell trait	Sickle cell trait	Sickle cell trait	Iron deficiency anemia	Anemia due to acute blood loss	Anemia due to acute blood loss
Anemia due to acute blood loss	Anemia due to acute blood loss	Anemia due to acute blood loss	Anemia of chronic disease	Iron deficiency anemia	Iron deficiency anemia
Hereditary spherocytosis	Ulcerative colitis	Thalassemia	Vitamin B12 deficiency	Anemia of chronic disease	Systemic lupus erythematosus
Anemia	Thalassemia	Hereditary spherocytosis	Folate deficiency	Systemic lupus erythematosus	Anemia of chronic disease
Babesiosis	Anemia	Ulcerative colitis	Acute leukemia	Vitamin B12 deficiency	Vitamin B12 deficiency
Celiac disease	Chronic renal failure	Anemia	Anemia	Folate deficiency	Folate deficiency
Chronic renal failure	Systemic lupus erythematosus	Systemic lupus erythematosus	Chronic lymphocytic leukemia	Gastric cancer	Gastric cancer
Bartonella infection (cat scratch disease)	Celiac disease	Acute leukemia	Chronic renal failure	Ulcerative colitis	Anemia
Systemic lupus erythematosus	Bladder tumor	Bartonella infection (cat scratch disease)	Babesiosis	Anemia	Chronic renal failure
Ulcerative colitis	Bartonella infection (cat scratch disease)	Chronic renal failure	Systemic lupus erythematosus	Chronic renal failure	Ulcerative colitis
Thalassemia	Babesiosis	Celiac disease	Ulcerative colitis	Babesiosis	Pancreatic cancer
Acute leukemia	Hereditary spherocytosis	Bladder tumor	Celiac disease	Pancreatic cancer	Chronic lymphocytic leukemia
Aplastic anemia	Acute leukemia	Babesiosis	Bladder tumor	Bladder tumor	Acute leukemia
Anemia of chronic disease	Aplastic anemia	Aplastic anemia	Chronic myelogenous leukemia	Aplastic anemia	Bartonella infection (cat scratch disease)
Folate deficiency	Anemia of chronic disease	Amebic dysentery	Bartonella infection (cat scratch disease)	Celiac disease	Babesiosis
Autoimmune hemolytic anemia	Folate deficiency	Ankylosing spondylitis	Sickle cell trait	Sideroblastic anemia	Celiac disease
Hypothyroidism	Autoimmune hemolytic anemia	Anemia of chronic disease		Bartonella infection (cat scratch disease)	Bladder tumor
Renal cell adenocarcinoma		Folate deficiency		Acute leukemia	

List continues on next page

Emergency Rule Out conditions shown in red. Entries in blue are for information only
Conditions are listed in approximate order of prevalence for this age range

23

List continued from previous page

Baby (0-1 yr)	Child (1-12 yr)	Adolescent (12-18 yr)	Adult (18-45 yr)	Middle Age Adult (45-65 yr)	Senior Adult (65+yr)
	Hypothyroidism	Autoimmune hemolytic	Ankylosing spondylitis	Chronic lymphocytic	Chronic myelogenous
	Renal cell adenocarcinoma	anemia	Thalassemia	leukemia	leukemia
		Chronic myelogenous	Amebic dysentery	Chronic myelogenous	Acute leukemia
		leukemia	Autoimmune hemolytic	leukemia	Aplastic anemia
		Chronic lymphocytic	anemia	Ankylosing spondylitis	Myelodysplastic syndromes
		leukemia	Sideroblastic anemia	Amebic dysentery	Ankylosing spondylitis
		Myelodysplastic syndromes	Aplastic anemia	Sickle cell trait	Sideroblastic anemia
		Hypothyroidism	Hereditary spherocytosis	Autoimmune hemolytic	Sickle cell trait
		Renal cell adenocarcinoma	Myelodysplastic syndromes	anemia	Autoimmune hemolytic
			Hypothyroidism	Hereditary spherocytosis	anemia
			Renal cell adenocarcinoma	Myelodysplastic syndromes	Hereditary spherocytosis
				Hypothyroidism	Hypothyroidism
				Renal cell adenocarcinoma	Renal cell adenocarcinoma

Baby (0-1 yr)	Child (1-12 yr)	Adolescent (12-18 yr)	Adult (18-45 yr)	Middle Age Adult (45-65 yr)	Senior Adult (65+yr)
Not relevant to this age group	Tendinitis Ankle injury Muscular strain Fracture	Tendinitis Ankle injury Muscular strain Fracture	Ankle injury Fracture Tendinitis Acute gout	Ankle injury Fracture Acute gout Tendinitis	Ankle injury Acute gout Fracture Tendinitis

Emergency Rule Out conditions shown in red. Entries in blue are for information only
Conditions are listed in approximate order of prevalence for this age range

Emergency Rule Out conditions shown in red. Entries in blue are for information only
Conditions are listed in approximate order of prevalence for this age range

Baby (0-1 yr)	Child (1-12 yr)	Adolescent (12-18 yr)	Adult (18-45 yr)	Middle Age Adult (45-65 yr)	Senior Adult (65+ yr)
Malignancy	Depression	Depression	Depression	Depression	Depression
Acute pancreatitis	Viral hepatitis	Anorexia nervosa	Anorexia nervosa	Congestive heart failure	Malignancy
Hypercalcemia	Chlamydia pneumoniae	Viral hepatitis	Viral hepatitis	Viral hepatitis	Congestive heart failure
Autism	Tuberculosis	Acute appendicitis	Typhoid fever	Typhoid fever	Chronic renal failure
Polyarteritis nodosa	Acute appendicitis	Sexual assault	Congestive heart failure	Sexual assault	Viral hepatitis
Sexual assault	Brucellosis	Chlamydia pneumoniae	Sexual assault	Infective endocarditis	Infective endocarditis
Systemic lupus erythematosus	Autism	Reiter's syndrome	Infective endocarditis	Acute pancreatitis	Hepatoma
Viral infection	Infective endocarditis	Hepatoma	Hepatoma	Chronic myelogenous leukemia	Primary lung malignancy
	Polyarteritis nodosa	Acute pancreatitis	Acute pancreatitis	Chlamydia pneumoniae	Chronic myelogenous leukemia
	Acute pancreatitis	Infective endocarditis	Chronic myelogenous leukemia	Reiter's syndrome	Acute pancreatitis
	Babesiosis	Brucellosis	Chlamydia pneumoniae	Primary lung malignancy	Sexual assault
	Sexual assault	Babesiosis	Polyarteritis nodosa	Brucellosis	Brucellosis
	Typhoid fever	Primary lung malignancy	Babesiosis	Babesiosis	Chlamydia pneumoniae
	Hypercalcemia	Autism	Brucellosis	Polyarteritis nodosa	Babesiosis
	Malignancy	Polyarteritis nodosa	Autism	Tuberculosis	Reiter's syndrome
	Anorexia nervosa	Typhoid fever	Primary lung malignancy	Alcoholic hepatitis	Polyarteritis nodosa
	Chronic renal failure	Tuberculosis	Reiter's syndrome	Hypercalcemia	Tuberculosis
	AIDS	Hypercalcemia	Tuberculosis	Malignancy	Typhoid fever
	Systemic lupus erythematosus	AIDS	Acute appendicitis	Chronic renal failure	Alcoholic hepatitis
		Chronic renal failure	Hypercalcemia	AIDS	Ankylosing spondylitis
		Ankylosing spondylitis	AIDS	Addison's disease	Addison's disease
		Addison's disease	Alcoholic hepatitis		Ischemic bowel disease
		Malignancy			

Baby (0-1 yr)	Child (1-12 yr)	Adolescent (12-18 yr)	Adult (18-45 yr)	Middle Age Adult (45-65 yr)	Senior Adult (65+ yr)
		Pancreatic cancer Systemic lupus erythematosus	Malignancy Ankylosing spondylitis Chronic renal failure Addison's disease Ischemic bowel disease Pancreatic cancer Systemic lupus erythematosus	Ischemic bowel disease Anorexia nervosa Ankylosing spondylitis Pancreatic cancer Systemic lupus erythematosus Autism	AIDS Hypercalcemia Pancreatic cancer Systemic lupus erythematosus

Emergency Rule Out conditions shown in red. Entries in blue are for information only
Conditions are listed in approximate order of prevalence for this age range

Anxiety

Baby (0-1 yr)	Child (1-12 yr)	Adolescent (12-18 yr)	Adult (18-45 yr)	Middle Age Adult (45-65 yr)	Senior Adult (65+ yr)
Not relevant to this age group	Drug withdrawal	Panic disorder	Panic disorder	Panic disorder	Depression
	Depression	Depression	Drug withdrawal	Drug withdrawal	Drug withdrawal
	Post-traumatic stress disorder	Post-traumatic stress disorder	Post-traumatic stress disorder	Post-traumatic stress disorder	Phobia
	Delirium	Allergic reactions and anaphylaxis	Delirium	Delirium	Delirium
	Obsessive compulsive disorder	Chronic fatigue syndrome	Chronic fatigue syndrome	Chronic fatigue syndrome	Allergic reactions and anaphylaxis
	Autism	Premenstrual syndrome	Anorexia nervosa	Autism	Chronic fatigue syndrome
	Anorexia nervosa	Obsessive compulsive disorder	Obsessive compulsive disorder	Obsessive compulsive disorder	Obsessive compulsive disorder
	Allergic reactions and anaphylaxis	Autism	Premenstrual syndrome	Anorexia nervosa	Autism
	Panic disorder	Delirium	Autism	Allergic reactions and anaphylaxis	Anorexia nervosa
	Phobia	Anorexia nervosa	Allergic reactions and anaphylaxis	Depression	Hyperthyroidism
	Hyperthyroidism	Phobia	Depression	Phobia	Panic disorder
	Diabetic hypoglycemia	Agoraphobia	Diabetic hypoglycemia	Diabetic hypoglycemia	Diabetic hypoglycemia
	Hepatic encephalopathy	Hyperthyroidism	Phobia	Agoraphobia	Agoraphobia
		Diabetic hypoglycemia	Agoraphobia	Hyperthyroidism	Hepatic encephalopathy
		Hepatic encephalopathy	Hyperthyroidism	Hepatic encephalopathy	
			Hepatic encephalopathy		

28

Baby (0-1 yr)	Child (1-12 yr)	Adolescent (12-18 yr)	Adult (18-45 yr)	Middle Age Adult (45-65 yr)	Senior Adult (65+ yr)
Not relevant to this age group	Developmental delay	Autism	Ischemic stroke	Ischemic stroke	Ischemic stroke
	Hearing loss	Psychosomatic	Transient ischemic attack	Transient ischemic attack	Transient ischemic attack
	Intracranial hemorrhage	Intracranial hemorrhage	Primary intracerebral hemorrhage stroke	Primary intracerebral hemorrhage stroke	Primary intracerebral hemorrhage stroke
	Autism	Primary intracerebral hemorrhage stroke	Brain tumor	Intracranial hemorrhage	Brain tumor
	Primary intracerebral hemorrhage stroke		Intracranial hemorrhage	Brain tumor	Intracranial hemorrhage
	Psychosomatic		Multiple sclerosis	Multiple sclerosis	Amyotrophic lateral sclerosis (motor neuron disease)
			Parkinson's disease	Parkinson's disease	Multiple sclerosis
			Migraine headache	Migraine headache	Parkinson's disease
			Amyotrophic lateral sclerosis (motor neuron disease)	Amyotrophic lateral sclerosis (motor neuron disease)	Migraine headache
			Depression	Depression	Dementia
				Dementia	Depression

Emergency Rule Out conditions shown in red. Entries in blue are for information only
Conditions are listed in approximate order of prevalence for this age range

29

Apneustic breathing

Emergency Rule Out conditions shown in red. Entries in blue are for information only
Conditions are listed in approximate order of prevalence for this age range

Baby (0-1 yr)	Child (1-12 yr)	Adolescent (12-18 yr)	Adult (18-45 yr)	Middle Age Adult (45-65 yr)	Senior Adult (65+ yr)
Hypoxia	Hypoxia	Hypoxia	Diabetic hypoglycemia	Primary intracerebral hemorrhage stroke	Primary intracerebral hemorrhage stroke
Bacterial meningitis	Bacterial meningitis	Bacterial meningitis	Hypoxia	Ischemic stroke	Subarachnoid hemorrhage and cerebral aneurysm stroke
Primary intracerebral hemorrhage stroke	Primary intracerebral hemorrhage stroke	Primary intracerebral hemorrhage stroke	Bacterial meningitis	Subarachnoid hemorrhage and cerebral aneurysm stroke	Ischemic stroke
Diabetic hypoglycemia	Diabetic hypoglycemia	Diabetic hypoglycemia	Primary intracerebral hemorrhage stroke	Bacterial meningitis	Diabetic hypoglycemia
			Ischemic stroke	Diabetic hypoglycemia	Hypoxia
			Subarachnoid hemorrhage and cerebral aneurysm stroke	Hypoxia	Bacterial meningitis

Baby (0-1 yr)	Child (1-12 yr)	Adolescent (12-18 yr)	Adult (18-45 yr)	Middle Age Adult (45-65 yr)	Senior Adult (65+ yr)
Not relevant to this age group	Parietal lobe lesion Hepatic encephalopathy Brain tumor Friedreich's ataxia	Parietal lobe lesion Hepatic encephalopathy Ataxia-telangiectasia Brain tumor Friedreich's ataxia	Parietal lobe lesion Hepatic encephalopathy Brain tumor Friedreich's ataxia	Parietal lobe lesion Hepatic encephalopathy Brain tumor	Parietal lobe lesion Hepatic encephalopathy Brain tumor

Emergency Rule Out conditions shown in red. Entries in blue are for information only
Conditions are listed in approximate order of prevalence for this age range

Apraxia in limb

Emergency Rule Out conditions shown in red. Entries in blue are for information only
Conditions are listed in approximate order of prevalence for this age range

Baby (0-1 yr)	Child (1-12 yr)	Adolescent (12-18 yr)	Adult (18-45 yr)	Middle Age Adult (45-65 yr)	Senior Adult (65+ yr)
Not relevant to this age group	Hydrocephalus Parietal lobe lesion	Hydrocephalus Parietal lobe lesion	Parietal lobe lesion Hydrocephalus	Parietal lobe lesion Hydrocephalus	Parietal lobe lesion Hydrocephalus

Baby (0-1 yr)	Child (1-12 yr)	Adolescent (12-18 yr)	Adult (18-45 yr)	Middle Age Adult (45-65 yr)	Senior Adult (65+ yr)
Not relevant to this age group	Trauma	Trauma	Trauma	Osteoarthritis	Osteoarthritis
	Viral infection	Viral infection	Viral infection	Trauma	Trauma
	Septic arthritis	Allergic reactions and anaphylaxis	Ulcerative colitis	Viral infection	Viral infection
	Hemarthrosis	Hemarthrosis	Psoriasis	Acute gout	Acute gout
	Allergic reactions and anaphylaxis	Septic arthritis	Acute gout	Polymyalgia rheumatica	Polymyalgia rheumatica
	Rubella	Avascular necrosis	Rheumatoid arthritis	Rheumatoid arthritis	Rheumatoid arthritis
	Serum sickness	Serum sickness	Septic arthritis	Septic arthritis	Septic arthritis
	Lyme disease	Osteochondrosis	Systemic lupus erythematosus	Ankylosing spondylitis	Rubella
	Juvenile idiopathic arthritis	Rubella	Rheumatic fever	Systemic lupus erythematosus	Systemic lupus erythematosus
	Babesiosis	Juvenile idiopathic arthritis	Rubella	Allergic reactions and anaphylaxis	Lyme disease
	Henoch-Schönlein purpura	Babesiosis	Lyme disease	Rubella	Pseudogout
	Rheumatic fever	Lyme disease	Reiter's syndrome	Ulcerative colitis	Henoch-Schönlein purpura
	Behçet's syndrome	Henoch-Schönlein purpura	Fibromyalgia	Fibromyalgia	Crohn's disease
	Brucellosis	Blastomycosis	Gonorrhea	Lyme disease	Brucellosis
	Infective endocarditis	Erythema nodosum	Henoch-Schönlein purpura	Babesiosis	Erythema nodosum
	Chronic lead poisoning	Brucellosis	Blastomycosis	Crohn's disease	Charcot's joint
	Charcot's joint	Charcot's joint	Erythema nodosum	Henoch-Schönlein purpura	Blastomycosis
	Blastomycosis	Crohn's disease	Charcot's joint	Brucellosis	Ulcerative colitis
	Fifth disease	Behçet's syndrome	Babesiosis	Blastomycosis	Babesiosis
	Crohn's disease	Ulcerative colitis	Allergic reactions and anaphylaxis	Charcot's joint	Behçet's syndrome
	Erythema nodosum	Chronic lead poisoning			Ankylosing spondylitis

List continues on next page

Emergency Rule Out conditions shown in red. Entries in blue are for information only
Conditions are listed in approximate order of prevalence for this age range

33

List continued from previous page

Baby (0-1 yr)	Child (1-12 yr)	Adolescent (12-18 yr)	Adult (18-45 yr)	Middle Age Adult (45-65 yr)	Senior Adult (65+yr)
	Osteochondrosis	Infective endocarditis	Brucellosis	Erythema nodosum	Psoriasis
	Ulcerative colitis	Fifth disease	Fifth disease	Rheumatic fever	Scleroderma
	Psoriasis	Chronic fatigue syndrome	Behçet's syndrome	Psoriasis	Allergic reactions and
	Avascular necrosis	Systemic lupus	Chronic lead poisoning	Behçet's syndrome	anaphylaxis
	Systemic lupus	erythematosus	Scleroderma	Scleroderma	Eosinophilic pneumonias
	erythematosus	Rheumatic fever	Crohn's disease	Pseudogout	Infective endocarditis
	Eosinophilic pneumonias	Eosinophilic pneumonias	Ankylosing spondylitis	Chronic lead poisoning	Reiter's syndrome
	Hypoxia	Hypoxia	Infective endocarditis	Eosinophilic pneumonias	Hemarthrosis
	Hurler's syndrome	Hurler's syndrome	Pseudogout	Gonorrhea	Avascular necrosis
	Scleroderma	Psoriasis	Huntington's disease	Reiter's syndrome	Osteochondrosis
		Reiter's syndrome	Eosinophilic pneumonias	Infective endocarditis	
		Ankylosing spondylitis	Hemarthrosis	Hemarthrosis	
		Scleroderma	Avascular necrosis	Avascular necrosis	
			Osteochondrosis	Osteochondrosis	

Arthritis & dermatitis

Baby (0-1 yr)	Child (1-12 yr)	Adolescent (12-18 yr)	Adult (18-45 yr)	Middle Age Adult (45-65 yr)	Senior Adult (65- yr)
Lyme disease	Juvenile idiopathic arthritis	Juvenile idiopathic arthritis	Psoriatic arthritis	Psoriatic arthritis	Rheumatoid arthritis
Rheumatic fever	Lyme disease	Psoriatic arthritis	Reiter's syndrome	Reiter's syndrome	Erythema nodosum
Psoriasis	Rheumatic fever	Lyme disease	Rheumatoid arthritis	Rheumatoid arthritis	Scleroderma
Erythema nodosum	Psoriasis	Erythema nodosum	Lyme disease	Lyme disease	Psoriasis
Vasculitis	Polymyositis/ dermatomyositis	Systemic lupus erythematosus	Systemic lupus erythematosus	Polymyositis/ dermatomyositis	Vasculitis
	Erythema nodosum	Psoriasis	Psoriasis	Psoriasis	Lyme disease
	Scleroderma	Rheumatic fever	Polymyositis/ dermatomyositis	Systemic lupus erythematosus	Gonorrhea
	Vasculitis	Gonorrhea	Rheumatic fever	Rheumatic fever	Rheumatic fever
		Scleroderma	Erythema nodosum	Erythema nodosum	Systemic lupus erythematosus
		Reiter's syndrome	Juvenile idiopathic arthritis	Juvenile idiopathic arthritis	
		Vasculitis	Gonorrhea	Gonorrhea	
			Vasculitis	Vasculitis	
			Scleroderma	Scleroderma	

Emergency Rule Out conditions shown in red. Entries in blue are for information only
Conditions are listed in approximate order of prevalence for this age range

Emergency Rule Out conditions shown in red. Entries in blue are for information only
Conditions are listed in approximate order of prevalence for this age range

Arthritis, monoarticular

Baby (0-1 yr)	Child (1-12 yr)	Adolescent (12-18 yr)	Adult (18-45 yr)	Middle Age Adult (45-65 yr)	Senior Adult (65+ yr)
Septic arthritis	Septic arthritis	Septic arthritis	Acute gout	Acute gout	Osteoarthritis
Tuberculosis	Tuberculosis	Tuberculosis	Lyme disease	Lyme disease	Acute gout
Mycoplasmal pneumonia	Mycoplasmal pneumonia	Mycoplasmal pneumonia	Gonorrhea	Osteoarthritis	Septic arthritis
Lyme disease	Lyme disease	Lyme disease	Septic bursitis	Septic arthritis	Lyme disease
Rheumatic fever	Rheumatic fever	Rheumatic fever	Septic arthritis	Septic bursitis	Pseudogout
Henoch-Schönlein purpura	Ulcerative colitis	Ulcerative colitis	Pseudogout	Gonorrhea	Septic bursitis
Kawasaki disease	Crohn's disease	Crohn's disease	Avascular necrosis	Pseudogout	Avascular necrosis
Sickle cell anemia	Henoch-Schönlein purpura	Henoch-Schönlein purpura	Ulcerative colitis	Avascular necrosis	Gonorrhea
Acute leukemia	Kawasaki disease	Kawasaki disease	Crohn's disease	Crohn's disease	Crohn's disease
Neuroblastoma	Sickle cell anemia	Sickle cell anemia		Ulcerative colitis	Ulcerative colitis
Juvenile idiopathic arthritis	Acute leukemia	Acute leukemia			
Connective tissue disease	Neuroblastoma	Neuroblastoma			
Cystic fibrosis	Juvenile idiopathic arthritis	Juvenile idiopathic arthritis			
	Connective tissue disease	Connective tissue disease			
	Cystic fibrosis	Cystic fibrosis			

Baby (0-1 yr)	Child (1-12 yr)	Adolescent (12-18 yr)	Adult (18-45 yr)	Middle Age Adult (45-65 yr)	Senior Adult (65+ yr)
Portal hypertension	Portal hypertension	Portal hypertension	Liver cirrhosis	Liver cirrhosis	Liver cirrhosis
Congenital abnormality of lymphatics	Portal vein thrombosis	Portal vein thrombosis	Malignancy	Peritonitis	Malignancy
Portal vein thrombosis	Acute pancreatitis	Budd-Chiari syndrome	Hypoalbuminemia	Malignancy	Hypoalbuminemia
Hypoalbuminemia	Hypoalbuminemia	Hypoalbuminemia	Peritonitis	Hypoalbuminemia	Peritonitis
Acute pancreatitis	Peritonitis	Acute pancreatitis	Acute pancreatitis	Acute pancreatitis	Acute pancreatitis
Mesenteric adenitis	Mesenteric adenitis	Alcoholic hepatitis	Alcoholic hepatitis	Alcoholic hepatitis	Alcoholic hepatitis
Peritonitis	Cardiomyopathy	Peritonitis	Epithelial cell ovarian cancer	Epithelial cell ovarian cancer	Epithelial cell ovarian cancer
Tuberculosis	Filariasis	Cardiomyopathy	Germ cell ovarian cancer	Germ cell ovarian cancer	Germ cell ovarian cancer
Filariasis	Tuberculosis	Mesenteric adenitis	Sex cord/stromal ovarian cancer	Sex cord/stromal ovarian cancer	Sex cord/stromal ovarian cancer
		Tuberculosis	Tuberculosis	Tuberculosis	Tuberculosis
		Filariasis	Filariasis	Filariasis	Filariasis
			Budd-Chiari syndrome	Budd-Chiari syndrome	Budd-Chiari syndrome

Emergency Rule Out conditions shown in red. Entries in blue are for information only
Conditions are listed in approximate order of prevalence for this age range

Emergency Rule Out conditions shown in red. Entries in blue are for information only
Conditions are listed in approximate order of prevalence for this age range

Baby (0-1 yr)	Child (1-12 yr)	Adolescent (12-18 yr)	Adult (18-45 yr)	Middle Age Adult (45-65 yr)	Senior Adult (65+yr)
Not relevant to this age group	Viral infection	Labyrinthitis	Labyrinthitis	Labyrinthitis	Labyrinthitis
	Head injury	Viral infection	Head injury	Head injury	Cerebellar hemorrhage
	Migraine headache	Head injury	Cerebellar hemorrhage	Cerebellar hemorrhage	Head injury
	Carbon monoxide poisoning	Migraine headache	Ischemic stroke	Ischemic stroke	Ischemic stroke
	Labyrinthitis	Carbon monoxide poisoning	Carbon monoxide poisoning	Migraine headache	Migraine headache
	Poisoning	Poisoning	Guillain-Barré syndrome (acute infective polyneuritis)	Carbon monoxide poisoning	Carbon monoxide poisoning
	Brain abscess	Brain abscess	Migraine headache	Guillain-Barré syndrome (acute infective polyneuritis)	Guillain-Barré syndrome (acute infective polyneuritis)
			Partial apraxia	Partial apraxia	Partial apraxia
			Poisoning	Poisoning	Poisoning
			Brain abscess	Brain abscess	Brain abscess
			Conversion disorder	Conversion disorder	Conversion disorder
			Brain tumor	Brain tumor	Brain tumor

Baby (0-1 yr)	Child (1-12 yr)	Adolescent (12-18 yr)	Adult (18-45 yr)	Middle Age Adult (45-65 yr)	Senior Adult (65+ yr)
Not relevant to this age group	Myopathy Hydrocephalus Creutzfeldt-Jakob disease Carbon monoxide poisoning Inborn errors of metabolism Brain tumor Chorea	Myopathy Hydrocephalus Carbon monoxide poisoning Creutzfeldt-Jakob disease Brain tumor Inborn errors of metabolism Multiple sclerosis	Parkinson's disease Hydrocephalus Creutzfeldt-Jakob disease Cervical spondylosis Multiple sclerosis Carbon monoxide poisoning Brain tumor Myopathy Huntington's disease Friedreich's ataxia	Parkinson's disease Hydrocephalus Cervical spondylosis Creutzfeldt-Jakob disease Carbon monoxide poisoning Multiple sclerosis Brain tumor Myopathy Huntington's disease Friedreich's ataxia	Parkinson's disease Brain tumor Hydrocephalus Creutzfeldt-Jakob disease Myopathy Carbon monoxide poisoning Cervical spondylosis Huntington's disease Multiple sclerosis Friedreich's ataxia

Emergency Rule Out conditions shown in red. Entries in blue are for information only
Conditions are listed in approximate order of prevalence for this age range

Emergency Rule Out conditions shown in red. Entries in blue are for information only
Conditions are listed in approximate order of prevalence for this age range

Baby (0-1 yr)	Child (1-12 yr)	Adolescent (12-18 yr)	Adult (18-45 yr)	Middle Age Adult (45-65 yr)	Senior Adult (65+ yr)
Lymphadenopathy	Lymphadenopathy	Lymphadenopathy	Lymphadenopathy	Lymphadenopathy	Lymphadenopathy
Congenital abnormality of lymphatics	Chronic lymphadenitis	Chronic lymphadenitis	Breast cancer	Breast cancer	Breast cancer
Pyogenic infection	Pyogenic infection	Pyogenic infection	Lipoma	Lipoma	Lipoma
	Lipoma	Lipoma	Chronic lymphadenitis	Chronic lymphadenitis	Chronic lymphadenitis
			Pyogenic infection	Pyogenic infection	Pyogenic infection
			Vascular aneurysm	Vascular aneurysm	Vascular aneurysm

Baby (0-1 yr)	Child (1-12 yr)	Adolescent (12-18 yr)	Adult (18-45 yr)	Middle Age Adult (45-65 yr)	Senior Adult (65- yr)
Acute glomerulonephritis	Acute glomerulonephritis	Acute glomerulonephritis	Dehydration	Dehydration	Dehydration
Acute renal failure	Acute renal failure	Acute renal failure	Congestive heart failure	Congestive heart failure	Congestive heart failure
Bladder trauma	Bladder trauma	Bladder trauma	Drug reaction	Drug reaction	Drug reaction
Acute tubular necrosis	Rhabdomyolysis	Rocky Mountain spotted fever	Sepsis	Sepsis	Sepsis
Rocky Mountain spotted fever	Rocky Mountain spotted fever	Rhabdomyolysis	Burns	Burns	Benign prostatic hyperplasia
Yellow fever	Yellow fever	Yellow fever	Acute tubular necrosis	Acute tubular necrosis	Renal artery stenosis
Bladder tumor	Acute tubular necrosis	Pelvic tumor	Acute glomerulonephritis	Acute glomerulonephritis	Prostatic cancer
Chronic renal failure	Bladder tumor	Bladder tumor	Liver failure	Rocky Mountain spotted fever	Liver failure
Dehydration	Chronic renal failure	Acute tubular necrosis	Rocky Mountain spotted fever	Liver failure	Rocky Mountain spotted fever
	Pelvic tumor	Chronic renal failure	Heat stroke and heat exhaustion	Heat stroke and heat exhaustion	Disseminated intravascular coagulation
	Dehydration	Dehydration	Disseminated intravascular coagulation	Disseminated intravascular coagulation	Acute glomerulonephritis
			Pelvic tumor	Benign prostatic hyperplasia	Acute tubular necrosis
			Prostatic cancer	Renal artery stenosis	Yellow fever
			Prostate calculus	Pelvic tumor	Post-prostatectomy
			Bladder trauma	Prostatic cancer	Heat stroke and heat exhaustion
			Yellow fever	Yellow fever	Burns
			Bladder tumor	Prostate calculus	Renal vein thrombosis
			Infiltrating renal fibrosis	Bladder trauma	Bladder tumor
			Prostatic abscess	Bladder tumor	Infiltrating renal fibrosis

List continues on next page

Emergency Rule Out conditions shown in red. Entries in blue are for information only
Conditions are listed in approximate order of prevalence for this age range

Baby (0-1 yr)	Child (1-12 yr)	Adolescent (12-18 yr)	Adult (18-45 yr)	Middle Age Adult (45-65 yr)	Senior Adult (65+ yr)
			Benign prostatic hyperplasia	Infiltrating renal fibrosis	Prostatic abscess
			Retroperitonial fibrosis	Prostatic abscess	**Retroperitonial fibrosis**
			Post-prostatectomy	**Retroperitonial fibrosis**	Bladder trauma
			Renal artery stenosis	Post-prostatectomy	**Prostate calculus**
			Renal vein thrombosis	Renal vein thrombosis	

Baby (0-1 yr)	Child (1-12 yr)	Adolescent (12-18 yr)	Adult (18-45 yr)	Middle Age Adult (45-65 yr)	Senior Adult (65+ yr)
Direct hyperbilirubinemia	Carbohydrate-rich meal	Carbohydrate-rich meal	Hepatocellular jaundice	Hepatocellular jaundice	Hepatocellular jaundice
Hepatocellular jaundice	Acid urine	Acid urine	Direct hyperbilirubinemia	Direct hyperbilirubinemia	Direct hyperbilirubinemia
Amino acidurea	Direct hyperbilirubinemia	Direct hyperbilirubinemia	Aplastic anemia	Aplastic anemia	Aplastic anemia
Acid urine	Hepatocellular jaundice	Hepatocellular jaundice	Acid urine	Acid urine	Acid urine
Hemorrhage into tissue	Hemorrhage into tissue	Hemorrhage into tissue	Carbohydrate-rich meal	Carbohydrate-rich meal	Carbohydrate-rich meal
Hemolytic disease of the newborn (erythroblastosis fetalis)	Autoimmune hemolytic anemia	Autoimmune hemolytic anemia	Dubin-Johnson syndrome	Dubin-Johnson syndrome	Dubin-Johnson syndrome
Autoimmune hemolytic anemia	Amino acidurea	Amino acidurea	Hemorrhage into tissue	Hemorrhage into tissue	Hemorrhage into tissue
Alpha-1-antitrypsin deficiency	Alpha-1-antitrypsin deficiency	Alpha-1-antitrypsin deficiency	Alpha-1-antitrypsin deficiency	Alpha-1-antitrypsin deficiency	Alpha-1-antitrypsin deficiency
Dubin-Johnson syndrome	Dubin-Johnson syndrome	Dubin-Johnson syndrome	Rotor syndrome	Rotor syndrome	Rotor syndrome
Rotor syndrome	Rotor syndrome	Rotor syndrome	Amino acidurea	Amino acidurea	Amino acidurea

Emergency Rule Out conditions shown in red. Entries in blue are for information only
Conditions are listed in approximate order of prevalence for this age range

43

Emergency Rule Out conditions shown in red. Entries in blue are for information only
Conditions are listed in approximate order of prevalence for this age range

Baby (0-1 yr)	Child (1-12 yr)	Adolescent (12-18 yr)	Adult (18-45 yr)	Middle Age Adult (45-65 yr)	Senior Adult (65+ yr)
Primary intracerebral hemorrhage stroke	Primary intracerebral hemorrhage stroke	Primary intracerebral hemorrhage stroke Subarachnoid hemorrhage and cerebral aneurysm stroke	Primary intracerebral hemorrhage stroke Subarachnoid hemorrhage and cerebral aneurysm stroke	Primary intracerebral hemorrhage stroke Subarachnoid hemorrhage and cerebral aneurysm stroke	Primary intracerebral hemorrhage stroke Subarachnoid hemorrhage and cerebral aneurysm stroke

Baby (0-1 yr)	Child (1-12 yr)	Adolescent (12-18 yr)	Adult (18-45 yr)	Middle Age Adult (45-65 yr)	Senior Adult (65+ yr)
Anal fissure	Anal fissure	Anal fissure	Anal fissure	Hemorrhoids	Hemorrhoids
Constipation	Constipation	Constipation	Hemorrhoids	Anal fissure	Anal carcinoma
Proctitis	Idiopathic thrombocytopenic purpura	Proctitis	Anal carcinoma	Anal carcinoma	Anal fissure
Idiopathic thrombocytopenic purpura	Proctitis	Idiopathic thrombocytopenic purpura	Malignancy	Amebic dysentery	Malignancy
Amebic dysentery	Amebic dysentery	Amebic dysentery	Proctitis	Colon cancer	Idiopathic thrombocytopenic purpura
Meckel's diverticulum	Encopresis	Hemorrhoids	Colon cancer	Idiopathic thrombocytopenic purpura	Colon cancer
	Crohn's disease	Ulcerative colitis	Idiopathic thrombocytopenic purpura	Proctitis	Cervical malignancy
	Meckel's diverticulum	Crohn's disease	Cervical malignancy	Cervical malignancy	Amebic dysentery
		Meckel's diverticulum	Amebic dysentery	Malignancy	Proctitis
			Vulvar malignancy	Vulvar malignancy	Vulvar malignancy
			Diverticular disease	Diverticular disease	Diverticular disease
			Crohn's disease	Crohn's disease	Crohn's disease
			Ulcerative colitis	Ulcerative colitis	Ulcerative colitis
			Arteriovenous malformation of the colon	Arteriovenous malformation of the colon	Arteriovenous malformation of the colon
			Acute mesenteric ischemia	Acute mesenteric ischemia	Acute mesenteric ischemia

Bleeding from anus

Emergency Rule Out conditions shown in red. Entries in blue are for information only
Conditions are listed in approximate order of prevalence for this age range

Bleeding from mouth

Emergency Rule Out conditions shown in red. Entries in blue are for information only
Conditions are listed in approximate order of prevalence for this age range

Baby (0-1 yr)	Child (1-12 yr)	Adolescent (12-18 yr)	Adult (18-45 yr)	Middle Age Adult (45-65 yr)	Senior Adult (65+ yr)
Trauma	Trauma	Trauma	Dental infection	Dental infection	Dental infection
Oral cavity cancer	Epistaxis	Epistaxis	Epistaxis	Epistaxis	Idiopathic thrombocytopenic purpura
Idiopathic thrombocytopenic purpura	Idiopathic thrombocytopenic purpura	Idiopathic thrombocytopenic purpura	Idiopathic thrombocytopenic purpura	Oral cavity cancer	Epistaxis
Epistaxis	Oral cavity cancer	Oral cavity cancer	Oral cavity cancer	Idiopathic thrombocytopenic purpura	Oral cavity cancer
	Tonsillitis	Tonsillitis	Gingivitis	Gingivitis	Gingivitis
	Dental infection	Dental infection	Trauma	Trauma	Trauma

46

Baby (0-1 yr)	Child (1-12 yr)	Adolescent (12-18 yr)	Adult (18-45 yr)	Middle Age Adult (45-65 yr)	Senior Adult (65+ yr)
Not relevant to this age group	Not relevant to this age group	Miscarriage Placenta previa Abruptio placentae Cervicitis Vaginal bleeding during pregnancy Ectopic pregnancy Retained products of gestation Cervical ectropion Gestational trophoblastic neoplasm Excessive anticoagulation	Miscarriage Ectopic pregnancy Cervical ectropion Cervicitis Vaginal bleeding during pregnancy Placenta previa Abruptio placentae Gestational trophoblastic neoplasm Excessive anticoagulation Retained products of gestation	Miscarriage Ectopic pregnancy Cervical ectropion Cervicitis Retained products of gestation Vaginal bleeding during pregnancy Abruptio placentae Placenta previa Excessive anticoagulation Gestational trophoblastic neoplasm	Not relevant to this age group

Emergency Rule Out conditions shown in red. Entries in blue are for information only
Conditions are listed in approximate order of prevalence for this age range

Bleeding in pregnancy

Emergency Rule Out conditions shown in red. Entries in blue are for information only
Conditions are listed in approximate order of prevalence for this age range

Baby (0-1 yr)	Child (1-12 yr)	Adolescent (12-18 yr)	Adult (18-45 yr)	Middle Age Adult (45-65 yr)	Senior Adult (65+yr)
Papilledema	Papilledema	Papilledema	Papilledema	Papilledema	Papilledema
Intracranial hemorrhage	Acute retinitis	Intracranial hemorrhage	Acute retinitis	Acute retinitis	Retinal tear
Acute retinitis	Retinal and vitreous hemorrhage	Acute retinitis	Retinal tear	Retinal tear	Retinal and vitreous hemorrhage
Retinal and vitreous hemorrhage	Retinal tear	Optic neuritis	Optic neuritis	Optic neuritis	Acute retinitis
Retinal tear	Optic neuritis	Retinal tear	Retinal and vitreous hemorrhage	Retinal and vitreous hemorrhage	Retinal artery occlusion
		Retinal and vitreous hemorrhage	Intracranial hemorrhage	Intracranial hemorrhage	Retinal vein occlusion
			Retinal artery occlusion	Retinal artery occlusion	Intracranial hemorrhage
			Retinal vein occlusion	Retinal vein occlusion	

Baby (0-1 yr)	Child (1-12 yr)	Adolescent (12-18 yr)	Adult (18-45 yr)	Middle Age Adult (45-65 yr)	Senior Adult (65+ yr)
Not relevant to this age group	Corneal abrasion	Myopia	Myopia	Myopia	Hypermetropia
	Vasovagal response	Vasovagal response	Hypermetropia	Hypermetropia	Myopia
	Myopia	Corneal abrasion	Diabetic retinopathy	Diabetic retinopathy	Diabetic retinopathy
	Hypermetropia	Hypermetropia	Diabetes mellitus type 2	Diabetes mellitus type 2	Diabetes mellitus type 2
	Orthostatic hypotension	Orthostatic hypotension	Vasovagal response	Vasovagal response	Vasovagal response
	Non-diabetic hypoglycemia	Cataract	Multiple myeloma	Glaucoma	Orthostatic hypotension
	Cavernous sinus thrombosis	Glaucoma	Cataract	Orthostatic hypotension	Glaucoma
	Retinal migraine	Cavernous sinus thrombosis	Glaucoma	Multiple myeloma	Multiple myeloma
	Botulism	Non-diabetic hypoglycemia	Migraine headache	Cataract	Cavernous sinus thrombosis
	Acute retinitis	Retinal detachment	Orthostatic hypotension	Cavernous sinus thrombosis	Cataract
	Retinal detachment	Botulism	Cavernous sinus thrombosis	Corneal abrasion	Corneal abrasion
	Uveitis	Acute retinitis	Corneal abrasion	Uveitis	Uveitis
	Retinal vein occlusion	Retinal migraine	Uveitis	Migraine headache	Acute retinitis
		Uveitis	Acute retinitis	Botulism	Botulism
		Retinal vein occlusion	Botulism	Acute retinitis	Retinal detachment
			Retinal detachment	Retinal detachment	Retinal migraine
			Retinal migraine	Retinal migraine	Retinal vein occlusion
			Retinal vein occlusion	Retinal vein occlusion	Migraine headache

Emergency Rule Out conditions shown in red. Entries in blue are for information only
Conditions are listed in approximate order of prevalence for this age range

Emergency Rule Out conditions shown in red. Entries in blue are for information only
Conditions are listed in approximate order of prevalence for this age range

Baby (0-1 yr)	Child (1-12 yr)	Adolescent (12-18 yr)	Adult (18-45 yr)	Middle Age Adult (45-65 yr)	Senior Adult (65+yr)
Chronic idiopathic neutropenia	Chronic idiopathic neutropenia	Chronic idiopathic neutropenia	Chronic idiopathic neutropenia	Chronic idiopathic neutropenia	Chronic idiopathic neutropenia
Aplastic anemia	Diabetes mellitus in children	Hidradenitis suppurativa	Hidradenitis suppurativa	Diabetes mellitus type 2	Diabetes mellitus type 2
Acute leukemia	Hidradenitis suppurativa	Diabetes mellitus type 2	Diabetes mellitus type 2	Hidradenitis suppurativa	Hidradenitis suppurativa
Diabetes mellitus in children	Acute leukemia	Acute leukemia	Acute leukemia	Acute leukemia	Chronic lymphocytic leukemia
Chronic lymphocytic leukemia	Aplastic anemia	Chronic lymphocytic leukemia	Chronic lymphocytic leukemia	Chronic lymphocytic leukemia	Chronic myelogenous leukemia
Chronic myelogenous leukemia	Metastatic cancer	Chronic myelogenous leukemia	Chronic myelogenous leukemia	Chronic myelogenous leukemia	Multiple myeloma
Hidradenitis suppurativa	Diabetes mellitus type 2	Aplastic anemia	Diabetes mellitus type 1	Diabetes mellitus type 1	Metastatic cancer
AIDS	Chronic lymphocytic leukemia	Metastatic cancer	Aplastic anemia	Aplastic anemia	Acute leukemia
Immunodeficiency diseases	Chronic myelogenous leukemia	Diabetes mellitus in children	Multiple myeloma	Multiple myeloma	Diabetes mellitus type 1
	AIDS	Myelodysplastic syndromes	Myelodysplastic syndromes	Myelodysplastic syndromes	Aplastic anemia
	Immunodeficiency diseases	Idiopathic myelofibrosis	Idiopathic myelofibrosis	Idiopathic myelofibrosis	Myelodysplastic syndromes
		AIDS	Metastatic cancer	Metastatic cancer	Idiopathic myelofibrosis
		Immunodeficiency diseases	AIDS	AIDS	AIDS
			Immunodeficiency diseases	Immunodeficiency diseases	Immunodeficiency diseases

Baby (0-1 yr)	Child (1-12 yr)	Adolescent (12-18 yr)	Adult (18-45 yr)	Middle Age Adult (45-65 yr)	Senior Adult (65+yr)
Fracture	Fracture	Fracture	Callus	Callus	Callus
Callus	Callus	Callus	Fracture	Osteoarthritis	Osteoarthritis
Exostosis (osteochondroma)	Exostosis (osteochondroma)	Exostosis (osteochondroma)	Paget's disease	Fracture	Fracture
Osgood-Schlatter disease	Osgood-Schlatter disease	Osgood-Schlatter disease	Metastatic cancer	Paget's disease	Paget's disease
Enchondroma	Osteoma	Osteoma	Osgood-Schlatter disease	Metastatic cancer	Metastatic cancer
Osteoma	Osteosarcoma	Enchondroma	Multiple myeloma	Osgood-Schlatter disease	Osgood-Schlatter disease
Osteosarcoma	Enchondroma	Osteosarcoma	Acromegaly (pituitary gigantism)	Multiple myeloma	Multiple myeloma
Acromegaly (pituitary gigantism)	Periosteal fibrosarcoma	Periosteal fibrosarcoma	Periosteal fibrosarcoma	Periosteal fibrosarcoma	Periosteal fibrosarcoma
	Acromegaly (pituitary gigantism)	Acromegaly (pituitary gigantism)	Exostosis (osteochondroma)	Exostosis (osteochondroma)	Exostosis (osteochondroma)
			Enchondroma	Acromegaly (pituitary gigantism)	Acromegaly (pituitary gigantism)
			Osteoma	Enchondroma	Enchondroma
			Osteosarcoma	Osteoma	Osteoma
				Osteosarcoma	Osteosarcoma

Emergency Rule Out conditions shown in red. Entries in blue are for information only
Conditions are listed in approximate order of prevalence for this age range

Emergency Rule Out conditions shown in red. Entries in blue are for information only
Conditions are listed in approximate order of prevalence for this age range

Bowel habits, change in

Baby (0-1 yr)	Child (1-12 yr)	Adolescent (12-18 yr)	Adult (18-45 yr)	Middle Age Adult (45-65 yr)	Senior Adult (65+yr)
Hypothyroidism	Anxiety	Anxiety	Irritable bowel syndrome	Depression	Depression
Drug reaction	Irritable bowel syndrome	Irritable bowel syndrome	Depression	Irritable bowel syndrome	Hypothyroidism
Hyperthyroidism	Drug reaction	Drug reaction	Hypothyroidism	Hypothyroidism	Irritable bowel syndrome
Pseudomembranous colitis	Hypothyroidism	Hypothyroidism	Hyperthyroidism	Hyperthyroidism	Colon cancer
	Pseudomembranous colitis	Hyperthyroidism	Acute pancreatitis	Colon cancer	Acute pancreatitis
	Hyperthyroidism	Anorexia nervosa	Anorexia nervosa	Acute pancreatitis	Pancreatic cancer
		Pseudomembranous colitis	Colon cancer	Pancreatic cancer	Hyperthyroidism
			Pancreatic cancer	Anorexia nervosa	Pseudomembranous colitis
			Ischemic bowel disease	Ischemic bowel disease	Anorexia nervosa
			Pseudomembranous colitis	Pseudomembranous colitis	Ischemic bowel disease
			Anxiety	Anxiety	Anxiety
			Epithelial cell ovarian cancer	Epithelial cell ovarian cancer	Epithelial cell ovarian cancer
			Germ cell ovarian cancer	Germ cell ovarian cancer	Germ cell ovarian cancer
			Sex cord/stromal ovarian cancer	Sex cord/stromal ovarian cancer	Sex cord/stromal ovarian cancer

Baby (0-1 yr)	Child (1-12 yr)	Adolescent (12-18 yr)	Adult (18-45 yr)	Middle Age Adult (45-65 yr)	Senior Adult (65-yr)
Paralytic ileus	Paralytic ileus	Paralytic ileus	Paralytic ileus	Paralytic ileus	Paralytic ileus
Peritonitis	Peritonitis	Peritonitis	Peritonitis	Peritonitis	Peritonitis
Hypokalemia	Hypokalemia	Hypokalemia	Hypokalemia	Hypokalemia	Hypokalemia
			Ischemic bowel disease	Ischemic bowel disease	Ischemic bowel disease

Emergency Rule Out conditions shown in red. Entries in blue are for information only
Conditions are listed in approximate order of prevalence for this age range

Bowel sounds, reduced

B

Emergency Rule Out conditions shown in red. Entries in blue are for information only
Conditions are listed in approximate order of prevalence for this age range

Baby (0-1 yr)	Child (1-12 yr)	Adolescent (12-18 yr)	Adult (18-45 yr)	Middle Age Adult (45-65 yr)	Senior Adult (65+ yr)
Allergic reactions and anaphylaxis	Vasovagal response	Vasovagal response	Hypothermia	Hypothyroidism	Hypothyroidism
Congenital heart disease	Healthy athlete	Healthy athlete	Hypothyroidism	Hypothermia	Hypothermia
Drug reaction	Fright	Drug reaction	Myocardial infarction	Myocardial infarction	Myocardial infarction
Congestive heart failure	Congenital heart disease	Fright	Psittacosis	Healthy athlete	Healthy athlete
Hypothyroidism	Allergic reactions and anaphylaxis	Allergic reactions and anaphylaxis	Healthy athlete	Typhoid fever	Psittacosis
Hypothermia	Congestive heart failure	Congestive heart failure	Vasovagal response	Psittacosis	Typhoid fever
Psittacosis	Drug reaction	Psittacosis	Typhoid fever	Vasovagal response	Vasovagal response
Typhoid fever	Psittacosis	Typhoid fever	Drug reaction	Drug reaction	Drug reaction
AV block, first degree	Typhoid fever	Hypothermia	AV block, first degree	AV block, first degree	AV block, first degree
AV block, second degree	Post-infection	Post-infection	AV block, second degree	AV block, second degree	AV block, second degree
AV block, third degree	Hypothermia	Hypothyroidism	AV block, third degree	AV block, third degree	AV block, third degree
Post-infection	Hypothyroidism	AV block, first degree			
	AV block, first degree	AV block, second degree			
	AV block, second degree	AV block, third degree			
	AV block, third degree				

54

Baby (0-1 yr)	Child (1-12 yr)	Adolescent (12-18 yr)	Adult (18-45 yr)	Middle Age Adult (45-65 yr)	Senior Adult (65+ yr)
Maternal estrogen	Precocious puberty Breast abscess	Fibrocystic breast disease Fibroadenosis Breast fibroadenoma Breast cyst Lactating mastitis Breast cancer	Breast cyst Breast fibroadenoma Fibrocystic breast disease Lactating mastitis Breast cancer Intraductal papilloma Thrombophlebitis Fibroadenosis	Breast fibroadenoma Breast cyst Breast cancer Fibrocystic breast disease Intraductal papilloma Thrombophlebitis Fibroadenosis	Breast cancer Breast fibroadenoma Breast cyst Intraductal papilloma Thrombophlebitis Fibrocystic breast disease Fibroadenosis

Emergency Rule Out conditions shown in red. Entries in blue are for information only
Conditions are listed in approximate order of prevalence for this age range

Breast tenderness

Emergency Rule Out conditions shown in red. Entries in blue are for information only
Conditions are listed in approximate order of prevalence for this age range

Baby (0-1 yr)	Child (1-12 yr)	Adolescent (12-18 yr)	Adult (18-45 yr)	Middle Age Adult (45-65 yr)	Senior Adult (65+ yr)
Not relevant to this age group	Not relevant to this age group	Fibrocystic breast disease Breast cancer Premenstrual syndrome Breast fibroadenoma	Fibrocystic breast disease Breast cancer Premenstrual syndrome Breast fibroadenoma	Fibrocystic breast disease Breast cancer Premenstrual syndrome Breast fibroadenoma	Fibrocystic breast disease Breast cancer Breast fibroadenoma

Baby (0-1 yr)	Child (1-12 yr)	Adolescent (12-18 yr)	Adult (18-45 yr)	Middle Age Adult (45-65 yr)	Senior Adult (65+ yr)
Behavioral problem in children	Behavioral problem in children	Anxiety	Not relevant to this age group	Not relevant to this age group	Not relevant to this age group
Sepsis	Sepsis	Sepsis			
		Chronic fatigue syndrome			

Emergency Rule Out conditions shown in red. Entries in blue are for information only
Conditions are listed in approximate order of prevalence for this age range

Emergency Rule Out conditions shown in red. Entries in blue are for information only
Conditions are listed in approximate order of prevalence for this age range

Baby (0-1 yr)	Child (1-12 yr)	Adolescent (12-18 yr)	Adult (18-45 yr)	Middle Age Adult (45-65 yr)	Senior Adult (65+yr)
Idiopathic Child abuse	Acute leukemia Child abuse Idiopathic	Acute leukemia Child abuse Idiopathic	Acute leukemia Idiopathic	Acute leukemia Idiopathic	Acute leukemia Idiopathic

Baby (0-1 yr)	Child (1-12 yr)	Adolescent (12-18 yr)	Adult (18-45 yr)	Middle Age Adult (45-65 yr)	Senior Adult (65+yr)
Aortic stenosis Peripheral vascular disease Renal artery stenosis	Aortic stenosis Renal artery stenosis Peripheral vascular disease Abdominal aortic aneurysm Hemangioma of the liver Thoracic aortic aneurysm	Aortic stenosis Renal artery stenosis Peripheral vascular disease Abdominal aortic aneurysm Thoracic aortic aneurysm Hemangioma of the liver	Asymptomatic carotid stenosis Abdominal aortic aneurysm Peripheral vascular disease Thoracic aortic aneurysm Renal artery stenosis	Asymptomatic carotid stenosis Abdominal aortic aneurysm Peripheral vascular disease Thoracic aortic aneurysm Renal artery stenosis	Asymptomatic carotid stenosis Peripheral vascular disease Abdominal aortic aneurysm Thoracic aortic aneurysm Renal artery stenosis

Bruit

Emergency Rule Out conditions shown in red. Entries in blue are for information only
Conditions are listed in approximate order of prevalence for this age range

Emergency Rule Out conditions shown in red. Entries in blue are for information only
Conditions are listed in approximate order of prevalence for this age range

Baby (0-1 yr)	Child (1-12 yr)	Adolescent (12-18 yr)	Adult (18-45 yr)	Middle Age Adult (45-65 yr)	Senior Adult (65-yr)
Patent ductus arteriosus	Atrial septal defect	Atrial septal defect	Mitral regurgitation	Mitral regurgitation	Mitral regurgitation
Atrial septal defect	Ventricular septal defect	Ventricular septal defect	Aortic stenosis	Aortic stenosis	Aortic stenosis
Ventricular septal defect	Idiopathic hypertrophic subaortic stenosis	Patent ductus arteriosus	Mitral valve prolapse	Mitral valve prolapse	Mitral valve prolapse
Coarctation of the aorta	Patent ductus arteriosus	Mitral regurgitation	Atrial septal defect	Atrial septal defect	Atrial septal defect
Infective endocarditis	Mitral regurgitation	Mitral stenosis	Aortic sclerosis	Infective endocarditis	Mitral stenosis
Mitral stenosis	Infective endocarditis	Infective endocarditis	Mitral stenosis	Aortic sclerosis	Infective endocarditis
Mitral regurgitation	Mitral stenosis	Aortic stenosis	Aortic regurgitation	Mitral stenosis	Aortic regurgitation
Idiopathic hypertrophic subaortic stenosis	Coarctation of the aorta	Aortic regurgitation	Infective endocarditis	Aortic regurgitation	Tricuspid stenosis
Aortic stenosis	Pulmonary valve stenosis	Pulmonary valve stenosis	Tricuspid stenosis	Tricuspid stenosis	Idiopathic hypertrophic subaortic stenosis
Arteriovenous fistula	Tricuspid regurgitation	Tricuspid stenosis	Idiopathic hypertrophic subaortic stenosis	Idiopathic hypertrophic subaortic stenosis	Pulmonary valve stenosis
Pulmonary valve stenosis	Tricuspid stenosis	Idiopathic hypertrophic subaortic stenosis	Pulmonary valve stenosis	Pulmonary valve stenosis	Pulmonic valve insufficiency (pulmonic regurgitation)
Tricuspid stenosis	Arteriovenous fistula	Arteriovenous fistula	Pulmonic valve insufficiency (pulmonic regurgitation)	Pulmonic valve insufficiency (pulmonic regurgitation)	Ventricular septal defect
Tricuspid regurgitation	Aortic sclerosis	Coarctation of the aorta	Ventricular septal defect	Ventricular septal defect	Cardiomyopathy
Aortic sclerosis		Aortic sclerosis	Cardiomyopathy	Cardiomyopathy	Tricuspid regurgitation
		Tricuspid regurgitation	Tricuspid regurgitation	Tricuspid regurgitation	Coarctation of the aorta
			Coarctation of the aorta	Coarctation of the aorta	Patent ductus arteriosus
			Patent ductus arteriosus	Patent ductus arteriosus	

Baby (0-1 yr)	Child (1-12 yr)	Adolescent (12-18 yr)	Adult (18-45 yr)	Middle Age Adult (45-65 yr)	Senior Adult (65+ yr)
Pericarditis	Pericarditis	Pericarditis	Myocardial infarction	Myocardial infarction	Myocardial infarction
Infective endocarditis	Infective endocarditis	Infective endocarditis	Trauma	Trauma	Trauma
Trauma	Trauma	Trauma	Infective endocarditis	Infective endocarditis	Infective endocarditis
Cardiac tamponade	Cardiac tamponade	Cardiac tamponade	Prosthetic valve failure	Prosthetic valve failure	Prosthetic valve failure
Pericardial effusion	Pericardial effusion	Pericardial effusion	Pulmonary thromboembolism	Pulmonary thromboembolism	Pulmonary thromboembolism
AV block, third degree	AV block, third degree	AV block, third degree	Abdominal aortic dissection	Thoracic aortic dissection	Abdominal aortic dissection
Ventricular tachycardia	Ventricular tachycardia	Ventricular tachycardia	Thoracic aortic dissection	Abdominal aortic dissection	Thoracic aortic dissection
		Myocardial infarction	Pericarditis	Pericarditis	Pericarditis
			Cardiac tamponade	Cardiac tamponade	Cardiac tamponade
			Pericardial effusion	Pericardial effusion	Pericardial effusion
			AV block, third degree	AV block, third degree	AV block, third degree
			Ventricular tachycardia	Ventricular tachycardia	Ventricular tachycardia

Emergency Rule Out conditions shown in red. Entries in blue are for information only
Conditions are listed in approximate order of prevalence for this age range

Emergency Rule Out conditions shown in red. Entries in blue are for information only
Conditions are listed in approximate order of prevalence for this age range

Baby (0-1 yr)	Child (1-12 yr)	Adolescent (12-18 yr)	Adult (18-45 yr)	Middle Age Adult (45-65 yr)	Senior Adult (65+ yr)
Congestive heart failure	Cardiomyopathy	Cardiomyopathy	Cardiomyopathy	Cardiomyopathy	Cardiomyopathy
Tetralogy of Fallot	Congestive heart failure	Congestive heart failure	Healthy athlete	Healthy athlete	Healthy athlete
Cardiomyopathy	Idiopathic hypertrophic	Healthy athlete	Kyphoscoliosis	Kyphoscoliosis	Kyphoscoliosis
Cor pulmonale	subaortic stenosis	Kyphosis	Kyphosis	Kyphosis	Kyphosis
Mitral regurgitation	Healthy athlete	Kyphoscoliosis	Congestive heart failure	Congestive heart failure	Congestive heart failure
Idiopathic hypertrophic	Mitral regurgitation	Mitral stenosis	Mitral regurgitation	Mitral regurgitation	Mitral regurgitation
subaortic stenosis	Cor pulmonale	Mitral regurgitation	Mitral stenosis	Mitral stenosis	Mitral stenosis
Iron deficiency anemia	Kyphosis	Idiopathic hypertrophic	Aortic stenosis	Aortic stenosis	Aortic stenosis
	Kyphoscoliosis	subaortic stenosis	Pulmonary hypertension	Pulmonary hypertension	Pulmonary hypertension
	Mitral stenosis	Cor pulmonale	Cor pulmonale	Cor pulmonale	Cor pulmonale
	Marfan's syndrome	Iron deficiency anemia	Marfan's syndrome	Marfan's syndrome	Marfan's syndrome
	Iron deficiency anemia	Aortic stenosis	Idiopathic hypertrophic	Idiopathic hypertrophic	Idiopathic hypertrophic
		Marfan's syndrome	subaortic stenosis	subaortic stenosis	subaortic stenosis

Baby (0-1 yr)	Child (1-12 yr)	Adolescent (12-18 yr)	Adult (18-45 yr)	Middle Age Adult (45-65 yr)	Senior Adult (65+ yr)
Hyperthyroidism Aortic stenosis Takayasu's syndrome	Hyperthyroidism Aortic stenosis Takayasu's syndrome	Hyperthyroidism Aortic stenosis Takayasu's syndrome	Aortic stenosis Hyperthyroidism Takayasu's syndrome	Aortic stenosis Hyperthyroidism Takayasu's syndrome	Aortic stenosis Hyperthyroidism Takayasu's syndrome

Carotid bruit

Emergency Rule Out conditions shown in red. Entries in blue are for information only
Conditions are listed in approximate order of prevalence for this age range

Emergency Rule Out conditions shown in red. Entries in blue are for information only
Conditions are listed in approximate order of prevalence for this age range

Baby (0-1 yr)	Child (1-12 yr)	Adolescent (12-18 yr)	Adult (18-45 yr)	Middle Age Adult (45-65 yr)	Senior Adult (65+yr)
Trauma	Sexual abuse	Sexual abuse	Sexual abuse	Sexual abuse	Sexual abuse
Foreign body	Cervicitis	Cervicitis	Cervicitis	Cervicitis	Cervical dysplasia
	Trauma	Oral contraception	Cervical ectropion	Cervical ectropion	Cervicitis
	Foreign body	Genital warts	Genital warts	Genital warts	Cervical ectropion
		Cervical dysplasia	Cervical dysplasia	Cervical dysplasia	Genital warts
		Cervical ectropion	Trauma	Trauma	Trauma
		Cervical malignancy	Foreign body	Foreign body	Foreign body
		Trauma			
		Foreign body			

Baby (0-1 yr)	Child (1-12 yr)	Adolescent (12-18 yr)	Adult (18-45 yr)	Middle Age Adult (45-65 yr)	Senior Adult (65+ yr)
Not relevant to this age group	Not relevant to this age group	Cervicitis Cervical dysplasia Genital warts Cervical ectropion Cervical malignancy	Cervicitis Genital warts Cervical ectropion Cervical dysplasia Cervical malignancy	Cervicitis Genital warts Cervical ectropion Cervical dysplasia Cervical malignancy	Genital warts Cervical dysplasia Cervical malignancy Cervicitis

Emergency Rule Out conditions shown in red. Entries in blue are for information only
Conditions are listed in approximate order of prevalence for this age range

Cervical smear, abnormal

Emergency Rule Out conditions shown in red. Entries in blue are for information only
Conditions are listed in approximate order of prevalence for this age range

Baby (0-1 yr)	Child (1-12 yr)	Adolescent (12-18 yr)	Adult (18-45 yr)	Middle Age Adult (45-65 yr)	Senior Adult (65+ yr)
Not relevant to this age group	Bacterial pneumonia	Bacterial pneumonia	Gastroesophageal reflux disease	Gastroesophageal reflux disease	Angina
	Viral pneumonia	Viral pneumonia	Bacterial pneumonia	Angina	Gastroesophageal reflux disease
	Mycoplasmal pneumonia	Mycoplasmal pneumonia	Viral pneumonia	Unstable angina	Unstable angina
	Costochondritis	Costochondritis	Angina	Bacterial pneumonia	Bacterial pneumonia
	Cough	Esophageal spasm	Unstable angina	Viral pneumonia	Viral pneumonia
	Pleurisy	Cough	Myocardial infarction	Myocardial infarction	Myocardial infarction
	Carbon monoxide poisoning	Pleurisy	Panic disorder	Mycoplasmal pneumonia	Mycoplasmal pneumonia
	Pneumothorax	Pneumothorax	Mycoplasmal pneumonia	Behçet's syndrome	Aspiration pneumonia
	Asthma	Asthma	Behçet's syndrome	Aspiration pneumonia	Aortic regurgitation
	Trauma	Trauma	Pleurisy	Aortic regurgitation	Carbon monoxide poisoning
	Behçet's syndrome	Aortic regurgitation	Pneumothorax	Pulmonary thromboembolism	Behçet's syndrome
	Aortic regurgitation	Carbon monoxide poisoning	Thoracic aortic dissection	Cardiac tamponade	Cardiac tamponade
	Muscular strain	Behçet's syndrome	Carbon monoxide poisoning	Carbon monoxide poisoning	Pulmonary thromboembolism
	Esophageal spasm	Muscular strain	Aortic regurgitation	Panic disorder	Panic disorder
	Cardiac tamponade	Cardiac tamponade	Cardiac tamponade	Pleurisy	Pleurisy
	Panic disorder	Panic disorder	Pulmonary thromboembolism	Thoracic aortic dissection	Thoracic aortic dissection
	Recreational drug abuse	Pulmonary thromboembolism	Recreational drug abuse	Biliary tract disease	Herpes zoster, shingles
	Pericarditis	Recreational drug abuse	Herpes zoster, shingles	Pneumothorax	Biliary tract disease
	Aortic stenosis	Pericarditis	Sickle cell anemia	Herpes zoster, shingles	Pneumothorax
	Mitral valve prolapse	Aortic stenosis	Pericarditis	Primary lung malignancy	Primary lung malignancy
	Gastroesophageal reflux disease	Mitral valve prolapse	Primary lung malignancy	Pericarditis	
	Foreign body				

Baby (0-1 yr)	Child (1-12 yr)	Adolescent (12-18 yr)	Adult (18-45 yr)	Middle Age Adult (45-65 yr)	Senior Adult (65-yr)
	Sickle cell anemia Herpes zoster, shingles	Gastroesophageal reflux disease Foreign body Sickle cell anemia Herpes zoster, shingles Biliary tract disease	Aspiration pneumonia Biliary tract disease Asthma	Sickle cell anemia Asthma	Pericarditis Asthma

Emergency Rule Out conditions shown in red. Entries in blue are for information only
Conditions are listed in approximate order of prevalence for this age range

Baby (0-1 yr)	Child (1-12 yr)	Adolescent (12-18 yr)	Adult (18-45 yr)	Middle Age Adult (45-65 yr)	Senior Adult (65+ yr)
Trauma	Trauma	Trauma	Lymphadenopathy	Lymphadenopathy	Lymphadenopathy
Lymphadenopathy	Lymphadenopathy	Lymphadenopathy	Fibrocystic breast disease	Lipoma	Lipoma
Soft tissue sarcoma	Lipoma	Fibrocystic breast disease	Lipoma	Fibrocystic breast disease	Fibrocystic breast disease
Scoliosis	Scoliosis	Breast fibroadenoma	Breast abscess	Breast abscess	Breast cancer
	Breast abscess	Scoliosis	Breast cancer	Breast cancer	Breast abscess
	Soft tissue sarcoma	Lipoma	Breast fibroadenoma	Breast fibroadenoma	Breast fibroadenoma
		Breast abscess	Scoliosis	Scoliosis	Scoliosis
		Soft tissue sarcoma	Soft tissue sarcoma	Soft tissue sarcoma	Soft tissue sarcoma

Cheyne-Stokes breathing

Baby (0-1 yr)	Child (1-12 yr)	Adolescent (12-18 yr)	Adult (18-45 yr)	Middle Age Adult (45-65 yr)	Senior Adult (65+ yr)
Primary intracerebral hemorrhage stroke	Primary intracerebral hemorrhage stroke	Primary intracerebral hemorrhage stroke	Brain tumor	Brain tumor	Brain tumor
Subarachnoid hemorrhage and cerebral aneurysm stroke	Subarachnoid hemorrhage and cerebral aneurysm stroke	Subarachnoid hemorrhage and cerebral aneurysm stroke	Bacterial meningitis	Bacterial meningitis	Bacterial meningitis
Brain tumor	Brain tumor	Brain tumor	Viral meningitis	Viral meningitis	Viral meningitis
Viral meningitis	Bacterial meningitis	Bacterial meningitis	Ischemic stroke	Ischemic stroke	Ischemic stroke
Bacterial meningitis	Viral meningitis	Viral meningitis	Primary intracerebral hemorrhage stroke	Primary intracerebral hemorrhage stroke	Primary intracerebral hemorrhage stroke
Hypoxia	Hypoxia	Hypoxia	Subarachnoid hemorrhage and cerebral aneurysm stroke	Subarachnoid hemorrhage and cerebral aneurysm stroke	Subarachnoid hemorrhage and cerebral aneurysm stroke
Congestive heart failure	Congestive heart failure	Congestive heart failure	Bacterial pneumonia	Bacterial pneumonia	Bacterial pneumonia
Bacterial pneumonia	Viral pneumonia	Bacterial pneumonia	Aspiration pneumonia	Aspiration pneumonia	Aspiration pneumonia
Viral pneumonia	Bacterial pneumonia	Viral pneumonia	Viral pneumonia	Viral pneumonia	Viral pneumonia
			Hypoxia	Hypoxia	Hypoxia
			Congestive heart failure	Congestive heart failure	Congestive heart failure

Emergency Rule Out conditions shown in red. Entries in blue are for information only
Conditions are listed in approximate order of prevalence for this age range

Emergency Rule Out conditions shown in red. Entries in blue are for information only
Conditions are listed in approximate order of prevalence for this age range

Baby (0-1 yr)	Child (1-12 yr)	Adolescent (12-18 yr)	Adult (18-45 yr)	Middle Age Adult (45-65 yr)	Senior Adult (65+ yr)
Urinary tract infection	Urinary tract infection	Urinary tract infection	Filariasis	Filariasis	Filariasis
Filariasis	Filariasis	Filariasis	Lymphatic obstruction	Lymphatic obstruction	Lymphatic obstruction
Lymphatic obstruction	Lymphatic obstruction	Lymphatic obstruction	Urinary tract infection	Urinary tract infection	Urinary tract infection
			Giardiasis	Giardiasis	Giardiasis

Baby (0-1 yr)	Child (1-12 yr)	Adolescent (12-18 yr)	Adult (18-45 yr)	Middle Age Adult (45-65 yr)	Senior Adult (65+ yr)
Not relevant to this age group	Muscular strain Coarctation of the aorta Peripheral vascular disease Thoracic outlet syndrome Deep vein thrombosis Arterial embolus and thrombosis	Muscular strain Coarctation of the aorta Peripheral vascular disease Thoracic outlet syndrome Deep vein thrombosis Arterial embolus and thrombosis	Arteriosclerosis Muscular strain Deep vein thrombosis Peripheral vascular disease Thoracic outlet syndrome Lumbar disc disorders Arterial embolus and thrombosis Spinal stenosis and neurogenic claudication Thoracic aortic dissection	Arteriosclerosis Muscular strain Deep vein thrombosis Thoracic outlet syndrome Peripheral vascular disease Lumbar disc disorders Arterial embolus and thrombosis Spinal stenosis and neurogenic claudication Thoracic aortic dissection	Arteriosclerosis Muscular strain Deep vein thrombosis Peripheral vascular disease Lumbar disc disorders Thoracic outlet syndrome Arterial embolus and thrombosis Spinal stenosis and neurogenic claudication Thoracic aortic dissection

Emergency Rule Out conditions shown in red. Entries in blue are for information only
Conditions are listed in approximate order of prevalence for this age range

Emergency Rule Out conditions shown in red. Entries in blue are for information only
Conditions are listed in approximate order of prevalence for this age range

Baby (0-1 yr)	Child (1-12 yr)	Adolescent (12-18 yr)	Adult (18-45 yr)	Middle Age Adult (45-65 yr)	Senior Adult (65+yr)
Hypoxia	Head injury	Head injury	Head injury	Bacterial meningitis	Cerebellar hemorrhage
Head injury	Bacterial meningitis	Bacterial meningitis	Diabetic hypoglycemia	Head injury	Diabetic hypoglycemia
Salicylate poisoning	Salicylate poisoning	Salicylate poisoning	Alcohol abuse	Hypoxia	Acute mesenteric ischemia
Bacterial meningitis	Encephalitis	Encephalitis	Antidepressant overdose	Diabetic hypoglycemia	Heat stroke and heat exhaustion
Encephalitis	Hypoxia	Hypoxia	Recreational drug abuse	Psychosomatic	Hypothermia
Poisoning	Hypothermia	Chronic lead poisoning	Psychosomatic	Alcohol abuse	Bacterial meningitis
Chronic lead poisoning	Chronic lead poisoning	Diabetic ketoacidosis	Ischemic stroke	Pontine hemorrhage	Head injury
Hypothermia	Carbon monoxide poisoning	Diabetic hypoglycemia	Primary intracerebral hemorrhage stroke	Heat stroke and heat exhaustion	Ischemic encephalopathy
Non-diabetic hypoglycemia	Acute iron toxicity	Carbon monoxide poisoning		Ischemic encephalopathy	Hypoxia
Viral meningitis	Diabetic hypoglycemia	Acute iron toxicity	Thrombotic thrombocytopenic purpura	Thrombotic thrombocytopenic purpura	Salicylate poisoning
Carcinoid syndrome	Viral meningitis	Viral meningitis	Salicylate poisoning		Hepatic encephalopathy
Carbon monoxide poisoning	Thrombotic thrombocytopenic purpura	Subdural hematoma	Subarachnoid hemorrhage and cerebral aneurysm stroke	Viral meningitis	Thrombotic thrombocytopenic purpura
Thrombotic thrombocytopenic purpura	Poisoning	Thrombotic thrombocytopenic purpura		Salicylate poisoning	Chronic lead poisoning
	Carcinoid syndrome	Metabolic encephalopathy	Brain tumor	Antidepressant overdose	Psychosomatic
Subdural hematoma	Addison's disease	Carcinoid syndrome	Chronic lead poisoning	Chronic lead poisoning	Viral meningitis
Addison's disease	Subdural hematoma	Addison's disease	Hepatic encephalopathy	Recreational drug abuse	Carbon monoxide poisoning
Diabetic hypoglycemia	Diabetic ketoacidosis	Ischemic encephalopathy	Metabolic encephalopathy	Carbon monoxide poisoning	Brain tumor
Diabetic ketoacidosis	Metabolic encephalopathy	Poisoning	Acute iron toxicity	Acute iron toxicity	Acute iron toxicity
Inborn errors of metabolism	Ischemic encephalopathy	Hypothermia	Brain abscess	Hepatic encephalopathy	Carcinoid syndrome
Metabolic encephalopathy	Inborn errors of metabolism	Rocky Mountain spotted fever	Hypothermia	Metabolic encephalopathy	Addison's disease
Ischemic encephalopathy	Arteriovenous malformation	Arteriovenous malformation	Carbon monoxide poisoning	Subdural hematoma	Brain abscess
Arteriovenous malformation				Ischemic stroke	

72

Baby (0-1 yr)	Child (1-12 yr)	Adolescent (12-18 yr)	Adult (18-45 yr)	Middle Age Adult (45-65 yr)	Senior Adult (65+ yr)
Primary intracerebral hemorrhage stroke	Rocky Mountain spotted fever	Subarachnoid hemorrhage and cerebral aneurysm stroke	Viral meningitis	Carcinoid syndrome	Brainstem disorders
Subarachnoid hemorrhage and cerebral aneurysm stroke	Ischemic stroke	Primary intracerebral hemorrhage stroke	Carcinoid syndrome	Addison's disease	Subdural hematoma
Ischemic stroke	Primary intracerebral hemorrhage stroke	Ischemic stroke	Subdural hematoma	Primary intracerebral hemorrhage stroke	Alcohol abuse
Rocky Mountain spotted fever	Subarachnoid hemorrhage and cerebral aneurysm stroke	Inborn errors of metabolism	Brainstem disorders	Subarachnoid hemorrhage and cerebral aneurysm stroke	Antidepressant overdose
Reye's syndrome	Reye's syndrome	Reye's syndrome	Addison's disease	Encephalitis	Recreational drug abuse
Brain injury	Brain injury	Brain injury	Heat stroke and heat exhaustion	Brain tumor	Ischemic stroke
			Myxedema	Cerebellar hemorrhage	Primary intracerebral hemorrhage stroke
			Bacterial meningitis	Brain abscess	Subarachnoid hemorrhage and cerebral aneurysm stroke
			Hypoxia	Hypothermia	Myxedema
			Encephalitis	Brainstem disorders	Poisoning
			Cerebellar hemorrhage	Myxedema	Metabolic encephalopathy
			Ischemic encephalopathy	Poisoning	Reye's syndrome
			Poisoning	Reye's syndrome	Brain injury
			Reye's syndrome	Brain injury	
			Brain injury		

Coma (continued)

73

Emergency Rule Out conditions shown in red. Entries in blue are for information only
Conditions are listed in approximate order of prevalence for this age range

Baby (0-1 yr)	Child (1-12 yr)	Adolescent (12-18 yr)	Adult (18-45 yr)	Middle Age Adult (45-65 yr)	Senior Adult (65+ yr)
Not relevant to this age group	Dementia	Dementia	Dementia Korsakoff's syndrome	Dementia Korsakoff's syndrome	Dementia Korsakoff's syndrome

Baby (0-1 yr)	Child (1-12 yr)	Adolescent (12-18 yr)	Adult (18-45 yr)	Middle Age Adult (45-65 yr)	Senior Adult (65+ yr)
Non-diabetic hypoglycemia	Diabetic ketoacidosis	Non-diabetic hypoglycemia	Alcohol abuse	Alcohol abuse	Alcohol abuse
Drug withdrawal	Non-diabetic hypoglycemia	Diabetic ketoacidosis	Drug reaction, delirium and confusional states	Drug reaction, delirium and confusional states	Drug reaction, delirium and confusional states
Hypothermia	Trauma	Alcohol abuse	Non-diabetic hypoglycemia	Non-diabetic hypoglycemia	Non-diabetic hypoglycemia
Hydrocephalus	Drug withdrawal	Recreational drug abuse	Hypoxia	Hypoxia	Hypoxia
Hypoxia	Hydrocephalus	Trauma	Hypothermia	Hypothermia	Hypothermia
Bacterial meningitis	Hypoxia	Drug withdrawal	Conversion disorder	Conversion disorder	Conversion disorder
Viral meningitis	Chronic fatigue syndrome	Hydrocephalus	Bacterial meningitis	Bacterial meningitis	Bacterial meningitis
Meningococcemia	Bacterial meningitis	Hypothermia	Viral meningitis	Viral meningitis	Viral meningitis
Transient ischemic attack	Viral meningitis	Hypoxia	Hypercalcemia	Hypercalcemia	Hypercalcemia
Thrombotic thrombocytopenic purpura	Meningococcemia	Chronic fatigue syndrome	Hyperkalemia	Hyperkalemia	Hyperkalemia
Diabetic ketoacidosis	Hypercalcemia	Bacterial meningitis	Transient ischemic attack	Hypernatremia	Hypernatremia
Behçet's syndrome	Hyperkalemia	Viral meningitis	Thrombotic thrombocytopenic purpura	Typhoid fever	Transient ischemic attack
Hepatic encephalopathy	Transient ischemic attack	Meningococcemia	Hypernatremia	Transient ischemic attack	Typhoid fever
Typhoid fever	Typhoid fever	Hypercalcemia	Behçet's syndrome	Thrombotic thrombocytopenic purpura	Behçet's syndrome
Creutzfeldt-Jakob disease	Thrombotic thrombocytopenic purpura	Typhoid fever	Hepatic encephalopathy	Hypernatremia	Hypocalcemia
Hypercalcemia	Hypernatremia	Transient ischemic attack	Typhoid fever	Hepatic encephalopathy	Hepatic encephalopathy
Hyperkalemia	Hepatic encephalopathy	Behçet's syndrome	Creutzfeldt-Jakob disease	Behçet's syndrome	Creutzfeldt-Jakob disease
Hypernatremia	Hypocalcemia	Thrombotic thrombocytopenic purpura	Hypocalcemia	Hypocalcemia	Thrombotic thrombocytopenic purpura
Hypocalcemia	Behçet's syndrome	Hepatic encephalopathy	Hypokalemia	Creutzfeldt-Jakob disease	Carbon monoxide poisoning
Hypokalemia	Creutzfeldt-Jakob disease	Hyperkalemia	Essential hypertension	Hypokalemia	Hypokalemia
Carbon monoxide poisoning	Hypokalemia	Creutzfeldt-Jakob disease		Carbon monoxide poisoning	

List continues on next page

Emergency Rule Out conditions shown in red. Entries in blue are for information only
Conditions are listed in approximate order of prevalence for this age range

List continued from previous page

Baby (0-1 yr)	Child (1-12 yr)	Adolescent (12-18 yr)	Adult (18-45 yr)	Middle Age Adult (45-65 yr)	Senior Adult (65+ yr)
Hyponatremia	Hyponatremia	Hypernatremia	Carbon monoxide poisoning	Essential hypertension	Essential hypertension
Acute renal failure	Carbon monoxide poisoning	Carbon monoxide poisoning	Acute renal failure	Acute renal failure	Acute renal failure
Chronic renal failure	Hypothermia	Hypocalcemia	Chronic renal failure	Chronic renal failure	Chronic renal failure
Hypothyroidism	Acute renal failure	Hypokalemia	Hypochondriasis	Hypochondriasis	Hypochondriasis
Pituitary hypothyroidism	Chronic renal failure	Hyponatremia	Hypothyroidism	Hypothyroidism	Hypothyroidism
Orthostatic hypotension	Hypochondriasis	Acute renal failure	Intracranial hemorrhage	Intracranial hemorrhage	Intracranial hemorrhage
Essential hypertension	Hypothyroidism	Chronic renal failure	Orthostatic hypotension	Orthostatic hypotension	Orthostatic hypotension
Intracranial hemorrhage	Pituitary hypothyroidism	Hypochondriasis	Hyponatremia	Hyponatremia	Hyponatremia
Poisoning	Orthostatic hypotension	Hypothyroidism	Meningococcemia	Meningococcemia	Meningococcemia
Febrile seizure	Salicylate poisoning	Pituitary hypothyroidism	Salicylate poisoning	Salicylate poisoning	Salicylate poisoning
Reye's syndrome	Essential hypertension	Salicylate poisoning	Pituitary hypothyroidism	Pituitary hypothyroidism	Pituitary hypothyroidism
	Poisoning	Orthostatic hypotension	Malaria	Malaria	Malaria
	Migraine headache	Essential hypertension	Porphyria	Porphyria	Porphyria
	Febrile seizure	Intracranial hemorrhage	Reye's syndrome	Reye's syndrome	Reye's syndrome
	Reye's syndrome	Poisoning			
		Migraine headache			
		Reye's syndrome			

Baby (0-1 yr)	Child (1-12 yr)	Adolescent (12-18 yr)	Adult (18-45 yr)	Middle Age Adult (45-65 yr)	Senior Adult (65+ yr)
Sepsis	von Willebrand's disease	von Willebrand's disease	Hemophilia A	Hemophilia A	Hemophilia A
Premature baby	Hemophilia A	Hemophilia A	Hemophilia B	Hemophilia B	Hemophilia B
Disseminated intravascular coagulation	Down syndrome	Down syndrome	von Willebrand's disease	von Willebrand's disease	von Willebrand's disease
Idiopathic thrombocytopenic purpura	Factor II deficiency	Factor II deficiency	Factor V deficiency	Factor V deficiency	Factor V deficiency
Down syndrome	Hemophilia B	Hemophilia B	Factor VII deficiency	Factor VII deficiency	Factor VII deficiency
Biliary atresia	Factor V deficiency	Factor V deficiency	Factor X deficiency	Factor X deficiency	Factor X deficiency
von Willebrand's disease	Factor VII deficiency	Factor VII deficiency	Factor II deficiency	Factor II deficiency	Factor II deficiency
Factor II deficiency	Factor X deficiency	Factor X deficiency			
Hemophilia B					
Factor V deficiency					
Factor VII deficiency					
Hemophilia A					
Factor X deficiency					

Emergency Rule Out conditions shown in red. Entries in blue are for information only
Conditions are listed in approximate order of prevalence for this age range

Congenital coagulopathy

Constipation

Emergency Rule Out conditions shown in red. Entries in blue are for information only
Conditions are listed in approximate order of prevalence for this age range

Baby (0-1 yr)	Child (1-12 yr)	Adolescent (12-18 yr)	Adult (18-45 yr)	Middle Age Adult (45-65 yr)	Senior Adult (65+yr)
Hypothyroidism	Hypothyroidism	Hypothyroidism	Hypothyroidism	Hypothyroidism	Hypothyroidism
Henoch-Schönlein purpura	Sedentary lifestyle	Sedentary lifestyle	Sedentary lifestyle	Sedentary lifestyle	Sedentary lifestyle
Fecal impaction	Muscular strain	Muscular strain	Muscular strain	Muscular strain	Muscular strain
Hemorrhoids	Depression	Dysmenorrhea	Dysmenorrhea	Depression	Depression
Genital herpes	Fecal impaction	Depression	Depression	Fecal impaction	Fecal impaction
Uterine myomas	Diverticular disease	Fecal impaction	Irritable bowel syndrome	Diverticular disease	Diverticular disease
Diverticular disease	Hypokalemia	Diverticular disease	Fecal impaction	Hypokalemia	Hypokalemia
Hypokalemia	Anorectal problems	Hypokalemia	Diverticular disease	Colon cancer	Colon cancer
Anorectal problems	Congenital megacolon	Irritable bowel syndrome	Hypokalemia	Anorectal problems	Anorectal problems
Congenital megacolon	Intestinal obstruction	Anorectal problems	Colon cancer	Congenital megacolon	Henoch-Schönlein purpura
Chronic lead poisoning	Henoch-Schönlein purpura	Congenital megacolon	Anorectal problems	Irritable bowel syndrome	Congenital megacolon
Intestinal obstruction	Genital herpes	Hemorrhoids	Congenital megacolon	Acute appendicitis	Intestinal obstruction
Poliomyelitis	Uterine myomas	Genital herpes	Acute appendicitis	Hemorrhoids	Genital herpes
Hypocalcemia	Hemorrhoids	Uterine myomas	Henoch-Schönlein purpura	Henoch-Schönlein purpura	Uterine myomas
Hypercalcemia	Hypocalcemia	Henoch-Schönlein purpura	Genital herpes	Uterine myomas	Hemorrhoids
Spinal cord compression	Acute appendicitis	Acute appendicitis	Hemorrhoids	Genital herpes	Hypercalcemia
Cerebral palsy	Hypercalcemia	Intestinal obstruction	Uterine myomas	Intestinal obstruction	Acute appendicitis
Myelodysplastic syndromes	Poliomyelitis	Hypocalcemia	Intestinal obstruction	Hypercalcemia	Poliomyelitis
Volvulus	Laxative abuse	Hypercalcemia	Hypercalcemia	Poliomyelitis	Laxative abuse
Hirschsprung's disease	Chronic lead poisoning	Poliomyelitis	Laxative abuse	Laxative abuse	Parkinson's disease
Ambiguous genitalia	Spinal cord compression	Laxative abuse	Parkinson's disease	Parkinson's disease	Spinal cord compression
Typhoid fever	Cerebral palsy	Chronic lead poisoning	Chronic lead poisoning	Spinal cord compression	Cerebral palsy
Proctitis	Volvulus	Spinal cord compression	Poliomyelitis	Cerebral palsy	Volvulus

List continues on next page

78

Baby (0-1 yr)	Child (1-12 yr)	Adolescent (12-18 yr)	Adult (18-45 yr)	Middle Age Adult (45-65 yr)	Senior Adult (65+ yr)
	Myelodysplastic syndromes	Cerebral palsy	Spinal cord compression	Volvulus	Irritable bowel syndrome
	Irritable bowel syndrome	Myelodysplastic syndromes	Cerebral palsy	Chronic lead poisoning	Brain tumor
	Brain tumor	Volvulus	Volvulus	Brain tumor	Dementia
	Polymyositis/ dermatomyositis	Brain tumor	Multiple sclerosis	Dementia	Chagas' disease
	Ambiguous genitalia	Multiple sclerosis	Brain tumor	Chagas' disease	Scleroderma
	Encopresis	Ambiguous genitalia	Dementia	Scleroderma	Multiple sclerosis
	Typhoid fever	Encopresis	Chagas' disease	Multiple sclerosis	Typhoid fever
	Proctitis	Typhoid fever	Polymyositis/ dermatomyositis	Polymyositis/ dermatomyositis	Proctitis
		Proctitis	Scleroderma	Typhoid fever	
			Typhoid fever	Proctitis	
			Proctitis		

Emergency Rule Out conditions shown in red. Entries in blue are for information only
Conditions are listed in approximate order of prevalence for this age range

Baby (0-1 yr)	Child (1-12 yr)	Adolescent (12-18 yr)	Adult (18-45 yr)	Middle Age Adult (45-65 yr)	Senior Adult (65+yr)
Febrile seizure	Epilepsy	Epilepsy	Epilepsy	Epilepsy	Epilepsy
Epilepsy	Diabetic hypoglycemia	Diabetic hypoglycemia	Diabetic hypoglycemia	Diabetic hypoglycemia	Diabetic hypoglycemia
Diabetic hypoglycemia	Hypercapnia	Hypercapnia	Hypoxia	Hypoxia	Hypoxia
Hypercapnia	Hyperventilation	Hyperventilation	Brain tumor	Brain tumor	Alcohol abuse
Hyperventilation	Hypothermia	Alcohol abuse	Alcohol abuse	Alcohol abuse	Ischemic stroke
Hypothermia	Diabetic ketoacidosis	Metabolic encephalopathy	Ischemic stroke	Ischemic stroke	Subarachnoid hemorrhage and cerebral aneurysm stroke
Poisoning	Poisoning	Diabetic ketoacidosis	Subarachnoid hemorrhage and cerebral aneurysm stroke	Subarachnoid hemorrhage and cerebral aneurysm stroke	Primary intracerebral hemorrhage stroke
Chronic lead poisoning	Chronic lead poisoning	Bacterial meningitis	Primary intracerebral hemorrhage stroke	Primary intracerebral hemorrhage stroke	Brain tumor
Diabetic ketoacidosis	Bacterial meningitis	Encephalitis	Bacterial meningitis	Liver failure	Bacterial meningitis
Encephalitis	Viral meningitis	Viral meningitis	Viral meningitis	Bacterial meningitis	Viral meningitis
Bacterial meningitis	Encephalitis	Meningococcemia	Head injury	Viral meningitis	Head injury
Viral meningitis	Metabolic encephalopathy	Hypoxia	Hypercapnia	Head injury	Hypercapnia
Meningococcemia	Meningococcemia	Trauma	Encephalitis	Encephalitis	Encephalitis
Viral infection	Viral infection	Primary intracerebral hemorrhage stroke	Hyperventilation	Hypercapnia	Hyperventilation
Hypoxia	Hypoxia	Brain tumor	Encephalopathy	Hyperventilation	Encephalopathy
Trauma	Trauma	Poisoning	Poisoning	Encephalopathy	Poisoning
Metabolic encephalopathy	Brain tumor	Chronic lead poisoning	Liver failure	Poisoning	Hypothermia
Primary intracerebral hemorrhage stroke	Primary intracerebral hemorrhage stroke	Hypothermia	Hypothermia	Hypothermia	Chronic renal failure
Subarachnoid hemorrhage and cerebral aneurysm stroke	Subarachnoid hemorrhage and cerebral aneurysm stroke	Subarachnoid hemorrhage and cerebral aneurysm stroke	Chronic renal failure	Chronic renal failure	Acute renal failure
Brain tumor	Sturge-Weber disease	Sturge-Weber disease	Meningococcemia	Acute renal failure	Meningococcemia

Baby (0-1 yr)	Child (1-12 yr)	Adolescent (12-18 yr)	Adult (18-45 yr)	Middle Age Adult (45-65 yr)	Senior Adult (65+ yr)
Sturge-Weber disease Tuberous sclerosis complex Neurofibromatosis	Tuberous sclerosis complex Neurofibromatosis Migraine headache Brain abscess	Pyridoxin deficiency Tuberous sclerosis complex Neurofibromatosis Migraine headache	Acute renal failure Cerebellar hemorrhage Carcinomatous meningitis Pyridoxin deficiency Ischemic encephalopathy Metabolic encephalopathy Hyperthyroidism Hepatic encephalopathy Porphyria	Meningococcemia Hepatic encephalopathy Cerebellar hemorrhage Carcinomatous meningitis Pyridoxin deficiency Ischemic encephalopathy Metabolic encephalopathy Hyperthyroidism Porphyria	Carcinomatous meningitis Hepatic encephalopathy Cerebellar hemorrhage Liver failure Pyridoxin deficiency Ischemic encephalopathy Metabolic encephalopathy Hyperthyroidism Porphyria

82

Emergency Rule Out conditions shown in red. Entries in blue are for information only
Conditions are listed in approximate order of prevalence for this age range

Baby (0-1 yr)	Child (1-12 yr)	Adolescent (12-18 yr)	Adult (18-45 yr)	Middle Age Adult (45-65 yr)	Senior Adult (65+ yr)
Upper respiratory tract infections	Upper respiratory tract infections	Upper respiratory tract infections	Upper respiratory tract infections	Upper respiratory tract infections	Upper respiratory tract infections
Acute bronchitis	Acute bronchitis	Acute bronchitis	Smoker's cough	Smoker's cough	Smoker's cough
Bronchiectasis	Airway irritants	Allergic rhinitis	Acute bronchitis	Acute bronchitis	Acute bronchitis
Epiglottitis	Cystic fibrosis	Vasomotor rhinitis	Allergic rhinitis	Allergic rhinitis	Airway irritants
Influenza	Gastroesophageal reflux disease	Acute sinusitis	Airway irritants	Vasomotor rhinitis	Influenza
Acute allergic alveolitis	Acute sinusitis	Airway irritants	Influenza	Airway irritants	Gastroesophageal reflux disease
Chlamydia pneumoniae	Influenza	Cystic fibrosis	Acute sinusitis	Influenza	Drug reaction, ACE inhibitors
Chronic allergic alveolitis	Allergic reactions and anaphylaxis	Allergic reactions and anaphylaxis	Gastroesophageal reflux disease	Drug reaction, ACE inhibitors	Primary lung malignancy
Primary lung malignancy	Acute allergic alveolitis	Influenza	Acute sinusitis	Gastroesophageal reflux disease	Congestive heart failure
Blastomycosis	Tuberculosis	Gastroesophageal reflux disease	Allergic reactions and anaphylaxis	Primary lung malignancy	Tuberculosis
Croup	Chronic allergic alveolitis	Acute allergic alveolitis	Primary lung malignancy	Congestive heart failure	Acute allergic alveolitis
Respiratory syncytial virus infection	Measles	Tuberculosis	Acute allergic alveolitis	Tuberculosis	Tularemia
Chronic fatigue syndrome	Croup	Chronic allergic alveolitis	Chronic allergic alveolitis	Syphilis	Chronic allergic alveolitis
Brucellosis	Chronic fatigue syndrome	Laryngeal cancer	Tuberculosis	Acute allergic alveolitis	Bronchiectasis
Laryngeal cancer	Brucellosis	Tularemia	Pulmonary thromboembolism	Chronic allergic alveolitis	Acute sinusitis
Allergic reactions and anaphylaxis	Pertussis	Croup	Croup	Tularemia	Croup
Typhoid fever	Laryngeal cancer	Chronic fatigue syndrome	Chronic fatigue syndrome	Bronchiectasis	Chronic fatigue syndrome
Laryngitis	Pulmonary thromboembolism	Bronchiectasis	Laryngeal cancer	Chronic fatigue syndrome	Laryngeal cancer
Legionnaires' disease	Syphilis	Brucellosis	Brucellosis	Croup	Chronic sinusitis
Measles		Primary lung malignancy		Laryngeal cancer	Brucellosis

Baby (0-1 yr)	Child (1-12 yr)	Adolescent (12-18 yr)	Adult (18-45 yr)	Middle Age Adult (45-65 yr)	Senior Adult (65+ yr)
Pertussis	Tularemia	Chronic sinusitis	Syphilis	Brucellosis	Psittacosis
Pulmonary thromboembolism	Bronchiectasis	Chlamydia pneumoniae	Tularemia	Acute sinusitis	Blastomycosis
Syphilis	Psittacosis	Typhoid fever	Drug reaction, ACE inhibitors	Psittacosis	Ankylosing spondylitis
Tuberculosis	Primary lung malignancy	Respiratory syncytial virus infection	Bronchiectasis	Chronic sinusitis	Respiratory syncytial virus infection
Tularemia	Blastomycosis	Psittacosis	Psittacosis	Respiratory syncytial virus infection	Chlamydia pneumoniae
Psittacosis	Chronic sinusitis	Blastomycosis	Chronic sinusitis	Chlamydia pneumoniae	Allergic reactions and anaphylaxis
Acute sinusitis	Ankylosing spondylitis	Ankylosing spondylitis	Respiratory syncytial virus infection	Allergic reactions and anaphylaxis	Typhoid fever
Chronic sinusitis	Chlamydia pneumoniae	Laryngitis	Chlamydia pneumoniae	Blastomycosis	Laryngitis
Poliomyelitis	Respiratory syncytial virus infection	Legionnaires' disease	Blastomycosis	Ankylosing spondylitis	Legionnaires' disease
	Typhoid fever	Measles	Ankylosing spondylitis	Laryngitis	Measles
	Laryngitis	Pertussis	Typhoid fever	Typhoid fever	Pertussis
	Legionnaires' disease	Pulmonary thromboembolism	Laryngitis	Legionnaires' disease	Pulmonary thromboembolism
	Poliomyelitis	Syphilis	Legionnaires' disease	Measles	Syphilis
		Poliomyelitis	Measles	Pertussis	Poliomyelitis
			Pertussis	Pulmonary thromboembolism	
			Poliomyelitis	Poliomyelitis	

Emergency Rule Out conditions shown in red. Entries in blue are for information only
Conditions are listed in approximate order of prevalence for this age range

Baby (0-1 yr)	Child (1-12 yr)	Adolescent (12-18 yr)	Adult (18-45 yr)	Middle Age Adult (45-65 yr)	Senior Adult (65+ yr)
Atopic dermatitis	Atopic dermatitis	Contact dermatitis	Drug reaction, skin	Drug reaction, skin	Drug reaction, skin
Seborrheic dermatitis	Drug reaction, allergic	Drug reaction, allergic	Contact dermatitis	Contact dermatitis	Contact dermatitis
Contact dermatitis	Contact dermatitis	Allergic reactions and anaphylaxis	Seborrheic dermatitis	Seborrheic dermatitis	Seborrheic dermatitis
Drug reaction, allergic	Urticaria	Urticaria	Urticaria	Urticaria	Urticaria
Allergic reactions and anaphylaxis	Seborrheic dermatitis	Atopic dermatitis	Allergic reactions and anaphylaxis	Allergic reactions and anaphylaxis	Allergic reactions and anaphylaxis
Diaper dermatitis	Allergic reactions and anaphylaxis	Seborrheic dermatitis	Atopic dermatitis	Atopic dermatitis	Atopic dermatitis
Scabies	Angioedema	Angioedema	Scabies	Scabies	Angioedema
Urticaria	Scabies	Scabies	Angioedema	Angioedema	Scabies
Angioedema			Schistosomiasis	Schistosomiasis	Schistosomiasis
			Intestinal parasites	Intestinal parasites	Intestinal parasites

Baby (0-1 yr)	Child (1-12 yr)	Adolescent (12-18 yr)	Adult (18-45 yr)	Middle Age Adult (45-65 yr)	Senior Adult (65+ yr)
Atrial septal defect	Atrial septal defect	Atrial septal defect	Asthma	Asthma	Asthma
Ventricular septal defect	Ventricular septal defect	Ventricular septal defect	Chronic obstructive pulmonary disease	Chronic obstructive pulmonary disease	Chronic obstructive pulmonary disease
Patent ductus arteriosus	Asthma	Asthma	Extrinsic airway compression	Reflex sympathetic dystrophy	Pulmonary thromboembolism
Tetralogy of Fallot	Thoracic outlet syndrome	Bacterial pneumonia	Pulmonary thromboembolism	Pulmonary thromboembolism	Reflex sympathetic dystrophy
Neonatal respiratory distress syndrome	Congestive heart failure	Viral pneumonia	Bacterial pneumonia	Bacterial pneumonia	Aortic regurgitation
Thoracic outlet syndrome	Reflex sympathetic dystrophy	Reflex sympathetic dystrophy	Reflex sympathetic dystrophy	Aortic regurgitation	Bacterial pneumonia
Reflex sympathetic dystrophy	Bacterial pneumonia	Respiratory syncytial virus infection	Mycoplasmal pneumonia	Viral pneumonia	Viral pneumonia
Aortic regurgitation	Bronchiolitis	Aortic regurgitation	Aortic regurgitation	Respiratory syncytial virus infection	Respiratory syncytial virus infection
Bronchiolitis	Respiratory syncytial virus infection	Thoracic outlet syndrome	Respiratory syncytial virus infection	Mycoplasmal pneumonia	Mycoplasmal pneumonia
Respiratory syncytial virus infection	Aortic regurgitation	Mycoplasmal pneumonia	Thoracic outlet syndrome	Thoracic outlet syndrome	Thoracic outlet syndrome
Bacterial pneumonia	Viral pneumonia	Congestive heart failure	Viral pneumonia	Extrinsic airway compression	Extrinsic airway compression
Viral pneumonia	Mycoplasmal pneumonia	Pulmonary thromboembolism	Congestive heart failure	Congestive heart failure	Congestive heart failure
Asthma	Pulmonary thromboembolism	Methemoglobinemia	Liver cirrhosis	Polycythemia vera	Superior vena cava syndrome
Congestive heart failure	Methemoglobinemia	Extrinsic airway compression	Methemoglobinemia	Superior vena cava syndrome	Polycythemia vera
Pulmonary thromboembolism	Extrinsic airway compression	Polycythemia vera	Polycythemia vera	Liver cirrhosis	Liver cirrhosis
Methemoglobinemia	Polycythemia vera		Patent ductus arteriosus	Idiopathic pulmonary interstitial fibrosis	
Extrinsic airway compression			Ventricular septal defect	Trench fever	
Polycythemia vera					

List continues on next page

Emergency Rule Out conditions shown in red. Entries in blue are for information only
Conditions are listed in approximate order of prevalence for this age range

85

List continued from previous page

Baby (0-1 yr)	Child (1-12 yr)	Adolescent (12-18 yr)	Adult (18-45 yr)	Middle Age Adult (45-65 yr)	Senior Adult (65+ yr)
			Idiopathic pulmonary interstitial fibrosis Superior vena cava syndrome Trench fever Atrial septal defect	Methemoglobinemia Atrial septal defect	Idiopathic pulmonary interstitial fibrosis Trench fever Methemoglobinemia Atrial septal defect

Baby (0-1 yr)	Child (1-12 yr)	Adolescent (12-18 yr)	Adult (18-45 yr)	Middle Age Adult (45-65 yr)	Senior Adult (65+ yr)
Mumps	Mumps	Mumps	Blepharitis	Blepharitis	Blepharitis
Blepharitis	Blepharitis	Blepharitis	Dry eye	Dry eye	Dry eye
Ectodermal dysplasia	Ectodermal dysplasia	Ectodermal dysplasia	Mumps	Sjögren's syndrome	Sjögren's syndrome
Dry eye	Dry eye	Dry eye	Hemochromatosis	Amyloidosis	Amyloidosis
Acute leukemia	Acute leukemia	Acute leukemia	Acute leukemia	Mumps	Mumps
Familial dysautonomia	Hodgkin's disease	Hodgkin's disease	Hodgkin's disease	Hemochromatosis	Hemochromatosis
	Familial dysautonomia	Familial dysautonomia	Non-Hodgkin's lymphoma	Acute leukemia	Acute leukemia
			Sjögren's syndrome	Hodgkin's disease	Hodgkin's disease
			Amyloidosis	Non-Hodgkin's lymphoma	Non-Hodgkin's lymphoma

Emergency Rule Out conditions shown in red. Entries in blue are for information only
Conditions are listed in approximate order of prevalence for this age range

Decreased tearing, abnormal

Emergency Rule Out conditions shown in red. Entries in blue are for information only
Conditions are listed in approximate order of prevalence for this age range

Baby (0-1 yr)	Child (1-12 yr)	Adolescent (12-18 yr)	Adult (18-45 yr)	Middle Age Adult (45-65 yr)	Senior Adult (65+yr)
Diabetic ketoacidosis	Diabetic ketoacidosis	Diabetic ketoacidosis	Heat stroke and heat exhaustion	Heat stroke and heat exhaustion	Heat stroke and heat exhaustion
Salmonella infection	Salmonella infection	Salmonella infection	Campylobacter infection	Campylobacter infection	Campylobacter infection
Campylobacter infection	Heat stroke and heat exhaustion	Campylobacter infection	Salmonella infection	Salmonella infection	Salmonella infection
Hypercalcemia	Sialadenitis	Migraine headache	Addison's disease	Giardiasis	Pyloric stenosis
Migraine headache	Hypercalcemia	Hypercalcemia	Hypercalcemia	Sialadenitis	Hypercalcemia
Pyloric stenosis	Migraine headache	Pyloric stenosis	Pyloric stenosis	Hypercalcemia	Giardiasis
Sialadenitis	Addison's disease	Sialadenitis	Sialadenitis	Migraine headache	Migraine headache
Heat stroke and heat exhaustion	Pyloric stenosis	Addison's disease	Migraine headache	Pyloric stenosis	Sialadenitis
Giardiasis	Giardiasis	Heat stroke and heat exhaustion	Giardiasis	Addison's disease	Addison's disease
Cholera	Campylobacter infection	Giardiasis	Diabetic ketoacidosis	Diabetic ketoacidosis	Diabetic ketoacidosis
Pseudomembranous colitis	Cholera	Cholera	Diuretic abuse	Diuretic abuse	Diuretic abuse
	Pseudomembranous colitis	Pseudomembranous colitis	Cholera	Cholera	Cholera
			Gastric cancer	Gastric cancer	Gastric cancer
			Pseudomembranous colitis	Pseudomembranous colitis	Pseudomembranous colitis

Baby (0-1 yr)	Child (1-12 yr)	Adolescent (12-18 yr)	Adult (18-45 yr)	Middle Age Adult (45-65 yr)	Senior Adult (65+ yr)
Carbon monoxide poisoning	Carbon monoxide poisoning	Carbon monoxide poisoning	Diabetic hypoglycemia	Pyridoxin deficiency	Diabetic hypoglycemia
Post-concussive syndrome	Post-concussive syndrome	Post-concussive syndrome	Alcohol abuse	Diabetic hypoglycemia	Alcohol abuse
Sepsis	Sepsis	Sepsis	Drug reaction	Alcohol abuse	Drug reaction
Diabetic hypoglycemia	Diabetic hypoglycemia	Diabetic hypoglycemia	Post-concussive syndrome	Drug reaction	Post-concussive syndrome
Hypercalcemia	Hypercalcemia	Hypercalcemia	Sepsis	Post-concussive syndrome	Sepsis
Postictal/postseizure phase	Postictal/postseizure phase	Postictal/postseizure phase	Postictal/postseizure phase	Sepsis	Postictal/postseizure phase
Typhoid fever	Typhoid fever	Typhoid fever	Bacterial meningitis	Postictal/postseizure phase	Bacterial meningitis
Pyridoxin deficiency	Pyridoxin deficiency	Pyridoxin deficiency	Hypoxia	Bacterial meningitis	Hypoxia
Hyponatremia	Hyponatremia	Hyponatremia	Typhoid fever	Typhoid fever	Ischemic stroke
Bacterial meningitis	Bacterial meningitis	Bacterial meningitis	Ischemic stroke	Hypoxia	Typhoid fever
Chronic lead poisoning	Hypoxia	Hypoxia	Hypercalcemia	Ischemic stroke	Hypercalcemia
Hypoxia	Hypercapnia	Hypercapnia	Hyperthyroidism	Hypercalcemia	Hyperthyroidism
Hypercapnia	Hyperthyroidism	Hyperthyroidism	Metabolic encephalopathy	Hyperthyroidism	Metabolic encephalopathy
Hyperthyroidism	Acute renal failure	Acute renal failure	Tularemia	Metabolic encephalopathy	Hepatic encephalopathy
Acute renal failure	Hypothermia	Hypothermia	Hepatic encephalopathy	Hepatic encephalopathy	Encephalitis
Hypothermia	Chronic lead poisoning	Heat stroke and heat exhaustion	Encephalitis	Encephalitis	Heat stroke and heat exhaustion
Heat stroke and heat exhaustion	Heat stroke and heat exhaustion	Encephalitis	Heat stroke and heat exhaustion	Heat stroke and heat exhaustion	Hypothermia
Encephalitis	Encephalitis	Tularemia	Hypothermia	Tularemia	Acute renal failure
Tularemia	Tularemia	Recreational drug abuse	Acute renal failure	Hypothermia	Tularemia
Reye's syndrome	Recreational drug abuse	Reye's syndrome	Malignant hypertension	Acute renal failure	Malignant hypertension
	Reye's syndrome		Hyponatremia	Malignant hypertension	Hyponatremia

List continues on next page

Emergency Rule Out conditions shown in red. Entries in blue are for information only
Conditions are listed in approximate order of prevalence for this age range

89

List continued from previous page

D

Delirium (continued)

Baby (0-1 yr)	Child (1-12 yr)	Adolescent (12-18 yr)	Adult (18-45 yr)	Middle Age Adult (45-65 yr)	Senior Adult (65+yr)
			Hypercapnia Carcinomatous meningitis Carbon monoxide poisoning **Pyridoxin deficiency** Reye's syndrome	Hyponatremia Hypercapnia Carcinomatous meningitis Carbon monoxide poisoning Reye's syndrome	Hypercapnia Carcinomatous meningitis Carbon monoxide poisoning **Pyridoxin deficiency** Reye's syndrome

90

Baby (0-1 yr)	Child (1-12 yr)	Adolescent (12-18 yr)	Adult (18-45 yr)	Middle Age Adult (45-65 yr)	Senior Adult (65+ yr)
Not relevant to this age group	Delirium Depression Obsessive compulsive disorder Manic depression Dementia Schizophrenia	Delirium Depression Alcohol abuse Obsessive compulsive disorder Recreational drug abuse Manic depression Dementia Schizophrenia	Delirium Schizophrenia Manic depression Obsessive compulsive disorder Dementia Depression Alcohol abuse Recreational drug abuse	Delirium Schizophrenia Manic depression Obsessive compulsive disorder Dementia Depression Alcohol abuse Recreational drug abuse	Delirium Dementia Schizophrenia Obsessive compulsive disorder Manic depression Depression Alcohol abuse Recreational drug abuse

Delusions

Emergency Rule Out conditions shown in red. Entries in blue are for information only
Conditions are listed in approximate order of prevalence for this age range

Emergency Rule Out conditions shown in red. Entries in blue are for information only
Conditions are listed in approximate order of prevalence for this age range

Baby (0-1 yr)	Child (1-12 yr)	Adolescent (12-18 yr)	Adult (18-45 yr)	Middle Age Adult (45-65 yr)	Senior Adult (65+ yr)
AIDS	AIDS	Dementia	AIDS	Alzheimer's disease	Alzheimer's disease
Brain tumor	Brain tumor	AIDS	Hydrocephalus	Arteriosclerosis	Arteriosclerosis
Hydrocephalus	Hydrocephalus	Brain tumor	Head injury	Hydrocephalus	Brain tumor
	Vitamin B12 deficiency	Metastatic cancer	Brain tumor	Brain tumor	Metastatic cancer
		Hydrocephalus	Metastatic cancer	AIDS	Hydrocephalus
		Vitamin B12 deficiency	Alzheimer's disease	Head injury	Head injury
			Arteriosclerosis	Korsakoff's syndrome	AIDS
			Korsakoff's syndrome	Creutzfeldt-Jakob disease	Korsakoff's syndrome
			Creutzfeldt-Jakob disease	Down syndrome	Creutzfeldt-Jakob disease
			Huntington's disease	Subacute sclerosing panencephalitis	Parkinson's disease
			Down syndrome	Parkinson's disease	Vitamin B12 deficiency
			Subacute sclerosing panencephalitis	Vitamin B12 deficiency	
			Parkinson's disease	Metastatic cancer	
			Vitamin B12 deficiency		

Baby (0-1 yr)	Child (1-12 yr)	Adolescent (12-18 yr)	Adult (18-45 yr)	Middle Age Adult (45-65 yr)	Senior Adult (65+ yr)
Not relevant to this age group	Depression	Depression	Depression	Depression	Depression
	Child abuse	Seasonal affective disorder	Seasonal affective disorder	Seasonal affective disorder	Seasonal affective disorder
	Post-traumatic stress disorder	Chronic fatigue syndrome	Hypothyroidism	Hypothyroidism	Hypothyroidism
	Autism	Post-traumatic stress disorder	Chronic fatigue syndrome	Premenstrual syndrome	Dementia
	Post-infection	Anorexia nervosa	Brucellosis	Post-traumatic stress disorder	Brucellosis
	Creutzfeldt-Jakob disease	Brucellosis	Bulimia nervosa	Celiac disease	Creutzfeldt-Jakob disease
	Bulimia nervosa	Premenstrual syndrome	Creutzfeldt-Jakob disease	Creutzfeldt-Jakob disease	Autism
	Brucellosis	Creutzfeldt-Jakob disease	Behçet's syndrome	Brucellosis	Celiac disease
	Behçet's syndrome	Bulimia nervosa	Autism	Bulimia nervosa	Bulimia nervosa
	Celiac disease	Child abuse	Celiac disease	Behçet's syndrome	Behçet's syndrome
	Seasonal affective disorder	Celiac disease	Premenstrual syndrome	Hyperthyroidism	Hyperthyroidism
	Hypothyroidism	Behçet's syndrome	Post-traumatic stress disorder	Autism	Manic depression
	Hyperthyroidism	Autism	Anorexia nervosa	Hyperthyroidism	Chronic fatigue syndrome
	Chronic fatigue syndrome	Post-infection	Manic depression	Dementia	Post-traumatic stress disorder
	Manic depression	Hypothyroidism	Hyperthyroidism	Chronic fatigue syndrome	Anorexia nervosa
	Dementia	Hyperthyroidism	Dementia	Manic depression	Polymyalgia rheumatica
	Polymyalgia rheumatica	Manic depression	Polymyalgia rheumatica	Anorexia nervosa	
		Dementia		Polymyalgia rheumatica	
		Polymyalgia rheumatica			

Emergency Rule Out conditions shown in red. Entries in blue are for information only
Conditions are listed in approximate order of prevalence for this age range

93

Emergency Rule Out conditions shown in red. Entries in blue are for information only
Conditions are listed in approximate order of prevalence for this age range

Baby (0-1 yr)	Child (1-12 yr)	Adolescent (12-18 yr)	Adult (18-45 yr)	Middle Age Adult (45-65 yr)	Senior Adult (65+yr)
Gastroenteritis	Gastroenteritis	Gastroenteritis	Gastroenteritis	Gastroenteritis	Gastroenteritis
Intestinal obstruction	Fecal impaction	Fecal impaction	Campylobacter infection	Campylobacter infection	Campylobacter infection
Legionnaires' disease	Intestinal obstruction	Intestinal obstruction	Legionnaires' disease	Legionnaires' disease	Fecal impaction
Giardiasis	Legionnaires' disease	Proctitis	Salmonella infection	Salmonella infection	Intestinal obstruction
Fecal impaction	Giardiasis	Giardiasis	Giardiasis	Giardiasis	Giardiasis
Campylobacter infection	Tularemia	Legionnaires' disease	Shellfish poisoning	Shellfish poisoning	Legionnaires' disease
Salmonella infection	Rocky Mountain spotted fever	Campylobacter infection	Fecal impaction	Fecal impaction	Colon cancer
Rocky Mountain spotted fever	Campylobacter infection	Salmonella infection	Rocky Mountain spotted fever	Intestinal obstruction	Salmonella infection
Proctitis	Salmonella infection	Rocky Mountain spotted fever	Intestinal obstruction	Addison's disease	Tularemia
Amebic dysentery	Proctitis	Amebic dysentery	Tularemia	Rocky Mountain spotted fever	Rocky Mountain spotted fever
Tularemia	Amebic dysentery	Addison's disease	Proctitis	Proctitis	Proctitis
Yersinia	Addison's disease	Tularemia	Addison's disease	Shigellosis	Addison's disease
Typhoid fever	Yersinia	Yersinia	Yersinia	Tularemia	Pseudomembranous colitis
Shigellosis	Typhoid fever	Typhoid fever	Typhoid fever	Yersinia	Shigellosis
Cholera	Shigellosis	Cholera	Cholera	Typhoid fever	Shellfish poisoning
Intestinal parasites	Cholera	Shigellosis	Shigellosis	Intestinal parasites	Yersinia
Pseudomembranous colitis	Intestinal parasites	Intestinal parasites	Intestinal parasites	Cholera	Intestinal parasites
Hirschsprung's disease	Pseudomembranous colitis	Pseudomembranous colitis	Amebic dysentery	Pseudomembranous colitis	Typhoid fever
Malignancy	Shellfish poisoning	Shellfish poisoning	Pseudomembranous colitis	Colon cancer	Cholera
	Malignancy	Malignancy	Colon cancer	Amebic dysentery	Amebic dysentery

Baby (0-1 yr)	Child (1-12 yr)	Adolescent (12-18 yr)	Adult (18-45 yr)	Middle Age Adult (45-65 yr)	Senior Adult (65+ yr)
Gastroenteritis	Gastroenteritis	Gastroenteritis	Irritable bowel syndrome	Irritable bowel syndrome	Irritable bowel syndrome
Lactose intolerance	Lactose intolerance	Irritable bowel syndrome	Diabetic enteropathy	Diabetic enteropathy	Diabetic enteropathy
Intestinal parasites	Intestinal parasites	Lactose intolerance	Hypothyroidism	Hypothyroidism	Hypothyroidism
Drug reaction	Irritable bowel syndrome	Intestinal parasites	Pancreatic insufficiency	Pancreatic insufficiency	Pancreatic insufficiency
Hirschsprung's disease	Ulcerative colitis	Drug reaction	Secretory villous adenoma	Secretory villous adenoma	Secretory villous adenoma
Proctitis	Crohn's disease	Tularemia	Fecal impaction	Fecal impaction	Fecal impaction
Tularemia	Tularemia	Proctitis	Laxative abuse	Laxative abuse	Laxative abuse
Cystic fibrosis	Proctitis	Crohn's disease	Proctitis	Tularemia	Proctitis
Allergic reactions and anaphylaxis	Celiac disease	Ulcerative colitis	Tularemia	Proctitis	Tularemia
Hyperthyroidism	Drug reaction	Cystic fibrosis	Crohn's disease	Crohn's disease	Crohn's disease
Hypothyroidism	Allergic reactions and anaphylaxis	Celiac disease	Ulcerative colitis	Ulcerative colitis	Ulcerative colitis
AIDS	Cystic fibrosis	Constipation	Celiac disease	Celiac disease	Intestinal parasites
Celiac disease	AIDS	Hypoparathyroidism	Intestinal parasites	Intestinal parasites	Celiac disease
	Hirschsprung's disease	Hyperthyroidism	Hodgkin's disease	Hodgkin's disease	Hodgkin's disease
	Hyperthyroidism	Hirschsprung's disease	AIDS	AIDS	AIDS
	Hypothyroidism	AIDS	Non-Hodgkin's lymphoma	Non-Hodgkin's lymphoma	Non-Hodgkin's lymphoma
		Zollinger-Ellison syndrome	Zollinger-Ellison syndrome	Zollinger-Ellison syndrome	Zollinger-Ellison syndrome
		Lassa fever	Scleroderma	Scleroderma	Scleroderma
			Carcinoid syndrome	Carcinoid syndrome	Carcinoid syndrome

Emergency Rule Out conditions shown in red. Entries in blue are for information only
Conditions are listed in approximate order of prevalence for this age range

Disequilibrium

Emergency Rule Out conditions shown in red. Entries in blue are for information only
Conditions are listed in approximate order of prevalence for this age range

Baby (0-1 yr)	Child (1-12 yr)	Adolescent (12-18 yr)	Adult (18-45 yr)	Middle Age Adult (45-65 yr)	Senior Adult (65+yr)
Cerebellar hemorrhage	Cerebellar hemorrhage	Cerebellar hemorrhage	Cerebellar hemorrhage	Cerebellar hemorrhage	Cerebellar hemorrhage
Charcot-Marie-Tooth disease	Brain tumor	Brain tumor	Brain tumor	Charcot-Marie-Tooth disease	Charcot-Marie-Tooth disease
Behçet's syndrome	Behçet's syndrome	Behçet's syndrome	Charcot-Marie-Tooth disease	Behçet's syndrome	Brain tumor
Brain tumor	Charcot-Marie-Tooth disease	Post-infection	Behçet's syndrome	Brain tumor	Behçet's syndrome
Post-infection	Post-infection	Poisoning	Acoustic neuroma	Acoustic neuroma	Acoustic neuroma
Poisoning	Poisoning	Charcot-Marie-Tooth disease	Ischemic stroke	Ischemic stroke	Ischemic stroke
Inborn errors of metabolism	Inborn errors of metabolism	Inborn errors of metabolism	Poisoning	Poisoning	Poisoning

Baby (0-1 yr)	Child (1-12 yr)	Adolescent (12-18 yr)	Adult (18-45 yr)	Middle Age Adult (45-65 yr)	Senior Adult (65+ yr)
Dry eye	Down syndrome	Down syndrome	Keratoconjunctivitis sicca	Dry eye	Keratoconjunctivitis sicca
Chronic fatigue syndrome	Chronic fatigue syndrome	Dry eye	Chronic fatigue syndrome	Chronic fatigue syndrome	Chronic fatigue syndrome
Down syndrome	Dry eye	Chronic fatigue syndrome	Dry eye	Keratoconjunctivitis sicca	Dry eye
Keratoconjunctivitis sicca	Keratoconjunctivitis sicca	Keratoconjunctivitis sicca	Down syndrome	Sjögren's syndrome	Sjögren's syndrome
		Sjögren's syndrome	Sjögren's syndrome		

Emergency Rule Out conditions shown in red. Entries in blue are for information only
Conditions are listed in approximate order of prevalence for this age range

Emergency Rule Out conditions shown in red. Entries in blue are for information only
Conditions are listed in approximate order of prevalence for this age range

Baby (0-1 yr)	Child (1-12 yr)	Adolescent (12-18 yr)	Adult (18-45 yr)	Middle Age Adult (45-65 yr)	Senior Adult (65+yr)
Not relevant to this age group	Aphthous ulcers	Aphthous ulcers	Aphthous ulcers	Aphthous ulcers	Ischemic stroke
	Cerebral palsy	Cerebral palsy	Ischemic stroke	Ischemic stroke	Aphthous ulcers
	Dental infection	Dental infection	Cerebral palsy	Hepatic encephalopathy	Hepatic encephalopathy
	Hepatic encephalopathy	Subarachnoid hemorrhage and cerebral aneurysm stroke	Dental infection	Cerebral palsy	Dental infection
	Friedreich's ataxia	Friedreich's ataxia	Hepatic encephalopathy	Dental infection	Pseudobulbar palsy
	Brainstem disorders	Hepatic encephalopathy	Parkinson's disease	Parkinson's disease	Parkinson's disease
	Oculopharyngeal muscular dystrophy	Brainstem disorders	Pseudobulbar palsy	Friedreich's ataxia	Myasthenia gravis
	Botulism	Oculopharyngeal muscular dystrophy	Subarachnoid hemorrhage and cerebral aneurysm stroke	Subarachnoid hemorrhage and cerebral aneurysm stroke	Friedreich's ataxia
	Pseudobulbar palsy	Botulism	Friedreich's ataxia	Pseudobulbar palsy	Subarachnoid hemorrhage and cerebral aneurysm stroke
	Muscular dystrophy	Pseudobulbar palsy	Myasthenia gravis	Myasthenia gravis	Cerebellar degeneration
	Oro-facial dyskinesia	Muscular dystrophy	Oculopharyngeal muscular dystrophy	Botulism	Oro-facial dyskinesia
	Stutter	Oro-facial dyskinesia	Multiple sclerosis	Oculopharyngeal muscular dystrophy	Botulism
	Hypothermia	Stutter	Muscular dystrophy	Muscular dystrophy	Amyotrophic lateral sclerosis (motor neuron disease)
		Hypothermia	Botulism	Cerebellar degeneration	Cerebral palsy
			Cerebellar degeneration	Oro-facial dyskinesia	Chorea
			Oro-facial dyskinesia	Athetosis	Muscular dystrophy
			Athetosis	Brainstem disorders	Athetosis
			Chorea	Amyotrophic lateral sclerosis (motor neuron disease)	Oculopharyngeal muscular dystrophy
			Amyotrophic lateral sclerosis (motor neuron disease)		

Baby (0-1 yr)	Child (1-12 yr)	Adolescent (12-18 yr)	Adult (18-45 yr)	Middle Age Adult (45-65 yr)	Senior Adult (65+yr)
			Brainstem disorders	Huntington's disease	Brainstem disorders
			Huntington's disease	Chorea	Huntington's disease
			Hypothermia	Hypothermia	Hypothermia

Emergency Rule Out conditions shown in red. Entries in blue are for information only
Conditions are listed in approximate order of prevalence for this age range

Baby (0-1 yr)	Child (1-12 yr)	Adolescent (12-18 yr)	Adult (18-45 yr)	Middle Age Adult (45-65 yr)	Senior Adult (65+ yr)
Not relevant to this age group	Not relevant to this age group	Mucocutaneous candidiasis	Mucocutaneous candidiasis	Estrogen deficient vulvovaginitis	Estrogen deficient vulvovaginitis
		Estrogen deficient vulvovaginitis	Bacterial vulvovaginitis	Mucocutaneous candidiasis	Mucocutaneous candidiasis
		Bacterial vulvovaginitis	Estrogen deficient vulvovaginitis	Bacterial vulvovaginitis	Bacterial vulvovaginitis
		Sexual dysfunction in men	Menopause	Pelvic inflammatory disease	Sexual dysfunction in men
		Uterine myomas	Endometriosis	Uterine myomas	Sexual dysfunction in women
		Endometriosis	Sexual dysfunction in men	Dyspareunia	Degenerative arthritis of hip
		Dyspareunia	Dyspareunia	Sexual dysfunction in men	Chancroid
		Chancroid	Uterine myomas	Menopause	Uterine myomas
		Pelvic inflammatory disease	Pelvic inflammatory disease	Chlamydia trachomatis infection	Dyspareunia
		Urethritis	Vaginal malignancy	Sexual dysfunction in women	Cervical malignancy
		Benign ovarian tumor	Sexual dysfunction in women	Sexual assault	Benign ovarian tumor
		Cervical malignancy	Cervical malignancy	Chancroid	Sexual assault
		Sexual dysfunction in women	Benign ovarian tumor	Cervical malignancy	Vaginal malignancy
		Sexual assault	Chancroid	Urethritis	Muscular back pain
		Vaginal malignancy	Sexual assault	Benign ovarian tumor	Bartholin cyst
		Chlamydia trachomatis infection	Chlamydia trachomatis infection	Genital herpes	Psychosomatic
		Genital herpes	Urethritis	Vaginal malignancy	Perineal laceration
		Bartholin cyst	Genital herpes	Bartholin cyst	Retroverted uterus
		Muscular back pain	Bartholin cyst	Degenerative arthritis of hip	Uterine prolapse
		Psychosomatic	Muscular back pain	Muscular back pain	Puerperal infection (endometritis)

List continues on next page

Baby (0-1 yr)	Child (1-12 yr)	Adolescent (12-18 yr)	Adult (18-45 yr)	Middle Age Adult (45-65 yr)	Senior Adult (65+ yr)
		Perineal laceration Retroverted uterus Uterine prolapse Puerperal infection (endometritis)	Degenerative arthritis of hip Psychosomatic Perineal laceration Retroverted uterus Uterine prolapse Puerperal infection (endometritis)	Perineal laceration Psychosomatic Retroverted uterus Uterine prolapse Puerperal infection (endometritis)	

Emergency Rule Out conditions shown in red. Entries in blue are for information only
Conditions are listed in approximate order of prevalence for this age range

Baby (0-1 yr)	Child (1-12 yr)	Adolescent (12-18 yr)	Adult (18-45 yr)	Middle Age Adult (45-65 yr)	Senior Adult (65-yr)
Gastroesophageal reflux disease	Gastroesophageal reflux disease	Gastroesophageal reflux disease	Gastroesophageal reflux disease	Gastroesophageal reflux disease	Gastroesophageal reflux disease
Primary intracerebral hemorrhage stroke	Tonsillitis	Tonsillitis	Esophageal candidiasis	Esophageal candidiasis	Esophageal candidiasis
Esophageal cancer	Primary intracerebral hemorrhage stroke	Primary intracerebral hemorrhage stroke	Ischemic stroke	Ischemic stroke	Ischemic stroke
Thyroiditis	Transient ischemic attack	Esophageal cancer	Primary intracerebral hemorrhage stroke	Primary intracerebral hemorrhage stroke	Primary intracerebral hemorrhage stroke
Gastritis	Iron deficiency anemia	Iron deficiency anemia	Subarachnoid hemorrhage and cerebral aneurysm stroke	Subarachnoid hemorrhage and cerebral aneurysm stroke	Subarachnoid hemorrhage and cerebral aneurysm stroke
Esophagitis	Esophagitis	Epiglottitis	Diabetic neuropathy	Diabetic neuropathy	Diabetic neuropathy
Epiglottitis	Epiglottitis	Thyroiditis	Thoracic aortic aneurysm	Thoracic aortic aneurysm	Thoracic aortic aneurysm
Oral cavity cancer	Laryngeal cancer	Esophagitis	Transient ischemic attack	Transient ischemic attack	Transient ischemic attack
Reflux laryngitis	Reflux laryngitis	Gastritis	Achalasia	Thyroiditis	Achalasia
Laryngeal cancer	Gastritis	Oral cavity cancer	Thyroiditis	Achalasia	Esophageal cancer
Iron deficiency anemia	Oral cavity cancer	Reflux laryngitis	Esophageal cancer	Esophageal cancer	Thyroiditis
Transient ischemic attack	Thyroiditis	Laryngeal cancer	Foreign body	Foreign body	Foreign body
Foreign body	Esophageal cancer	Transient ischemic attack	Reflux laryngitis	Reflux laryngitis	Esophagitis
Achalasia	Foreign body	Foreign body	Esophagitis	Esophagitis	Reflux laryngitis
Brain tumor	Achalasia	Achalasia	Scleroderma	Acoustic neuroma	Laryngeal cancer
Poliomyelitis	Brain tumor	Brain tumor	Iron deficiency anemia	Iron deficiency anemia	Iron deficiency anemia
Thyroid carcinoma	Hodgkin's disease	Hodgkin's disease	Acoustic neuroma	Scleroderma	Acoustic neuroma
	Non-Hodgkin's lymphoma	Non-Hodgkin's lymphoma	Oral cavity cancer	Oral cavity cancer	Epiglottitis
	Poliomyelitis	Poliomyelitis	Epiglottitis	Laryngeal cancer	Gastritis
	Thyroid carcinoma	Thyroid carcinoma			

List continues on next page

Baby (0-1 yr)	Child (1-12 yr)	Adolescent (12-18 yr)	Adult (18-45 yr)	Middle Age Adult (45-65 yr)	Senior Adult (65+ yr)
			Laryngeal cancer	Epiglottitis	Scleroderma
			Gastritis	Gastritis	Oral cavity cancer
			Acute left ventricular failure	Acute left ventricular failure	Acute left ventricular failure
			Hodgkin's disease	Hodgkin's disease	Hodgkin's disease
			Myasthenia gravis	Myasthenia gravis	Myasthenia gravis
			Non-Hodgkin's lymphoma	Non-Hodgkin's lymphoma	Non-Hodgkin's lymphoma
			Brain tumor	Brain tumor	Brain tumor
			Schistosomiasis	Schistosomiasis	Schistosomiasis
			Blastomycosis	Blastomycosis	Blastomycosis
			Acute mesenteric adenitis	Acute mesenteric adenitis	Acute mesenteric adenitis
			Empyema	Empyema	Empyema
			Amyloidosis	Amyloidosis	Amyloidosis
			Botulism	Botulism	Botulism
			Poliomyelitis	Poliomyelitis	Poliomyelitis
			Thyroid carcinoma	Thyroid carcinoma	Thyroid carcinoma

Emergency Rule Out conditions shown in red. Entries in blue are for information only
Conditions are listed in approximate order of prevalence for this age range

Baby (0-1 yr)	Child (1-12 yr)	Adolescent (12-18 yr)	Adult (18-45 yr)	Middle Age Adult (45-65 yr)	Senior Adult (65+ yr)
Asthma	Asthma	Anxiety	Asthma	Asthma	Asthma
Croup	Croup	Asthma	Chronic obstructive pulmonary disease	Chronic obstructive pulmonary disease	Chronic obstructive pulmonary disease
Bronchiolitis	Bronchiolitis	Bacterial pneumonia	Anxiety	Acute left ventricular failure	Acute left ventricular failure
Viral pneumonia	Congestive heart failure	Viral pneumonia	Bacterial pneumonia	Congestive heart failure	Congestive heart failure
Bacterial pneumonia	Viral pneumonia	Mycoplasmal pneumonia	Acute bronchitis	Acute bronchitis	Acute bronchitis
Superior vena cava syndrome	Bacterial pneumonia	Acute bronchitis	Viral pneumonia	Bacterial pneumonia	Bacterial pneumonia
Thyroiditis	Mycoplasmal pneumonia	Superior vena cava syndrome	Mycoplasmal pneumonia	Viral pneumonia	Viral pneumonia
Congenital heart disease	Acute bronchitis	Thyroiditis	Anemia	Mycoplasmal pneumonia	Mycoplasmal pneumonia
Mitral stenosis	Superior vena cava syndrome	Respiratory syncytial virus infection	Pulmonary thromboembolism	Anxiety	Anxiety
Anemia	Thyroiditis	Anemia	Pleural effusion	Primary lung malignancy	Pulmonary thromboembolism
Iron deficiency anemia	Anemia	Pneumothorax	Pneumothorax	Pulmonary thromboembolism	Primary lung malignancy
Chronic allergic alveolitis	Respiratory syncytial virus infection	Iron deficiency anemia	Congestive heart failure	Anemia	Anemia
Laryngeal cancer	Iron deficiency anemia	Chronic allergic alveolitis	Acute left ventricular failure	Pneumothorax	Pneumothorax
Myocardial infarction	Foreign body	Myocardial infarction	Primary lung malignancy	Mitral stenosis	Mitral stenosis
Respiratory syncytial virus infection	Laryngeal cancer	Cardiomyopathy	Mitral stenosis	Thyroiditis	Adult respiratory distress syndrome
Congestive heart failure	Myocardial infarction	Laryngeal cancer	Thyroiditis	Superior vena cava syndrome	Superior vena cava syndrome
Cystic fibrosis	Chronic allergic alveolitis	Congestive heart failure	Superior vena cava syndrome	Amyloidosis	Thyroiditis
Chlamydia pneumoniae	Congenital heart disease	Chlamydia pneumoniae	Cardiomyopathy	Myocardial infarction	Respiratory syncytial virus infection
Bronchiectasis	Chlamydia pneumoniae	Carbon monoxide poisoning	Amyloidosis	Pleural effusion	
Cardiomyopathy	Pleural effusion	Congenital heart disease	Ankylosing spondylitis	Chronic allergic alveolitis	
Carbon monoxide poisoning	Acute left ventricular failure	Ankylosing spondylitis			

List continues on next page

Baby (0-1 yr)	Child (1-12 yr)	Adolescent (12-18 yr)	Adult (18-45 yr)	Middle Age Adult (45-65 yr)	Senior Adult (65+yr)
AV block, second degree	Carbon monoxide poisoning	Mitral stenosis	Myocardial infarction	Iron deficiency anemia	Amyloidosis
AV block, third degree	Cardiac tamponade	AV block, second degree	Iron deficiency anemia	Aortic stenosis	Iron deficiency anemia
Carcinoid syndrome	Cystic fibrosis	AV block, third degree	Chronic allergic alveolitis	Laryngeal cancer	Chronic allergic alveolitis
Behçet's syndrome	AV block, second degree	Behçet's syndrome	Laryngeal cancer	Respiratory syncytial virus infection	Myocardial infarction
Mycoplasmal pneumonia	AV block, third degree	Carcinoid syndrome	Cardiac tamponade	Adult respiratory distress syndrome	Laryngeal cancer
Pleural effusion	Behçet's syndrome	Pleural effusion	Respiratory syncytial virus infection	Chlamydia pneumoniae	Aortic stenosis
Pneumothorax	Carcinoid syndrome	Cardiac tamponade	Adult respiratory distress syndrome	Cardiomyopathy	Carbon monoxide poisoning
Cardiac tamponade	Bronchiectasis	Foreign body	Atrial septal defect	Carbon monoxide poisoning	Ankylosing spondylitis
Diaphragmatic paralysis	Mitral stenosis	Extrinsic airway compression	Chlamydia pneumoniae	Ankylosing spondylitis	Chlamydia pneumoniae
Foreign body	Cardiomyopathy	Acute left ventricular failure	Carbon monoxide poisoning	Carcinoid syndrome	Pleural effusion
Extrinsic airway compression	Pneumothorax	Cystic fibrosis	Foreign body	Atrial septal defect	Cardiomyopathy
Acute left ventricular failure	Methemoglobinemia	Bronchiectasis	Kyphoscoliosis	AV block, second degree	Kyphosis
Methemoglobinemia	Anxiety	Methemoglobinemia	Kyphosis	AV block, third degree	Atrial septal defect
Poliomyelitis	Extrinsic airway compression	Diaphragmatic paralysis	AV block, second degree	Behçet's syndrome	AV block, second degree
Thyroid carcinoma	Diaphragmatic paralysis	Poliomyelitis	Behçet's syndrome	Cardiac tamponade	AV block, third degree
	Poliomyelitis	Thyroid carcinoma	AV block, third degree	Foreign body	Carcinoid syndrome
	Thyroid carcinoma		Extrinsic airway compression	Kyphosis	Behçet's syndrome
			Carcinoid syndrome	Kyphoscoliosis	Cardiac tamponade
			Methemoglobinemia	Myasthenia gravis	Foreign body
			Diaphragmatic paralysis	Bronchiectasis	Bronchiectasis
				Extrinsic airway compression	Kyphoscoliosis
					Myasthenia gravis
					Extrinsic airway compression

List continues on next page

Dyspnea (continued)

List continued from previous page

Baby (0-1 yr)	Child (1-12 yr)	Adolescent (12-18 yr)	Adult (18-45 yr)	Middle Age Adult (45-65 yr)	Senior Adult (65+ yr)
			Cystic fibrosis Bronchiectasis Myasthenia gravis Aspiration pneumonia Pulmonary hypertension Aortic stenosis Poliomyelitis Thyroid carcinoma	Methemoglobinemia Diaphragmatic paralysis Aspiration pneumonia Poliomyelitis Thyroid carcinoma	Methemoglobinemia Diaphragmatic paralysis Aspiration pneumonia Poliomyelitis Thyroid carcinoma

Baby (0-1 yr)	Child (1-12 yr)	Adolescent (12-18 yr)	Adult (18-45 yr)	Middle Age Adult (45-65 yr)	Senior Adult (65+yr)
Balanitis and balanoposthitis	Urinary tract infection	Urinary tract infection	Urinary tract infection	Urinary tract infection	Urinary tract infection
	Prepubescent vulvovaginitis	Mucocutaneous candidiasis	Mucocutaneous candidiasis	Mucocutaneous candidiasis	Mucocutaneous candidiasis
	Pyelonephritis	Bacterial vulvovaginitis	Bacterial vulvovaginitis	Bacterial vulvovaginitis	Bacterial vulvovaginitis
	Cystitis	Chemical irritant	Genital herpes	Estrogen deficient vulvovaginitis	Genital herpes
	Urethritis	Pyelonephritis	Cystitis	Uterine prolapse	Chlamydia trachomatis infection
	Balanitis and balanoposthitis	Cystitis	Uterine prolapse	Chemical irritant	Pyelonephritis
	Uterine prolapse	Genital herpes	Pyelonephritis	Cystitis	Gonorrhea
	Chemical irritant	Urethritis	Menopause	Urethritis	Urethritis
	Genital herpes	Balanitis and balanoposthitis	Balanitis and balanoposthitis	Pyelonephritis	Cystitis
		Uterine prolapse	Urethritis	Balanitis and balanoposthitis	Uterine prolapse
		Genital warts	Chlamydia trachomatis infection	Genital herpes	Balanitis and balanoposthitis
		Chlamydia trachomatis infection	Gonorrhea	Chlamydia trachomatis infection	Lymphogranuloma venereum
		Gonorrhea	Lymphogranuloma venereum	Gonorrhea	Syphilis
		Lymphogranuloma venereum	Syphilis	Lymphogranuloma venereum	Estrogen deficient vulvovaginitis
		Syphilis	Reiter's syndrome	Syphilis	Chemical irritant
			Chemical irritant	Bladder tumor	Catheter in-situ
			Crohn's disease	Urethral stricture	Bladder tumor
				Reiter's syndrome	Urethral stricture
				Crohn's disease	Diverticular disease
				Diverticular disease	

Emergency Rule Out conditions shown in red. Entries in blue are for information only
Conditions are listed in approximate order of prevalence for this age range

Emergency Rule Out conditions shown in red. Entries in blue are for information only
Conditions are listed in approximate order of prevalence for this age range

Baby (0-1 yr)	Child (1-12 yr)	Adolescent (12-18 yr)	Adult (18-45 yr)	Middle Age Adult (45-65 yr)	Senior Adult (65+yr)
Acute otitis media	Acute otitis media	Acute otitis media	Acute otitis media	Acute otitis media	Acute otitis media
Chronic otitis media	Chronic otitis media	Chronic otitis media	Chronic otitis media	Chronic otitis media	Chronic otitis media
Otitis externa	Otitis externa	Otitis externa	Otitis externa	Otitis externa	Otitis externa
Eustachian tube dysfunction	Eustachian tube dysfunction	Eustachian tube dysfunction	Eustachian tube dysfunction	Eustachian tube dysfunction	Eustachian tube dysfunction
Traumatic tympanic membrane rupture	Traumatic tympanic membrane rupture	Traumatic tympanic membrane rupture	Barotitis media	Temporomandibular joint syndrome	Temporomandibular joint syndrome
Barotitis media	Barotitis media	Barotitis media	Temporomandibular joint syndrome	Infectious myringitis	Infectious myringitis
Foreign body	Foreign body	Foreign body	Infectious myringitis	Barotitis media	Barotitis media
Mastoiditis	Dental infection	Dental infection	Traumatic tympanic membrane rupture	Traumatic tympanic membrane rupture	Traumatic tympanic membrane rupture
Trauma	Mastoiditis	Trauma	Foreign body	Foreign body	Foreign body
Herpes simplex	Trauma	Mastoiditis	Herpes zoster, shingles	Herpes zoster, shingles	Herpes zoster, shingles
Chickenpox	Herpes simplex	Herpes simplex	Mastoiditis	Mastoiditis	Mastoiditis
	Chickenpox	Chickenpox	Dental infection	Dental infection	Dental infection
			Erysipelas	Erysipelas	Erysipelas

Baby (0-1 yr)	Child (1-12 yr)	Adolescent (12-18 yr)	Adult (18-45 yr)	Middle Age Adult (45-65 yr)	Senior Adult (65+ yr)
Drug reaction	Drug reaction	Drug reaction	Venous insufficiency	Venous insufficiency	Venous insufficiency
Congestive heart failure	Congestive heart failure	Hypoalbuminemia	Deep vein thrombosis	Deep vein thrombosis	Congestive heart failure
Hypoalbuminemia	Hypoalbuminemia	Venous obstruction	Congestive heart failure	Congestive heart failure	Liver cirrhosis
Kawasaki disease	Venous obstruction	Cardiac tamponade	Liver cirrhosis	Liver cirrhosis	Rocky Mountain spotted fever
Hepatoma	Mitral stenosis	Nephrotic syndrome	Eclampsia	Rocky Mountain spotted fever	Nephritic syndrome
Mitral stenosis	Hepatoma	Kawasaki disease	Mitral stenosis	Kawasaki disease	Nephrotic syndrome
Cardiac tamponade	Kawasaki disease	Mitral stenosis	Kawasaki disease	Hepatoma	Mitral stenosis
Rocky Mountain spotted fever	Cardiac tamponade	Nephritic syndrome	Burns	Mitral stenosis	Kawasaki disease
Burns	Rocky Mountain spotted fever	Burns	Nephrotic syndrome	Eclampsia	Deep vein thrombosis
Cellulitis	Burns	Hepatoma	Hepatoma	Nephritic syndrome	Reflex sympathetic dystrophy
Cardiomyopathy	Nephritic syndrome	Rocky Mountain spotted fever	Nephritic syndrome	Hypoalbuminemia	Burns
Lymphatic obstruction	Nephrotic syndrome	Lymphatic obstruction	Rocky Mountain spotted fever	Nephrotic syndrome	Cellulitis
Reflex sympathetic dystrophy	Thoracic outlet syndrome	Thoracic outlet syndrome	Hypoalbuminemia	Acne rosacea	Lymphatic obstruction
Nephrotic syndrome	Cellulitis	Reflex sympathetic dystrophy	Cellulitis	Cellulitis	Thoracic outlet syndrome
Nephritic syndrome	Cardiomyopathy	Cellulitis	Thoracic outlet syndrome	Burns	Acute glomerulonephritis
Thoracic outlet syndrome	Reflex sympathetic dystrophy	Nutritional deficiencies	Reflex sympathetic dystrophy	Reflex sympathetic dystrophy	Acne rosacea
Nutritional deficiencies	Acute glomerulonephritis	Cardiomyopathy	Cardiomyopathy	Thoracic outlet syndrome	Hypoalbuminemia
Myxedema	Lymphatic obstruction	Acute glomerulonephritis	Acute glomerulonephritis	Cardiomyopathy	Superior vena cava syndrome
Anemia	Nutritional deficiencies	Myxedema	Acne rosacea	Acute glomerulonephritis	
Pericarditis	Myxedema	Acne rosacea	Cardiac tamponade	Cardiac tamponade	

List continues on next page

Emergency Rule Out conditions shown in red. Entries in blue are for information only
Conditions are listed in approximate order of prevalence for this age range

109

List continued from previous page

Baby (0-1 yr)	Child (1-12 yr)	Adolescent (12-18 yr)	Adult (18-45 yr)	Middle Age Adult (45-65 yr)	Senior Adult (65+ yr)
Hypothyroidism	Pericarditis	Eclampsia	Lymphatic obstruction	Lymphatic obstruction	Myxedema
Venous obstruction	Superior vena cava syndrome	Pericarditis	Myxedema	Myxedema	Cardiac tamponade
Allergic reactions and anaphylaxis	Cystic fibrosis	Superior vena cava syndrome	Nutritional deficiencies	Nutritional deficiencies	Nutritional deficiencies
Inappropriate secretion of antidiuretic hormone	Stevens-Johnson syndrome	Cystic fibrosis	Filariasis	Filariasis	Filariasis
	Allergic reactions and anaphylaxis	Stevens-Johnson syndrome	Superior vena cava syndrome	Superior vena cava syndrome	Millard-Gubler syndrome
	Inappropriate secretion of antidiuretic hormone	Allergic reactions and anaphylaxis	Millard-Gubler syndrome	Millard-Gubler syndrome	Inappropriate secretion of antidiuretic hormone
		Inappropriate secretion of antidiuretic hormone	Inappropriate secretion of antidiuretic hormone	Inappropriate secretion of antidiuretic hormone	Hepatoma

Baby (0-1 yr)	Child (1-12 yr)	Adolescent (12-18 yr)	Adult (18-45 yr)	Middle Age Adult (45-65 yr)	Senior Adult (65+ yr)
Elbow injury	Elbow injury	Muscular strain	Aseptic bursitis	Elbow injury	Elbow injury
Elbow dislocation	Elbow dislocation	Overuse	Elbow injury	Aseptic bursitis	Aseptic bursitis
Epicondylitis	Muscular strain	Tendinitis	Medial epicondylitis	Medial epicondylitis	Medial epicondylitis
Fracture	Tendinitis	Medial epicondylitis	Tendinitis	Epicondylitis	Tendinitis
Septic arthritis	Overuse	Epicondylitis	Epicondylitis	Tendinitis	Epicondylitis
	Epicondylitis	Elbow injury	Elbow dislocation	Acute gout	Acute gout
	Fracture	Elbow dislocation	Acute gout	Septic arthritis	Septic arthritis
	Aseptic bursitis	Fracture	Cubital tunnel syndrome	Fracture	Fracture
	Medial epicondylitis	Aseptic bursitis	Fracture	Cubital tunnel syndrome	Cubital tunnel syndrome
	Septic arthritis	Septic arthritis	Ruptured distal biceps tendon	Elbow dislocation	Elbow dislocation
	Epitrochlear lymphadenitis	Epitrochlear lymphadenitis	Epitrochlear lymphadenitis	Ruptured distal biceps tendon	Ruptured distal biceps tendon
		Cubital tunnel syndrome	Septic arthritis	Epitrochlear lymphadenitis	Epitrochlear lymphadenitis

Emergency Rule Out conditions shown in red. Entries in blue are for information only
Conditions are listed in approximate order of prevalence for this age range

Emergency Rule Out conditions shown in red. Entries in blue are for information only
Conditions are listed in approximate order of prevalence for this age range

Baby (0-1 yr)	Child (1-12 yr)	Adolescent (12-18 yr)	Adult (18-45 yr)	Middle Age Adult (45-65 yr)	Senior Adult (65+yr)
Not relevant to this age group	Constipation Fecal impaction Behavioral problem in children	Constipation Fecal impaction Behavioral problem in children	Constipation Fecal impaction	Constipation Fecal impaction	Constipation Fecal impaction

Baby (0-1 yr)	Child (1-12 yr)	Adolescent (12-18 yr)	Adult (18-45 yr)	Middle Age Adult (45-65 yr)	Senior Adult (65+ yr)
Dry mucous membranes	Dry mucous membranes	Dry mucous membranes	Dry mucous membranes	Dry mucous membranes	Dry mucous membranes
Hereditary hemorrhagic telangectasia	Trauma	Trauma	Trauma	Trauma	Trauma
Barotitis media	Chronic sinusitis	Allergic rhinitis	Allergic rhinitis	Allergic rhinitis	Allergic rhinitis
Trauma	Foreign body	Chronic sinusitis	Chronic sinusitis	Chronic sinusitis	Chronic sinusitis
	Allergic rhinitis	Foreign body	Essential hypertension	Essential hypertension	Essential hypertension
	Septal ulceration	Septal ulceration	Septal ulceration	Septal ulceration	Septal ulceration
	Thrombotic thrombocytopenic purpura	Thrombotic thrombocytopenic purpura	Foreign body	Foreign body	Foreign body
	Barotitis media	Barotitis media	Thrombotic thrombocytopenic purpura	Thrombotic thrombocytopenic purpura	Thrombotic thrombocytopenic purpura
	Hemophilia A	Hemophilia A	Barotitis media	Barotitis media	Hemophilia A
	Hemophilia B	Hemophilia B	Hemophilia A	Hemophilia A	Barotitis media
	Hereditary hemorrhagic telangectasia	Hereditary hemorrhagic telangectasia	Hemophilia B	Hemophilia B	Hemophilia B
	Excessive anticoagulation	Excessive anticoagulation	Hereditary hemorrhagic telangectasia	Hereditary hemorrhagic telangectasia	Hereditary hemorrhagic telangectasia
	Essential hypertension	Essential hypertension	Excessive anticoagulation	Excessive anticoagulation	Excessive anticoagulation

Emergency Rule Out conditions shown in red. Entries in blue are for information only
Conditions are listed in approximate order of prevalence for this age range

Erythema multiforme

Emergency Rule Out conditions shown in red. Entries in blue are for information only
Conditions are listed in approximate order of prevalence for this age range

Baby (0-1 yr)	Child (1-12 yr)	Adolescent (12-18 yr)	Adult (18-45 yr)	Middle Age Adult (45-65 yr)	Senior Adult (65+ yr)
Viral infection	Viral infection	Viral infection	Idiopathic	Idiopathic	Idiopathic
Idiopathic	Drug reaction, allergic	Drug reaction, allergic	Herpes simplex	Herpes simplex	Herpes simplex
Drug reaction, allergic	Mycoplasmal pneumonia	Mycoplasmal pneumonia	Mycoplasmal pneumonia	Mycoplasmal pneumonia	Mycoplasmal pneumonia
	Idiopathic	Idiopathic	Drug reaction, allergic	Drug reaction, allergic	Drug reaction, allergic
	Herpes simplex	Herpes simplex	Radiation sickness	Radiation sickness	Radiation sickness
			Occult cancer	Occult cancer	Occult cancer
			Psittacosis	Psittacosis	Psittacosis
			Histoplasmosis	Histoplasmosis	Histoplasmosis
			Zollinger-Ellison syndrome	Zollinger-Ellison syndrome	Zollinger-Ellison syndrome

Baby (0-1 yr)	Child (1-12 yr)	Adolescent (12-18 yr)	Adult (18-45 yr)	Middle Age Adult (45-65 yr)	Senior Adult (65-yr)
Behçet's syndrome	Idiopathic	Idiopathic	Streptococcal throat infection	Streptococcal throat infection	Streptococcal throat infection
Drug reaction	Streptococcal throat infection	Streptococcal throat infection	Drug reaction	Drug reaction	Sarcoidosis
	Tuberculosis	Tuberculosis	Sarcoidosis	Sarcoidosis	Drug reaction
	Behçet's syndrome	Behçet's syndrome	Behçet's syndrome	Behçet's syndrome	Tuberculosis
	Crohn's disease	Crohn's disease	Tuberculosis	Tuberculosis	Behçet's syndrome
	Drug reaction	Drug reaction	Crohn's disease	Crohn's disease	Crohn's disease
			Histoplasmosis	Histoplasmosis	Histoplasmosis
			Lymphogranuloma venereum	Lymphogranuloma venereum	Lymphogranuloma venereum
			Psittacosis	Psittacosis	Psittacosis

Emergency Rule Out conditions shown in red. Entries in blue are for information only
Conditions are listed in approximate order of prevalence for this age range

Emergency Rule Out conditions shown in red. Entries in blue are for information only
Conditions are listed in approximate order of prevalence for this age range

Baby (0-1 yr)	Child (1-12 yr)	Adolescent (12-18 yr)	Adult (18-45 yr)	Middle Age Adult (45-65 yr)	Senior Adult (65+ yr)
Viral infection	Viral infection	Viral infection	Pityriasis rosea	Pityriasis rosea	Pityriasis rosea
Chickenpox	Chickenpox	Chickenpox	Erythema multiforme	Erythema multiforme	Erythema multiforme
Scarlet fever	Scarlet fever	Fifth disease	Fifth disease	Rocky Mountain spotted fever	Rocky Mountain spotted fever
Erythema multiforme	Fifth disease	Scarlet fever	Mononucleosis	Meningococcemia	Fifth disease
Fifth disease	Erythema infectiosum	Erythema infectiosum	Rocky Mountain spotted fever	Fifth disease	Meningococcemia
Erythema infectiosum	Mononucleosis	Hand-foot-and-mouth disease	Primary HIV infection	Syphilis	Syphilis
Hand-foot-and-mouth disease	Hand-foot-and-mouth disease	Mononucleosis	AIDS	Hand-foot-and-mouth disease	Hand-foot-and-mouth disease
Rubella	Rubella	Rubella	Hand-foot-and-mouth disease	Primary HIV infection	Primary HIV infection
Meningococcemia	Pityriasis rosea	Pityriasis rosea	Meningococcemia	AIDS	AIDS
Syphilis	Meningococcemia	Meningococcemia	Syphilis	Toxic shock syndrome	Toxic shock syndrome
Mononucleosis	Toxic shock syndrome	Toxic shock syndrome	Toxic shock syndrome	Mononucleosis	Mononucleosis
Primary HIV infection	Typhoid fever	Typhoid fever	Scarlet fever	Scarlet fever	Scarlet fever
AIDS	Erythema multiforme	Erythema multiforme	Chickenpox	Rubella	Rubella
Rocky Mountain spotted fever	Rocky Mountain spotted fever	Rocky Mountain spotted fever	Erythema infectiosum	Typhoid fever	Typhoid fever
Toxic shock syndrome	Primary HIV infection	Primary HIV infection	Typhoid fever	Chickenpox	Chickenpox
Typhoid fever	AIDS	AIDS	Rubella	Ehrlichiosis	Ehrlichiosis
Ehrlichiosis	Syphilis	Syphilis	Ehrlichiosis	Erythema infectiosum	Erythema infectiosum
	Ehrlichiosis	Ehrlichiosis			

Baby (0-1 yr)	Child (1-12 yr)	Adolescent (12-18 yr)	Adult (18-45 yr)	Middle Age Adult (45-65 yr)	Senior Adult (65+ yr)
Graves' disease	Graves' disease	Graves' disease	Graves' disease	Graves' disease	Graves' disease
Cellulitis	Orbital cellulitis	Orbital cellulitis	Orbital tumor	Orbital tumor	Orbital tumor
Orbital cellulitis	Orbital tumor	Cellulitis	Periorbital cellulitis	Periorbital cellulitis	Periorbital cellulitis
	Cellulitis	Orbital tumor	Drug reaction, lithium	Drug reaction, lithium	Drug reaction, lithium
	Cavernous sinus thrombosis	Cavernous sinus thrombosis	Orbital hemorrhage	Orbital hemorrhage	Cellulitis
			Cellulitis	Cellulitis	Orbital hemorrhage
			Cavernous sinus thrombosis	Cavernous sinus thrombosis	Cavernous sinus thrombosis
			Arteriovenous fistula	Intracavernous carotid artery aneurysm	Intracavernous carotid artery aneurysm
			Intracavernous carotid artery aneurysm	Arteriovenous fistula	Arteriovenous fistula
			Carotid-cavernous sinus fistula	Carotid-cavernous sinus fistula	Carotid-cavernous sinus fistula
			Meningioma	Meningioma	Meningioma

Emergency Rule Out conditions shown in red. Entries in blue are for information only
Conditions are listed in approximate order of prevalence for this age range

Exophthalmos

Extravasation of urine

Emergency Rule Out conditions shown in red. Entries in blue are for information only
Conditions are listed in approximate order of prevalence for this age range

Baby (0-1 yr)	Child (1-12 yr)	Adolescent (12-18 yr)	Adult (18-45 yr)	Middle Age Adult (45-65 yr)	Senior Adult (65-yr)
Ectopic ureter	Ectopic ureter	Ectopic ureter	Trauma	Bladder tumor	Bladder tumor
Neurogenic bladder	Neurogenic bladder	Neurogenic bladder	Bladder tumor	Trauma	Colon cancer
Ureterocele	Ureterocele	Ureterocele	Colon cancer	Colon cancer	Pelvic tumor
Trauma	Trauma	Trauma	Pelvic tumor	Pelvic tumor	Trauma
Bladder tumor	Bladder tumor	Bladder tumor	Neurogenic bladder	Neurogenic bladder	Neurogenic bladder
Pelvic tumor	Pelvic tumor	Pelvic tumor			

Baby (0-1 yr)	Child (1-12 yr)	Adolescent (12-18 yr)	Adult (18-45 yr)	Middle Age Adult (45-65 yr)	Senior Adult (65+ yr)
Bacterial conjunctivitis	Bacterial conjunctivitis	Bacterial conjunctivitis	Bacterial conjunctivitis	Bacterial conjunctivitis	Bacterial conjunctivitis
Corneal abrasion	Corneal abrasion	Corneal abrasion	Corneal abrasion	Corneal abrasion	Corneal abrasion
Hordeolum, chalazion, blepharitis	Ocular trauma	Chronic sinusitis	Chronic sinusitis	Chronic sinusitis	Glaucoma
Cellulitis	Periorbital cellulitis	Retinal migraine	Ocular trauma	Ankylosing spondylitis	Chronic sinusitis
Dry eye	Orbital cellulitis	Ocular trauma	Dry eye	Herpes zoster, shingles	Ankylosing spondylitis
Viral meningitis	Dry eye	Dry eye	Viral meningitis	Dry eye	Dry eye
Periorbital cellulitis	Hordeolum, chalazion, blepharitis	Viral meningitis	Hordeolum, chalazion, blepharitis	Hordeolum, chalazion, blepharitis	Herpes zoster, shingles
Orbital cellulitis	Viral meningitis	Hordeolum, chalazion, blepharitis	Herpes simplex	Glaucoma	Hordeolum, chalazion, blepharitis
Ocular trauma	Ankylosing spondylitis	Periorbital cellulitis	Cellulitis	Cellulitis	Cellulitis
	Chronic sinusitis	Ankylosing spondylitis	Periorbital cellulitis	Viral meningitis	Giant cell arteritis
	Cellulitis	Orbital cellulitis	Ankylosing spondylitis	Ocular trauma	Viral meningitis
	Episcleritis	Cellulitis	Scleritis	Herpes simplex	Ocular trauma
	Scleritis	Episcleritis	Glaucoma	Periorbital cellulitis	Periorbital cellulitis
	Herpes zoster, shingles	Scleritis	Uveitis	Scleritis	Herpes simplex
	Herpes simplex	Herpes simplex	Herpes zoster, shingles	Uveitis	Scleritis
	Uveitis	Herpes zoster, shingles	Optic neuritis	Giant cell arteritis	Uveitis
	Optic neuritis	Optic neuritis	Retinal migraine	Optic neuritis	Retinal migraine
	Glaucoma	Uveitis		Retinal migraine	
		Glaucoma			

Emergency Rule Out conditions shown in red. Entries in blue are for information only
Conditions are listed in approximate order of prevalence for this age range

Facial paralysis

Emergency Rule Out conditions shown in red. Entries in blue are for information only
Conditions are listed in approximate order of prevalence for this age range

Baby (0-1 yr)	Child (1-12 yr)	Adolescent (12-18 yr)	Adult (18-45 yr)	Middle Age Adult (45-65 yr)	Senior Adult (65+yr)
Trauma	Bell's palsy	Bell's palsy	Bell's palsy	Bell's palsy	Bell's palsy
Cavernous sinus thrombosis	Dementia	Sarcoidosis	Dental infection	Ischemic stroke	Ischemic stroke
Congenital facial palsy	Trauma	Dementia	Parotitis	Dental infection	Dental infection
Dementia	Cavernous sinus thrombosis	Trauma	Mastoiditis	Parotitis	Dementia
	Dental infection	Cavernous sinus thrombosis	Dementia	Dementia	Parotitis
	Mastoiditis	Dental infection	Ischemic stroke	Mastoiditis	Mastoiditis
	Mumps	Mumps	Amyloidosis	Amyloidosis	Amyloidosis
	Ramsay Hunt syndrome	Ramsay Hunt syndrome	Ramsay Hunt syndrome	Cavernous sinus thrombosis	Cavernous sinus thrombosis
		Mastoiditis	Cavernous sinus thrombosis	Ramsay Hunt syndrome	Ramsay Hunt syndrome
			Mononucleosis	Mononucleosis	Mononucleosis
			Poliomyelitis	Poliomyelitis	Poliomyelitis
			Mumps	Mumps	Mumps
			Guillain-Barré syndrome (acute infective polyneuritis)	Guillain-Barré syndrome (acute infective polyneuritis)	Guillain-Barré syndrome (acute infective polyneuritis)
			Syphilis	Syphilis	Syphilis
			Sarcoidosis	Sarcoidosis	Sarcoidosis

Baby (0-1 yr)	Child (1-12 yr)	Adolescent (12-18 yr)	Adult (18-45 yr)	Middle Age Adult (45-65 yr)	Senior Adult (65-yr)
Not relevant to this age group	Chronic sinusitis	Chronic sinusitis	Dental infection	Dental infection	Dental infection
	Dental occlusion defects	Dental occlusion defects	Chronic sinusitis	Chronic sinusitis	Chronic sinusitis
	Dental infection	Dental infection	Temporomandibular joint syndrome	Temporomandibular joint syndrome	Temporomandibular joint syndrome
	Bruxism	Trigeminal neuralgia	Trigeminal neuralgia	Bruxism	Bruxism
	Acute sinusitis	Temporomandibular joint syndrome	Bruxism	Migraine headache	Migraine headache
	Sialadenitis	Sialadenitis	Dental occlusion defects	Fracture	Fracture
	Parotitis	Acute sinusitis	Sialadenitis	Acute sinusitis	Acute sinusitis
	Fracture	Parotitis	Acute sinusitis	Sialadenitis	Sialadenitis
	Connective tissue disease	Bruxism	Migraine headache	Myocardial infarction	Myocardial infarction
	Cavernous sinus thrombosis	Connective tissue disease	Acoustic neuroma	Acoustic neuroma	Acoustic neuroma
		Fracture	Ocular trauma	Ocular trauma	Ocular trauma
		Parotid calculus	Fracture	Trigeminal neuralgia	Trigeminal neuralgia
		Cavernous sinus thrombosis	Parotid calculus	Parotitis	Parotitis
			Connective tissue disease	Parotid calculus	Parotid calculus
			Giant cell arteritis	Connective tissue disease	Connective tissue disease
			Myocardial infarction	Giant cell arteritis	Giant cell arteritis
			Parotitis	Cavernous sinus thrombosis	Cavernous sinus thrombosis
			Cavernous sinus thrombosis	Dental occlusion defects	Dental occlusion defects

Emergency Rule Out conditions shown in red. Entries in blue are for information only
Conditions are listed in approximate order of prevalence for this age range

Facial/dental/temporomandibular pain

Emergency Rule Out conditions shown in red. Entries in blue are for information only
Conditions are listed in approximate order of prevalence for this age range

Baby (0-1 yr)	Child (1-12 yr)	Adolescent (12-18 yr)	Adult (18-45 yr)	Middle Age Adult (45-65 yr)	Senior Adult (65+ yr)
Idiopathic Spinal muscular atrophy	Idiopathic Poliomyelitis Spinal muscular atrophy	Idiopathic Poliomyelitis Spinal muscular atrophy	Idiopathic Lumbar disc disorders Amyotrophic lateral sclerosis (motor neuron disease) Poliomyelitis Ischemic stroke Spinal muscular atrophy	Idiopathic Lumbar disc disorders Amyotrophic lateral sclerosis (motor neuron disease) Poliomyelitis Ischemic stroke Spinal muscular atrophy	Idiopathic Lumbar disc disorders Amyotrophic lateral sclerosis (motor neuron disease) Poliomyelitis Ischemic stroke Spinal muscular atrophy

Baby (0-1 yr)	Child (1-12 yr)	Adolescent (12-18 yr)	Adult (18-45 yr)	Middle Age Adult (45-65 yr)	Senior Adult (65+ yr)
Malnutrition	Anemia	Anemia	Anxiety	Anxiety	Depression
Iron deficiency anemia	Chronic infection	Chronic infection	Depression	Depression	Insomnia
Congestive heart failure	Malnutrition	Malnutrition	Insomnia	Insomnia	Anemia
Atrial septal defect	Reiter's syndrome	Chronic fatigue syndrome	Anemia	Orthostatic hypotension	Menopause
Diabetes mellitus in children	Narcolepsy	Premenstrual syndrome	Hypothyroidism	Anemia	Manic depression
Hypercalcemia	Orthostatic hypotension	Hypercalcemia	Narcolepsy	Chronic infection	Narcolepsy
Thalassemia	Diabetes mellitus in children	Fibromyalgia	Orthostatic hypotension	Tularemia	Hypercalcemia
Orthostatic hypotension	Fibromyalgia	Menopause	Chronic infection	Babesiosis	Chronic infection
Behçet's syndrome	Congestive heart failure	Orthostatic hypotension	Chronic fatigue syndrome	Manic depression	Fibromyalgia
Babesiosis	Hypercalcemia	Diabetes mellitus in children	Manic depression	Hypercalcemia	Iron deficiency anemia
Chronic lymphocytic leukemia	Chronic myelogenous leukemia	Manic depression	Premenstrual syndrome	Menopause	Malignancy
Chronic myelogenous leukemia	Iron deficiency anemia	Chronic myelogenous leukemia	Hypercalcemia	Fibromyalgia	Chronic myelogenous leukemia
Cardiomyopathy	Manic depression	Congestive heart failure	Behçet's syndrome	Premenstrual syndrome	Congestive heart failure
Celiac disease	Chronic lymphocytic leukemia	Iron deficiency anemia	Fibromyalgia	Iron deficiency anemia	Chronic lymphocytic leukemia
	Celiac disease	Chronic myelogenous leukemia	Iron deficiency anemia	Congestive heart failure	Babesiosis
	Chronic fatigue syndrome	Narcolepsy	Menopause	Chronic myelogenous leukemia	Orthostatic hypotension
	Cardiomyopathy	Chronic lymphocytic leukemia	Chronic myelogenous leukemia	Narcolepsy	Tularemia
	Atrial septal defect	Reiter's syndrome	Congestive heart failure	Behçet's syndrome	Celiac disease
	Behçet's syndrome	Celiac disease	Reiter's syndrome	Chronic lymphocytic leukemia	Cardiomyopathy
	Babesiosis	Babesiosis	Babesiosis	Celiac disease	Atrial septal defect
		Atrial septal defect			

List continues on next page

Emergency Rule Out conditions shown in red. Entries in blue are for information only
Conditions are listed in approximate order of prevalence for this age range

List continued from previous page

Baby (0-1 yr)	Child (1-12 yr)	Adolescent (12-18 yr)	Adult (18-45 yr)	Middle Age Adult (45-65 yr)	Senior Adult (65+yr)
	Acute leukemia	Behçet's syndrome	Chronic lymphocytic leukemia	Malignancy	Behçet's syndrome
	Tularemia	Tularemia	Celiac disease	Amyloidosis	Amyloidosis
	Bulimia nervosa	Cardiomyopathy	Cardiomyopathy	Atrial septal defect	Reiter's syndrome
	Anorexia nervosa	Bulimia nervosa	Tularemia	Reiter's syndrome	Acute leukemia
	Hypothyroidism	Acute leukemia	Atrial septal defect	Acute leukemia	Malnutrition
	Bronchiectasis	Ankylosing spondylitis	Amyloidosis	Cardiomyopathy	Ankylosing spondylitis
	Depression	Anorexia nervosa	Acute leukemia	Malnutrition	Chronic pain disorder
	Polymyalgia rheumatica	Bronchiectasis	Ankylosing spondylitis	Ankylosing spondylitis	Bronchiectasis
	Thalassemia	Hypothyroidism	Malnutrition	Chronic pain disorder	Hypothyroidism
		Depression	Bulimia nervosa	Bronchiectasis	Chronic renal failure
		Polymyalgia rheumatica	Anorexia nervosa	Hypothyroidism	Diabetes mellitus type 1
		Thalassemia	Malignancy	Chronic fatigue syndrome	Polymyalgia rheumatica
			Bronchiectasis	Chronic renal failure	Thalassemia
			Chronic pain disorder	Diabetes mellitus type 1	
			Chronic renal failure	Polymyalgia rheumatica	
			Diabetes mellitus type 1	Thalassemia	
			Polymyalgia rheumatica		
			Thalassemia		

Baby (0-1 yr)	Child (1-12 yr)	Adolescent (12-18 yr)	Adult (18-45 yr)	Middle Age Adult (45-65 yr)	Senior Adult (65+yr)
Lymphadenopathy	Lymphadenopathy	Lymphadenopathy	Lymphadenopathy	Lymphadenopathy	Lymphadenopathy
Femoral hernia	Femoral hernia	Femoral hernia	Femoral hernia	Femoral hernia	Femoral hernia
			Bursal swelling	Bursal swelling	Bursal swelling
			Varicose veins	Lipoma	Lipoma
			Lipoma	Varicose veins	Varicose veins
			Femoral artery aneurysm	Femoral artery aneurysm	Femoral artery aneurysm
			Psoas abscess	Psoas abscess	Psoas abscess

Emergency Rule Out conditions shown in red. Entries in blue are for information only
Conditions are listed in approximate order of prevalence for this age range

Emergency Rule Out conditions shown in red. Entries in blue are for information only
Conditions are listed in approximate order of prevalence for this age range

Baby (0-1 yr)	Child (1-12 yr)	Adolescent (12-18 yr)	Adult (18-45 yr)	Middle Age Adult (45-65 yr)	Senior Adult (65+ yr)
Upper respiratory tract infections	Acute otitis media	Chronic otitis media	Sepsis	Sepsis	Sepsis
Myelodysplastic syndromes	Acute sinusitis	Acute sinusitis	Infective endocarditis	Infective endocarditis	Infective endocarditis
Tularemia	Urinary tract infection	Acute otitis media	Drug fever	Drug fever	Drug fever
Thrombotic thrombocytopenic purpura	Drug reaction	Urinary tract infection	Occult cancer	Occult cancer	Occult cancer
Rocky Mountain spotted fever	Tularemia	Tularemia	Tuberculosis	Tuberculosis	Tuberculosis
Measles	Bacterial pneumonia	Bacterial meningitis	Acute pancreatitis	Acute pancreatitis	Acute pancreatitis
Mastoiditis	Chronic otitis media	Drug reaction	Viral hepatitis	Hodgkin's disease	Hodgkin's disease
Legionnaires' disease	Thrombotic thrombocytopenic purpura	Thyroiditis	Hodgkin's disease	Lyme disease	Lyme disease
Influenza	Bacterial meningitis	Thrombotic thrombocytopenic purpura	Lyme disease	Non-Hodgkin's lymphoma	Non-Hodgkin's lymphoma
Pyelonephritis	Toxic shock syndrome	Tonsillitis	Non-Hodgkin's lymphoma	Primary HIV infection	Primary HIV infection
Acute allergic alveolitis	Salicylate poisoning	Salicylate poisoning	Primary HIV infection	AIDS	AIDS
Chronic allergic alveolitis	Tonsillitis	Toxic shock syndrome	AIDS	Viral hepatitis	Viral hepatitis
Hodgkin's disease	Reiter's syndrome	Scarlet fever	Osteomyelitis	Osteomyelitis	Osteomyelitis
Herpes zoster, shingles	Scarlet fever	Pelvic abscess	Munchausen syndrome	Munchausen syndrome	Giant cell arteritis
Herpes simplex	Pyelonephritis	Reiter's syndrome	Chronic sinusitis	Chronic sinusitis	Munchausen syndrome
Hepatoma	Polyarteritis nodosa	Pyelonephritis	Cytomegalovirus	Cytomegalovirus	Chronic sinusitis
Hand-foot-and-mouth disease	Rocky Mountain spotted fever	Puerperal infection (endometritis)	Metastatic neoplasm of the liver	Metastatic neoplasm of the liver	Cytomegalovirus
Genital herpes	Pharyngitis	Polyarteritis nodosa	Ulcerative colitis	Giant cell arteritis	Metastatic neoplasm of the liver
Febrile seizure	Upper respiratory tract infections	Pharyngitis	Renal calculi	Renal calculi	Renal calculi
	Idiopathic myelofibrosis	Upper respiratory tract infections	Typhoid fever	Alcoholic hepatitis	Typhoid fever
			Atrial myxoma	Acoustic neuroma	Acoustic neuroma
				Typhoid fever	Atrial myxoma

Baby (0-1 yr)	Child (1-12 yr)	Adolescent (12-18 yr)	Adult (18-45 yr)	Middle Age Adult (45-65 yr)	Senior Adult (65+yr)
Erythema nodosum	Bartonella infection (cat scratch disease)	Chlamydia pneumoniae	Systemic lupus erythematosus	Atrial myxoma	Systemic lupus erythematosus
Idiopathic myelofibrosis	Myelodysplastic syndromes	Bartonella infection (cat scratch disease)	Alcoholic hepatitis	Systemic lupus erythematosus	Hepatoma
Encephalitis	Acute iron toxicity	Blastomycosis	Acoustic neuroma	Acute iron toxicity	Acute iron toxicity
Cellulitis	Measles	Idiopathic myelofibrosis	Acute iron toxicity	Hepatoma	Syphilis
Cavernous sinus thrombosis	Blastomycosis	Myelodysplastic syndromes	Hepatoma	Viral meningitis	Upper respiratory tract infections
Chickenpox	Mastoiditis	Measles	Syphilis	Upper respiratory tract infections	Sarcoidosis
Cholecystitis	Influenza	Rocky Mountain spotted fever	Upper respiratory tract infections	Syphilis	Alcoholic hepatitis
Infective endocarditis	Legionnaires' disease	Mastoiditis	Crohn's disease	Tularemia	Viral meningitis
Blastomycosis	Acute allergic alveolitis	Legionnaires' disease	Toxic shock syndrome	Tonsillitis	Toxic shock syndrome
Behçet's syndrome	Chronic allergic alveolitis	Influenza	Tonsillitis	Thyroiditis	Thyroiditis
Poliomyelitis	Hodgkin's disease	Acute allergic alveolitis	Thyroiditis	Thrombotic thrombocytopenic purpura	Tonsillitis
Bartonella infection (cat scratch disease)	Herpes simplex	Chronic allergic alveolitis	Thrombotic thrombocytopenic purpura	Ulcerative colitis	Thrombotic thrombocytopenic purpura
Chlamydia pneumoniae	Hepatoma	Herpes zoster, shingles	Tularemia	Rocky Mountain spotted fever	Scarlet fever
Pharyngitis	Herpes zoster, shingles	Hodgkin's disease	Salicylate poisoning	Salicylate poisoning	Salicylate poisoning
Reiter's syndrome	Hand-foot-and-mouth disease	Herpes simplex	Scarlet fever	Scarlet fever	Rocky Mountain spotted fever
Polyarteritis nodosa	Febrile seizure	Hand-foot-and-mouth disease	Rocky Mountain spotted fever	Reiter's syndrome	Reiter's syndrome
Respiratory syncytial virus infection	Genital herpes	Acute allergic alveolitis	Malaria	Puerperal infection (endometritis)	Tularemia
Salicylate poisoning	Infective endocarditis	Infective endocarditis	Reiter's syndrome		Crohn's disease
Scarlet fever	Poliomyelitis	Febrile seizure	Salmonella infection		Polyarteritis nodosa
Thyroiditis	Encephalitis	Genital herpes			
Tonsillitis	Cavernous sinus thrombosis				

List continues on next page

Baby (0-1 yr)	Child (1-12 yr)	Adolescent (12-18 yr)	Adult (18-45 yr)	Middle Age Adult (45-65 yr)	Senior Adult (65+ yr)
Toxic shock syndrome	Erythema nodosum	Erythema nodosum	Puerperal infection (endometritis)	Pyelonephritis	Poliomyelitis
Fever	Cellulitis	Encephalitis	Pyelonephritis	Polyarteritis nodosa	Behçet's syndrome
Plague	Respiratory syncytial virus infection	Cavernous sinus thrombosis	Pharyngitis	Pharyngitis	Pharyngitis
Proctitis	Chickenpox	Alcoholic hepatitis	Polyarteritis nodosa	Poliomyelitis	Pyelonephritis
Wegener's granulomatosis	Cholecystitis	Cholecystitis	Bartonella infection (cat scratch disease)	Bartonella infection (cat scratch disease)	Bartonella infection (cat scratch disease)
	Behçet's syndrome	Chickenpox	Idiopathic myelofibrosis	Chlamydia pneumoniae	Myelodysplastic syndromes
	Thyroiditis	Cellulitis	Myelodysplastic syndromes	Myelodysplastic syndromes	Blastomycosis
	Chlamydia pneumoniae	Poliomyelitis	Brucellosis	Idiopathic myelofibrosis	Idiopathic myelofibrosis
	Fungal infection	Respiratory syncytial virus infection	Blastomycosis	Blastomycosis	Measles
	Viral meningitis	Gastroenteritis	Measles	Measles	Mastoiditis
	Gastroenteritis	Behçet's syndrome	Respiratory syncytial virus infection	Mastoiditis	Legionnaires' disease
	Kawasaki disease	Acute iron toxicity	Legionnaires' disease	Behçet's syndrome	Influenza
	Connective tissue disease	Malignancy	Mastoiditis	Legionnaires' disease	Acute allergic alveolitis
	Malignancy	Fungal infection	Influenza	Influenza	Chronic allergic alveolitis
	Munchausen syndrome	Viral meningitis	Acute allergic alveolitis	Acute allergic alveolitis	Herpes simplex
	Pelvic abscess	Kawasaki disease	Chronic allergic alveolitis	Chronic allergic alveolitis	Herpes zoster, shingles
	Malaria	Munchausen syndrome	Herpes zoster, shingles	Herpes simplex	Hand-foot-and-mouth disease
	Crohn's disease	Connective tissue disease	Herpes simplex	Herpes zoster, shingles	Febrile seizure
	Fever	Crohn's disease	Hand-foot-and-mouth disease	Hand-foot-and-mouth disease	Genital herpes
	Plague	Ulcerative colitis		Febrile seizure	Ulcerative colitis
	Proctitis	Malaria		Genital herpes	Erythema nodosum
	Wegener's granulomatosis	Fever			

Baby (0-1 yr)	Child (1-12 yr)	Adolescent (12-18 yr)	Adult (18-45 yr)	Middle Age Adult (45-65 yr)	Senior Adult (65+yr)
		Plague	Febrile seizure	Crohn's disease	Encephalitis
		Proctitis	Genital herpes	Erythema nodosum	Chlamydia pneumoniae
		Wegener's granulomatosis	Poliomyelitis	Malaria	Malaria
			Erythema nodosum	Encephalitis	Cholecystitis
			Encephalitis	Cholecystitis	Salmonella infection
			Cavernous sinus thrombosis	Salmonella infection	Respiratory syncytial virus infection
			Cellulitis	Chickenpox	Cellulitis
			Cholecystitis	Cellulitis	Gastroenteritis
			Chickenpox	Cavernous sinus thrombosis	Cavernous sinus thrombosis
			Viral meningitis	Brucellosis	Brucellosis
			Gastroenteritis	Respiratory syncytial virus infection	Endemic typhus
			Endemic typhus	Gastroenteritis	Familial Mediterranean fever
			Behçet's syndrome	Endemic typhus	Meningococcemia
			Chlamydia pneumoniae	Rheumatic fever	Psittacosis
			Rheumatic fever	Familial Mediterranean fever	Cyclic neutropenia
			Familial Mediterranean fever	Meningococcemia	Babesiosis
			Meningococcemia	Psittacosis	Mononucleosis
			Psittacosis	Cyclic neutropenia	Rheumatic fever
			Cyclic neutropenia	Babesiosis	Toxoplasmosis
			Babesiosis	Mononucleosis	Fever
			Mononucleosis	Toxoplasmosis	Chickenpox
			Toxoplasmosis		

List continues on next page

456

List continued from previous page

Baby (0-1 yr)	Child (1-12 yr)	Adolescent (12-18 yr)	Adult (18-45 yr)	Middle Age Adult (45-65 yr)	Senior Adult (65+yr)
			Sarcoidosis	Sarcoidosis	Plague
			Giant cell arteritis	Fever	Proctitis
			Fever	Plague	Wegener's granulomatosis
			Plague	Proctitis	
			Proctitis	Wegener's granulomatosis	
			Wegener's granulomatosis		

Finger clubbing

Baby (0-1 yr)	Child (1-12 yr)	Adolescent (12-18 yr)	Adult (18-45 yr)	Middle Age Adult (45-65 yr)	Senior Adult (65+ yr)
Congenital heart disease	Congenital heart disease	Congenital heart disease	Congenital heart disease	Congenital heart disease	Bronchiectasis
Chronic obstructive pulmonary disease	Cystic fibrosis	Cystic fibrosis	Chronic obstructive pulmonary disease	Chronic obstructive pulmonary disease	Chronic obstructive pulmonary disease
Cystic fibrosis	Chronic obstructive pulmonary disease	Bronchiectasis	Primary lung malignancy	Primary lung malignancy	Primary lung malignancy
	Bronchiectasis	Crohn's disease	Cystic fibrosis	Bronchiectasis	Congenital heart disease
	Liver cirrhosis	Lung abscess	Bronchiectasis	Fibrosing alveolitis	Liver cirrhosis
	Crohn's disease	Chronic obstructive pulmonary disease	Fibrosing alveolitis	Crohn's disease	Fibrosing alveolitis
	Lung abscess	Liver cirrhosis	Primary lung malignancy	Liver cirrhosis	Crohn's disease
	Tuberculosis	Tuberculosis	Crohn's disease	Primary biliary cirrhosis	Primary biliary cirrhosis
			Liver cirrhosis	Lung abscess	Lung abscess
			Primary biliary cirrhosis	Tuberculosis	Tuberculosis
			Lung abscess		
			Tuberculosis		

Emergency Rule Out conditions shown in red. Entries in blue are for information only
Conditions are listed in approximate order of prevalence for this age range

131

Emergency Rule Out conditions shown in red. Entries in blue are for information only
Conditions are listed in approximate order of prevalence for this age range

Baby (0-1 yr)	Child (1-12 yr)	Adolescent (12-18 yr)	Adult (18-45 yr)	Middle Age Adult (45-65 yr)	Senior Adult (65+ yr)
Not relevant to this age group	Migraine headache	Migraine headache	Retinal detachment	Retinal detachment	Vitreous opacities
	Retinal migraine	Retinal migraine	Vitreous opacities	Vitreous opacities	Amaurosis fugax
	Acute retinitis	Acute retinitis	Migraine headache	Amaurosis fugax	Occipital cortex lesion
	Retinal tear	Retinal tear	Amaurosis fugax	Migraine headache	Ocular trauma
	Optic neuritis	Optic neuritis	Ocular trauma	Ocular trauma	Retinal tear
	Retinal detachment	Retinal detachment	Occipital cortex lesion	Occipital cortex lesion	Migraine headache
	Retinal and vitreous hemorrhage	Retinal and vitreous hemorrhage	Optic neuritis	Optic neuritis	Retinal detachment
	Retinal vein occlusion	Retinal vein occlusion	Retinal and vitreous hemorrhage	Retinal and vitreous hemorrhage	Diabetic retinopathy
	Retinal artery occlusion	Retinal artery occlusion	Retinal artery occlusion	Retinal artery occlusion	Retinal and vitreous hemorrhage
	Diabetic retinopathy	Diabetic retinopathy	Retinal migraine	Diabetic retinopathy	Retinal artery occlusion
			Retinal tear	Retinal migraine	Retinal migraine
			Retinal vein occlusion	Retinal tear	Retinal vein occlusion
			Acute retinitis	Retinal vein occlusion	Acute retinitis
			Diabetic retinopathy	Acute retinitis	

Baby (0-1 yr)	Child (1-12 yr)	Adolescent (12-18 yr)	Adult (18-45 yr)	Middle Age Adult (45-65 yr)	Senior Adult (65-yr)
Colic	Lactose intolerance	Lactose intolerance	Carbohydrate-rich meal	Carbohydrate-rich meal	Carbohydrate-rich meal
Lactose intolerance	Carbohydrate-rich meal	Carbohydrate-rich meal	Irritable bowel syndrome	Irritable bowel syndrome	Fatty food intolerance
Celiac disease	Celiac disease	Celiac disease	Fatty food intolerance	Fatty food intolerance	Celiac disease
Giardiasis	Giardiasis	Giardiasis	Celiac disease	Celiac disease	Irritable bowel syndrome
			Premenstrual syndrome	Premenstrual syndrome	Giardiasis
			Giardiasis	Giardiasis	

Flatulence, eructation, and gas pain

Emergency Rule Out conditions shown in red. Entries in blue are for information only
Conditions are listed in approximate order of prevalence for this age range

Flushing of the face

Emergency Rule Out conditions shown in red. Entries in blue are for information only
Conditions are listed in approximate order of prevalence for this age range

Baby (0-1 yr)	Child (1-12 yr)	Adolescent (12-18 yr)	Adult (18-45 yr)	Middle Age Adult (45-65 yr)	Senior Adult (65+ yr)
Fever	Fever	Fever	Fever	Fever	Fever
Cluster headache	Heat stroke and heat exhaustion	Scarlet fever	Alcohol abuse	Menopause	Scarlet fever
Heat stroke and heat exhaustion	Cluster headache	Cluster headache	Scarlet fever	Scarlet fever	Heat stroke and heat exhaustion
Scarlet fever	Scarlet fever	Heat stroke and heat exhaustion	Cluster headache	Cluster headache	Cluster headache
		Pregnancy	Heat stroke and heat exhaustion	Heat stroke and heat exhaustion	Menopause
		Carcinoid syndrome	Pregnancy	Carcinoid syndrome	Carcinoid syndrome
			Menopause	Alcohol abuse	Alcohol abuse
			Carcinoid syndrome	Pheochromocytoma	Pheochromocytoma
			Pheochromocytoma		

Baby (0-1 yr)	Child (1-12 yr)	Adolescent (12-18 yr)	Adult (18-45 yr)	Middle Age Adult (45-65 yr)	Senior Adult (65+yr)
Charcot-Marie-Tooth disease	Charcot-Marie-Tooth disease	Charcot-Marie-Tooth disease	Charcot-Marie-Tooth disease	Charcot-Marie-Tooth disease	Charcot-Marie-Tooth disease
	Peroneal nerve palsy	Peroneal nerve palsy	Peroneal nerve palsy	Peroneal nerve palsy	Peroneal nerve palsy
	Trauma	Trauma	Trauma	Trauma	Trauma

Emergency Rule Out conditions shown in red. Entries in blue are for information only
Conditions are listed in approximate order of prevalence for this age range

Emergency Rule Out conditions shown in red. Entries in blue are for information only
Conditions are listed in approximate order of prevalence for this age range

Baby (0-1 yr)	Child (1-12 yr)	Adolescent (12-18 yr)	Adult (18-45 yr)	Middle Age Adult (45-65 yr)	Senior Adult (65+ yr)
Trauma	Trauma	Trauma	Plantar fasciitis	Acute gout	Acute gout
Foreign body in foot	Foreign body in foot	Foreign body in foot	Acute gout	Plantar fasciitis	Hallux valgus (bunion)
Hand-foot-and-mouth disease	Fracture	Fracture	Hallux valgus (bunion)	Hallux valgus (bunion)	Plantar fasciitis
Ingrown nail	Palmar-plantar warts	Palmar-plantar warts	Interdigital neuroma	Lumbar disc disorders	Lumbar disc disorders
Sickle cell anemia	Ingrown nail	Ingrown nail	Ingrown nail	Ingrown nail	Ingrown nail
Osteomyelitis	Plantar fasciitis	Plantar fasciitis	Lumbar disc disorders	Interdigital neuroma	Interdigital neuroma
	Osteomyelitis	Osteochondritis dissecans	Fracture	Metatarsalgia	Metatarsalgia
	Rheumatoid arthritis	Osteomyelitis	Metatarsalgia	Pes planus	Pes planus
	Metatarsalgia	Rheumatoid arthritis	Pes planus	Fracture	Fracture

Baby (0-1 yr)	Child (1-12 yr)	Adolescent (12-18 yr)	Adult (18-45 yr)	Middle Age Adult (45-65 yr)	Senior Adult (65+ yr)
Not relevant to this age group	Cerebral palsy	Cerebral palsy	Brain tumor Ischemic stroke	Brain tumor Ischemic stroke	Ischemic stroke Brain tumor

Gait apraxia

Emergency Rule Out conditions shown in red. Entries in blue are for information only
Conditions are listed in approximate order of prevalence for this age range

Emergency Rule Out conditions shown in red. Entries in blue are for information only
Conditions are listed in approximate order of prevalence for this age range

Baby (0-1 yr)	Child (1-12 yr)	Adolescent (12-18 yr)	Adult (18-45 yr)	Middle Age Adult (45-65 yr)	Senior Adult (65+yr)
Not relevant to this age group	Myotonia congenita	Myotonia congenita	Ankle injury	Myotonia congenita	Myotonia congenita
	Joint disorder	Corns	Corns	Corns	Corns
	Foreign body in foot	Joint disorder	Joint disorder	Joint disorder	Joint disorder
	Ankle injury	Foreign body in foot	Foreign body in foot	Foreign body in foot	Osteoarthritis
	Hip fracture	Ankle injury	Hip fracture	Ankle injury	Foreign body in foot
	Lumbar disc disorders	Hip fracture	Parkinson's disease	Hip fracture	Ankle injury
	Flat foot	Parkinson's disease	Lumbar disc disorders	Parkinson's disease	Hip fracture
	Hallux valgus (bunion)	Lumbar disc disorders	Flat foot	Lumbar disc disorders	Parkinson's disease
	Palmar-plantar warts	Flat foot	Hallux valgus (bunion)	Osteoarthritis	Lumbar disc disorders
	Postphlebitic syndrome	Hallux valgus (bunion)	Palmar-plantar warts	Flat foot	Flat foot
	Ankylosis of hip	Palmar-plantar warts	Postphlebitic syndrome	Hallux valgus (bunion)	Hallux valgus (bunion)
	Congenital dislocation of hip	Postphlebitic syndrome	Ankylosis of hip	Palmar-plantar warts	Palmar-plantar warts
	Huntington's disease	Ankylosis of hip	Congenital dislocation of hip	Postphlebitic syndrome	Postphlebitic syndrome
	Slipped femoral epiphysis	Slipped femoral epiphysis	Arterial insufficiency	Ankylosis of hip	Aseptic bursitis
	Hip injury	Congenital dislocation of hip	Malignancy	Congenital dislocation of hip	Ankylosis of hip
	Dementia	Arterial insufficiency	Osteomalacia	Slipped femoral epiphysis	Congenital dislocation of hip
	Charcot-Marie-Tooth disease	Huntington's disease	Slipped femoral epiphysis	Arterial insufficiency	Slipped femoral epiphysis
	Cushing's syndrome	Hip injury	Hip injury	Huntington's disease	Arterial insufficiency
	Osteomalacia	Dementia	Huntington's disease	Malignancy	Huntington's disease
	Arterial insufficiency	Charcot-Marie-Tooth disease	Cushing's syndrome	Dementia	Hip injury
	Malignancy	Cushing's syndrome	Dementia	Osteomalacia	Dementia
	Myopathy	Malignancy	Charcot-Marie-Tooth disease	Cushing's syndrome	Cushing's syndrome

Baby (0-1 yr)	Child (1-12 yr)	Adolescent (12-18 yr)	Adult (18-45 yr)	Middle Age Adult (45-65 yr)	Senior Adult (65-yr)
	Coxa valga	Osteomalacia	Myopathy	Charcot-Marie-Tooth disease	Charcot-Marie-Tooth disease
	Coxa vara	Myopathy	Coxa valga	Hip injury	Malignancy
	Occult cancer	Coxa valga	Coxa vara	Myopathy	Osteomalacia
	Extrapyramidal lesion	Coxa vara	Occult cancer	Coxa valga	Myopathy
	Conversion disorder	Occult cancer	Extrapyramidal lesion	Coxa vara	Coxa valga
	Cauda equina syndrome	Extrapyramidal lesion	Conversion disorder	Occult cancer	Coxa vara
	Myotonic dystrophy	Conversion disorder	Cauda equina syndrome	Extrapyramidal lesion	Occult cancer
	Head injury	Cauda equina syndrome	Myasthenia gravis	Conversion disorder	Extrapyramidal lesion
	Fracture	Myasthenia gravis	Myotonic dystrophy	Cauda equina syndrome	Conversion disorder
	Plantar fasciitis	Myotonic dystrophy	Head injury	Myasthenia gravis	Cauda equina syndrome
	Encephalitis lethargica	Head injury	Fracture	Aseptic bursitis	Myasthenia gravis
	Rickets in children	Fracture	Plantar fasciitis	Myotonic dystrophy	Myotonic dystrophy
		Plantar fasciitis	Encephalitis lethargica	Head injury	Head injury
		Encephalitis lethargica	Aseptic bursitis	Fracture	Fracture
		Eaton-Lambert (myasthenic) syndrome	Myotonia congenita	Plantar fasciitis	Plantar fasciitis
		Rickets in children	Eaton-Lambert (myasthenic) syndrome	Encephalitis lethargica	Eaton-Lambert (myasthenic) syndrome
				Eaton-Lambert (myasthenic) syndrome	Encephalitis lethargica

Emergency Rule Out conditions shown in red. Entries in blue are for information only
Conditions are listed in approximate order of prevalence for this age range

Baby (0-1 yr)	Child (1-12 yr)	Adolescent (12-18 yr)	Adult (18-45 yr)	Middle Age Adult (45-65 yr)	Senior Adult (65+ yr)
Cushing's syndrome	Cushing's syndrome	Cushing's syndrome	Diabetes mellitus type 1	Diabetes mellitus type 2	Diabetes mellitus type 2
Diabetes mellitus in children	Diabetes mellitus in children	Diabetes mellitus in children	Diabetes mellitus type 2	Diabetes mellitus type 1	Diabetes mellitus type 1
Renal tubular acidosis	Renal tubular acidosis	Renal tubular acidosis	Pregnancy	Drug reaction	Drug reaction
Fanconi's syndrome	Fanconi's syndrome	Fanconi's syndrome	Drug reaction	Hyperaldosteronism	Hyperaldosteronism
		Pregnancy	Hyperaldosteronism	Acute pancreatitis	Pancreatic cancer
		Diabetes mellitus type 2	Acute pancreatitis	Pancreatic cancer	Cushing's syndrome
			Cushing's syndrome	Cushing's syndrome	Acute pancreatitis
			Pancreatic cancer		

Baby (0-1 yr)	Child (1-12 yr)	Adolescent (12-18 yr)	Adult (18-45 yr)	Middle Age Adult (45-65 yr)	Senior Adult (65+yr)
Hypothyroidism Hyperthyroidism	Hypothyroidism Hyperthyroidism Thyroiditis	Hyperthyroidism Hypothyroidism Thyroiditis	Hypothyroidism Thyroiditis Hyperthyroidism Multinodular goiter Myxedema Riedel's disease	Hypothyroidism Thyroiditis Hyperthyroidism Multinodular goiter Riedel's disease Myxedema	Hypothyroidism Thyroiditis Hyperthyroidism Multinodular goiter Riedel's disease Myxedema

Emergency Rule Out conditions shown in red. Entries in blue are for information only
Conditions are listed in approximate order of prevalence for this age range

Emergency Rule Out conditions shown in red. Entries in blue are for information only
Conditions are listed in approximate order of prevalence for this age range

Baby (0-1 yr)	Child (1-12 yr)	Adolescent (12-18 yr)	Adult (18-45 yr)	Middle Age Adult (45-65 yr)	Senior Adult (65- yr)
Maternal estrogen	Klinefelter's syndrome Chronic renal failure	Klinefelter's syndrome Chronic renal failure Testicular malignancy Recreational drug abuse	Liver cirrhosis Hyperthyroidism Testicular malignancy Chronic renal failure Pituitary eosinophilic adenoma (prolactinoma) Klinefelter's syndrome	Liver cirrhosis Hyperthyroidism Chronic renal failure Testicular malignancy Pituitary eosinophilic adenoma (prolactinoma) Klinefelter's syndrome	Liver cirrhosis Hyperthyroidism Chronic renal failure Testicular malignancy Pituitary eosinophilic adenoma (prolactinoma) Klinefelter's syndrome

Baby (0-1 yr)	Child (1-12 yr)	Adolescent (12-18 yr)	Adult (18-45 yr)	Middle Age Adult (45-65 yr)	Senior Adult (65+ yr)
Not relevant to this age group	Drug withdrawal Delirium Dementia Brain tumor Recreational drug abuse Schizophrenia	Drug withdrawal Recreational drug abuse Dementia Brain tumor Delirium Schizophrenia Narcolepsy	Schizophrenia Delirium Dementia Brain tumor Drug withdrawal Recreational drug abuse	Drug withdrawal Delirium Dementia Brain tumor Schizophrenia Recreational drug abuse	Drug withdrawal Delirium Dementia Brain tumor Schizophrenia Recreational drug abuse

Emergency Rule Out conditions shown in red. Entries in blue are for information only
Conditions are listed in approximate order of prevalence for this age range

Emergency Rule Out conditions shown in red. Entries in blue are for information only
Conditions are listed in approximate order of prevalence for this age range

Baby (0-1 yr)	Child (1-12 yr)	Adolescent (12-18 yr)	Adult (18-45 yr)	Middle Age Adult (45-65 yr)	Senior Adult (65-yr)
Not relevant to this age group	Migraine headache Glaucoma Cataract	Migraine headache Drug reaction Cataract Glaucoma	Migraine headache Cataract Glaucoma Drug reaction	Cataract Migraine headache Glaucoma Drug reaction	Cataract Migraine headache Glaucoma Drug reaction

Baby (0-1 yr)	Child (1-12 yr)	Adolescent (12-18 yr)	Adult (18-45 yr)	Middle Age Adult (45-65 yr)	Senior Adult (65+ yr)
Bennet's fracture	Bennet's fracture	Bennet's fracture	Carpal tunnel syndrome	Carpal tunnel syndrome	Carpal tunnel syndrome
Ganglion	Ganglion	Ganglion	Ganglion	Ganglion	Dupuytren's contracture
Hand injury	de Quervain's contracture	de Quervain's contracture	Paronychia	Paronychia	Hand injury
Colles' fracture	Hand injury	Colles' fracture	Hand injury	Felon	Paronychia
Lichen planus	Colles' fracture	Hand injury	Felon	Hand injury	Fracture
Fracture	Lichen planus	Lichen planus	Lichen planus	Lichen planus	Lichen planus
Navicular fracture	Fracture	Fracture	Fracture	Fracture	Mallet finger
Lunate dislocation	Navicular fracture	Navicular fracture	Mallet finger	Mallet finger	Reflex sympathetic dystrophy
	Reflex sympathetic dystrophy	Reflex sympathetic dystrophy	de Quervain's contracture	de Quervain's contracture	Lunate dislocation
	Lunate dislocation	Lunate dislocation	Reflex sympathetic dystrophy	Reflex sympathetic dystrophy	de Quervain's contracture
			Lunate dislocation	Lunate dislocation	Ganglion
			Dupuytren's contracture	Dupuytren's contracture	

Emergency Rule Out conditions shown in red. Entries in blue are for information only
Conditions are listed in approximate order of prevalence for this age range

Hand and wrist phenomena

Emergency Rule Out conditions shown in red. Entries in blue are for information only
Conditions are listed in approximate order of prevalence for this age range

Baby (0-1 yr)	Child (1-12 yr)	Adolescent (12-18 yr)	Adult (18-45 yr)	Middle Age Adult (45-65 yr)	Senior Adult (65+yr)
Bartonella infection (cat scratch disease)	Tension headache	Tension headache	Tension headache	Tension headache	Tension headache
Intracranial hemorrhage	Migraine headache	Migraine headache	Migraine headache	Migraine headache	Head injury
Heat stroke and heat exhaustion	Tonsillitis	Cluster headache	Cluster headache	Temporomandibular joint syndrome	Malignant hypertension
Herpes simplex	Poliomyelitis	Tonsillitis	Temporomandibular joint syndrome	Cluster headache	Giant cell arteritis
Chronic lead poisoning	Daily headache	Poliomyelitis	Acute sinusitis	Poliomyelitis	Poliomyelitis
Carbon monoxide poisoning	Cluster headache	Scarlet fever	Head injury	Premenstrual syndrome	Thrombotic thrombocytopenic purpura
Chronic fatigue syndrome	Orthostatic hypotension	Orthostatic hypotension	Premenstrual syndrome	Malignant hypertension	Hyperprolactinemia
Cervical hyperextension injuries	Scarlet fever	Menopause	Poliomyelitis	Hyperprolactinemia	Temporomandibular joint syndrome
Cavernous sinus thrombosis	Legionnaires' disease	Hyperprolactinemia	Brain injury	Orthostatic hypotension	Orthostatic hypotension
Hyponatremia	Intracranial hemorrhage	Legionnaires' disease	Rocky Mountain spotted fever	Scarlet fever	Acute sinusitis
Campylobacter infection	Influenza	Intracranial hemorrhage	Orthostatic hypotension	Menopause	Bartonella infection (cat scratch disease)
Brucellosis	Hyponatremia	Influenza	Malignant hypertension	Rocky Mountain spotted fever	Legionnaires' disease
Influenza	Ischemic stroke	Hyponatremia	Thrombotic thrombocytopenic purpura	Legionnaires' disease	Intracranial hemorrhage
Legionnaires' disease	Brucellosis	Herpes simplex	Hyperprolactinemia	Intracranial hemorrhage	Hyponatremia
Behçet's syndrome	Heat stroke and heat exhaustion	Ischemic stroke	Menopause	Hyponatremia	Herpes simplex
Campylobacter infection	Behçet's syndrome	Heat stroke and heat exhaustion	Behçet's syndrome	Herpes simplex	Influenza
Diabetes insipidus	Campylobacter infection	Behçet's syndrome	Intracranial hemorrhage	Influenza	Campylobacter infection
Plague	Carbon monoxide poisoning	Campylobacter infection	Hyponatremia	Bartonella infection (cat scratch disease)	Heat stroke and heat exhaustion
Sarcoidosis	Hyperprolactinemia	Premenstrual syndrome	Influenza	Campylobacter infection	Behçet's syndrome
	Bartonella infection (cat scratch disease)	Cavernous sinus thrombosis			
		Cervical hyperextension			

Baby (0-1 yr)	Child (1-12 yr)	Adolescent (12-18 yr)	Adult (18-45 yr)	Middle Age Adult (45-65 yr)	Senior Adult (65+ yr)
	Cervical hyperextension injuries	injuries	Herpes simplex	Heat stroke and heat exhaustion	Carbon monoxide poisoning
	Herpes simplex	Carbon monoxide poisoning	Heat stroke and heat exhaustion	Brucellosis	Cervical hyperextension injuries
	Chronic fatigue syndrome	Chronic fatigue syndrome	Campylobacter infection	Behçet's syndrome	Chronic lead poisoning
	Chronic lead poisoning	Chronic lead poisoning	Legionnaires' disease	Cavernous sinus thrombosis	Cavernous sinus thrombosis
	Cavernous sinus thrombosis	Brucellosis	Carbon monoxide poisoning	Carbon monoxide poisoning	Chronic fatigue syndrome
	Chlamydia pneumoniae	Bartonella infection (cat scratch disease)	Cavernous sinus thrombosis	Cervical hyperextension injuries	Rocky Mountain spotted fever
	Rocky Mountain spotted fever	Rocky Mountain spotted fever	Cervical hyperextension injuries	Chronic fatigue syndrome	Brucellosis
	Sexual assault	Chlamydia pneumoniae	Sexual assault	Chronic lead poisoning	Sexual assault
	Acute sinusitis	Sexual assault	Bartonella infection (cat scratch disease)	Head injury	Chlamydia pneumoniae
	Temporomandibular joint syndrome	Acute sinusitis	Scarlet fever	Thrombotic thrombocytopenic purpura	Ischemic stroke
	Thrombotic thrombocytopenic purpura	Temporomandibular joint syndrome	Chronic fatigue syndrome	Sexual assault	Brain injury
	Brain injury	Thrombotic thrombocytopenic purpura	Chronic lead poisoning	Chlamydia pneumoniae	Benign intracranial hypertension
	Head injury	Brain injury	Brucellosis	Acute sinusitis	Subdural hematoma
	Bacterial meningitis	Head injury	Ischemic stroke	Ischemic stroke	Brain tumor
	Viral meningitis	Bacterial meningitis	Chlamydia pneumoniae	Brain injury	Migraine headache
	Brain tumor	Viral meningitis	Menstrual headache	Benign intracranial hypertension	Bacterial meningitis
	Diabetes insipidus	Brain tumor	Bacterial meningitis		Diabetes insipidus
		Diabetes insipidus	Viral meningitis		Plague
			Subarachnoid hemorrhage		Sarcoidosis

List continues on next page

Headache (continued)

147

List continued from previous page

Baby (0-1 yr)	Child (1-12 yr)	Adolescent (12-18 yr)	Adult (18-45 yr)	Middle Age Adult (45-65 yr)	Senior Adult (65+ yr)
	Plague **Sarcoidosis** Psittacosis	Plague **Sarcoidosis** Psittacosis	and cerebral aneurysm stroke Subdural hematoma **Brain tumor** Diabetes insipidus Plague **Sarcoidosis** **Psittacosis**	Subarachnoid hemorrhage and cerebral aneurysm stroke Subdural hematoma Bacterial meningitis Diabetes insipidus Plague Sarcoidosis	**Scarlet fever** Psittacosis

Baby (0-1 yr)	Child (1-12 yr)	Adolescent (12-18 yr)	Adult (18-45 yr)	Middle Age Adult (45-65 yr)	Senior Adult (65+yr)
Acute otitis media	Acute otitis media	Acute otitis media	Hearing loss	Hearing loss	Hearing loss
Chronic otitis media	Chronic otitis media	Chronic otitis media	Wax in ear	Wax in ear	Wax in ear
Congenital middle ear defect	Congenital middle ear defect	Congenital middle ear defect	Acute otitis media	Acute otitis media	Acute otitis media
Drug reaction	Salicylate poisoning	Drug reaction	Chronic otitis media	Chronic otitis media	Chronic otitis media
Mastoiditis	Mastoiditis	Salicylate poisoning	Salicylate poisoning	Otitis externa	Temporomandibular joint syndrome
Salicylate poisoning	Barotitis media	Mastoiditis	Mastoiditis	Mastoiditis	Salicylate poisoning
Behçet's syndrome	Behçet's syndrome	Behçet's syndrome	Otitis externa	Salicylate poisoning	Mastoiditis
Temporomandibular joint syndrome	Drug reaction	Temporomandibular joint syndrome	Temporomandibular joint syndrome	Temporomandibular joint syndrome	Barotitis media
Barotitis media	Temporomandibular joint syndrome	Barotitis media	Behçet's syndrome	Barotitis media	Otitis externa
Bacterial meningitis	Bacterial meningitis	Bacterial meningitis	Barotitis media	Behçet's syndrome	Behçet's syndrome
Foreign body	Foreign body	Foreign body	Ménière's disease	Ménière's disease	Ménière's disease
Direct hyperbilirubinemia	Direct hyperbilirubinemia	Direct hyperbilirubinemia	Otosclerosis	Otosclerosis	Otosclerosis
Congenital rubella syndrome	Congenital rubella syndrome	Congenital rubella syndrome	Trauma	Trauma	Trauma
Viral meningitis	Viral meningitis	Viral meningitis	Foreign body	Foreign body	Foreign body
Hypothyroidism	Hypothyroidism	Hypothyroidism	Aural atresia	Acoustic neuroma	Dysbarism and barotrauma
Cleft lip and palate			Dysbarism and barotrauma	Dysbarism and barotrauma	Acoustic neuroma
			Acoustic neuroma	Aural atresia	Aural atresia
			Hypothyroidism	Hypothyroidism	Hypothyroidism

Emergency Rule Out conditions shown in red. Entries in blue are for information only
Conditions are listed in approximate order of prevalence for this age range

Heart sounds, diastolic murmur

Emergency Rule Out conditions shown in red. Entries in blue are for information only
Conditions are listed in approximate order of prevalence for this age range

Baby (0-1 yr)	Child (1-12 yr)	Adolescent (12-18 yr)	Adult (18-45 yr)	Middle Age Adult (45-65 yr)	Senior Adult (65+ yr)
Patent ductus arteriosus	Patent ductus arteriosus	Patent ductus arteriosus	Mitral stenosis	Mitral stenosis	Aortic regurgitation
Aortic regurgitation	Aortic regurgitation	Aortic regurgitation	Aortic regurgitation	Aortic regurgitation	Mitral stenosis

Baby (0-1 yr)	Child (1-12 yr)	Adolescent (12-18 yr)	Adult (18-45 yr)	Middle Age Adult (45-65 yr)	Senior Adult (65+ yr)
Congestive heart failure	Congestive heart failure	Congestive heart failure	Cardiomyopathy	Cardiomyopathy	Cardiomyopathy
Congenital heart disease	Cardiomyopathy	Cardiomyopathy	Essential hypertension	Essential hypertension	Essential hypertension
			Aortic stenosis	Aortic stenosis	Congestive heart failure
			Congestive heart failure	Congestive heart failure	Angina
			Angina	Angina	Aortic stenosis
			Myocardial infarction	Myocardial infarction	Myocardial infarction
			Pulmonary valve stenosis	Pulmonary valve stenosis	Pulmonary valve stenosis

Emergency Rule Out conditions shown in red. Entries in blue are for information only
Conditions are listed in approximate order of prevalence for this age range

Emergency Rule Out conditions shown in red. Entries in blue are for information only
Conditions are listed in approximate order of prevalence for this age range

Heart sounds, loud aortic S2

	Baby (0-1 yr)	Child (1-12 yr)	Adolescent (12-18 yr)	Adult (18-45 yr)	Middle Age Adult (45-65 yr)	Senior Adult (65+yr)
Congenital heart disease		Sinus tachycardia	Essential hypertension	Essential hypertension Sinus tachycardia	Essential hypertension Sinus tachycardia	Essential hypertension Sinus tachycardia

Baby (0-1 yr)	Child (1-12 yr)	Adolescent (12-18 yr)	Adult (18-45 yr)	Middle Age Adult (45-65 yr)	Senior Adult (65+ yr)
Atrial septal defect	Pulmonary hypertension Atrial septal defect	Pulmonary hypertension Atrial septal defect	Pulmonary hypertension Atrial septal defect	Pulmonary hypertension Atrial septal defect	Pulmonary hypertension Atrial septal defect

Heart sounds, loud pulmonary S2

Emergency Rule Out conditions shown in red. Entries in blue are for information only
Conditions are listed in approximate order of prevalence for this age range

Emergency Rule Out conditions shown in red. Entries in blue are for information only
Conditions are listed in approximate order of prevalence for this age range

Heart sounds, loud S1

Baby (0-1 yr)	Child (1-12 yr)	Adolescent (12-18 yr)	Adult (18-45 yr)	Middle Age Adult (45-65 yr)	Senior Adult (65+ yr)
Mitral stenosis Atrial septal defect	Ventricular tachycardia Sinus tachycardia Atrial septal defect Mitral stenosis	Ventricular tachycardia Sinus tachycardia Atrial septal defect Hyperaldosteronism	Sinus tachycardia Hyperthyroidism Mitral stenosis Atrial septal defect Wolff-Parkinson-White syndrome	Sinus tachycardia Hyperthyroidism Mitral stenosis Atrial septal defect Wolff-Parkinson-White syndrome	Sinus tachycardia Hyperthyroidism Mitral stenosis Atrial septal defect Wolff-Parkinson-White syndrome

Baby (0-1 yr)	Child (1-12 yr)	Adolescent (12-18 yr)	Adult (18-45 yr)	Middle Age Adult (45-65 yr)	Senior Adult (65+ yr)
Pericardial effusion Congestive heart failure	Obesity Congestive heart failure Pericardial effusion AV block, first degree	Obesity Congestive heart failure Pericardial effusion AV block, first degree	Congestive heart failure AV block, first degree Pericardial effusion	Congestive heart failure AV block, first degree Pericardial effusion	Congestive heart failure AV block, first degree Pericardial effusion

Emergency Rule Out conditions shown in red. Entries in blue are for information only
Conditions are listed in approximate order of prevalence for this age range

Heart sounds, soft S1

Emergency Rule Out conditions shown in red. Entries in blue are for information only
Conditions are listed in approximate order of prevalence for this age range

Baby (0-1 yr)	Child (1-12 yr)	Adolescent (12-18 yr)	Adult (18-45 yr)	Middle Age Adult (45-65 yr)	Senior Adult (65+ yr)
Physiological	Physiological	Physiological	Physiological	Aortic stenosis	Aortic stenosis
Atrial septal defect	Atrial septal defect	Atrial septal defect	Essential hypertension	Essential hypertension	Essential hypertension
Pulmonary valve stenosis	Pulmonary valve stenosis	Pulmonary valve stenosis	Aortic stenosis	Atrial septal defect	Atrial septal defect
Pulmonary valve insufficiency (pulmonic regurgitation)	Pulmonary valve insufficiency (pulmonic regurgitation)	Pulmonary valve insufficiency (pulmonic regurgitation)	Atrial septal defect	Pulmonary valve stenosis	Pulmonary valve stenosis
Aortic stenosis	Aortic stenosis	Aortic stenosis	Pulmonary hypertension		
			Pulmonary valve stenosis		

Baby (0-1 yr)	Child (1-12 yr)	Adolescent (12-18 yr)	Adult (18-45 yr)	Middle Age Adult (45-65 yr)	Senior Adult (65+ yr)
Flow murmur	Flow murmur	Flow murmur	Flow murmur	Flow murmur	Flow murmur
Atrial septal defect	Atrial septal defect	Atrial septal defect	Aortic stenosis	Aortic stenosis	Aortic stenosis
Cardiomyopathy	Ventricular septal defect	Ventricular septal defect	Pregnancy	Mitral regurgitation	Mitral regurgitation
Ventricular septal defect	Cardiomyopathy	Aortic stenosis	Mitral regurgitation	Tricuspid regurgitation	Tricuspid regurgitation
Aortic stenosis	Aortic stenosis	Cardiomyopathy	Mitral valve prolapse	Pulmonary valve stenosis	Pulmonary valve stenosis
Pulmonary valve stenosis	Pulmonary valve stenosis	Anemia	Cardiomyopathy	Cardiomyopathy	Angina
Anemia	Anemia	Pregnancy	Pericarditis	Prosthetic valve failure	Prosthetic valve failure
		Pulmonary valve stenosis	Tricuspid regurgitation	Angina	Cardiomyopathy
		Mitral valve prolapse	Angina	Pericarditis	Pericarditis
			Pulmonary valve stenosis	Mitral valve prolapse	Mitral valve prolapse
			Prosthetic valve failure	Atrial septal defect	Atrial septal defect
			Ventricular septal defect	Ventricular septal defect	Ventricular septal defect
			Atrial septal defect	Anemia	Anemia
			Anemia		

Emergency Rule Out conditions shown in red. Entries in blue are for information only
Conditions are listed in approximate order of prevalence for this age range

Heart sounds, systolic murmur

Emergency Rule Out conditions shown in red. Entries in blue are for information only
Conditions are listed in approximate order of prevalence for this age range

Baby (0-1 yr)	Child (1-12 yr)	Adolescent (12-18 yr)	Adult (18-45 yr)	Middle Age Adult (45-65 yr)	Senior Adult (65+yr)
Congestive heart failure	Congestive heart failure	Congestive heart failure	Pregnancy	Cardiomyopathy	Cardiomyopathy
Cardiomyopathy	Ventricular septal defect	Ventricular septal defect	Cardiomyopathy	Congestive heart failure	Congestive heart failure
	Cardiomyopathy	Pericarditis	Congestive heart failure	Tricuspid regurgitation	Tricuspid regurgitation
		Pregnancy	Tricuspid regurgitation	Angina	Angina
		Cardiomyopathy	Angina	Pericarditis	Pericarditis
			Pericarditis	Ventricular septal defect	Ventricular septal defect
			Ventricular septal defect		

Baby (0-1 yr)	Child (1-12 yr)	Adolescent (12-18 yr)	Adult (18-45 yr)	Middle Age Adult (45-65 yr)	Senior Adult (65+ yr)
Reflux laryngitis	Gastroesophageal reflux disease Gastritis Reflux laryngitis Hiatal hernia	Gastroesophageal reflux disease Esophagitis Gastritis Reflux laryngitis Hiatal hernia Pregnancy	Gastritis Gastroesophageal reflux disease Hiatal hernia Reflux laryngitis Peptic ulcer Esophageal candidiasis Scleroderma Gastric cancer	Gastritis Gastroesophageal reflux disease Hiatal hernia Reflux laryngitis Peptic ulcer Esophageal candidiasis Scleroderma Gastric cancer	Gastritis Gastroesophageal reflux disease Hiatal hernia Reflux laryngitis Peptic ulcer Esophageal candidiasis Scleroderma Gastric cancer

Emergency Rule Out conditions shown in red. Entries in blue are for information only
Conditions are listed in approximate order of prevalence for this age range

159

Emergency Rule Out conditions shown in red. Entries in blue are for information only
Conditions are listed in approximate order of prevalence for this age range

Baby (0-1 yr)	Child (1-12 yr)	Adolescent (12-18 yr)	Adult (18-45 yr)	Middle Age Adult (45-65 yr)	Senior Adult (65+ yr)
Swallowed maternal blood	Gastritis	Gastritis	Gastritis	Gastritis	Gastritis
Gastroesophageal reflux disease	Gastroesophageal reflux disease	Peptic ulcer	Esophageal candidiasis	Esophageal candidiasis	Esophageal candidiasis
Volvulus	Peptic ulcer	Gastroesophageal reflux disease	Esophageal varices	Esophageal varices	Esophageal varices
Drug reaction, peptic ulcer	Drug reaction, peptic ulcer	Drug reaction, peptic ulcer	Gastroesophageal reflux disease	Gastroesophageal reflux disease	Gastroesophageal reflux disease
Hemorrhagic disease of newborn	Acute iron toxicity	Acute iron toxicity	Mallory-Weiss tear	Mallory-Weiss tear	Mallory-Weiss tear
Yellow fever	Esophageal varices	Mallory-Weiss tear	Gastric cancer	Gastric cancer	Gastric cancer
	Yellow fever	Esophageal varices	Esophageal cancer	Esophageal cancer	Esophageal cancer
		Yellow fever	Peptic ulcer	Peptic ulcer	Peptic ulcer
			Drug reaction, peptic ulcer	Drug reaction, peptic ulcer	Drug reaction, peptic ulcer
			Yellow fever	Yellow fever	Yellow fever

Baby (0-1 yr)	Child (1-12 yr)	Adolescent (12-18 yr)	Adult (18-45 yr)	Middle Age Adult (45-65 yr)	Senior Adult (65+ yr)
Urinary tract infection	Urinary tract infection	Urinary tract infection	Urinary tract infection	Urinary tract infection	Urinary tract infection
Acute glomerulonephritis	Acute glomerulonephritis	Acute glomerulonephritis	Trauma	Trauma	Trauma
Trauma	Trauma	Trauma	Renal calculi	Renal calculi	Renal calculi
Sickle cell anemia	Sickle cell anemia	Sickle cell anemia	Acute glomerulonephritis	Acute glomerulonephritis	Prostatic cancer
Nephroblastoma (Wilms' tumor)	Hemophilia A	Nephroblastoma (Wilms' tumor)	Urethritis	Excessive anticoagulation	Excessive anticoagulation
Hemophilia A	Drug reaction	Urethritis	Bladder tumor	Bladder tumor	Bladder tumor
Drug reaction		Hemophilia A	Renal cell adenocarcinoma	Renal cell adenocarcinoma	Renal cell adenocarcinoma
		Drug reaction	Drug reaction	Drug reaction	Drug reaction
			Polycystic kidney disease	Polycystic kidney disease	Acute glomerulonephritis
				Renal infarction	Polycystic kidney disease
					Renal infarction

Emergency Rule Out conditions shown in red. Entries in blue are for information only
Conditions are listed in approximate order of prevalence for this age range

Hemidiaphragm, elevated

Emergency Rule Out conditions shown in red. Entries in blue are for information only
Conditions are listed in approximate order of prevalence for this age range

Baby (0-1 yr)	Child (1-12 yr)	Adolescent (12-18 yr)	Adult (18-45 yr)	Middle Age Adult (45-65 yr)	Senior Adult (65+yr)
Atelectasis Phrenic nerve palsy	Atelectasis Phrenic nerve palsy Subdiaphragmatic abscess Traumatic ruptured diaphragm	Atelectasis Phrenic nerve palsy Subdiaphragmatic abscess Traumatic ruptured diaphragm	Atelectasis Primary lung malignancy Subdiaphragmatic abscess Traumatic ruptured diaphragm Phrenic nerve palsy	Atelectasis Primary lung malignancy Subdiaphragmatic abscess Traumatic ruptured diaphragm Phrenic nerve palsy	Atelectasis Primary lung malignancy Subdiaphragmatic abscess Traumatic ruptured diaphragm Phrenic nerve palsy

Baby (0-1 yr)	Child (1-12 yr)	Adolescent (12-18 yr)	Adult (18-45 yr)	Middle Age Adult (45-65 yr)	Senior Adult (65+ yr)
Idiopathic	Idiopathic	Idiopathic	Migraine headache	Ischemic stroke	Ischemic stroke
Intracranial hemorrhage	Intracranial hemorrhage	Intracranial hemorrhage	Epilepsy	Subarachnoid hemorrhage and cerebral aneurysm stroke	Subarachnoid hemorrhage and cerebral aneurysm stroke
Spina bifida	Brain tumor	Brain tumor	Brain tumor		
Cerebral palsy	Ischemic stroke	Ischemic stroke	Brain abscess	Brain tumor	Brain tumor
Transient ischemic attack	Transient ischemic attack	Transient ischemic attack	Encephalitis	Epilepsy	Brain abscess
Brain abscess	Cerebral palsy	Cerebral palsy	Transient ischemic attack	Migraine headache	Transient ischemic attack
Brain tumor	Brain abscess	Brain abscess	Multiple sclerosis	Brain tumor	Encephalitis
Ischemic stroke	Spina bifida	Spina bifida	Ischemic stroke	Transient ischemic attack	Migraine headache
	Migraine headache	Migraine headache	Subarachnoid hemorrhage and cerebral aneurysm stroke	Brain abscess	Epilepsy
	Encephalitis	Encephalitis		Encephalitis	Spinal cord lesion
			Spinal cord lesion	Multiple sclerosis	Vasculitis
			Vasculitis	Spinal cord lesion	Multiple sclerosis
			Cerebral palsy	Vasculitis	Cerebral palsy
				Cerebral palsy	

Emergency Rule Out conditions shown in red. Entries in blue are for information only
Conditions are listed in approximate order of prevalence for this age range

Emergency Rule Out conditions shown in red. Entries in blue are for information only
Conditions are listed in approximate order of prevalence for this age range

Baby (0-1 yr)	Child (1-12 yr)	Adolescent (12-18 yr)	Adult (18-45 yr)	Middle Age Adult (45-65 yr)	Senior Adult (65+yr)
Hemolysis	Hemolysis	Trauma	Hemolysis	Hemolysis	Hemolysis
Henoch-Schönlein purpura	Trauma	Hemolysis	Autoimmune hemolytic anemia	Autoimmune hemolytic anemia	Autoimmune hemolytic anemia
Trauma	Henoch-Schönlein purpura	Henoch-Schönlein purpura	Disseminated intravascular coagulation	Disseminated intravascular coagulation	Disseminated intravascular coagulation
Hemolytic disease of the newborn (erythroblastosis fetalis)	Hemolytic uremic syndrome	Paroxysmal nocturnal hemoglobinuria	Hemolytic transfusion reaction	Hemolytic transfusion reaction	Henoch-Schönlein purpura
Malaria	Disseminated intravascular coagulation	Hemolytic uremic syndrome	Henoch-Schönlein purpura	Henoch-Schönlein purpura	Hemolytic transfusion reaction
	Hemolytic transfusion reaction	Disseminated intravascular coagulation	Malaria	Malaria	Malaria
	Malaria	Hemolytic transfusion reaction	Hemolytic uremic syndrome	Hemolytic uremic syndrome	Hemolytic uremic syndrome
	Drug reaction	Malaria	Thrombotic thrombocytopenic purpura	Thrombotic thrombocytopenic purpura	Thrombotic thrombocytopenic purpura
	Snake and reptile bites	Drug reaction	Snake and reptile bites	Snake and reptile bites	Snake and reptile bites
	Prosthetic cardiac valve	Prosthetic cardiac valve	Insect and spider bites and stings	Insect and spider bites and stings	Insect and spider bites and stings
	Paroxysmal hemoglobinuria following exercise		Drug reaction	Drug reaction	Drug reaction
			Trauma	Trauma	Trauma
			Prosthetic cardiac valve	Prosthetic cardiac valve	Prosthetic cardiac valve

Baby (0-1 yr)	Child (1-12 yr)	Adolescent (12-18 yr)	Adult (18-45 yr)	Middle Age Adult (45-65 yr)	Senior Adult (65+ yr)
Behçet's syndrome	Trauma	Trauma	Bacterial pneumonia	Bacterial pneumonia	Bacterial pneumonia
Laryngeal cancer	Bronchiectasis	Bronchiectasis	Acute bronchitis	Acute bronchitis	Excessive anticoagulation
Blastomycosis	Bacterial pneumonia	Bacterial pneumonia	Tuberculosis	Tuberculosis	Primary lung malignancy
Epistaxis	Foreign body	Foreign body	Congestive heart failure	Congestive heart failure	Tuberculosis
Thrombotic thrombocytopenic purpura	Ulcerative colitis	Blastomycosis	Primary lung malignancy	Primary lung malignancy	Congestive heart failure
Acute leukemia	Blastomycosis	Cystic fibrosis	Pulmonary infarction	Ulcerative colitis	Ulcerative colitis
	Laryngeal cancer	Laryngeal cancer	Ulcerative colitis	Pulmonary infarction	Acute bronchitis
	Cystic fibrosis	Ulcerative colitis	Foreign body	Foreign body	Mitral stenosis
	Behçet's syndrome	Behçet's syndrome	Acute leukemia	Blastomycosis	Pulmonary infarction
	Tuberculosis	Tuberculosis	Mitral stenosis	Acute leukemia	Lung abscess
	Arteriovenous malformation	Arteriovenous malformation	Lung abscess	Mitral stenosis	Wegener's granulomatosis
	Aspergillosis	Aspergillosis	Blastomycosis	Lung abscess	Goodpasture's syndrome
	Hereditary hemorrhagic telangiectasia	Hereditary hemorrhagic telangiectasia	Wegener's granulomatosis	Wegener's granulomatosis	Blastomycosis
	Pulmonary hemosiderosis	Pulmonary hemosiderosis	Excessive anticoagulation	Behçet's syndrome	Behçet's syndrome
	Epistaxis	Epistaxis	Behçet's syndrome	Excessive anticoagulation	Aspergillosis
	Thrombotic thrombocytopenic purpura	Thrombotic thrombocytopenic purpura	Laryngeal cancer	Laryngeal cancer	Laryngeal cancer
	Acute leukemia	Acute leukemia	Goodpasture's syndrome	Goodpasture's syndrome	Bronchiectasis
			Aspergillosis	Aspergillosis	Foreign body
			Bronchiectasis	Bronchiectasis	Metastatic cancer
			Metastatic cancer	Metastatic cancer	Acute leukemia
			Pulmonary valve stenosis	Pulmonary valve stenosis	Pulmonary valve stenosis
			Echinococcosis	Echinococcosis	Echinococcosis

List continues on next page

Emergency Rule Out conditions shown in red. Entries in blue are for information only
Conditions are listed in approximate order of prevalence for this age range

List continued from previous page

Baby (0-1 yr)	Child (1-12 yr)	Adolescent (12-18 yr)	Adult (18-45 yr)	Middle Age Adult (45-65 yr)	Senior Adult (65+yr)
			Hereditary hemorrhagic telangectasia Schistosomiasis Chronic obstructive pulmonary disease Pulmonary hemosiderosis Epistaxis Thrombotic thrombocytopenic purpura	Hereditary hemorrhagic telangectasia Schistosomiasis Chronic obstructive pulmonary disease Pulmonary hemosiderosis Epistaxis Thrombotic thrombocytopenic purpura	Hereditary hemorrhagic telangectasia Schistosomiasis Chronic obstructive pulmonary disease Epistaxis Thrombotic thrombocytopenic purpura

Baby (0-1 yr)	Child (1-12 yr)	Adolescent (12-18 yr)	Adult (18-45 yr)	Middle Age Adult (45-65 yr)	Senior Adult (65+ yr)
Congestive heart failure	Congestive heart failure	Congestive heart failure	Viral hepatitis	Viral hepatitis	Viral hepatitis
Viral hepatitis	Viral hepatitis	Viral hepatitis	Alcoholic hepatitis	Alcoholic hepatitis	Alcoholic hepatitis
Sickle cell trait	Mononucleosis	Mononucleosis	Mononucleosis	Congestive heart failure	Congestive heart failure
Sickle cell anemia	Cytomegalovirus	Cytomegalovirus	Fatty liver	Fatty liver	Chronic lymphocytic leukemia
Thalassemia	Bartonella infection (cat scratch disease)	Chronic lymphocytic leukemia	Congestive heart failure	Liver cirrhosis	Fatty liver
Hemolytic disease of the newborn (erythroblastosis fetalis)	Chronic lymphocytic leukemia	Thalassemia	Liver cirrhosis	Chronic lymphocytic leukemia	Liver cirrhosis
Chronic lymphocytic leukemia	Thalassemia	Typhoid fever	Hodgkin's disease	Metastatic neoplasm of the liver	Metastatic neoplasm of the liver
Hepatoma	Sickle cell anemia	Bartonella infection (cat scratch disease)	Chronic lymphocytic leukemia	Hepatoma	Bartonella infection (cat scratch disease)
Typhoid fever	Typhoid fever	Sickle cell anemia	Typhoid fever	Typhoid fever	Typhoid fever
Bartonella infection (cat scratch disease)	Acute leukemia	Acute leukemia	Acute leukemia	Hodgkin's disease	Hepatoma
Cytomegalovirus	Neuroblastoma	Neuroblastoma	Bartonella infection (cat scratch disease)	Bartonella infection (cat scratch disease)	Hodgkin's disease
Mononucleosis	Hepatoma	Hepatoma	Hemochromatosis	Acute leukemia	Acute leukemia
Gaucher's disease	Sickle cell trait	Sickle cell trait	Hepatoma	Non-Hodgkin's lymphoma	Non-Hodgkin's lymphoma
Mucopolysaccharidosis	Crohn's disease	Crohn's disease	Non-Hodgkin's lymphoma	Pyogenic liver abscess	Pyogenic liver abscess
Congenital rubella syndrome	Mucopolysaccharidosis	Mucopolysaccharidosis	Amyloidosis	Hemochromatosis	Hemochromatosis
Neuroblastoma	Gaucher's disease	Gaucher's disease	Cytomegalovirus	Amyloidosis	Amyloidosis
Acute leukemia			Crohn's disease	Cytomegalovirus	Cytomegalovirus
			Pyogenic liver abscess	Crohn's disease	Budd-Chiari syndrome
			Budd-Chiari syndrome	Budd-Chiari syndrome	Crohn's disease

List continues on next page

Emergency Rule Out conditions shown in red. Entries in blue are for information only
Conditions are listed in approximate order of prevalence for this age range

167

List continued from previous page

Baby (0-1 yr)	Child (1-12 yr)	Adolescent (12-18 yr)	Adult (18-45 yr)	Middle Age Adult (45-65 yr)	Senior Adult (65+yr)
			Metastatic neoplasm of the liver		

Baby (0-1 yr)	Child (1-12 yr)	Adolescent (12-18 yr)	Adult (18-45 yr)	Middle Age Adult (45-65 yr)	Senior Adult (65+ yr)
Idiopathic	Idiopathic	Idiopathic	Idiopathic	Idiopathic	Idiopathic
Bacterial meningitis	Drug reaction	Drug reaction	Bacterial pneumonia	Bacterial pneumonia	Bacterial pneumonia
Viral meningitis	Postoperative	Postoperative	Subdiaphragmatic abscess	Subdiaphragmatic abscess	Postoperative
	Chronic renal failure	Chronic renal failure	Postoperative	Postoperative	Subdiaphragmatic abscess
	Subdiaphragmatic abscess	Subdiaphragmatic abscess	Aspiration pneumonia	Aspiration pneumonia	Aspiration pneumonia
	Bacterial meningitis	Bacterial meningitis	Mycoplasmal pneumonia	Mycoplasmal pneumonia	Mycoplasmal pneumonia
	Viral meningitis	Viral meningitis	Viral pneumonia	Viral pneumonia	Viral pneumonia
	Foreign body	Encephalitis	Primary lung malignancy	Primary lung malignancy	Primary lung malignancy
	Excess laughter	Foreign body	Esophageal cancer	Esophageal cancer	Esophageal cancer
		Excess laughter	Chronic renal failure	Chronic renal failure	Chronic renal failure
			Somatization disorder	Somatization disorder	Somatization disorder
			Splenic infarct	Splenic infarct	Splenic infarct
			Pericarditis	Pericarditis	Pericarditis
			Encephalitis	Encephalitis	Encephalitis
			Abdominal aortic aneurysm	Abdominal aortic aneurysm	Abdominal aortic aneurysm
			Thoracic aortic aneurysm	Thoracic aortic aneurysm	Thoracic aortic aneurysm
			Metastatic neoplasm of the liver	Metastatic neoplasm of the liver	Metastatic neoplasm of the liver
			Sarcoidosis	Sarcoidosis	Sarcoidosis
			Zollinger-Ellison syndrome	Zollinger-Ellison syndrome	Zollinger-Ellison syndrome
			Tobacco smoking	Tabes dorsalis	Tabes dorsalis
			Excess laughter	Tobacco smoking	Tobacco smoking
				Excess laughter	Excess laughter

Emergency Rule Out conditions shown in red. Entries in blue are for information only
Conditions are listed in approximate order of prevalence for this age range

Emergency Rule Out conditions shown in red. Entries in blue are for information only
Conditions are listed in approximate order of prevalence for this age range

Baby (0-1 yr)	Child (1-12 yr)	Adolescent (12-18 yr)	Adult (18-45 yr)	Middle Age Adult (45-65 yr)	Senior Adult (65+yr)
Congenital dislocation of hip	Trauma	Trauma	Hip injury	Aseptic bursitis	Osteoarthritis
Trauma	Hip fracture	Hip fracture	Aseptic bursitis	Hip injury	Aseptic bursitis
Septic arthritis	Septic arthritis	Septic arthritis	Nerve root compression	Nerve root compression	Hip fracture
Osteomyelitis	Osteomyelitis	Osteomyelitis	Iliac apophysitis	Osteoarthritis	Hip injury
Hip fracture	Sickle cell anemia	Sickle cell anemia	Obturator inflammation	Ankylosing spondylitis	Nerve root compression
	Slipped femoral epiphysis	Slipped femoral epiphysis	Meralgia paresthetica	Polymyalgia rheumatica	Avascular necrosis
	Perthes' disease	Perthes' disease	Septic arthritis	Hip fracture	Septic arthritis
	Hip synovitis	Hip synovitis	Avascular necrosis	Obturator inflammation	Obturator inflammation
	Congenital dislocation of hip	Congenital dislocation of hip	Ankylosing spondylitis	Avascular necrosis	Polymyalgia rheumatica
		Tuberculosis	Hip fracture	Septic arthritis	Meralgia paresthetica
			Arterial embolus and thrombosis	Meralgia paresthetica	Arterial embolus and thrombosis
			Congenital dislocation of hip	Iliac apophysitis	Iliac apophysitis
			Tuberculosis	Arterial embolus and thrombosis	Congenital dislocation of hip
				Congenital dislocation of hip	Tuberculosis
				Tuberculosis	

Baby (0-1 yr)	Child (1-12 yr)	Adolescent (12-18 yr)	Adult (18-45 yr)	Middle Age Adult (45-65 yr)	Senior Adult (65+ yr)
Cushing's syndrome Adrenocortical carcinoma/ adenoma Benign ovarian tumor	Cushing's syndrome Adrenocortical carcinoma/ adenoma Benign ovarian tumor	Idiopathic Cushing's syndrome Benign ovarian tumor Polycystic ovarian disease Adrenocortical carcinoma/ adenoma	Idiopathic Polycystic ovarian disease Hyperprolactinemia Benign ovarian tumor Cushing's syndrome Epithelial cell ovarian cancer Germ cell ovarian cancer Sex cord/stromal ovarian cancer Adrenocortical carcinoma/ adenoma Acromegaly (pituitary gigantism)	Idiopathic Hyperprolactinemia Cushing's syndrome Epithelial cell ovarian cancer Benign ovarian tumor Germ cell ovarian cancer Sex cord/stromal ovarian cancer Polycystic ovarian disease Adrenocortical carcinoma/ adenoma Acromegaly (pituitary gigantism)	Cushing's syndrome Hyperprolactinemia Epithelial cell ovarian cancer Benign ovarian tumor Germ cell ovarian cancer Sex cord/stromal ovarian cancer Adrenocortical carcinoma/ adenoma Acromegaly (pituitary gigantism)

Emergency Rule Out conditions shown in red. Entries in blue are for information only
Conditions are listed in approximate order of prevalence for this age range

171

Emergency Rule Out conditions shown in red. Entries in blue are for information only
Conditions are listed in approximate order of prevalence for this age range

Baby (0-1 yr)	Child (1-12 yr)	Adolescent (12-18 yr)	Adult (18-45 yr)	Middle Age Adult (45-65 yr)	Senior Adult (65+ yr)
Laryngitis	Laryngitis	Laryngitis	Laryngitis	Laryngitis	Laryngitis
Thyroiditis	Vocal cord nodules	Vocal cord nodules	Hypothyroidism	Hypothyroidism	Hypothyroidism
Recurrent laryngeal nerve injury	Thyroiditis	Thyroiditis	Vocal cord nodules	Vocal cord nodules	Vocal cord nodules
Thyroid carcinoma	Recurrent laryngeal nerve injury	Vocal cord polyp	Vocal cord polyp	Thyroiditis	Thyroiditis
	Hypothyroidism	Recurrent laryngeal nerve injury	Thyroiditis	Gastroesophageal reflux disease	Gastroesophageal reflux disease
	Thyroid carcinoma	Hypothyroidism	Gastroesophageal reflux disease	Recurrent laryngeal nerve injury	Recurrent laryngeal nerve injury
		Thyroid carcinoma	Recurrent laryngeal nerve injury	Angioedema	Vocal cord polyp
		Retrosternal goiter	Angioedema	Vocal cord polyp	Laryngeal cancer
		Multinodular goiter	Laryngeal cancer	Laryngeal cancer	Angioedema
		Overuse	Thyroid carcinoma	Thyroid carcinoma	Thyroid carcinoma
			Retrosternal goiter	Retrosternal goiter	Retrosternal goiter
			Multinodular goiter	Multinodular goiter	Multinodular goiter
			Overuse	Overuse	Overuse
			Myxedema	Myxedema	Myxedema

Baby (0-1 yr)	Child (1-12 yr)	Adolescent (12-18 yr)	Adult (18-45 yr)	Middle Age Adult (45-65 yr)	Senior Adult (65+ yr)
Malignancy Reflex sympathetic dystrophy Nutritional deficiencies Chronic renal failure	Malignancy Nutritional deficiencies Reflex sympathetic dystrophy Chronic renal failure	Malignancy Reflex sympathetic dystrophy Nutritional deficiencies Chronic renal failure	Diabetes mellitus type 2 Diabetes mellitus type 1 Reflex sympathetic dystrophy Malignancy Amyloidosis Nutritional deficiencies Chronic renal failure	Diabetes mellitus type 2 Diabetes mellitus type 1 Malignancy Reflex sympathetic dystrophy Amyloidosis Nutritional deficiencies Chronic renal failure	Diabetes mellitus type 2 Diabetes mellitus type 1 Reflex sympathetic dystrophy Amyloidosis Malignancy Nutritional deficiencies Chronic renal failure

Emergency Rule Out conditions shown in red. Entries in blue are for information only
Conditions are listed in approximate order of prevalence for this age range

Emergency Rule Out conditions shown in red. Entries in blue are for information only
Conditions are listed in approximate order of prevalence for this age range

Baby (0-1 yr)	Child (1-12 yr)	Adolescent (12-18 yr)	Adult (18-45 yr)	Middle Age Adult (45-65 yr)	Senior Adult (65+yr)
Hyperparathyroidism	Hyperparathyroidism	Hyperparathyroidism	Hyperparathyroidism	Hyperparathyroidism	Malignancy
Vitamin D excess	Vitamin D excess	Vitamin D excess	Malignancy	Malignancy	Multiple myeloma
Williams syndrome	Williams syndrome	Williams syndrome	Multiple myeloma	Multiple myeloma	Hyperparathyroidism
Malignancy	Malignancy	Malignancy	Tuberculosis	Tuberculosis	Tuberculosis
Hyperthyroidism	Hyperthyroidism	Hyperthyroidism	Williams syndrome	Williams syndrome	Vitamin D excess
Rhabdomyolysis	Rhabdomyolysis	Rhabdomyolysis	Vitamin D excess	Vitamin D excess	Williams syndrome
			Hyperthyroidism	Hyperthyroidism	Hyperthyroidism
			Milk-alkali syndrome	Milk-alkali syndrome	Milk-alkali syndrome
			Sarcoidosis	Sarcoidosis	Paget's disease
			Rhabdomyolysis	Acute renal failure	Metastatic cancer
				Addison's disease	Acute renal failure
				Rhabdomyolysis	Addison's disease
					Prolonged immobilization
					Rhabdomyolysis

174

Baby (0-1 yr)	Child (1-12 yr)	Adolescent (12-18 yr)	Adult (18-45 yr)	Middle Age Adult (45-65 yr)	Senior Adult (65+ yr)
Neonatal respiratory distress syndrome	Asthma	Asthma	Asthma	Chronic obstructive pulmonary disease	Chronic obstructive pulmonary disease
Bronchiolitis	Bacterial pneumonia	Bacterial pneumonia	Chronic obstructive pulmonary disease	Bacterial pneumonia	Bacterial pneumonia
Asthma	Pneumothorax	Pneumothorax	Bacterial pneumonia	Asthma	Congestive heart failure
Bacterial pneumonia	Bronchiolitis	Atelectasis	Congestive heart failure	Congestive heart failure	Asthma
Atelectasis	Kyphoscoliosis	Kyphoscoliosis	Pneumothorax	Pneumothorax	Obstructive sleep apnea
Obstructive sleep apnea	Obstructive sleep apnea	Obstructive sleep apnea	Obstructive sleep apnea	Obstructive sleep apnea	Pneumothorax
Pneumothorax	Atelectasis	Congestive heart failure	Myasthenia gravis	Myasthenia gravis	Kyphoscoliosis
Congestive heart failure	Congestive heart failure	Muscular dystrophy	Kyphoscoliosis	Kyphoscoliosis	Idiopathic pulmonary interstitial fibrosis
Spinal muscular atrophy	Guillain-Barré syndrome (acute infective polyneuritis)	Myasthenia gravis	Idiopathic pulmonary interstitial fibrosis	Idiopathic pulmonary interstitial fibrosis	Myasthenia gravis
Kyphoscoliosis	Spinal muscular atrophy	Guillain-Barré syndrome (acute infective polyneuritis)	Guillain-Barré syndrome (acute infective polyneuritis)	Guillain-Barré syndrome (acute infective polyneuritis)	Amyotrophic lateral sclerosis (motor neuron disease)
Myasthenia gravis	Muscular dystrophy	Spinal muscular atrophy	Amyotrophic lateral sclerosis (motor neuron disease)	Amyotrophic lateral sclerosis (motor neuron disease)	Guillain-Barré syndrome (acute infective polyneuritis)
Guillain-Barré syndrome (acute infective polyneuritis)	Myasthenia gravis		Spinal muscular atrophy	Spinal muscular atrophy	Atelectasis
			Atelectasis	Atelectasis	

Emergency Rule Out conditions shown in red. Entries in blue are for information only
Conditions are listed in approximate order of prevalence for this age range

Emergency Rule Out conditions shown in red. Entries in blue are for information only
Conditions are listed in approximate order of prevalence for this age range

Baby (0-1 yr)	Child (1-12 yr)	Adolescent (12-18 yr)	Adult (18-45 yr)	Middle Age Adult (45-65 yr)	Senior Adult (65-yr)
Burns	Burns	Burns	Burns	Burns	Burns
Sleeping sickness (African trypanosomiasis)	Sleeping sickness (African trypanosomiasis)	Sleeping sickness (African trypanosomiasis)	Sleeping sickness (African trypanosomiasis)	Sleeping sickness (African trypanosomiasis)	Sleeping sickness (African trypanosomiasis)
Post-traumatic stress disorder	Post-traumatic stress disorder	Post-traumatic stress disorder	Diabetes mellitus type 2	Diabetes mellitus type 2	Poliomyelitis
Poliomyelitis	Poliomyelitis	Poliomyelitis	Poliomyelitis	Post-traumatic stress disorder	Diabetes mellitus type 2
Trauma	Trauma	Diabetes mellitus type 2	Post-traumatic stress disorder	Poliomyelitis	Post-traumatic stress disorder
Reflex sympathetic dystrophy	Reflex sympathetic dystrophy	Trauma	Diabetes mellitus type 1	Diabetes mellitus type 1	Diabetes mellitus type 1
		Reflex sympathetic dystrophy	Trauma	Trauma	Trauma
			Reflex sympathetic dystrophy	Reflex sympathetic dystrophy	Reflex sympathetic dystrophy

Baby (0-1 yr)	Child (1-12 yr)	Adolescent (12-18 yr)	Adult (18-45 yr)	Middle Age Adult (45-65 yr)	Senior Adult (65+yr)
Acromegaly (pituitary gigantism)	Anxiety	Anxiety	Anxiety	Anxiety	Anxiety
Heat stroke and heat exhaustion	Hyperthyroidism	Hyperthyroidism	Hyperthyroidism	Menopause	Hyperthyroidism
Insect and spider bites and stings	Congestive heart failure	Congestive heart failure	Menopause	Hyperthyroidism	Alcohol abuse
Infective endocarditis	Pheochromocytoma	Recreational drug abuse	Alcohol abuse	Insect and spider bites and stings	Congestive heart failure
Brucellosis	Malaria	Ménière's disease	Insect and spider bites and stings	Pheochromocytoma	Malaria
Ménière's disease	Infective endocarditis	Insect and spider bites and stings	Infective endocarditis	Heat stroke and heat exhaustion	Brucellosis
Malaria	Heat stroke and heat exhaustion	Heat stroke and heat exhaustion	Ménière's disease	Infective endocarditis	Heat stroke and heat exhaustion
Motion sickness	Insect and spider bites and stings	Brucellosis	Heat stroke and heat exhaustion	Motion sickness	Insect and spider bites and stings
Orthostatic hypotension	Brucellosis	Infective endocarditis	Brucellosis	Brucellosis	Infective endocarditis
Hypothyroidism	Ménière's disease	Malaria	Malaria	Malaria	Orthostatic hypotension
	Motion sickness	Orthostatic hypotension	Motion sickness	Ménière's disease	Ménière's disease
	Orthostatic hypotension	Motion sickness	Orthostatic hypotension	Orthostatic hypotension	Motion sickness
	Acromegaly (pituitary gigantism)	Alcohol abuse	Acromegaly (pituitary gigantism)	Alcohol abuse	Acromegaly (pituitary gigantism)
	Spinal cord lesion	Acromegaly (pituitary gigantism)	Congestive heart failure	Congestive heart failure	Pheochromocytoma
	Recreational drug abuse	Pheochromocytoma	Pheochromocytoma	Spinal cord lesion	Spinal cord lesion
	Familial dysautonomia	Spinal cord lesion	Spinal cord lesion	Acromegaly (pituitary gigantism)	Menopause
	Hypothyroidism	Familial dysautonomia	Drug reaction	Drug reaction	Drug reaction
		Drug reaction	Hypothyroidism	Hypothyroidism	Hypothyroidism
		Hypothyroidism			

Emergency Rule Out conditions shown in red. Entries in blue are for information only
Conditions are listed in approximate order of prevalence for this age range

177

Emergency Rule Out conditions shown in red. Entries in blue are for information only
Conditions are listed in approximate order of prevalence for this age range

Baby (0-1 yr)	Child (1-12 yr)	Adolescent (12-18 yr)	Adult (18-45 yr)	Middle Age Adult (45-65 yr)	Senior Adult (65+yr)
Not relevant to this age group	Viral meningitis Bacterial meningitis Ischemic stroke Guillain-Barré syndrome (acute infective polyneuritis) Myasthenia gravis Malignancy Poliomyelitis Syringomyelia	Viral meningitis Bacterial meningitis Ischemic stroke Guillain-Barré syndrome (acute infective polyneuritis) Myasthenia gravis Malignancy Poliomyelitis Syringomyelia	Ischemic stroke Viral meningitis Bacterial meningitis Myasthenia gravis Amyotrophic lateral sclerosis (motor neuron disease) Malignancy Poliomyelitis Syringomyelia	Ischemic stroke Viral meningitis Bacterial meningitis Myasthenia gravis Amyotrophic lateral sclerosis (motor neuron disease) Malignancy Poliomyelitis Syringomyelia	Ischemic stroke Viral meningitis Malignancy Amyotrophic lateral sclerosis (motor neuron disease) Bacterial meningitis Myasthenia gravis Poliomyelitis Syringomyelia

Baby (0-1 yr)	Child (1-12 yr)	Adolescent (12-18 yr)	Adult (18-45 yr)	Middle Age Adult (45-65 yr)	Senior Adult (65+ yr)
Dehydration	Dehydration	Dehydration	Diabetic ketoacidosis	Diabetic ketoacidosis	Diabetic ketoacidosis
Gastroenteritis	Gastroenteritis	Gastroenteritis	Gastroenteritis	Gastroenteritis	Gastroenteritis
Diabetic ketoacidosis	Diabetic ketoacidosis	Diabetic ketoacidosis	Dehydration	Dehydration	Dehydration
Chronic renal failure	Chronic renal failure	Chronic renal failure	Chronic renal failure	Chronic renal failure	Chronic renal failure
Diabetes insipidus	Diabetes insipidus	Diabetes insipidus	Burns	Burns	Burns
			Diabetes insipidus	Diabetes insipidus	Diabetes insipidus
			Hyperaldosteronism	Hyperaldosteronism	Hyperaldosteronism
			Cushing's syndrome	Cushing's syndrome	Cushing's syndrome

Emergency Rule Out conditions shown in red. Entries in blue are for information only
Conditions are listed in approximate order of prevalence for this age range

Hypernatremia

Emergency Rule Out conditions shown in red. Entries in blue are for information only
Conditions are listed in approximate order of prevalence for this age range

Hyperpigmentation

Baby (0-1 yr)	Child (1-12 yr)	Adolescent (12-18 yr)	Adult (18-45 yr)	Middle Age Adult (45-65 yr)	Senior Adult (65-yr)
Neurofibromatosis	Addison's disease	Addison's disease	Addison's disease	Addison's disease	Addison's disease
Melanoma	Neurofibromatosis	Cushing's syndrome	Hemochromatosis	Hemochromatosis	Hemochromatosis
	Scarlet fever	Melanoma	Cafe au lait spot	Cafe au lait spot	Cafe au lait spot
	Melanoma	Neurofibromatosis	Primary biliary cirrhosis	Primary biliary cirrhosis	Primary biliary cirrhosis
	Cushing's syndrome	Scarlet fever	Metastatic cancer	Metastatic cancer	Metastatic cancer
	Hemochromatosis	Hemochromatosis	Primary lung malignancy	Scarlet fever	Neurofibromatosis
	Peutz-Jeghers syndrome	Peutz-Jeghers syndrome	Scarlet fever	Melanoma	Scarlet fever
			Melanoma	Neurofibromatosis	Primary lung malignancy
			Neurofibromatosis	Primary lung malignancy	Melanoma
			Thyroid carcinoma	Thyroid carcinoma	Thyroid carcinoma
			Heavy metal poisoning	Heavy metal poisoning	Heavy metal poisoning
			Pellagra	Pellagra	Pellagra
			Whipple's disease	Whipple's disease	Whipple's disease
			Porphyria	Porphyria	Porphyria
			Chloasma	Chloasma	Wilson's disease
			Wilson's disease	Wilson's disease	Acromegaly (pituitary gigantism)
			Oral contraception	Acromegaly (pituitary gigantism)	Malnutrition
				Malnutrition	

Hyperreflexia

Baby (0-1 yr)	Child (1-12 yr)	Adolescent (12-18 yr)	Adult (18-45 yr)	Middle Age Adult (45-65 yr)	Senior Adult (65+ yr)
Cerebral palsy	Cerebral palsy	Cerebral palsy	Cervical spondylosis	Cervical spondylosis	Ischemic stroke
Dementia	Dementia	Dementia	Hyperthyroidism	Hyperthyroidism	Hepatic encephalopathy
Hyperthyroidism	Hyperthyroidism	Hyperthyroidism	Multiple sclerosis	Multiple sclerosis	Uremic encephalopathy
Spinal cord lesion	Spinal cord lesion	Spinal cord lesion	Dementia	Dementia	Dementia
			Metabolic encephalopathy	Ischemic stroke	Spinal cord compression
			Hepatic encephalopathy	Metabolic encephalopathy	Cervical spondylosis
			Uremic encephalopathy	Hepatic encephalopathy	Multiple sclerosis
			Spinal cord compression	Uremic encephalopathy	Amyotrophic lateral sclerosis (motor neuron disease)
			Ischemic stroke	Spinal cord compression	
			Amyotrophic lateral sclerosis (motor neuron disease)	Amyotrophic lateral sclerosis (motor neuron disease)	

Emergency Rule Out conditions shown in red. Entries in blue are for information only
Conditions are listed in approximate order of prevalence for this age range

Emergency Rule Out conditions shown in red. Entries in blue are for information only
Conditions are listed in approximate order of prevalence for this age range

Baby (0-1 yr)	Child (1-12 yr)	Adolescent (12-18 yr)	Adult (18-45 yr)	Middle Age Adult (45-65 yr)	Senior Adult (65+ yr)
Not relevant to this age group	Prader-Willi syndrome Manic depression Hypothyroidism Narcolepsy	Depression Manic depression Hypothyroidism Prader-Willi syndrome Narcolepsy	Depression Hypothyroidism Manic depression Obstructive sleep apnea Narcolepsy	Depression Hypothyroidism Manic depression Obstructive sleep apnea Narcolepsy	Depression Hypothyroidism Manic depression Obstructive sleep apnea Narcolepsy Dementia

Baby (0-1 yr)	Child (1-12 yr)	Adolescent (12-18 yr)	Adult (18-45 yr)	Middle Age Adult (45-65 yr)	Senior Adult (65+ yr)
Renal artery stenosis	Renal artery stenosis	Renal artery stenosis	Essential hypertension	Essential hypertension	Essential hypertension
Coarctation of the aorta	Coarctation of the aorta	Coarctation of the aorta	Pregnancy-induced hypertension	Renal artery stenosis	Renal artery stenosis
Nephroblastoma (Wilms' tumor)	Nephroblastoma (Wilms' tumor)	Neuroblastoma	Alcohol abuse	Alcohol abuse	Alcohol abuse
Essential hypertension	Insect and spider bites and stings	Pregnancy-induced hypertension	Renal artery stenosis	Insect and spider bites and stings	Acute glomerulonephritis
Insect and spider bites and stings	Essential hypertension	Acute glomerulonephritis	Acute glomerulonephritis	Systemic lupus erythematosus	Polyarteritis nodosa
Malignant hypertension	Cushing's syndrome	Nephritic syndrome	Nephritic syndrome	Acute glomerulonephritis	Malignant hypertension
Polyarteritis nodosa	Malignant hypertension	Essential hypertension	Malignant hypertension	Polyarteritis nodosa	Insect and spider bites and stings
Classic congenital adrenal hyperplasia	Polyarteritis nodosa	Malignant hypertension	Insect and spider bites and stings	Malignant hypertension	Nephritic syndrome
Nephritic syndrome	Nephritic syndrome	Insect and spider bites and stings	Polyarteritis nodosa	Carcinoid syndrome	Systemic lupus erythematosus
Systemic lupus erythematosus	Systemic lupus erythematosus	Polyarteritis nodosa	Systemic lupus erythematosus	Chronic renal failure	Chronic renal failure
Pheochromocytoma	Acute glomerulonephritis	Systemic lupus erythematosus	Chronic renal failure	Cushing's syndrome	Hyperaldosteronism
Cushing's syndrome	Pheochromocytoma	Cushing's syndrome	Cushing's syndrome	Hyperaldosteronism	Cushing's syndrome
Chronic renal failure	Renal cell adenocarcinoma	Pheochromocytoma	Hyperaldosteronism	Pheochromocytoma	Pheochromocytoma
Renal cell adenocarcinoma	Chronic renal failure	Chronic renal failure	Pheochromocytoma	Nephritic syndrome	Carcinoid syndrome
	Polycystic kidney disease	Renal cell adenocarcinoma	Polycystic kidney disease		
		Polycystic kidney disease	Carcinoid syndrome		

Emergency Rule Out conditions shown in red. Entries in blue are for information only
Conditions are listed in approximate order of prevalence for this age range

Hypertensive emergencies

Emergency Rule Out conditions shown in red. Entries in blue are for information only
Conditions are listed in approximate order of prevalence for this age range

Baby (0-1 yr)	Child (1-12 yr)	Adolescent (12-18 yr)	Adult (18-45 yr)	Middle Age Adult (45-65 yr)	Senior Adult (65+ yr)
Renal artery stenosis	Renal artery stenosis	Renal artery stenosis	Pregnancy-induced hypertension	Renal artery stenosis	Renal artery stenosis
Malignant hypertension	Malignant hypertension	Vasculitis	Renal artery stenosis	Vasculitis	Vasculitis
	Hyperaldosteronism	Malignant hypertension	Malignant hypertension	Malignant hypertension	Malignant hypertension
	Vasculitis	Hyperaldosteronism	Vasculitis	Pheochromocytoma	Pheochromocytoma
	Pheochromocytoma	Pheochromocytoma	Pheochromocytoma	Hyperaldosteronism	Hyperaldosteronism
		Pregnancy-induced hypertension	Hyperaldosteronism		

Baby (0-1 yr)	Child (1-12 yr)	Adolescent (12-18 yr)	Adult (18-45 yr)	Middle Age Adult (45-65 yr)	Senior Adult (65+ yr)
Metabolic acidosis	Diabetic ketoacidosis	Diabetic ketoacidosis	Fever	Fever	Fever
Birth asphyxia	Hepatic encephalopathy	Hepatic encephalopathy	Anxiety	Anxiety	Anxiety
Inborn errors of metabolism	Chronic renal failure	Acute renal failure	Asthma	Asthma	Asthma
Hepatic encephalopathy	Metabolic acidosis	Chronic renal failure	Chronic obstructive pulmonary disease	Chronic obstructive pulmonary disease	Hepatic encephalopathy
Diabetic ketoacidosis			Bacterial pneumonia	Bacterial pneumonia	Chronic obstructive pulmonary disease
Acute renal failure			Metabolic acidosis	Metabolic acidosis	Bacterial pneumonia
Chronic renal failure			Pulmonary thromboembolism	Pulmonary thromboembolism	Metabolic acidosis
			Congestive heart failure	Congestive heart failure	Pulmonary thromboembolism
			Pneumothorax	Hepatic encephalopathy	Congestive heart failure
			Hepatic encephalopathy	Pneumothorax	Pneumothorax
			Pleural effusion	Pleural effusion	Pleural effusion
			Kyphosis	Kyphosis	Kyphosis
			Primary lung malignancy	Primary lung malignancy	Primary lung malignancy
			Salicylate poisoning	Salicylate poisoning	Salicylate poisoning
			Ankylosing spondylitis	Ankylosing spondylitis	Ankylosing spondylitis
			Cardiac tamponade	Cardiac tamponade	Cardiac tamponade
			Idiopathic pulmonary interstitial fibrosis	Idiopathic pulmonary interstitial fibrosis	Idiopathic pulmonary interstitial fibrosis
			Viral hepatitis	Viral hepatitis	Viral hepatitis
			Alcoholic hepatitis	Alcoholic hepatitis	Alcoholic hepatitis
			Poisoning	Poisoning	Poisoning

Emergency Rule Out conditions shown in red. Entries in blue are for information only
Conditions are listed in approximate order of prevalence for this age range

185

Emergency Rule Out conditions shown in red. Entries in blue are for information only
Conditions are listed in approximate order of prevalence for this age range

Baby (0-1 yr)	Child (1-12 yr)	Adolescent (12-18 yr)	Adult (18-45 yr)	Middle Age Adult (45-65 yr)	Senior Adult (65+yr)
Not relevant to this age group	Anxiety Depression	Anxiety Depression	Anxiety Depression Munchausen syndrome	Anxiety Depression Munchausen syndrome	Anxiety Depression Munchausen syndrome

Baby (0-1 yr)	Child (1-12 yr)	Adolescent (12-18 yr)	Adult (18-45 yr)	Middle Age Adult (45-65 yr)	Senior Adult (65+ yr)
Not relevant to this age group	Bell's palsy	Bell's palsy	Bell's palsy	Bell's palsy	Bell's palsy
	Trauma	Trauma	Ischemic stroke	Ischemic stroke	Ischemic stroke
	Acute otitis media	Acute otitis media	Acute otitis media	Acute otitis media	Acute otitis media
	Chronic otitis media	Chronic otitis media	Chronic otitis media	Chronic otitis media	Chronic otitis media
	Herpes zoster, shingles	Herpes zoster, shingles	Head injury	Herpes zoster, shingles	Herpes zoster, shingles
	Ramsay Hunt syndrome	Ramsay Hunt syndrome	Herpes zoster, shingles	Head injury	Head injury
	Mastoiditis	Mastoiditis	Myasthenia gravis	Myasthenia gravis	Myasthenia gravis
			Parkinson's disease	Parkinson's disease	Parkinson's disease

Emergency Rule Out conditions shown in red. Entries in blue are for information only
Conditions are listed in approximate order of prevalence for this age range

Emergency Rule Out conditions shown in red. Entries in blue are for information only
Conditions are listed in approximate order of prevalence for this age range

Baby (0-1 yr)	Child (1-12 yr)	Adolescent (12-18 yr)	Adult (18-45 yr)	Middle Age Adult (45-65 yr)	Senior Adult (65+ yr)
Gastroenteritis	Gastroenteritis	Vomiting	Diarrhea	Diarrhea	Diarrhea
Diarrhea	Vomiting	Bulimia nervosa	Vomiting	Vomiting	Vomiting
Vomiting	Pyloric stenosis	Diarrhea	Bulimia nervosa	Drug reaction	Diabetic ketoacidosis
Pyloric stenosis	Diabetic ketoacidosis	Gastroenteritis	Drug reaction	Diabetic ketoacidosis	Drug reaction
Hypokalemia	Hypokalemia	Hypokalemia	Diabetic ketoacidosis	Bulimia nervosa	Cushing's syndrome
Cushing's syndrome	Cushing's syndrome	Diabetic ketoacidosis	Cushing's syndrome	Cushing's syndrome	Hyperaldosteronism
Celiac disease	Celiac disease	Celiac disease	Celiac disease	Hypokalemia	Congestive heart failure
Hyperaldosteronism	Diarrhea	Hyperaldosteronism	Hypokalemia	Hyperaldosteronism	Hypokalemia
Acute renal failure	Hyperaldosteronism	Cushing's syndrome	Hyperaldosteronism	Celiac disease	Liver cirrhosis
Chronic renal failure	Acute renal failure	Acute renal failure	Congestive heart failure	Congestive heart failure	Celiac disease
Renal tubular acidosis	Chronic renal failure	Chronic renal failure	Liver cirrhosis	Liver cirrhosis	Nephrotic syndrome
Diabetic ketoacidosis	Renal tubular acidosis	Renal tubular acidosis	Burns	Nephrotic syndrome	Renal tubular acidosis
			Nephrotic syndrome	Renal tubular acidosis	Burns
			Renal tubular acidosis	Burns	Bartter's syndrome
			Bartter's syndrome	Bartter's syndrome	Altitude sickness
			Altitude sickness	Altitude sickness	Laxative abuse
			Secretory villous adenoma	Secretory villous adenoma	Secretory villous adenoma

Baby (0-1 yr)	Child (1-12 yr)	Adolescent (12-18 yr)	Adult (18-45 yr)	Middle Age Adult (45-65 yr)	Senior Adult (65+ yr)
Albinism	Albinism	Vitiligo	Vitiligo	Vitiligo	Vitiligo
Vitiligo	Vitiligo	Albinism	Albinism	Albinism	Albinism
Tuberous sclerosis complex	Tuberous sclerosis complex	Tuberous sclerosis complex	Tuberous sclerosis complex	Tuberous sclerosis complex	Tuberous sclerosis complex
		Pityriasis versicolor	Pityriasis versicolor	Pityriasis versicolor	Post-inflammatory reaction
			Post-inflammatory reaction	Post-inflammatory reaction	

Emergency Rule Out conditions shown in red. Entries in blue are for information only
Conditions are listed in approximate order of prevalence for this age range

Emergency Rule Out conditions shown in red. Entries in blue are for information only
Conditions are listed in approximate order of prevalence for this age range

Baby (0-1 yr)	Child (1-12 yr)	Adolescent (12-18 yr)	Adult (18-45 yr)	Middle Age Adult (45-65 yr)	Senior Adult (65+yr)
Hypothyroidism	Diabetes mellitus in children	Diabetes mellitus in children	Hypothyroidism	Hypothyroidism	Hypothyroidism
Diabetes mellitus in children	Hypothyroidism	Nerve root compression	Nerve root compression	Nerve root compression	Nerve root compression
Vitamin B12 deficiency	Muscular dystrophy	Hypothyroidism	Diabetes mellitus type 1	Diabetes mellitus type 1	Ischemic stroke
Megaloblastic anemias	Vitamin B12 deficiency	Vitamin B12 deficiency	Diabetes mellitus type 2	Diabetes mellitus type 2	Diabetes mellitus type 2
Cervical disk syndrome	Nerve root compression	Megaloblastic anemias	Charcot-Marie-Tooth disease	Vitamin B12 deficiency	Vitamin B12 deficiency
Nerve root compression	Cervical disk syndrome	Muscular dystrophy	Myasthenia gravis	Ischemic stroke	Chronic renal failure
Myopathy	Megaloblastic anemias	Cervical disk syndrome	Friedreich's ataxia	Cervical disk syndrome	Megaloblastic anemias
Inborn errors of metabolism	Myasthenia gravis	Charcot-Marie-Tooth disease	Megaloblastic anemias	Megaloblastic anemias	Cervical disk syndrome
Botulism	Friedreich's ataxia	Myasthenia gravis	Cervical disk syndrome	Chronic renal failure	Charcot-Marie-Tooth disease
	Guillain-Barré syndrome (acute infective polyneuritis)	Diabetes mellitus type 2	Alcohol abuse	Charcot-Marie-Tooth disease	Occult cancer
	Botulism	Alcohol abuse	Muscular dystrophy	Myasthenia gravis	Guillain-Barré syndrome (acute infective polyneuritis)
		Friedreich's ataxia	Vitamin B12 deficiency	Occult cancer	Amyloidosis
		Guillain-Barré syndrome (acute infective polyneuritis)	Ischemic stroke	Guillain-Barré syndrome (acute infective polyneuritis)	Alcohol abuse
		Botulism	Occult cancer	Amyloidosis	Botulism
			Guillain-Barré syndrome (acute infective polyneuritis)	Alcohol abuse	Myopathy
			Amyloidosis	Botulism	
			Chronic renal failure	Myopathy	
			Myopathy		
			Botulism		

Baby (0-1 yr)	Child (1-12 yr)	Adolescent (12-18 yr)	Adult (18-45 yr)	Middle Age Adult (45-65 yr)	Senior Adult (65+ yr)
Sepsis	Sepsis	Sepsis	Alcohol abuse	Sepsis	Sepsis
Hypothyroidism	**Hypothyroidism**	**Hypothyroidism**	Burns	Alcohol abuse	Hypothyroidism
Hypothermia	Hypothermia	Burns	**Hypothyroidism**	Hypothyroidism	Alcohol abuse
Burns	Burns	Hypothermia	Sepsis	Burns	**Dementia**
Malnutrition	**Malnutrition**	**Malnutrition**	Hypothermia	**Dementia**	Ischemic stroke
Near drowning	Near drowning	Near drowning	**Dementia**	Hypothermia	Hypothermia
Autonomic dysfunction	Autonomic dysfunction	Autonomic dysfunction	Ischemic stroke	Ischemic stroke	Autonomic dysfunction
Diabetic ketoacidosis	Myxedema	Myxedema	Autonomic dysfunction	Autonomic dysfunction	Burns
Diabetic hypoglycemia	Diabetic ketoacidosis	Diabetic ketoacidosis	Malnutrition	Malnutrition	Malnutrition
	Diabetic hypoglycemia	Diabetic hypoglycemia	Erythroderma	Erythroderma	Erythroderma
			Near drowning	Near drowning	Near drowning
			Myxedema	Myxedema	Myxedema
			Diabetic ketoacidosis	Diabetic ketoacidosis	Diabetic ketoacidosis
			Diabetic hypoglycemia	Diabetic hypoglycemia	Diabetic hypoglycemia

Emergency Rule Out conditions shown in red. Entries in blue are for information only
Conditions are listed in approximate order of prevalence for this age range

Emergency Rule Out conditions shown in red. Entries in blue are for information only
Conditions are listed in approximate order of prevalence for this age range

Baby (0-1 yr)	Child (1-12 yr)	Adolescent (12-18 yr)	Adult (18-45 yr)	Middle Age Adult (45-65 yr)	Senior Adult (65+ yr)
Hypoxia	Muscular dystrophy	Muscular dystrophy	Ischemic stroke	Ischemic stroke	Ischemic stroke
Sepsis	Guillain-Barré syndrome (acute infective polyneuritis)	Guillain-Barré syndrome (acute infective polyneuritis)	Cerebral palsy	Cerebral palsy	Cerebral palsy
Viral infection	Hyponatremia	Myasthenia gravis	Rheumatic fever	Rheumatic fever	Osteomalacia
Bacterial meningitis	Viral meningitis	Cerebral palsy	Osteomalacia	Hyponatremia	Hyponatremia
Hyponatremia	Inborn errors of metabolism	Down syndrome	Hyponatremia	Osteomalacia	Rheumatic fever
Viral meningitis	Hypothyroidism	Hyponatremia	Amyotrophic lateral sclerosis (motor neuron disease)	Amyotrophic lateral sclerosis (motor neuron disease)	Amyotrophic lateral sclerosis (motor neuron disease)
Inborn errors of metabolism	Cerebral palsy	Osteomalacia	Guillain-Barré syndrome (acute infective polyneuritis)	Guillain-Barré syndrome (acute infective polyneuritis)	Guillain-Barré syndrome (acute infective polyneuritis)
Hypothyroidism	Down syndrome	Prader-Willi syndrome	Huntington's disease	Huntington's disease	Porphyria
Cerebral palsy	Prader-Willi syndrome	Marfan's syndrome	Porphyria	Porphyria	
Down syndrome	Marfan's syndrome	Rickets in children	Inborn errors of metabolism	Spinal muscular atrophy	
Muscular dystrophy	Osteomalacia	Celiac disease	Myotonic dystrophy		
Guillain-Barré syndrome (acute infective polyneuritis)	Rickets in children	Hypothyroidism	Spinal muscular atrophy		
Prader-Willi syndrome	Celiac disease	Inborn errors of metabolism			
Marfan's syndrome	Hypothyroidism	Myotonic dystrophy			
Rickets in children	Inborn errors of metabolism	Spinal muscular atrophy			
Celiac disease	Myotonic dystrophy				
Myotonic dystrophy	Spinal muscular atrophy				
Spinal muscular atrophy	Mucopolysaccharidosis				
Mucopolysaccharidosis	Sepsis				
Encephalitis	Bacterial meningitis				
Osteomalacia	Viral meningitis				
	Encephalitis				

192

Baby (0-1 yr)	Child (1-12 yr)	Adolescent (12-18 yr)	Adult (18-45 yr)	Middle Age Adult (45-65 yr)	Senior Adult (65+ yr)
Trauma	Trauma	Trauma	Trauma	Trauma	Lower GI bleeding
Lower GI bleeding	Snake and reptile bites	Dysfunctional uterine bleeding	Dysfunctional uterine bleeding	Lower GI bleeding	Upper GI bleeding
Rocky Mountain spotted fever	Rocky Mountain spotted fever	Lower GI bleeding	Lower GI bleeding	Upper GI bleeding	Fracture
Snake and reptile bites	Lower GI bleeding	Rocky Mountain spotted fever	Upper GI bleeding	Snake and reptile bites	Snake and reptile bites
Upper GI bleeding	Upper GI bleeding	Snake and reptile bites	Snake and reptile bites	Rocky Mountain spotted fever	Rocky Mountain spotted fever
Hemolytic disease of the newborn (erythroblastosis fetalis)	Pseudomembranous colitis	Upper GI bleeding	Rocky Mountain spotted fever	Fracture	Trauma
Pseudomembranous colitis		Pseudomembranous colitis	Fracture	Retroperitoneal hemorrhage	Abdominal aortic aneurysm
			Retroperitoneal hemorrhage	Abdominal aortic aneurysm	Thoracic aortic aneurysm
			Abdominal aortic aneurysm	Thoracic aortic aneurysm	Retroperitoneal hemorrhage
			Thoracic aortic aneurysm	Pseudomembranous colitis	Pseudomembranous colitis
			Pseudomembranous colitis		

Emergency Rule Out conditions shown in red. Entries in blue are for information only
Conditions are listed in approximate order of prevalence for this age range

Emergency Rule Out conditions shown in red. Entries in blue are for information only
Conditions are listed in approximate order of prevalence for this age range

Baby (0-1 yr)	Child (1-12 yr)	Adolescent (12-18 yr)	Adult (18-45 yr)	Middle Age Adult (45-65 yr)	Senior Adult (65+ yr)
Trauma	Trauma	Trauma	Trauma	Trauma	Trauma
Dehydration	Dehydration	Dehydration	Upper GI bleeding	Upper GI bleeding	Upper GI bleeding
Gastroenteritis	Gastroenteritis	Gastroenteritis	Lower GI bleeding	Lower GI bleeding	Lower GI bleeding
Pyloric stenosis	Salmonella infection	Salmonella infection	Dehydration	Dehydration	Dehydration
Snake and reptile bites	Shigellosis	Shigellosis	Burns	Burns	Burns
Shigellosis	Snake and reptile bites	Snake and reptile bites	Snake and reptile bites	Snake and reptile bites	Snake and reptile bites
Salmonella infection	Cholera	Abruptio placentae	Abruptio placentae	Abruptio placentae	Diabetic ketoacidosis
Cholera	Upper GI bleeding	Cholera	Diabetic ketoacidosis	Diabetic ketoacidosis	Salmonella infection
Upper GI bleeding	Lower GI bleeding	Upper GI bleeding	Salmonella infection	Salmonella infection	Shigellosis
Lower GI bleeding	Burns	Lower GI bleeding	Shigellosis	Shigellosis	Gastroenteritis
Burns	Diabetic ketoacidosis	Burns	Gastroenteritis	Gastroenteritis	Cholera
Diabetes mellitus in children	Diabetes mellitus in children	Diabetic ketoacidosis	Cholera	Cholera	

Baby (0-1 yr)	Child (1-12 yr)	Adolescent (12-18 yr)	Adult (18-45 yr)	Middle Age Adult (45-65 yr)	Senior Adult (65+ yr)
Birth asphyxia	Bronchiolitis	Asthma	Asthma	Asthma	Asthma
Neonatal respiratory distress syndrome	Asthma	Congestive heart failure	Chronic obstructive pulmonary disease	Chronic obstructive pulmonary disease	Chronic obstructive pulmonary disease
Bacteremia	Congestive heart failure	Congenital heart disease	Bacterial pneumonia	Bacterial pneumonia	Bacterial pneumonia
Congestive heart failure	Congenital heart disease	Bacterial pneumonia	Congestive heart failure	Congestive heart failure	Congestive heart failure
Congenital heart disease	Bacterial pneumonia	Mycoplasmal pneumonia	Pneumothorax	Pneumothorax	Pneumothorax
Extrinsic airway compression	Viral pneumonia	Viral pneumonia	Pleural effusion	Pleural effusion	Pleural effusion
Foreign body	Mycoplasmal pneumonia	Bacteremia	Pulmonary thromboembolism	Pulmonary thromboembolism	Pulmonary thromboembolism
Croup	Pertussis	Tonsillar hypertrophy	Primary lung malignancy	Allergic reactions and anaphylaxis	Primary lung malignancy
Epiglottitis	Bacteremia	Extrinsic airway compression	Smoke inhalation injury	Primary lung malignancy	Smoke inhalation injury
Bronchiolitis	Tonsillar hypertrophy	Foreign body	Tuberculosis	Smoke inhalation injury	Tuberculosis
Allergic reactions and anaphylaxis	Extrinsic airway compression	Croup	Allergic reactions and anaphylaxis	Tuberculosis	Extrinsic airway compression
Foreign body	Allergic reactions and anaphylaxis	Epiglottitis	Extrinsic airway compression	Extrinsic airway compression	Allergic reactions and anaphylaxis
Bacterial pneumonia	Foreign body	Epilepsy	Idiopathic pulmonary interstitial fibrosis	Allergic reactions and anaphylaxis	Idiopathic pulmonary interstitial fibrosis
Mycoplasmal pneumonia	Croup	Allergic reactions and anaphylaxis	Kyphosis	Idiopathic pulmonary interstitial fibrosis	Kyphosis
Viral pneumonia	Epiglottitis	Febrile seizure	Kyphoscoliosis	Kyphosis	Kyphoscoliosis
Pertussis	Epilepsy	Bronchiectasis	Near drowning	Kyphoscoliosis	Near drowning
Epilepsy	Febrile seizure	Muscular dystrophy		Near drowning	
Febrile seizure	Bronchiectasis	Guillain-Barré syndrome (acute infective polyneuritis)			
Obstructive sleep apnea	Guillain-Barré syndrome (acute infective polyneuritis)				
Asthma					

List continues on next page

Emergency Rule Out conditions shown in red. Entries in blue are for information only
Conditions are listed in approximate order of prevalence for this age range

195

Baby (0-1 yr)	Child (1-12 yr)	Adolescent (12-18 yr)	Adult (18-45 yr)	Middle Age Adult (45-65 yr)	Senior Adult (65+ yr)
Atelectasis	Muscular dystrophy	Myasthenia gravis	Guillain-Barré syndrome (acute infective polyneuritis)	Guillain-Barré syndrome (acute infective polyneuritis)	Guillain-Barré syndrome (acute infective polyneuritis)
Raised intracranial pressure	Myasthenia gravis	Atelectasis	Myasthenia gravis	Myasthenia gravis	Myasthenia gravis
Pleural effusion	Atelectasis	Pleural effusion	Adult respiratory distress syndrome	Adult respiratory distress syndrome	Adult respiratory distress syndrome
Pneumothorax	Pleural effusion	Pneumothorax	Atelectasis	Atelectasis	Atelectasis
Sepsis	Pneumothorax	Raised intracranial pressure	Foreign body	Foreign body	Foreign body
Choanal atresia	Raised intracranial pressure	Pertussis	Raised intracranial pressure	Raised intracranial pressure	Raised intracranial pressure
	Cystic fibrosis	Cystic fibrosis	Amyotrophic lateral sclerosis (motor neuron disease)	Amyotrophic lateral sclerosis (motor neuron disease)	Amyotrophic lateral sclerosis (motor neuron disease)

Baby (0-1 yr)	Child (1-12 yr)	Adolescent (12-18 yr)	Adult (18-45 yr)	Middle Age Adult (45-65 yr)	Senior Adult (65+ yr)
Urinary tract infection	Urinary tract infection	Urinary tract infection	Prostatitis	Prostatitis	Benign prostatic hyperplasia
Distended urinary bladder	Constipation	Distended urinary bladder	Urinary tract infection	Urinary tract infection	Prostatic cancer
Posterior urethral valves	Distended urinary bladder	Constipation	Distended urinary bladder	Benign prostatic hyperplasia	Distended urinary bladder
Constipation	Posterior urethral valves	Pelvic tumor	Drug reaction	Drug reaction	Drug reaction
Pelvic tumor	Pelvic tumor	Prostatitis	Diabetic neuropathy	Distended urinary bladder	Diabetic neuropathy
		Posterior urethral valves	Constipation	Diabetic neuropathy	Urinary tract infection
			Prostatic cancer	Constipation	Prostatitis
			Retroverted uterus in pregnancy	Prostatic cancer	Constipation
			Genital herpes	Genital herpes	Pelvic tumor
			Pelvic tumor	Pelvic tumor	Herpes zoster, shingles
			Benign prostatic hyperplasia	Prostatic abscess	Post-prostatectomy
			Prostatic abscess	Prostate calculus	Prostate calculus
			Prostate calculus	Post-prostatectomy	Prostatic abscess
			Post-prostatectomy	Herpes zoster, shingles	Genital herpes
			Herpes zoster, shingles	Retroverted uterus in pregnancy	

Incomplete bladder emptying

Emergency Rule Out conditions shown in red. Entries in blue are for information only
Conditions are listed in approximate order of prevalence for this age range

Emergency Rule Out conditions shown in red. Entries in blue are for information only
Conditions are listed in approximate order of prevalence for this age range

Baby (0-1 yr)	Child (1-12 yr)	Adolescent (12-18 yr)	Adult (18-45 yr)	Middle Age Adult (45-65 yr)	Senior Adult (65- yr)
Urinary tract infection	Cystitis	Cystitis	Cystitis	Cystitis	Female stress incontinence
Carbon monoxide poisoning	Enuresis	Enuresis	Female stress incontinence	Female stress incontinence	Cystitis
Dementia	Urinary tract infection	Neurogenic bladder	Urinary tract infection	Urinary tract infection	Urinary tract infection
Lumbar disc disorders	Neurogenic bladder	Lumbar disc disorders	Drug reaction	Benign prostatic hyperplasia	Drug reaction
	Ectopic ureter	Drug reaction	Prostatitis	Drug reaction	Benign prostatic hyperplasia
	Dementia	Dementia	Lumbar disc disorders	Prostatitis	Post-prostatectomy
	Diabetes mellitus in children	Urinary tract infection	Dementia	Dementia	Dementia
	Cough	Carbon monoxide poisoning	Decreased cortical inhibition	Post-prostatectomy	Lumbar disc disorders
	Bladder outlet obstruction	Bladder diverticula	Carbon monoxide poisoning	Lumbar disc disorders	Carbon monoxide poisoning
	Lumbar disc disorders	Ectopic ureter	Multiple sclerosis	Decreased cortical inhibition	Prostatitis
	Carbon monoxide poisoning	Cough	Spinal cord compression	Carbon monoxide poisoning	Spinal cord compression
	Drug reaction	Decreased cortical inhibition	Benign prostatic hyperplasia	Multiple sclerosis	Decreased cortical inhibition
	Decreased cortical inhibition	Diabetes mellitus in children	Bladder outlet obstruction	Spinal cord compression	Multiple sclerosis
	Bladder diverticula	Bladder outlet obstruction	Bladder diverticula	Bladder outlet obstruction	Bladder outlet obstruction
		Prostatitis	Post-prostatectomy	Bladder diverticula	Bladder diverticula
		Prostatic abscess			Normal pressure hydrocephalus

Baby (0-1 yr)	Child (1-12 yr)	Adolescent (12-18 yr)	Adult (18-45 yr)	Middle Age Adult (45-65 yr)	Senior Adult (65+yr)
Gastroenteritis	Anxiety	Anxiety	Anxiety	Anxiety	Anxiety
Constipation	Gastroenteritis	Gastroenteritis	Gastroenteritis	Gastroenteritis	Gastroenteritis
Intussusception	Constipation	Drug reaction	Drug reaction	Drug reaction	Drug reaction
Intestinal obstruction	Intestinal obstruction	Constipation	Constipation	Constipation	Constipation
Incarcerated hernia	Incarcerated hernia	Intestinal obstruction	Intestinal obstruction	Intestinal obstruction	Intestinal obstruction
Volvulus	Intussusception	Incarcerated hernia	Incarcerated hernia	Incarcerated hernia	Incarcerated hernia
	Volvulus	Volvulus	Volvulus	Volvulus	Volvulus
		Intussusception	Intussusception	Intussusception	Intussusception
			Carcinoid syndrome	Carcinoid syndrome	Carcinoid syndrome
			Peutz-Jeghers syndrome	Peutz-Jeghers syndrome	Peutz-Jeghers syndrome

Increased bowel sounds

Emergency Rule Out conditions shown in red. Entries in blue are for information only
Conditions are listed in approximate order of prevalence for this age range

Emergency Rule Out conditions shown in red. Entries in blue are for information only
Conditions are listed in approximate order of prevalence for this age range

Baby (0-1 yr)	Child (1-12 yr)	Adolescent (12-18 yr)	Adult (18-45 yr)	Middle Age Adult (45-65 yr)	Senior Adult (65+ yr)
Foreign body	Foreign body	Foreign body	Foreign body	Foreign body	Foreign body
Viral conjunctivitis	Viral conjunctivitis	Hordeolum, chalazion, blepharitis	Bacterial conjunctivitis	Bacterial conjunctivitis	Bacterial conjunctivitis
Hordeolum, chalazion, blepharitis	Episcleritis	Dry eye	Cluster headache	Cluster headache	Cluster headache
Upper respiratory tract infections	Upper respiratory tract infections	Chlamydial conjunctivitis	Upper respiratory tract infections	Chlamydial conjunctivitis	Dry eye
Episcleritis	Dry eye	Upper respiratory tract infections	Chlamydial conjunctivitis	Upper respiratory tract infections	Chlamydial conjunctivitis
Chlamydial conjunctivitis	Chlamydial conjunctivitis	Episcleritis	Dry eye	Dry eye	Upper respiratory tract infections
Dry eye	Cluster headache	Cluster headache	Episcleritis	Episcleritis	Episcleritis
Cluster headache	Hordeolum, chalazion, blepharitis	Viral conjunctivitis	Hordeolum, chalazion, blepharitis	Hordeolum, chalazion, blepharitis	Hordeolum, chalazion, blepharitis
Corneal abrasion	Corneal abrasion	Corneal abrasion	Corneal abrasion	Corneal abrasion	Corneal abrasion
Congenital nasolacrimal duct stenosis	Uveitis	Uveitis	Glaucoma	Glaucoma	Glaucoma
Uveitis	Pertussis	Pertussis	Uveitis	Uveitis	Uveitis
Pertussis			Pertussis	Pertussis	Pertussis

Baby (0-1 yr)	Child (1-12 yr)	Adolescent (12-18 yr)	Adult (18-45 yr)	Middle Age Adult (45-65 yr)	Senior Adult (65+ yr)
Inguinal hernia	Inguinal hernia	Inguinal hernia	Inguinal hernia	Inguinal hernia	Inguinal hernia
Hydrocele	Hydrocele	Hydrocele	Hydrocele	Hydrocele	Chancroid
Lymphadenopathy	Chancroid	Chancroid	Chancroid	Chancroid	Hydrocele
Malignant lymphadenopathy	Lymphadenopathy	Lymphadenopathy	Lymphadenopathy	Lymphadenopathy	Lymphadenopathy
Trauma	Malignant lymphadenopathy	Malignant lymphadenopathy	Malignant lymphadenopathy	Malignant lymphadenopathy	Malignant lymphadenopathy
	Trauma	Trauma	Trauma	Trauma	Trauma

Inguinal swelling

Emergency Rule Out conditions shown in red. Entries in blue are for information only
Conditions are listed in approximate order of prevalence for this age range

Emergency Rule Out conditions shown in red. Entries in blue are for information only
Conditions are listed in approximate order of prevalence for this age range

Baby (0-1 yr)	Child (1-12 yr)	Adolescent (12-18 yr)	Adult (18-45 yr)	Middle Age Adult (45-65 yr)	Senior Adult (65+ yr)
Meatal stenosis	Urethral stricture	Urethral stricture	Benign prostatic hyperplasia	Benign prostatic hyperplasia	Benign prostatic hyperplasia
Posterior urethral valves	Meatal stenosis	Meatal stenosis	Prostatic cancer	Prostatic cancer	Prostatic cancer
Neurogenic bladder	Bladder outlet obstruction	Bladder outlet obstruction	Urethral stricture	Urethral stricture	Urethral stricture
Megaureter	Ectopic ureter	Ectopic ureter	Meatal stenosis	Meatal stenosis	Meatal stenosis
Ectopic ureter	Neurogenic bladder	Neurogenic bladder	Bladder outlet obstruction	Bladder outlet obstruction	Bladder outlet obstruction
Bladder diverticula	Ureterocele	Ureterocele	Ectopic ureter	Ectopic ureter	Ectopic ureter
Ureterocele	Megaureter	Megaureter	Neurogenic bladder	Neurogenic bladder	Neurogenic bladder
Bladder outlet obstruction	Bladder diverticula	Bladder diverticula	Ureterocele	Ureterocele	Ureterocele
	Posterior urethral valves	Posterior urethral valves	Megaureter	Megaureter	Megaureter
			Bladder diverticula	Bladder diverticula	Bladder diverticula

Baby (0-1 yr)	Child (1-12 yr)	Adolescent (12-18 yr)	Adult (18-45 yr)	Middle Age Adult (45-65 yr)	Senior Adult (65+ yr)
Fecal impaction	Fecal impaction	Fecal impaction	Fecal impaction	Fecal impaction	Fecal impaction
Imperforate anus	Intussusception	Paralytic ileus	Paralytic ileus	Paralytic ileus	Paralytic ileus
Meconium ileus	Volvulus	Volvulus	Adhesions	Adhesions	Malignancy
Hirschsprung's disease	Paralytic ileus	Intussusception	Acute iron toxicity	Acute iron toxicity	Adhesions
Paralytic ileus	Acute iron toxicity	Carcinoid syndrome	Carcinoid syndrome	Malignancy	Acute iron toxicity
Carcinoid syndrome	Carcinoid syndrome	Acute iron toxicity	Malignancy	Abdominal hernias	Foreign body
Volvulus	Cystic fibrosis	Acute appendicitis	Abdominal hernias	Carcinoid syndrome	Abdominal hernias
Intussusception	Acute appendicitis	Hirschsprung's disease	Foreign body	Foreign body	Carcinoid syndrome
Duodenal atresia	Hirschsprung's disease	Cystic fibrosis	Crohn's disease	Crohn's disease	Volvulus
Pyloric stenosis	Ulcerative colitis	Ulcerative colitis	Ulcerative colitis	Ulcerative colitis	Intussusception
Peritonitis	Crohn's disease	Crohn's disease	Volvulus	Volvulus	Crohn's disease
	Peritonitis	Peritonitis			Ulcerative colitis

Emergency Rule Out conditions shown in red. Entries in blue are for information only
Conditions are listed in approximate order of prevalence for this age range

203

Emergency Rule Out conditions shown in red. Entries in blue are for information only
Conditions are listed in approximate order of prevalence for this age range

Baby (0-1 yr)	Child (1-12 yr)	Adolescent (12-18 yr)	Adult (18-45 yr)	Middle Age Adult (45-65 yr)	Senior Adult (65+ yr)
Febrile seizure	Febrile seizure	Epilepsy	Drug reaction	Drug reaction	Drug reaction
Epilepsy	Cerebral palsy	Benign essential/familial tremor syndrome	Alcohol abuse	Alcohol abuse	Alcohol abuse
Cerebral palsy	Epilepsy	Cerebral palsy	Epilepsy	Epilepsy	Epilepsy
Carbon monoxide poisoning	Tourette's syndrome	Tourette's syndrome	Benign essential/familial tremor syndrome	Benign essential/familial tremor syndrome	Benign essential/familial tremor syndrome
Chorea	Chorea	Febrile seizure	Hyperthyroidism	Hyperthyroidism	Hyperthyroidism
Dystonia	Carbon monoxide poisoning	Chorea	Parkinson's disease	Parkinson's disease	Parkinson's disease
Ataxia-telangiectasia	Brain tumor	Carbon monoxide poisoning	Encephalopathy	Encephalopathy	Encephalopathy
	Friedreich's ataxia	Brain tumor	Multiple sclerosis	Multiple sclerosis	Chorea
	Ataxia-telangiectasia	Dystonia	Chorea	Brain tumor	Torticollis
	Dystonia	Ataxia-telangiectasia	Brain tumor	Chorea	Brain tumor
	Wilson's disease	Friedreich's ataxia	Torticollis	Carbon monoxide poisoning	Huntington's disease
		Wilson's disease	Carbon monoxide poisoning	Torticollis	Liver failure
			Parkinson's disease	Huntington's disease	Carbon monoxide poisoning
			Huntington's disease	Liver failure	Systemic lupus erythematosus
			Liver failure	Systemic lupus erythematosus	Polycythemia vera
			Systemic lupus erythematosus	Polycythemia vera	Multiple sclerosis
			Polycythemia vera	Amyotrophic lateral sclerosis (motor neuron disease)	Amyotrophic lateral sclerosis (motor neuron disease)
			Amyotrophic lateral sclerosis (motor neuron disease)	Wilson's disease	Wilson's disease
			Wilson's disease	Tourette's syndrome	Tourette's syndrome
			Tourette's syndrome		

Baby (0-1 yr)	Child (1-12 yr)	Adolescent (12-18 yr)	Adult (18-45 yr)	Middle Age Adult (45-65 yr)	Senior Adult (65+ yr)
Rh incompatibility	Viral hepatitis	Viral hepatitis	Viral hepatitis	Viral hepatitis	Viral hepatitis
Drug reaction	Drug reaction	Drug reaction	Cholecystitis	Pancreatic cancer	Pancreatic cancer
Newborn jaundice	Hemolytic transfusion reaction	Hepatoma	Alcoholic hepatitis	Cholecystitis	Cholecystitis
Indirect neonatal hyperbilirubinemia	Liver cirrhosis	Liver cirrhosis	Drug reaction	Alcoholic hepatitis	Alcoholic hepatitis
Liver cirrhosis	Budd-Chiari syndrome	Budd-Chiari syndrome	Hemolysis	Drug reaction	Liver cirrhosis
Hepatoma	Hepatoma	Hemolytic transfusion reaction	Liver cirrhosis	Liver cirrhosis	Drug reaction
Hemolytic disease of the newborn (erythroblastosis fetalis)	Leptospirosis	Leptospirosis	Budd-Chiari syndrome	Yellow fever	Hepatoma
Budd-Chiari syndrome	Yellow fever	Yellow fever	Leptospirosis	Budd-Chiari syndrome	Hemolytic transfusion reaction
Kernicterus	Bartonella infection (cat scratch disease)	Bartonella infection (cat scratch disease)	Hemolytic transfusion reaction	Leptospirosis	Leptospirosis
Leptospirosis	Thalassemia	Thalassemia	Yellow fever	Hemolytic transfusion reaction	Budd-Chiari syndrome
Yellow fever			Hepatoma	Hepatoma	Hemolysis
Breast-feeding			Bartonella infection (cat scratch disease)	Hemolysis	Yellow fever
Biliary atresia			Metastatic neoplasm of the liver	Gilbert's disease	Gilbert's disease
Hypothyroidism			Gilbert's disease	Metastatic neoplasm of the liver	Metastatic neoplasm of the liver
Thalassemia			Mononucleosis	Mononucleosis	Mononucleosis
			Acute leukemia	Acute leukemia	Acute leukemia
			Amyloidosis	Amyloidosis	Amyloidosis
			Malaria	Malaria	Malaria
				Schistosomiasis	Schistosomiasis
				Thalassemia	Thalassemia

List continues on next page

Emergency Rule Out conditions shown in red. Entries in blue are for information only
Conditions are listed in approximate order of prevalence for this age range

205

List continued from previous page

Baby (0-1 yr)	Child (1-12 yr)	Adolescent (12-18 yr)	Adult (18-45 yr)	Middle Age Adult (45-65 yr)	Senior Adult (65+ yr)
			Schistosomiasis Thalassemia		

Baby (0-1 yr)	Child (1-12 yr)	Adolescent (12-18 yr)	Adult (18-45 yr)	Middle Age Adult (45-65 yr)	Senior Adult (65+ yr)
Not relevant to this age group	Congestive heart failure Cardiac tamponade Fluid overload Pericarditis Tricuspid regurgitation Superior vena cava syndrome	Congestive heart failure Cardiac tamponade Fluid overload Pneumothorax Pericarditis Tricuspid regurgitation Superior vena cava syndrome	Congestive heart failure Sinus bradycardia Pericarditis Pneumothorax Pulmonary hypertension Tricuspid regurgitation Superior vena cava syndrome Cardiac tamponade	Congestive heart failure Sinus bradycardia Pericarditis Tricuspid regurgitation Pneumothorax Superior vena cava syndrome Cardiac tamponade	Congestive heart failure Sinus bradycardia Pericarditis Tricuspid regurgitation Pneumothorax Superior vena cava syndrome Cardiac tamponade

Emergency Rule Out conditions shown in red. Entries in blue are for information only
Conditions are listed in approximate order of prevalence for this age range

Jugular venous distension

Emergency Rule Out conditions shown in red. Entries in blue are for information only
Conditions are listed in approximate order of prevalence for this age range

Baby (0-1 yr)	Child (1-12 yr)	Adolescent (12-18 yr)	Adult (18-45 yr)	Middle Age Adult (45-65 yr)	Senior Adult (65+ yr)
Trauma	Chondromalacia patellae (patellofemoral pain syndrome)	Chondromalacia patellae (patellofemoral pain syndrome)	Chondromalacia patellae (patellofemoral pain syndrome)	Collateral ligament sprain	Osteoarthritis
	Collateral ligament sprain	Collateral ligament sprain	Collateral ligament sprain	Chondromalacia patellae (patellofemoral pain syndrome)	Collateral ligament sprain
	Meniscal tear	Meniscal tear	Meniscal tear	Meniscal tear	Meniscal tear
	Slipped femoral epiphysis	Anterior cruciate ligament tear	Anterior cruciate ligament tear	Anterior cruciate ligament tear	Septic arthritis
	Anterior cruciate ligament tear	Tendinitis	Tendinitis	Tendinitis	Anterior cruciate ligament tear
	Tendinitis	Slipped femoral epiphysis	Baker's cyst	Baker's cyst	Tendinitis
	Fracture	Muscular strain	Slipped femoral epiphysis	Aseptic bursitis	Slipped femoral epiphysis
	Patellar dislocation	Fracture	Aseptic bursitis	Slipped femoral epiphysis	Muscular strain
	Osteochondritis dissecans	Patellar dislocation	Muscular strain	Muscular strain	Baker's cyst
	Septic arthritis	Osteochondritis dissecans	Fracture	Osteoarthritis	Chondromalacia patellae (patellofemoral pain syndrome)
	Osgood-Schlatter disease	Hemarthrosis	Patellar dislocation	Fracture	Hemarthrosis
	Trauma	Septic arthritis	Hemarthrosis	Patellar dislocation	Patellar dislocation
		Osgood-Schlatter disease	Septic arthritis	Hemarthrosis	Aseptic bursitis
			Osteonecrosis	Septic arthritis	Fracture
			Osteoarthritis	Osteonecrosis	Osteonecrosis
			Osgood-Schlatter disease	Osgood-Schlatter disease	Osgood-Schlatter disease

Baby (0-1 yr)	Child (1-12 yr)	Adolescent (12-18 yr)	Adult (18-45 yr)	Middle Age Adult (45-65 yr)	Senior Adult (65+yr)
Inborn errors of metabolism Metabolic acidosis Diabetes mellitus in children Diabetic ketoacidosis Ischemic encephalopathy Chronic renal failure	Metabolic acidosis Diabetic ketoacidosis Inborn errors of metabolism Diabetes mellitus in children Ischemic encephalopathy Chronic renal failure Peritonitis Hemorrhage into tissue	Metabolic acidosis Chronic renal failure Diabetic ketoacidosis Hemorrhage into tissue	Metabolic acidosis Diabetic ketoacidosis Chronic renal failure Hemorrhage into tissue	Metabolic acidosis Chronic renal failure Diabetic ketoacidosis Aspiration pneumonia Bacterial pneumonia	Metabolic acidosis Chronic renal failure Aspiration pneumonia Bacterial pneumonia

Emergency Rule Out conditions shown in red. Entries in blue are for information only
Conditions are listed in approximate order of prevalence for this age range

Kussmaul breathing

Emergency Rule Out conditions shown in red. Entries in blue are for information only
Conditions are listed in approximate order of prevalence for this age range

Lack of normal physiological development

Baby (0-1 yr)	Child (1-12 yr)	Adolescent (12-18 yr)	Adult (18-45 yr)	Middle Age Adult (45-65 yr)	Senior Adult (65+yr)
Developmental delay	Developmental delay	Developmental delay	Congenital heart disease	Congenital heart disease	Congenital heart disease
Congenital heart disease	Congenital heart disease	Congenital heart disease	Nutritional deficiencies	Nutritional deficiencies	Nutritional deficiencies
Nutritional deficiencies	Hypothyroidism	Hypothyroidism	Chronic infection	Chronic infection	Chronic infection
Chronic infection	Chronic renal failure	Chronic renal failure	Malabsorption	Hyperprolactinemia	Malabsorption
Malabsorption	Nutritional deficiencies	Fragile X syndrome	Fragile X syndrome	Malabsorption	Hyperprolactinemia
Hyperprolactinemia	Fragile X syndrome	Nutritional deficiencies	Chronic renal failure	Fragile X syndrome	Fragile X syndrome
Fragile X syndrome	Precocious puberty	Hyperprolactinemia	Hyperprolactinemia	Chronic renal failure	Chronic renal failure
Precocious puberty	Hyperprolactinemia	Chronic infection	Congenital megacolon	Hypothyroidism	Hypothyroidism
Diabetes mellitus in children	Chronic infection	Child abuse	Hypothyroidism	Congenital megacolon	Immunodeficiency diseases
Child abuse	Child abuse	Malabsorption	Immunodeficiency diseases	Immunodeficiency diseases	Congenital megacolon
Hypothyroidism	Malabsorption	Diabetes mellitus in children	Classic congenital adrenal hyperplasia	Classic congenital adrenal hyperplasia	Classic congenital adrenal hyperplasia
Classic congenital adrenal hyperplasia	Diabetes mellitus in children	Congenital megacolon	Late onset congenital adrenal hyperplasia	Late onset congenital adrenal hyperplasia	Late onset congenital adrenal hyperplasia
Immunodeficiency diseases	Congenital megacolon	Classic congenital adrenal hyperplasia	Hypopituitarism	Hypopituitarism	Hypopituitarism
Congenital megacolon	Classic congenital adrenal hyperplasia	Immunodeficiency diseases	Thalassemia	Thalassemia	Thalassemia
Chronic renal failure	Immunodeficiency diseases	Diabetes insipidus			
Diabetes insipidus	Diabetes insipidus	Late onset congenital adrenal hyperplasia			
Late onset congenital adrenal hyperplasia	Late onset congenital adrenal hyperplasia	Hypopituitarism			
Hypopituitarism	Hypopituitarism	Thalassemia			
Thalassemia	Thalassemia				

Baby (0-1 yr)	Child (1-12 yr)	Adolescent (12-18 yr)	Adult (18-45 yr)	Middle Age Adult (45-65 yr)	Senior Adult (65+ yr)
Allergic reactions and anaphylaxis	Allergic reactions and anaphylaxis	Allergic reactions and anaphylaxis	Allergic reactions and anaphylaxis	Allergic reactions and anaphylaxis	Allergic reactions and anaphylaxis
Smoke inhalation injury	Smoke inhalation injury	Smoke inhalation injury	Angioedema	Angioedema	Angioedema
Burns	Burns	Burns	Smoke inhalation injury	Smoke inhalation injury	Smoke inhalation injury
Foreign body	Foreign body	Angioedema	Burns	Burns	Burns
Epiglottitis	Angioedema	Foreign body	Foreign body	Foreign body	Foreign body
Angioedema	Epiglottitis	Epiglottitis	Corrosive acid ingestion	Corrosive acid ingestion	Corrosive acid ingestion
Post-tracheostomy	Post-tracheostomy	Post-tracheostomy	Neck injury	Neck injury	Neck injury
Corrosive acid ingestion	Corrosive acid ingestion	Corrosive acid ingestion	Laryngeal cancer	Laryngeal cancer	Laryngeal cancer
Neck injury	Neck injury	Neck injury	Epiglottitis	Epiglottitis	Epiglottitis
			Post-tracheostomy	Post-tracheostomy	Post-tracheostomy

Emergency Rule Out conditions shown in red. Entries in blue are for information only
Conditions are listed in approximate order of prevalence for this age range

Laryngeal edema

Emergency Rule Out conditions shown in red. Entries in blue are for information only
Conditions are listed in approximate order of prevalence for this age range

Learning disorders in children

Baby (0-1 yr)	Child (1-12 yr)	Adolescent (12-18 yr)	Adult (18-45 yr)	Middle Age Adult (45-65 yr)	Senior Adult (65+ yr)
Attention deficit hyperactivity disorder	Down syndrome	Down syndrome	Not relevant to this age group	Not relevant to this age group	Not relevant to this age group
Chronic lead poisoning	Dyslexia	Dyslexia			
Muscular dystrophy	Fragile X syndrome	Fragile X syndrome			
Autism	Turner's syndrome	Turner's syndrome			
	Cerebral palsy	Tuberous sclerosis complex			
	Tuberous sclerosis complex	Autism			
	Muscular dystrophy	Chronic lead poisoning			
	Chronic lead poisoning	Muscular dystrophy			
	Autism	Cerebral palsy			
	Attention deficit hyperactivity disorder	Attention deficit hyperactivity disorder			
	Williams syndrome	Williams syndrome			
	Metabolic acidosis	Metabolic acidosis			
	Metabolic encephalopathy	Metabolic encephalopathy			
	Post-infection	Post-infection			
	Idiopathic	Idiopathic			
	Trauma	Trauma			

Baby (0-1 yr)	Child (1-12 yr)	Adolescent (12-18 yr)	Adult (18-45 yr)	Middle Age Adult (45-65 yr)	Senior Adult (65+ yr)
Lymphatic obstruction	Muscular strain	Cellulitis	Deep vein thrombosis	Deep vein thrombosis	Deep vein thrombosis
Muscular strain	Baker's cyst	Muscular strain	Muscular strain	Muscular strain	Baker's cyst
Cellulitis	Lymphatic obstruction	Deep vein thrombosis	Cellulitis	Cellulitis	Venous insufficiency
Thrombophlebitis	Cellulitis	Baker's cyst	Thrombophlebitis	Baker's cyst	Cellulitis
	Deep vein thrombosis	Venous insufficiency	Postphlebitic syndrome	Venous insufficiency	Muscular strain
	Venous insufficiency	Postphlebitic syndrome	Baker's cyst	Thrombophlebitis	Thrombophlebitis
	Thrombophlebitis	Lymphatic obstruction	Venous insufficiency	Postphlebitic syndrome	Postphlebitic syndrome
		Thrombophlebitis	Lymphatic obstruction	Lymphatic obstruction	Lymphatic obstruction

Emergency Rule Out conditions shown in red. Entries in blue are for information only
Conditions are listed in approximate order of prevalence for this age range

L

Leg ulcer

Emergency Rule Out conditions shown in red. Entries in blue are for information only
Conditions are listed in approximate order of prevalence for this age range

Baby (0-1 yr)	Child (1-12 yr)	Adolescent (12-18 yr)	Adult (18-45 yr)	Middle Age Adult (45-65 yr)	Senior Adult (65+ yr)
Systemic lupus erythematosus	Sickle cell anemia	Sickle cell anemia	Diabetic neuropathy	Diabetic neuropathy	Diabetic neuropathy
Varicose veins	Varicose veins	Varicose veins	Arterial insufficiency	Arterial insufficiency	Arterial insufficiency
	Systemic lupus erythematosus	Systemic lupus erythematosus	Furunculosis	Pressure ulcer	Pressure ulcer
			Lymphangitis	Lymphangitis	Lymphangitis
			Syphilis	Furunculosis	Furunculosis
			Varicose veins	Squamous cell carcinoma	Varicose veins
			Pressure ulcer	Varicose veins	Squamous cell carcinoma
			Squamous cell carcinoma	Acute leukemia	Acute leukemia
			Acute leukemia	Syphilis	Syphilis
			Polycythemia vera	Polycythemia vera	Polycythemia vera
			Scleroderma	Scleroderma	Scleroderma
			Venous insufficiency	Venous insufficiency	Venous insufficiency
			Stasis dermatitis	Stasis dermatitis	Stasis dermatitis
			Systemic lupus erythematosus	Systemic lupus erythematosus	Systemic lupus erythematosus

214

Baby (0-1 yr)	Child (1-12 yr)	Adolescent (12-18 yr)	Adult (18-45 yr)	Middle Age Adult (45-65 yr)	Senior Adult (65+ yr)
Atopic dermatitis	Atopic dermatitis Psoriasis Palmar-plantar warts	Atopic dermatitis Psoriasis Palmar-plantar warts	Palmar-plantar warts Atopic dermatitis Psoriasis Lichen planus	Palmar-plantar warts Atopic dermatitis Psoriasis Lichen planus	Palmar-plantar warts Atopic dermatitis Psoriasis Lichen planus

Emergency Rule Out conditions shown in red. Entries in blue are for information only
Conditions are listed in approximate order of prevalence for this age range

Emergency Rule Out conditions shown in red. Entries in blue are for information only
Conditions are listed in approximate order of prevalence for this age range

Baby (0-1 yr)	Child (1-12 yr)	Adolescent (12-18 yr)	Adult (18-45 yr)	Middle Age Adult (45-65 yr)	Senior Adult (65+ yr)
Not relevant to this age group	Anxiety	Anxiety	Orthostatic hypotension	Orthostatic hypotension	Orthostatic hypotension
	Syncope	Syncope	Anxiety	Anxiety	Anxiety
	Carcinoid syndrome	Orthostatic hypotension	Hyperventilation	Myocardial infarction	Myocardial infarction
	Orthostatic hypotension	Myocardial infarction	Myocardial infarction	Hyperventilation	Hyperventilation
	Myocardial infarction	Carcinoid syndrome	Carcinoid syndrome	Carcinoid syndrome	Carcinoid syndrome
	Hyperventilation	Hyperventilation	Conversion disorder	Conversion disorder	Conversion disorder
	Anemia	Panic disorder	Panic disorder	Panic disorder	Panic disorder
	Panic disorder	Anemia	Syncope	Syncope	Chronic fatigue syndrome
	Chronic fatigue syndrome	Conversion disorder	Anemia	Anemia	Anemia
	Conversion disorder	Alcohol abuse	Agoraphobia	Chronic fatigue syndrome	Syncope
	Agoraphobia	Chronic fatigue syndrome	Chronic fatigue syndrome	Agoraphobia	Agoraphobia
	AV block, second degree	Agoraphobia	AV block, second degree	AV block, second degree	AV block, second degree
	AV block, third degree	AV block, second degree	AV block, third degree	AV block, third degree	AV block, third degree
	Carbon monoxide poisoning	AV block, third degree	Carbon monoxide poisoning	Carbon monoxide poisoning	Carbon monoxide poisoning
	Multiple myeloma	Carbon monoxide poisoning	Multiple myeloma	Multiple myeloma	Multiple myeloma
		Multiple myeloma			

Baby (0-1 yr)	Child (1-12 yr)	Adolescent (12-18 yr)	Adult (18-45 yr)	Middle Age Adult (45-65 yr)	Senior Adult (65- yr)
Epilepsy	Epilepsy	Epilepsy Migraine headache	Temporal lobe epilepsy Migraine headache Epilepsy Transient ischemic attack	Transient ischemic attack Temporal lobe epilepsy Migraine headache Epilepsy	Transient ischemic attack Temporal lobe epilepsy Migraine headache Epilepsy

Emergency Rule Out conditions shown in red. Entries in blue are for information only
Conditions are listed in approximate order of prevalence for this age range

Limb paralysis, transient

Emergency Rule Out conditions shown in red. Entries in blue are for information only
Conditions are listed in approximate order of prevalence for this age range

Baby (0-1 yr)	Child (1-12 yr)	Adolescent (12-18 yr)	Adult (18-45 yr)	Middle Age Adult (45-65 yr)	Senior Adult (65+ yr)
Trauma	Trauma	Trauma	Insect and spider bites and stings	Insect and spider bites and stings	Insect and spider bites and stings
Congestive heart failure	Congestive heart failure	Congestive heart failure	Deep vein thrombosis	Congestive heart failure	Congestive heart failure
Insect and spider bites and stings	Insect and spider bites and stings	Insect and spider bites and stings	Lymphedema	Deep vein thrombosis	Deep vein thrombosis
Cavernous hemangioma	Lymphedema	Lymphedema	Venous insufficiency	Lymphedema	Lymphedema
	Lipoma	Lipoma	Cellulitis	Venous insufficiency	Venous insufficiency
	Cavernous hemangioma	Cavernous hemangioma	Stasis dermatitis	Cellulitis	Cellulitis
			Lipoma	Stasis dermatitis	Stasis dermatitis
			Congestive heart failure	Lipoma	Thrombophlebitis
			Gangrene	Gangrene	
				Thrombophlebitis	

218

Baby (0-1 yr)	Child (1-12 yr)	Adolescent (12-18 yr)	Adult (18-45 yr)	Middle Age Adult (45-65 yr)	Senior Adult (65+ yr)
Muscular strain	Muscular strain	Muscular strain	Muscular strain	Muscular strain	Muscular strain
Uterine prolapse	Idiopathic	Idiopathic	Lumbar disc disorders	Lumbar disc disorders	Lumbar disc disorders
Cervical malignancy	Trauma	Trauma	Pyelonephritis	Osteoarthritis	Osteoarthritis
Cervical hyperextension injuries	Fracture	Addison's disease	Kyphoscoliosis	Pyelonephritis	Osteoporosis
Guillain-Barré syndrome (acute infective polyneuritis)	Guillain-Barré syndrome (acute infective polyneuritis)	Guillain-Barré syndrome (acute infective polyneuritis)	Sacroiliitis	Sacroiliitis	Pyelonephritis
Benign ovarian tumor	Cervical hyperextension injuries	Cervical hyperextension injuries	Guillain-Barré syndrome (acute infective polyneuritis)	Addison's disease	Guillain-Barré syndrome (acute infective polyneuritis)
	Cervical malignancy	Benign ovarian tumor	Cervical hyperextension injuries	Guillain-Barré syndrome (acute infective polyneuritis)	Cervical malignancy
	Benign ovarian tumor	Cervical malignancy	Addison's disease	Cervical hyperextension injuries	Cervical hyperextension injuries
	Addison's disease	Fracture	Ankylosing spondylitis	Benign ovarian tumor	Benign ovarian tumor
	Osteochondritis dissecans	Osteochondritis dissecans	Cervical malignancy	Cervical malignancy	Sacroiliitis
	Osteomyelitis	Osteomyelitis	Benign ovarian tumor	Kyphoscoliosis	Addison's disease
	Spinal cord compression	Spinal cord compression	Epidural abscess	Ankylosing spondylitis	Metastatic cancer
	Uterine prolapse	Uterine prolapse	Metastatic cancer	Metastatic cancer	Abdominal aortic dissection
			Abdominal aortic dissection	Abdominal aortic dissection	Pancreatic cancer
			Cauda equina syndrome	Cauda equina syndrome	Cauda equina syndrome
			Pancreatic cancer	Epidural abscess	Epidural abscess
			Trauma	Pancreatic cancer	Trauma
			Uterine prolapse	Trauma	Uterine prolapse
				Uterine prolapse	

Emergency Rule Out conditions shown in red. Entries in blue are for information only
Conditions are listed in approximate order of prevalence for this age range

Low back pain

Emergency Rule Out conditions shown in red. Entries in blue are for information only
Conditions are listed in approximate order of prevalence for this age range

Lymphadenopathy, generalized

Baby (0-1 yr)	Child (1-12 yr)	Adolescent (12-18 yr)	Adult (18-45 yr)	Middle Age Adult (45-65 yr)	Senior Adult (65+yr)
Mononucleosis	Mononucleosis	Mononucleosis	Mononucleosis	AIDS	Hodgkin's disease
Congenital rubella syndrome	Rubella	Rubella	AIDS	Hodgkin's disease	Non-Hodgkin's lymphoma
Tuberculosis	Tuberculosis	Tuberculosis	Hodgkin's disease	Primary HIV infection	Tuberculosis
Primary HIV infection	Primary HIV infection	Primary HIV infection	Primary HIV infection	Acute leukemia	Rheumatoid arthritis
Systemic lupus erythematosus	AIDS	AIDS	Acute leukemia	Tuberculosis	Primary HIV infection
Chronic lymphocytic leukemia	Sarcoidosis	Sarcoidosis	Tuberculosis	Chronic lymphadenitis	AIDS
Lymphogranuloma venereum	Toxoplasmosis	Systemic lupus erythematosus	Chronic lymphadenitis	Non-Hodgkin's lymphoma	Acute leukemia
Brucellosis	Acute leukemia	Lymphogranuloma venereum	Non-Hodgkin's lymphoma	Hyperthyroidism	Chronic lymphadenitis
Erythema nodosum	Brucellosis	Chronic lymphocytic leukemia	Hyperthyroidism	Polymyositis/ dermatomyositis	Systemic lupus erythematosus
Oral cavity cancer	Chronic lymphocytic leukemia	Toxoplasmosis	Polymyositis/ dermatomyositis	Rheumatoid arthritis	Hyperthyroidism
AIDS	Systemic lupus erythematosus	Acute leukemia	Systemic lupus erythematosus	Systemic lupus erythematosus	Lymphogranuloma venereum
Bartonella infection (cat scratch disease)	Lymphogranuloma venereum	Non-Hodgkin's lymphoma	Rheumatoid arthritis	Mononucleosis	Exfoliative dermatitis
Sarcoidosis	Oral cavity cancer	Bartonella infection (cat scratch disease)	Lymphogranuloma venereum	Lymphogranuloma venereum	Chronic lymphocytic leukemia
Acute leukemia	Non-Hodgkin's lymphoma	Brucellosis	Syphilis	Chronic lymphocytic leukemia	Autoimmune hemolytic anemia
Cellulitis	Bartonella infection (cat scratch disease)	Oral cavity cancer	Bartonella infection (cat scratch disease)	Syphilis	Serum sickness
Osteomyelitis	Hodgkin's disease	Hodgkin's disease	Chronic lymphocytic leukemia	Tularemia	Toxoplasmosis
	Neuroblastoma	Erythema nodosum	Tularemia	Cutaneous T cell lymphoma	Bartonella infection (cat scratch disease)
	Erythema nodosum	Neuroblastoma	Brucellosis	Serum sickness	Oral cavity cancer
	Burkitt's lymphoma	Burkitt's lymphoma			

Baby (0-1 yr)	Child (1-12 yr)	Adolescent (12-18 yr)	Adult (18-45 yr)	Middle Age Adult (45-65 yr)	Senior Adult (65+ yr)
	Cutaneous T cell lymphoma	Cutaneous T cell lymphoma	Cutaneous T cell lymphoma	Granuloma inguinale (donovanosis)	Brucellosis
	Chronic lymphadenitis	Chronic lymphadenitis	Serum sickness	Brucellosis	Syphilis
	Kawasaki disease	Kawasaki disease	Granuloma inguinale (donovanosis)	Oral cavity cancer	Hypopituitarism
	Juvenile idiopathic arthritis	Juvenile idiopathic arthritis	Oral cavity cancer	Bartonella infection (cat scratch disease)	Erythema nodosum
	Cellulitis	Cellulitis	Toxoplasmosis	Toxoplasmosis	Kawasaki disease
	Osteomyelitis	Osteomyelitis	Hypopituitarism	Hypopituitarism	Tularemia
	Serum sickness	Serum sickness	Exfoliative dermatitis	Erythema nodosum	Granuloma inguinale (donovanosis)
			Erythema nodosum	Exfoliative dermatitis	Whipple's disease
			Kawasaki disease	Kawasaki disease	Burkitt's lymphoma
			Whipple's disease	Whipple's disease	Cutaneous T cell lymphoma
			Burkitt's lymphoma	Burkitt's lymphoma	Mononucleosis
			Autoimmune hemolytic anemia	Autoimmune hemolytic anemia	Sarcoidosis
			Sarcoidosis	Sarcoidosis	

Lymphadenopathy, generalized (continued)

221

Emergency Rule Out conditions shown in red. Entries in blue are for information only
Conditions are listed in approximate order of prevalence for this age range

Baby (0-1 yr)	Child (1-12 yr)	Adolescent (12-18 yr)	Adult (18-45 yr)	Middle Age Adult (45-65 yr)	Senior Adult (65+yr)
Viral infection	Viral infection	Viral infection	Drug reaction, skin	Drug reaction, skin	Drug reaction, skin
Drug reaction, allergic	Drug reaction, allergic	Drug reaction, allergic	Allergic reactions and anaphylaxis	Allergic reactions and anaphylaxis	Allergic reactions and anaphylaxis
Parvovirus B19 infection	Gastroenteritis	Gastroenteritis	Acne rosacea	Acne rosacea	Seborrheic keratosis
Insect and spider bites and stings	Parvovirus B19 infection	Parvovirus B19 infection	Acne vulgaris	Acne vulgaris	Acne rosacea
Allergic reactions and anaphylaxis	Erythema multiforme	Allergic reactions and anaphylaxis	Seborrheic keratosis	Seborrheic keratosis	Erythema multiforme
Erythema multiforme	Hand-foot-and-mouth disease	Erythema multiforme	Erythema multiforme	Erythema multiforme	Basal cell carcinoma
Hand-foot-and-mouth disease	Pityriasis rosea	Hand-foot-and-mouth disease	Mononucleosis	Hand-foot-and-mouth disease	Hand-foot-and-mouth disease
Allergic reactions and anaphylaxis	Mononucleosis	Mononucleosis	Hand-foot-and-mouth disease	Pityriasis rosea	Mononucleosis
Mononucleosis	Allergic reactions and anaphylaxis	Pityriasis rosea	Pityriasis rosea	Mononucleosis	Pityriasis rosea
Pityriasis rosea	Insect and spider bites and stings	Insect and spider bites and stings	Scabies	Scabies	Scabies
Gastroenteritis	Upper respiratory tract infections	Upper respiratory tract infections	Melanoma	Melanoma	Tuberculosis
Upper respiratory tract infections	Rubella	Rubella	Lichen planus	Lichen planus	Melanoma
Rubella	Measles	Measles	Tuberculosis	Tuberculosis	Lichen planus
Measles	Henoch-Schönlein purpura	Henoch-Schönlein purpura	Neurofibromatosis	Neurofibromatosis	Neurofibromatosis
Henoch-Schönlein purpura	Stevens-Johnson syndrome	Tinea versicolor	Basal cell carcinoma	Basal cell carcinoma	Tuberous sclerosis complex
Stevens-Johnson syndrome		Stevens-Johnson syndrome	Tuberous sclerosis complex	Tuberous sclerosis complex	
			Tinea versicolor	Tinea versicolor	
			Stevens-Johnson syndrome		

Baby (0-1 yr)	Child (1-12 yr)	Adolescent (12-18 yr)	Adult (18-45 yr)	Middle Age Adult (45-65 yr)	Senior Adult (65+ yr)
Chlamydia pneumoniae	Mononucleosis	Mononucleosis	Viral infection	Viral infection	Viral infection
Herpes zoster, shingles	Chronic fatigue syndrome	Depression	Depression	Depression	Depression
Brucellosis	Depression	Poliomyelitis	Chronic fatigue syndrome	Chronic fatigue syndrome	Hypothyroidism
Crohn's disease	Poliomyelitis	Chronic fatigue syndrome	Mononucleosis	Hypothyroidism	Hyperthyroidism
Encephalitis	Malignancy	Tularemia	Hypothyroidism	Hyperthyroidism	Acute renal failure
Erythema nodosum	Tularemia	Chronic infection	Hyperthyroidism	Primary lung malignancy	Polyarteritis nodosa
Heat stroke and heat exhaustion	Polyarteritis nodosa	Typhoid fever	Poliomyelitis	Poliomyelitis	Poliomyelitis
Genital herpes	Chronic infection	Chlamydia pneumoniae	Tularemia	Acute renal failure	Chronic renal failure
Herpes simplex	Pertussis	Herpes zoster, shingles	Scarlet fever	Polyarteritis nodosa	Reiter's syndrome
Babesiosis	Reiter's syndrome	Herpes simplex	Polyarteritis nodosa	Tularemia	Alcoholic hepatitis
Behçet's syndrome	Herpes simplex	Pertussis	Chlamydia pneumoniae	Pertussis	Pertussis
Diabetes mellitus in children	Brucellosis	Heat stroke and heat exhaustion	Herpes zoster, shingles	Reiter's syndrome	Scarlet fever
Systemic lupus erythematosus	Heat stroke and heat exhaustion	Genital herpes	Pertussis	Herpes zoster, shingles	Herpes simplex
	Erythema nodosum	Erythema nodosum	Herpes simplex	Herpes simplex	Herpes zoster, shingles
	Genital herpes	Crohn's disease	Heat stroke and heat exhaustion	Heat stroke and heat exhaustion	Heat stroke and heat exhaustion
	Encephalitis	Encephalitis	Primary lung malignancy	Alcoholic hepatitis	Genital herpes
	Herpes zoster, shingles	Brucellosis	Brucellosis	Behçet's syndrome	Erythema nodosum
	Babesiosis	Behçet's syndrome	Encephalitis	Erythema nodosum	Encephalitis
	Primary lung malignancy	Scarlet fever	Crohn's disease	Crohn's disease	Crohn's disease
	Behçet's syndrome	Babesiosis	Erythema nodosum	Encephalitis	Brucellosis
	Chlamydia pneumoniae	Polyarteritis nodosa	Genital herpes	Genital herpes	Babesiosis

List continues on next page

Emergency Rule Out conditions shown in red. Entries in blue are for information only
Conditions are listed in approximate order of prevalence for this age range

List continued from previous page

Baby (0-1 yr)	Child (1-12 yr)	Adolescent (12-18 yr)	Adult (18-45 yr)	Middle Age Adult (45-65 yr)	Senior Adult (65+ yr)
	Crohn's disease	Primary lung malignancy	Bartonella infection (cat scratch disease)	Brucellosis	Behçet's syndrome
	Typhoid fever	Cellulitis	Behçet's syndrome	Scarlet fever	Primary lung malignancy
	Cellulitis	Reiter's syndrome	Babesiosis	Cellulitis	Tularemia
	Scarlet fever	Alcoholic hepatitis	Cellulitis	Babesiosis	Cellulitis
	Viral hepatitis	Tuberculosis	Alcoholic hepatitis	Chlamydia pneumoniae	Chlamydia pneumoniae
	Bartonella infection (cat scratch disease)	Bartonella infection (cat scratch disease)	Reiter's syndrome	Chronic renal failure	Mononucleosis
	Tuberculosis	Viral hepatitis	Typhoid fever	Typhoid fever	Viral hepatitis
	Acute renal failure	Malignancy	Recreational drug abuse	Viral hepatitis	Liver failure
	Chronic renal failure	Acute renal failure	Viral hepatitis	Mononucleosis	Typhoid fever
	Liver failure	Chronic renal failure	Acute renal failure	Liver failure	Malignancy
	Hypothyroidism	Liver failure	Chronic renal failure	Malignancy	Chronic infection
	Hyperthyroidism	Hypothyroidism	Liver failure	Chronic infection	Congestive heart failure
	Connective tissue disease	Systemic lupus erythematosus	Malignancy	Recreational drug abuse	Recreational drug abuse
	Systemic lupus erythematosus		Chronic infection	Congestive heart failure	Temporal arteritis
			Congestive heart failure	Temporal arteritis	Polymyalgia rheumatica
			Rheumatoid arthritis	Polymyalgia rheumatica	Systemic lupus erythematosus
			Systemic lupus erythematosus	Systemic lupus erythematosus	

Baby (0-1 yr)	Child (1-12 yr)	Adolescent (12-18 yr)	Adult (18-45 yr)	Middle Age Adult (45-65 yr)	Senior Adult (65+ yr)
Not relevant to this age group	Mammary duct ectasia Breast cyst	Fibrocystic breast disease Breast cyst Breast fibroadenoma Fibroadenosis Lactating mastitis Mammary duct ectasia	Fibroadenosis Pregnancy Mastalgia Breast fibroadenoma Breast cancer Fibrocystic breast disease Galactorrhea Phyllode tumor Intraductal papilloma Mammary duct ectasia Lactating mastitis Lipoma Soft tissue sarcoma Breast cyst	Fibroadenosis Mastalgia Breast fibroadenoma Breast cancer Fibrocystic breast disease Phyllode tumor Lipoma Intraductal papilloma Galactorrhea Mammary duct ectasia Lactating mastitis Soft tissue sarcoma Breast cyst	Breast cancer Fibroadenosis Breast fibroadenoma Fibrocystic breast disease Phyllode tumor Mastalgia Lipoma Intraductal papilloma Mammary duct ectasia Lactating mastitis Soft tissue sarcoma Breast cyst

Emergency Rule Out conditions shown in red. Entries in blue are for information only
Conditions are listed in approximate order of prevalence for this age range

Emergency Rule Out conditions shown in red. Entries in blue are for information only
Conditions are listed in approximate order of prevalence for this age range

Baby (0-1 yr)	Child (1-12 yr)	Adolescent (12-18 yr)	Adult (18-45 yr)	Middle Age Adult (45-65 yr)	Senior Adult (65+ yr)
Tuberculosis	Tuberculosis	Tuberculosis	Hiatal hernia	Hiatal hernia	Hiatal hernia
Acute leukemia	Acute leukemia	Acute leukemia	Hodgkin's disease	Hodgkin's disease	Non-Hodgkin's lymphoma
Hodgkin's disease	Hodgkin's disease	Hodgkin's disease	Non-Hodgkin's lymphoma	Non-Hodgkin's lymphoma	Malignancy
Non-Hodgkin's lymphoma	Non-Hodgkin's lymphoma	Non-Hodgkin's lymphoma	Retrosternal goiter	Retrosternal goiter	Thoracic aortic aneurysm
Dermoid cyst	Dermoid cyst	Retrosternal goiter	Malignancy	Malignancy	Hodgkin's disease
		Dermoid cyst	Thoracic aortic aneurysm	Thoracic aortic aneurysm	Retrosternal goiter
			Malignant thymoma	Malignant thymoma	Malignant thymoma
			Tuberculosis	Tuberculosis	Tuberculosis
			Sarcoidosis	Sarcoidosis	Sarcoidosis
			Neurofibroma	Neurofibroma	

Baby (0-1 yr)	Child (1-12 yr)	Adolescent (12-18 yr)	Adult (18-45 yr)	Middle Age Adult (45-65 yr)	Senior Adult (65+yr)
Intussusception	Intussusception	Campylobacter infection	Hemorrhoids	Hemorrhoids	Hemorrhoids
Volvulus	Campylobacter infection	Peptic ulcer	Anal fissure	Anal fissure	Anal fissure
Hemolytic disease of the newborn (erythroblastosis fetalis)	Volvulus	Crohn's disease	Colonic polyp	Diverticular disease	Diverticular disease
	Meckel's diverticulum	Ulcerative colitis	Peptic ulcer	Crohn's disease	Crohn's disease
Salmonella infection	Peptic ulcer	Anal fissure	Crohn's disease	Ischemic bowel disease	Ischemic bowel disease
Campylobacter infection	Anal fissure	Hemorrhoids	Gastritis	Peptic ulcer	Peptic ulcer
Behçet's syndrome	Behçet's syndrome	Salmonella infection	Ulcerative colitis	Colonic polyp	Colonic polyp
Liver cirrhosis	Salmonella infection	Behçet's syndrome	Diverticular disease	Colon cancer	Gastritis
Meckel's diverticulum	Liver cirrhosis	Liver cirrhosis	Colon cancer	Gastritis	Colon cancer
Anal fissure	Crohn's disease	Intussusception	Arterial-intestinal fistula	Ulcerative colitis	Ulcerative colitis
Malignancy	Ischemic bowel disease	Ischemic bowel disease	Ischemic bowel disease	Arterial-intestinal fistula	Arterial-intestinal fistula
Ischemic bowel disease	Malignancy	Malignancy	Hereditary hemorrhagic telangectasia	Hereditary hemorrhagic telangectasia	Liver cirrhosis
Ulcerative colitis	Ulcerative colitis	Mallory-Weiss tear	Amyloidosis	Amyloidosis	Behçet's syndrome
			Campylobacter infection	Behçet's syndrome	Hereditary hemorrhagic telangectasia
			Behçet's syndrome	Liver cirrhosis	Amyloidosis
			Liver cirrhosis	Campylobacter infection	Campylobacter infection
			Angiodysplasia	Angiodysplasia	Angiodysplasia
			Salmonella infection	Malignancy	Malignancy
			Malignancy	Salmonella infection	Salmonella infection
			Intussusception	Intussusception	Intussusception
			Mallory-Weiss tear	Mallory-Weiss tear	
				Esophageal varices	

Emergency Rule Out conditions shown in red. Entries in blue are for information only
Conditions are listed in approximate order of prevalence for this age range

Melena, lower GI bleeding

Emergency Rule Out conditions shown in red. Entries in blue are for information only
Conditions are listed in approximate order of prevalence for this age range

Baby (0-1 yr)	Child (1-12 yr)	Adolescent (12-18 yr)	Adult (18-45 yr)	Middle Age Adult (45-65 yr)	Senior Adult (65+ yr)
Not relevant to this age group	Depression	Depression	Depression	Depression	Alzheimer's disease
	Hypothyroidism	Hypothyroidism	Parkinson's disease	Parkinson's disease	Depression
	Brain tumor	AIDS	Hydrocephalus	Hypothyroidism	Dementia
	Subdural hematoma	Brain tumor	Korsakoff's syndrome	Brain tumor	Brain tumor
	Chronic fatigue syndrome	Post-traumatic stress disorder	Vitamin B12 deficiency	Subdural hematoma	Vitamin B12 deficiency
	Post-traumatic stress disorder	Chronic fatigue syndrome	Post-traumatic stress disorder	Post-traumatic stress disorder	Hypothyroidism
	Hydrocephalus	Subdural hematoma	Hypothyroidism	Alzheimer's disease	Post-traumatic stress disorder
	Wilson's disease	Hydrocephalus	AIDS	Korsakoff's syndrome	Subdural hematoma
	Mucopolysaccharidosis	Wilson's disease	Brain tumor	Vitamin B12 deficiency	Hydrocephalus
	Creutzfeldt-Jakob disease	Creutzfeldt-Jakob disease	Drug reaction, delirium and confusional states	Drug reaction, delirium and confusional states	Drug reaction, delirium and confusional states
			Subdural hematoma	Chronic fatigue syndrome	AIDS
			Syphilis	Hydrocephalus	Korsakoff's syndrome
			Chronic fatigue syndrome	AIDS	Chronic fatigue syndrome
			Alzheimer's disease	Syphilis	Parkinson's disease
			Wilson's disease	Dementia	Syphilis
			Creutzfeldt-Jakob disease	Huntington's disease	Wilson's disease
			Dementia	Wilson's disease	Creutzfeldt-Jakob disease
			Huntington's disease	Creutzfeldt-Jakob disease	Frontotemporal lobe degeneration (Pick's disease)

228

Baby (0-1 yr)	Child (1-12 yr)	Adolescent (12-18 yr)	Adult (18-45 yr)	Middle Age Adult (45-65 yr)	Senior Adult (65+ yr)
Viral meningitis	Bacterial meningitis	Bacterial meningitis	Influenza	Influenza	Influenza
Encephalitis	Viral meningitis	Viral meningitis	Viral meningitis	Viral meningitis	Viral meningitis
Bacterial meningitis	Encephalitis	Encephalitis	Bacterial meningitis	Bacterial meningitis	Bacterial meningitis
Subarachnoid hemorrhage and cerebral aneurysm	Influenza	Influenza	Encephalitis	Encephalitis	Subarachnoid hemorrhage and cerebral aneurysm
stroke	Tonsillitis	Tonsillitis	Subarachnoid hemorrhage and cerebral aneurysm	Subarachnoid hemorrhage and cerebral aneurysm	stroke
Kernicterus	Subarachnoid hemorrhage and cerebral aneurysm	Subarachnoid hemorrhage and cerebral aneurysm	stroke	stroke	Encephalitis
	stroke	stroke	Porphyria	Porphyria	Porphyria
		Cervical spine injury	Cervical spine injury	Cervical spine injury	

Emergency Rule Out conditions shown in red. Entries in blue are for information only
Conditions are listed in approximate order of prevalence for this age range

Emergency Rule Out conditions shown in red. Entries in blue are for information only
Conditions are listed in approximate order of prevalence for this age range

Baby (0-1 yr)	Child (1-12 yr)	Adolescent (12-18 yr)	Adult (18-45 yr)	Middle Age Adult (45-65 yr)	Senior Adult (65+ yr)
Iron deficiency anemia	Iron deficiency anemia	Iron deficiency anemia	Iron deficiency anemia	Iron deficiency anemia	Iron deficiency anemia
Thalassemia	Thalassemia	Thalassemia	Sickle cell anemia	Chronic infection	Chronic infection
Chronic lead poisoning	Chronic lead poisoning	Sickle cell anemia	Chronic infection	Sickle cell anemia	Sickle cell anemia
Sickle cell anemia	Sickle cell anemia	Hemoglobin C disease	Hemoglobin C disease	Hemoglobin C disease	Hemoglobin C disease
Hemoglobin C disease	Hemoglobin C disease	Chronic infection	Thalassemia	Thalassemia	Thalassemia
Chronic infection	Chronic infection	Chronic lead poisoning			

Baby (0-1 yr)	Child (1-12 yr)	Adolescent (12-18 yr)	Adult (18-45 yr)	Middle Age Adult (45-65 yr)	Senior Adult (65+ yr)
Congenital heart disease	Congenital heart disease	Congenital heart disease	Mitral valve prolapse	Mitral valve prolapse	Cardiomyopathy
Mitral valve prolapse	Mitral valve prolapse	Mitral valve prolapse	Cardiomyopathy	Cardiomyopathy	Mitral valve prolapse
Cardiomyopathy	Cardiomyopathy	Cardiomyopathy	Systemic lupus erythematosus	Systemic lupus erythematosus	Infective endocarditis
	Infective endocarditis	Infective endocarditis	Congenital heart disease	Congenital heart disease	Ruptured chordae tendinae
	Marfan's syndrome	Marfan's syndrome	Infective endocarditis	Infective endocarditis	Ruptured mitral papillary muscle
	Rheumatic fever	Rheumatic fever	Ruptured chordae tendinae	Ruptured chordae tendinae	Rheumatoid arthritis
			Ruptured mitral papillary muscle	Ruptured mitral papillary muscle	Congenital heart disease
			Rheumatic fever	Rheumatic fever	Rheumatic fever
			Rheumatoid arthritis	Rheumatoid arthritis	Systemic lupus erythematosus

Emergency Rule Out conditions shown in red. Entries in blue are for information only
Conditions are listed in approximate order of prevalence for this age range

Emergency Rule Out conditions shown in red. Entries in blue are for information only
Conditions are listed in approximate order of prevalence for this age range

Baby (0-1 yr)	Child (1-12 yr)	Adolescent (12-18 yr)	Adult (18-45 yr)	Middle Age Adult (45-65 yr)	Senior Adult (65+ yr)
Fibromyalgia Epicondylitis	Juvenile idiopathic arthritis Fibromyalgia Epicondylitis Psoriatic arthritis	Ankylosing spondylitis Epicondylitis Fibromyalgia Juvenile idiopathic arthritis Psoriatic arthritis	Ankylosing spondylitis Fibromyalgia Epicondylitis Rheumatoid arthritis Polymyalgia rheumatica	Rheumatoid arthritis Epicondylitis Fibromyalgia Ankylosing spondylitis Polymyalgia rheumatica	Rheumatoid arthritis Fibromyalgia Epicondylitis Polymyalgia rheumatica

Baby (0-1 yr)	Child (1-12 yr)	Adolescent (12-18 yr)	Adult (18-45 yr)	Middle Age Adult (45-65 yr)	Senior Adult (65+ yr)
Foreign body Choanal atresia Deviated nasal septum Anxiety Drug reaction, allergic Drug reaction Tonsilitis	Allergic rhinitis Foreign body Lymphadenopathy Nasal polyp Anxiety Drug reaction, allergic Drug reaction Deviated nasal septum Tonsillitis	Allergic rhinitis Lymphadenopathy Foreign body Deviated nasal septum Anxiety Nasal polyp Drug reaction, allergic Drug reaction Tonsillitis	Allergic rhinitis Nasal polyp Deviated nasal septum Anxiety	Allergic rhinitis Nasal polyp Anxiety	Allergic rhinitis Malignancy Anxiety

Mouth breathing

Emergency Rule Out conditions shown in red. Entries in blue are for information only
Conditions are listed in approximate order of prevalence for this age range

233

Emergency Rule Out conditions shown in red. Entries in blue are for information only
Conditions are listed in approximate order of prevalence for this age range

Baby (0-1 yr)	Child (1-12 yr)	Adolescent (12-18 yr)	Adult (18-45 yr)	Middle Age Adult (45-65 yr)	Senior Adult (65-yr)
Tetanus	Overuse	Overuse	Overuse	Overuse	Overuse
Celiac disease	Dehydration	Dehydration	Dehydration	Dehydration	Dehydration
	Drug reaction	Drug reaction	Drug reaction	Drug reaction	Drug reaction
	Celiac disease	Hyperventilation	Hyperventilation	Hyperventilation	Hyperventilation
	Hyperventilation	Hypokalemia	Hypokalemia	Hypokalemia	Hypokalemia
	Hypokalemia	Dystonia	Hypocalcemia	Hypocalcemia	Hypocalcemia
	Dystonia	Celiac disease	Hyponatremia	Hyponatremia	Hyponatremia
	Restless leg syndrome	Restless leg syndrome	Celiac disease	Celiac disease	Celiac disease
	Myotonic dystrophy	Myotonic dystrophy	Dystonia	Dystonia	Dystonia
	Fibromyalgia	Fibromyalgia	Restless leg syndrome	Restless leg syndrome	Restless leg syndrome
			Hemifacial spasm	Celiac disease	Hemifacial spasm
			Myotonic dystrophy	Hemifacial spasm	Myotonic dystrophy
			Amyotrophic lateral sclerosis (motor neuron disease)	Myotonic dystrophy	Amyotrophic lateral sclerosis (motor neuron disease)
			Black widow spider bite	Amyotrophic lateral sclerosis (motor neuron disease)	Black widow spider bite
			Fibromyalgia	Black widow spider bite	Fibromyalgia
				Fibromyalgia	

234

Baby (0-1 yr)	Child (1-12 yr)	Adolescent (12-18 yr)	Adult (18-45 yr)	Middle Age Adult (45-65 yr)	Senior Adult (65+ yr)
Not relevant to this age group	**Chickenpox** Post-infection **Herpes zoster, shingles** **Guillain-Barré syndrome** (acute infective polyneuritis) **Poliomyelitis** **Spinal cord lesion**	**Chickenpox** Post-infection **Herpes zoster, shingles** **Guillain-Barré syndrome** (acute infective polyneuritis) **Spinal cord lesion** **Poliomyelitis** **AIDS**	Encephalitis **Cytomegalovirus** Multiple sclerosis Syphilis Poliomyelitis Radiation sickness **AIDS** Spinal cord lesion Epidural abscess **Chickenpox** Malignancy Trauma Systemic lupus erythematosus Idiopathic	Encephalitis **Cytomegalovirus** Multiple sclerosis Syphilis Poliomyelitis Radiation sickness **AIDS** Spinal cord lesion Epidural abscess **Chickenpox** Malignancy Trauma Systemic lupus erythematosus Idiopathic	Encephalitis **Cytomegalovirus** Multiple sclerosis Syphilis Poliomyelitis Radiation sickness **AIDS** Spinal cord lesion Epidural abscess **Chickenpox** Malignancy Trauma Systemic lupus erythematosus Idiopathic

Emergency Rule Out conditions shown in red. Entries in blue are for information only
Conditions are listed in approximate order of prevalence for this age range

235

Emergency Rule Out conditions shown in red. Entries in blue are for information only
Conditions are listed in approximate order of prevalence for this age range

Baby (0-1 yr)	Child (1-12 yr)	Adolescent (12-18 yr)	Adult (18-45 yr)	Middle Age Adult (45-65 yr)	Senior Adult (65+ yr)
Benign essential myoclonus	Benign essential myoclonus	Benign essential myoclonus	Benign essential myoclonus	Benign essential myoclonus	Benign essential myoclonus
Epilepsy	Epilepsy	Epilepsy	Encephalopathy	Encephalopathy	Encephalopathy
			Hepatic encephalopathy	Hepatic encephalopathy	Hepatic encephalopathy
			Uremic encephalopathy	Uremic encephalopathy	Uremic encephalopathy
			Epilepsy	Epilepsy	Alzheimer's disease
			Head injury	Head injury	Epilepsy
			Creutzfeldt-Jakob disease	Creutzfeldt-Jakob disease	Head injury
			Subacute sclerosing panencephalitis	Subacute sclerosing panencephalitis	Creutzfeldt-Jakob disease
					Subacute sclerosing panencephalitis

Baby (0-1 yr)	Child (1-12 yr)	Adolescent (12-18 yr)	Adult (18-45 yr)	Middle Age Adult (45-65 yr)	Senior Adult (65+ yr)
Burns	Burns	Burns	Burns	Burns	Burns
Trauma	Trauma	Trauma	Trauma	Trauma	Trauma
Rhabdomyolysis	Epilepsy	Sepsis	Rhabdomyolysis	Rhabdomyolysis	Rhabdomyolysis
	Sepsis	Hypokalemia	Epilepsy	Epilepsy	Epilepsy
	Metabolic acidosis	Metabolic acidosis	Sepsis	Sepsis	Sepsis
		Epilepsy	Hypokalemia	Hypokalemia	Hypokalemia
			Post-prostatectomy	Post-prostatectomy	Post-prostatectomy

Emergency Rule Out conditions shown in red. Entries in blue are for information only
Conditions are listed in approximate order of prevalence for this age range

Nail abnormalities

Emergency Rule Out conditions shown in red. Entries in blue are for information only
Conditions are listed in approximate order of prevalence for this age range

Baby (0-1 yr)	Child (1-12 yr)	Adolescent (12-18 yr)	Adult (18-45 yr)	Middle Age Adult (45-65 yr)	Senior Adult (65+yr)
Congenital heart disease	Congenital heart disease	Fungal infection	Fungal infection	Fungal infection	Fungal infection
Psoriatic arthritis	Fungal infection	Psoriasis	Psoriasis	Iron deficiency anemia	Hypothyroidism
Onychomycosis	Reiter's syndrome	Paronychia	Iron deficiency anemia	Hypothyroidism	Liver cirrhosis
Ingrown nail	Paronychia	Ingrown nail	Hypothyroidism	Psoriasis	Iron deficiency anemia
Paronychia	Ingrown nail	Onychomycosis	Liver cirrhosis	Liver cirrhosis	Crohn's disease
Reiter's syndrome	Onychomycosis	Psoriatic arthritis	Crohn's disease	Crohn's disease	Malabsorption
Reflex sympathetic dystrophy	Psoriatic arthritis	Reiter's syndrome	Malabsorption	Malabsorption	Reiter's syndrome
	Psoriasis	Vasculitis	Vasculitis	Vasculitis	Psoriatic arthritis
	Vasculitis	Infective endocarditis	Onychomycosis	Onychomycosis	Onychomycosis
	Infective endocarditis	Trauma	Reiter's syndrome	Psoriatic arthritis	Psoriasis
	Trauma	Reflex sympathetic dystrophy	Ingrown nail	Ingrown nail	Ingrown nail
	Reflex sympathetic dystrophy		Psoriatic arthritis	Paronychia	Bronchiectasis
			Mesothelioma	Bronchiectasis	Vasculitis
			Paronychia	Reiter's syndrome	Paronychia
			Congenital heart disease	Mesothelioma	Primary lung malignancy
			Bronchiectasis	Congenital heart disease	Idiopathic pulmonary interstitial fibrosis
			Infective endocarditis	Primary lung malignancy	Mesothelioma
			Primary lung malignancy	Idiopathic pulmonary interstitial fibrosis	Congenital heart disease
			Idiopathic pulmonary interstitial fibrosis	Infective endocarditis	Infective endocarditis
			Hyperthyroidism	Hyperthyroidism	Hyperthyroidism
			Pituitary hypothyroidism	Pituitary hypothyroidism	Pituitary hypothyroidism
			Thyroid carcinoma	Thyroid carcinoma	Thyroid carcinoma

Baby (0-1 yr)	Child (1-12 yr)	Adolescent (12-18 yr)	Adult (18-45 yr)	Middle Age Adult (45-65 yr)	Senior Adult (65+ yr)
			Thyroiditis Trauma Polycystic kidney disease Reflex sympathetic dystrophy	Thyroiditis Polycystic kidney disease Trauma Reflex sympathetic dystrophy	Thyroiditis Trauma Polycystic kidney disease Reflex sympathetic dystrophy

Nail abnormalities (continued)

Emergency Rule Out conditions shown in red. Entries in blue are for information only
Conditions are listed in approximate order of prevalence for this age range

Baby (0-1 yr)	Child (1-12 yr)	Adolescent (12-18 yr)	Adult (18-45 yr)	Middle Age Adult (45-65 yr)	Senior Adult (65+yr)
Paronychia	Fungal infection	Fungal infection	Fungal infection	Fungal infection	Fungal infection
Onychomycosis	Psoriasis	Psoriasis	Psoriasis	Psoriasis	Paronychia
Hyperthyroidism	Onychomycosis	Onychomycosis	Hypothyroidism	Onychomycosis	Onychomycosis
	Paronychia	Paronychia	Onychomycosis	Paronychia	Psoriasis
	Trauma	Trauma	Paronychia	Hypothyroidism	Hypothyroidism
	Hyperthyroidism	Contact dermatitis	Trauma	Trauma	Trauma
		Hyperthyroidism	Contact dermatitis	Contact dermatitis	Hyperthyroidism
			Hyperthyroidism	Hyperthyroidism	

Baby (0-1 yr)	Child (1-12 yr)	Adolescent (12-18 yr)	Adult (18-45 yr)	Middle Age Adult (45-65 yr)	Senior Adult (65+ yr)
Upper respiratory tract infections	Upper respiratory tract infections	Upper respiratory tract infections	Upper respiratory tract infections	Upper respiratory tract infections	Upper respiratory tract infections
Allergic rhinitis	Allergic rhinitis	Allergic rhinitis	Allergic rhinitis	Allergic rhinitis	Allergic rhinitis
Respiratory syncytial virus infection	Acute sinusitis	Acute sinusitis	Acute sinusitis	Acute sinusitis	Acute sinusitis
Cluster headache	Chronic sinusitis	Chronic sinusitis	Chronic sinusitis	Chronic sinusitis	Chronic sinusitis
Laryngitis	Cluster headache	Cluster headache	Laryngitis	Laryngitis	Respiratory syncytial virus infection
Foreign body	Laryngitis	Laryngitis	Cluster headache	Cluster headache	Laryngitis
Cerebrospinal fluid leak	Respiratory syncytial virus infection	Respiratory syncytial virus infection	Respiratory syncytial virus infection	Respiratory syncytial virus infection	Cluster headache
Primary ciliary dysplasia	Nasal polyp	Nasal polyp	Vasomotor rhinitis	Vasomotor rhinitis	Vasomotor rhinitis
	Foreign body	Foreign body	Nasal polyp	Nasal polyp	Nasal polyp
	Cerebrospinal fluid leak	Cerebrospinal fluid leak	Deviated nasal septum	Deviated nasal septum	Deviated nasal septum
	Primary ciliary dysplasia	Wegener's granulomatosis	Foreign body	Foreign body	Foreign body
		Primary ciliary dysplasia	Wegener's granulomatosis	Wegener's granulomatosis	Wegener's granulomatosis
			Cerebrospinal fluid leak	Cerebrospinal fluid leak	Cerebrospinal fluid leak
			Sarcoidosis	Sarcoidosis	Sarcoidosis

Emergency Rule Out conditions shown in red. Entries in blue are for information only
Conditions are listed in approximate order of prevalence for this age range

Nasal congestion, discharge

Emergency Rule Out conditions shown in red. Entries in blue are for information only
Conditions are listed in approximate order of prevalence for this age range

Baby (0-1 yr)	Child (1-12 yr)	Adolescent (12-18 yr)	Adult (18-45 yr)	Middle Age Adult (45-65 yr)	Senior Adult (65+yr)
Hypercalcemia	Gastroenteritis	Food poisoning	Food poisoning	Food poisoning	Food poisoning
Babesiosis	Cough	Gastroenteritis	Gastroenteritis	Gastroenteritis	Gastroenteritis
Encephalitis	Acute appendicitis	Migraine headache	Pregnancy	Migraine headache	Gastroesophageal reflux disease
Chronic fatigue syndrome	Gastroesophageal reflux disease	Diabetes mellitus in children	Migraine headache	Gastroesophageal reflux disease	Drug reaction
Diabetes mellitus in children	Head injury	Chronic fatigue syndrome	Drug reaction	Drug reaction	Encephalitis
Diabetic ketoacidosis	Encephalitis	Motion sickness	Alcohol abuse	Encephalitis	Intestinal obstruction
Carcinoid syndrome	Motion sickness	Gastroesophageal reflux disease	Motion sickness	Motion sickness	Motion sickness
Carbon monoxide poisoning	Diabetes mellitus in children	Diabetic ketoacidosis	Encephalitis	Diabetic ketoacidosis	Chronic fatigue syndrome
Lactose intolerance	Chronic fatigue syndrome	Acute appendicitis	Diabetic ketoacidosis	Chronic fatigue syndrome	Diabetic ketoacidosis
Campylobacter infection	Diabetic ketoacidosis	Encephalitis	Chronic fatigue syndrome	Alcohol abuse	Labyrinthitis
Insect and spider bites and stings	Carbon monoxide poisoning	Babesiosis	Babesiosis	Carbon monoxide poisoning	Carbon monoxide poisoning
Hypernatremia	Carcinoid syndrome	Chlamydia pneumoniae	Carbon monoxide poisoning	Campylobacter infection	Hypercalcemia
Malaria	Babesiosis	Carcinoid syndrome	Carcinoid syndrome	Carcinoid syndrome	Babesiosis
Ménière's disease	Campylobacter infection	Carbon monoxide poisoning	Hypercalcemia	Acute appendicitis	Carcinoid syndrome
Orthostatic hypotension	Migraine headache	Campylobacter infection	Campylobacter infection	Babesiosis	Campylobacter infection
Pancreatic cancer	Hypercalcemia	Intestinal obstruction	Labyrinthitis	Hypercalcemia	Alcohol abuse
Salicylate poisoning	Raised intracranial pressure	Hypercalcemia	Acute appendicitis	Labyrinthitis	Head injury
Sarcoidosis	Insect and spider bites and stings	Head injury	Intestinal obstruction	Intestinal obstruction	Raised intracranial pressure
Toxic shock syndrome	Lactose intolerance	Insect and spider bites and stings	Head injury	Head injury	Benign paroxysmal positional vertigo
	Bacterial meningitis	Alcohol abuse	Pyelonephritis	Raised intracranial pressure	Insect and spider bites and stings
	Viral meningitis	Lactose intolerance	Insect and spider bites and stings	Insect and spider bites and stings	
			Lactose intolerance		

Baby (0-1 yr)	Child (1-12 yr)	Adolescent (12-18 yr)	Adult (18-45 yr)	Middle Age Adult (45-65 yr)	Senior Adult (65+yr)
	Reye's syndrome	Pyelonephritis	Renal calculi	Lactose intolerance	Lactose intolerance
	Hypernatremia	Bacterial meningitis	Bacterial meningitis	Benign paroxysmal positional vertigo	Acute renal failure
	Malaria	Viral meningitis	Benign paroxysmal positional vertigo	Pyelonephritis	Chronic renal failure
	Ménière's disease	Hypernatremia	Metabolic acidosis	Renal calculi	Renal calculi
	Orthostatic hypotension	Malaria	Hypernatremia	Metabolic acidosis	Metabolic acidosis
	Pancreatic cancer	Ménière's disease	Malaria	Hypernatremia	Hypernatremia
	Salicylate poisoning	Orthostatic hypotension	Ménière's disease	Malaria	Malaria
	Sarcoidosis	Pancreatic cancer	Orthostatic hypotension	Ménière's disease	Ménière's disease
	Toxic shock syndrome	Salicylate poisoning	Pancreatic cancer	Orthostatic hypotension	Orthostatic hypotension
		Sarcoidosis	Salicylate poisoning	Pancreatic cancer	Pancreatic cancer
		Toxic shock syndrome	Sarcoidosis	Salicylate poisoning	Salicylate poisoning
			Toxic shock syndrome	Sarcoidosis	Sarcoidosis
				Toxic shock syndrome	Toxic shock syndrome

Nausea (continued)

243

Emergency Rule Out conditions shown in red. Entries in blue are for information only
Conditions are listed in approximate order of prevalence for this age range

Baby (0-1 yr)	Child (1-12 yr)	Adolescent (12-18 yr)	Adult (18-45 yr)	Middle Age Adult (45-65 yr)	Senior Adult (65+ yr)
Branchial cyst	Lymphadenopathy	Lymphadenopathy	Lymphadenopathy	Lymphadenopathy	Lymphadenopathy
Thyroglossal duct cyst	Branchial cyst	Thyroglossal duct cyst	Parotitis	Parotitis	Parotitis
Skin abscess	Thyroglossal duct cyst	Skin abscess	Laryngeal cancer	Laryngeal cancer	Skin abscess
Laryngeal cancer	Skin abscess	Parotitis	Skin abscess	Skin abscess	Laryngeal cancer
Thyroiditis	Laryngeal cancer	Laryngeal cancer	Hodgkin's disease	Hodgkin's disease	Hodgkin's disease
Parotitis	Thyroiditis	Thyroiditis	Non-Hodgkin's lymphoma	Non-Hodgkin's lymphoma	Non-Hodgkin's lymphoma
Malignancy	Parotitis	Branchial cyst			
	Hodgkin's disease	Hodgkin's disease			
	Malignancy	Non-Hodgkin's lymphoma			
	Non-Hodgkin's lymphoma	Malignancy			

Baby (0-1 yr)	Child (1-12 yr)	Adolescent (12-18 yr)	Adult (18-45 yr)	Middle Age Adult (45-65 yr)	Senior Adult (65+ yr)
Viral meningitis	Muscular strain	Muscular strain	Muscular strain	Muscular strain	Muscular strain
Bacterial meningitis	Lymphadenopathy	Lymphadenopathy	Lymphadenopathy	Lymphadenopathy	Lymphadenopathy
Poliomyelitis	Torticollis	Tonsillitis	Nerve root compression	Torticollis	Nerve root compression
Orthostatic hypotension	Thyroiditis	Torticollis	Tonsillitis	Nerve root compression	Torticollis
Cervical disk syndrome	Poliomyelitis	Polymyalgia rheumatica	Posterior cervical lymphadenopathy	Posterior cervical lymphadenopathy	Posterior cervical lymphadenopathy
Laryngeal cancer	Thoracic outlet syndrome	Cervical disk syndrome	Thoracic outlet syndrome	Poliomyelitis	Thoracic outlet syndrome
Polymyalgia rheumatica	Cervical disk syndrome	Cervical hyperextension injuries	Orthostatic hypotension	Laryngeal cancer	Orthostatic hypotension
Thoracic outlet syndrome	Laryngeal cancer	Orthostatic hypotension	Laryngeal cancer	Cervical disk syndrome	Cervical disk syndrome
Cervical hyperextension injuries	Cervical hyperextension injuries	Laryngeal cancer	Poliomyelitis	Thoracic outlet syndrome	Poliomyelitis
Thyroiditis	Orthostatic hypotension	Poliomyelitis	Cervical disk syndrome	Orthostatic hypotension	Laryngeal cancer
Cervical spine injury	Polymyalgia rheumatica	Thoracic outlet syndrome	Polymyalgia rheumatica	Cervical hyperextension injuries	Polymyalgia rheumatica
	Tonsillitis	Thyroiditis	Cervical hyperextension injuries	Polymyalgia rheumatica	Cervical hyperextension injuries
	Fracture	Skin abscess	Thyroiditis	Thyroiditis	Thyroiditis
	Skin abscess	Fracture	Torticollis	Cervical spondylosis	Cervical spondylosis
	Nerve root compression	Nerve root compression	Cervical spondylosis	Myocardial infarction	Fracture
	Cervical spine injury	Cervical spondylosis	Myocardial infarction	Fracture	Myocardial infarction
		Cervical spine injury	Fracture	Atlantoaxial subluxation	Atlantoaxial subluxation
			Atlantoaxial subluxation	Cervical spine injury	Cervical spine injury
			Cervical spine injury		

Emergency Rule Out conditions shown in red. Entries in blue are for information only
Conditions are listed in approximate order of prevalence for this age range

Nervousness

Emergency Rule Out conditions shown in red. Entries in blue are for information only
Conditions are listed in approximate order of prevalence for this age range

Baby (0-1 yr)	Child (1-12 yr)	Adolescent (12-18 yr)	Adult (18-45 yr)	Middle Age Adult (45-65 yr)	Senior Adult (65+ yr)
Not relevant to this age group	Anxiety Phobia Depression Hyperthyroidism Recreational drug abuse	Anxiety Phobia Depression Hyperthyroidism Recreational drug abuse Alcohol abuse	Anxiety Depression Schizophrenia Phobia Alcohol abuse Recreational drug abuse Hyperthyroidism Pheochromocytoma Dementia	Anxiety Depression Phobia Alcohol abuse Schizophrenia Hyperthyroidism Dementia Recreational drug abuse Pheochromocytoma	Anxiety Alcohol abuse Depression Phobia Dementia Hyperthyroidism Schizophrenia Pheochromocytoma Recreational drug abuse

Baby (0-1 yr)	Child (1-12 yr)	Adolescent (12-18 yr)	Adult (18-45 yr)	Middle Age Adult (45-65 yr)	Senior Adult (65+ yr)
Not relevant to this age group	Not relevant to this age group	Not relevant to this age group	Ischemic stroke Brain tumor Encephalitis Subdural hematoma Brain abscess Multiple sclerosis Tuberculosis Vasculitis	Ischemic stroke Brain tumor Encephalitis Subdural hematoma Brain abscess Tuberculosis Vasculitis Multiple sclerosis	Ischemic stroke Brain tumor Encephalitis Subdural hematoma Brain abscess Tuberculosis Vasculitis Multiple sclerosis

Emergency Rule Out conditions shown in red. Entries in blue are for information only
Conditions are listed in approximate order of prevalence for this age range

Neurological neglect syndrome

Emergency Rule Out conditions shown in red. Entries in blue are for information only
Conditions are listed in approximate order of prevalence for this age range

Baby (0-1 yr)	Child (1-12 yr)	Adolescent (12-18 yr)	Adult (18-45 yr)	Middle Age Adult (45-65 yr)	Senior Adult (65+yr)
Bacterial pneumonia	Pyelonephritis	Anxiety	Anxiety	Anxiety	Anxiety
Viral pneumonia	Bacterial pneumonia	Chronic infection	Chronic infection	Chronic infection	Chronic infection
Idiopathic myelofibrosis	Idiopathic myelofibrosis	Pyelonephritis	Idiopathic myelofibrosis	Pyelonephritis	Bacterial pneumonia
Pyelonephritis	Chronic fatigue syndrome	Myelodysplastic syndromes	Chronic fatigue syndrome	Idiopathic myelofibrosis	Chronic fatigue syndrome
Chronic fatigue syndrome	Myelodysplastic syndromes	Chronic fatigue syndrome	Myelodysplastic syndromes	Bacterial pneumonia	Myelodysplastic syndromes
Blastomycosis	Blastomycosis	Menopause	Menopause	Blastomycosis	Menopause
Myelodysplastic syndromes	Viral pneumonia	Blastomycosis	Pyelonephritis	Chronic fatigue syndrome	Blastomycosis
Tuberculosis	Tuberculosis	Idiopathic myelofibrosis	Blastomycosis	Menopause	Idiopathic myelofibrosis
Acute leukemia	Acute leukemia	Bacterial pneumonia	Bacterial pneumonia	Myelodysplastic syndromes	Viral pneumonia
	Malaria	Viral pneumonia	Viral pneumonia	Viral pneumonia	Myeloproliferative disorders
		Hyperthyroidism	Hyperthyroidism	Hyperthyroidism	Tuberculosis
		Tuberculosis	Tuberculosis	Tuberculosis	Malaria
		Acute leukemia	Acute leukemia	Myeloproliferative disorders	Pyelonephritis
		Malaria	Malaria	Malaria	

248

Baby (0-1 yr)	Child (1-12 yr)	Adolescent (12-18 yr)	Adult (18-45 yr)	Middle Age Adult (45-65 yr)	Senior Adult (65+ yr)
Maternal estrogen	Malignancy	Fibroadenosis	Breast-feeding	Breast cancer	Breast cancer
Galactorrhea	Galactorrhea	Malignancy	Pituitary eosinophilic adenoma (prolactinoma)	Pituitary eosinophilic adenoma (prolactinoma)	Pituitary eosinophilic adenoma (prolactinoma)
		Galactorrhea	Breast cancer	Breast fibroadenoma	Intraductal papilloma
			Breast fibroadenoma	Fibrocystic breast disease	Breast fibroadenoma
			Fibrocystic breast disease	Fibroadenosis	Fibrocystic breast disease
			Fibroadenosis	Mammary duct ectasia	Fibroadenosis
			Mammary duct ectasia	Intraductal papilloma	Mammary duct ectasia
			Intraductal papilloma	Galactorrhea	Galactorrhea
			Galactorrhea	Drug reaction	Drug reaction
			Drug reaction		

Emergency Rule Out conditions shown in red. Entries in blue are for information only
Conditions are listed in approximate order of prevalence for this age range

Nipple discharge

Emergency Rule Out conditions shown in red. Entries in blue are for information only
Conditions are listed in approximate order of prevalence for this age range

Baby (0-1 yr)	Child (1-12 yr)	Adolescent (12-18 yr)	Adult (18-45 yr)	Middle Age Adult (45-65 yr)	Senior Adult (65+ yr)
All babies have nocturia	Urinary tract infection	Urinary tract infection	Urinary tract infection	Urinary tract infection	Benign prostatic hyperplasia
	Psychosomatic	Urethritis	Diabetes mellitus type 2	Benign prostatic hyperplasia	Urinary tract infection
	Urethritis	Psychosomatic	Diabetes mellitus type 1	Diabetes mellitus type 2	Diabetes mellitus type 2
	Diabetes mellitus in children	Diabetes mellitus in children	Diabetes insipidus	Diabetes mellitus type 1	Diabetes mellitus type 1
	Diabetes insipidus	Diabetes insipidus	Benign prostatic hyperplasia	Diabetes insipidus	Prostatic cancer
	Insomnia	Insomnia	Prostatic cancer	Prostatic cancer	Dementia
			Psychosomatic	Psychosomatic	Psychosomatic
			Dementia	Dementia	Diabetes insipidus
			Congestive heart failure	Congestive heart failure	Congestive heart failure
			Insomnia	Insomnia	Insomnia

Baby (0-1 yr)	Child (1-12 yr)	Adolescent (12-18 yr)	Adult (18-45 yr)	Middle Age Adult (45-65 yr)	Senior Adult (65+ yr)
Idiopathic	Idiopathic	Idiopathic	Hypokalemia	Hypokalemia	Hypokalemia
Hypocalcemia	Hypocalcemia	Hypocalcemia	Hyponatremia	Hyponatremia	Hyponatremia
Hyponatremia	Hyponatremia	Hyponatremia	Drug reaction	Drug reaction	Drug reaction
Deep vein thrombosis	Deep vein thrombosis	Deep vein thrombosis	Diabetic hypoglycemia	Diabetic hypoglycemia	Diabetic hypoglycemia
	Dehydration	Dehydration	Hyperthyroidism	Hypoparathyroidism	Hyperthyroidism
		Recreational drug abuse	Deep vein thrombosis	Deep vein thrombosis	Deep vein thrombosis
			Diabetic neuropathy	Diabetic neuropathy	Diabetic neuropathy
			Arteriosclerosis	Arteriosclerosis	Arteriosclerosis
			Hypocalcemia	Hypocalcemia	Hypocalcemia
			Hyperkalemia	Hyperkalemia	Hyperkalemia
			Chronic renal failure	Chronic renal failure	Chronic renal failure
			Vitamin B12 deficiency	Vitamin B12 deficiency	Vitamin B12 deficiency
			Amyotrophic lateral sclerosis (motor neuron disease)	Amyotrophic lateral sclerosis (motor neuron disease)	Amyotrophic lateral sclerosis (motor neuron disease)
			Muscular dystrophy		
			Dehydration	Dehydration	Dehydration
			Restless leg syndrome	Restless leg syndrome	Restless leg syndrome

Emergency Rule Out conditions shown in red. Entries in blue are for information only
Conditions are listed in approximate order of prevalence for this age range

Nocturnal leg cramps

251

Emergency Rule Out conditions shown in red. Entries in blue are for information only
Conditions are listed in approximate order of prevalence for this age range

Baby (0-1 yr)	Child (1-12 yr)	Adolescent (12-18 yr)	Adult (18-45 yr)	Middle Age Adult (45-65 yr)	Senior Adult (65+ yr)
Congenital nystagmus	Congenital nystagmus	Congenital nystagmus	Labyrinthitis	Labyrinthitis	Labyrinthitis
Friedreich's ataxia	Head injury	Drug reaction	Benign paroxysmal positional vertigo	Drug reaction	Drug reaction
Head injury	Friedreich's ataxia	Friedreich's ataxia	Drug reaction	Benign paroxysmal positional vertigo	Friedreich's ataxia
Cataract	Drug reaction	Head injury	Friedreich's ataxia	Friedreich's ataxia	Brain tumor
Cerebral palsy	Cataract	Cataract	Cataract	Brain tumor	Cataract
Labyrinthine dysfunction	Labyrinthine dysfunction	Brain tumor	Brain tumor	Cataract	Benign paroxysmal positional vertigo
	Brain tumor	Labyrinthine dysfunction	Multiple sclerosis	Multiple sclerosis	Multiple sclerosis
	Cerebral palsy	Cerebral palsy	Congenital nystagmus	Congenital nystagmus	Congenital nystagmus
			Heavy metal poisoning	Heavy metal poisoning	Heavy metal poisoning
			Head injury	Head injury	Head injury

Baby (0-1 yr)	Child (1-12 yr)	Adolescent (12-18 yr)	Adult (18-45 yr)	Middle Age Adult (45-65 yr)	Senior Adult (65+ yr)
Overfeeding	Overfeeding	Dietary weight gain	Dietary weight gain	Dietary weight gain	Dietary weight gain
Cushing's syndrome	Cushing's syndrome	Hypothyroidism	Depression	Depression	Hypothyroidism
Hypothyroidism	Hypothyroidism	Cushing's syndrome	Hypothyroidism	Hypothyroidism	Depression
Prader-Willi syndrome	Prader-Willi syndrome	Prader-Willi syndrome	Diabetes mellitus type 2	Diabetes mellitus type 2	Diabetes mellitus type 2
Turner's syndrome	Turner's syndrome	Turner's syndrome	Polycystic ovarian disease	Polycystic ovarian disease	Cushing's syndrome
Laurence-Moon syndrome	Laurence-Moon syndrome	Laurence-Moon syndrome	Bulimia nervosa	Bulimia nervosa	Insulinoma
Growth hormone deficiency in children	Growth hormone deficiency in children	Growth hormone deficiency in children	Cushing's syndrome	Cushing's syndrome	
			Insulinoma	Insulinoma	

Emergency Rule Out conditions shown in red. Entries in blue are for information only
Conditions are listed in approximate order of prevalence for this age range

253

Emergency Rule Out conditions shown in red. Entries in blue are for information only
Conditions are listed in approximate order of prevalence for this age range

Baby (0-1 yr)	Child (1-12 yr)	Adolescent (12-18 yr)	Adult (18-45 yr)	Middle Age Adult (45-65 yr)	Senior Adult (65+ yr)
Esophageal candidiasis	Esophageal candidiasis	Esophageal candidiasis	Pharyngitis	Pharyngitis	Pharyngitis
Esophageal spasm	Esophageal spasm	Gastroesophageal reflux disease	Esophageal candidiasis	Esophageal candidiasis	Esophageal candidiasis
Gastroesophageal reflux disease	Gastroesophageal reflux disease	Esophageal spasm	Gastroesophageal reflux disease	Gastroesophageal reflux disease	Gastroesophageal reflux disease
Foreign body	Foreign body	Foreign body	Esophageal spasm	Esophageal spasm	Esophageal spasm
Laryngeal cancer	Laryngeal cancer	Laryngeal cancer	Foreign body	Laryngeal cancer	Achalasia
			Laryngeal cancer	Foreign body	Foreign body
			Esophageal cancer	Esophageal cancer	Esophageal cancer
			Head and neck carcinoma	Head and neck carcinoma	Laryngeal cancer
			Scleroderma	Scleroderma	Head and neck carcinoma
			Esophageal diverticulum	Esophageal diverticulum	Scleroderma
			Schatzki's ring	Schatzki's ring	Schatzki's ring
			Plummer-Vinson syndrome	Plummer-Vinson syndrome	Esophageal diverticulum
					Plummer-Vinson syndrome

Baby (0-1 yr)	Child (1-12 yr)	Adolescent (12-18 yr)	Adult (18-45 yr)	Middle Age Adult (45-65 yr)	Senior Adult (65+ yr)
Mucocutaneous candidiasis	Aphthous ulcers	Aphthous ulcers	Aphthous ulcers	Aphthous ulcers	Angular cheilitis
Aphthous ulcers	Trauma	Trauma	Angular cheilitis	Angular cheilitis	Aphthous ulcers
Glossitis	Herpes simplex	Herpes simplex	Stomatitis	Stomatitis	Stomatitis
Reiter's syndrome	Hand-foot-and-mouth disease	Hand-foot-and-mouth disease	Herpes simplex	Herpes simplex	Herpes simplex
Systemic lupus erythematosus	Glossitis	Gingivitis	Reiter's syndrome	Erythema multiforme	Crohn's disease
Hand-foot-and-mouth disease	Systemic lupus erythematosus	Glossitis	Erythema multiforme	Glossitis	Glossitis
Herpes simplex	Reiter's syndrome	Systemic lupus erythematosus	Glossitis	Systemic lupus erythematosus	Reiter's syndrome
	Herpangina	Reiter's syndrome	Systemic lupus erythematosus	Reiter's syndrome	Herpes zoster, shingles
	Burns	Herpangina	Primary HIV infection	Crohn's disease	Systemic lupus erythematosus
	Corrosive acid ingestion	Burns	AIDS	Herpes zoster, shingles	Squamous cell carcinoma
	Behçet's syndrome	Corrosive acid ingestion	Impetigo	Behçet's syndrome	Erythema multiforme
	Acute leukemia	Behçet's syndrome	Crohn's disease	Acute leukemia	Acute leukemia
	Crohn's disease	Acute leukemia	Behçet's syndrome	Squamous cell carcinoma	Syphilis
		Crohn's disease	Lichen planus	Primary HIV infection	Bullous pemphigoid
			Syphilis	AIDS	Primary HIV infection
			Squamous cell carcinoma	Syphilis	AIDS
			Herpes zoster, shingles	Lichen planus	Lichen planus
			Acute leukemia	Bullous pemphigoid	Behçet's syndrome
			Bullous pemphigoid	Impetigo	

Emergency Rule Out conditions shown in red.   Entries in blue are for information only
Conditions are listed in approximate order of prevalence for this age range

Emergency Rule Out conditions shown in red. Entries in blue are for information only
Conditions are listed in approximate order of prevalence for this age range

Baby (0-1 yr)	Child (1-12 yr)	Adolescent (12-18 yr)	Adult (18-45 yr)	Middle Age Adult (45-65 yr)	Senior Adult (65+yr)
Congenital heart disease Aortic regurgitation Cardiomyopathy	Congenital heart disease Congestive heart failure Cardiomyopathy Aortic regurgitation	Congestive heart failure Cardiomyopathy Aortic regurgitation	Congestive heart failure Pleural effusion Cardiomyopathy Aortic regurgitation Aortic stenosis	Congestive heart failure Aortic regurgitation Cardiomyopathy Pleural effusion Aortic stenosis	Congestive heart failure Aortic regurgitation Cardiomyopathy Pleural effusion Aortic stenosis

Baby (0-1 yr)	Child (1-12 yr)	Adolescent (12-18 yr)	Adult (18-45 yr)	Middle Age Adult (45-65 yr)	Senior Adult (65+ yr)
Acute otitis media	Acute otitis media	Acute otitis media	Otitis externa	Otitis externa	Otitis externa
Chronic otitis media	Chronic otitis media	Chronic otitis media	Cellulitis	Acute otitis media	Cellulitis
Otitis externa	Otitis externa	Otitis externa	Acute otitis media	Cellulitis	Influenza
Laryngeal cancer	Temporomandibular joint syndrome	Temporomandibular joint syndrome	Chronic otitis media	Chronic otitis media	Furunculosis
	Laryngeal cancer	Laryngeal cancer	Influenza	Furunculosis	Dysbarism and barotrauma
			Furunculosis	Influenza	Acute otitis media
			Mastoiditis	Dysbarism and barotrauma	Chronic otitis media
			Dysbarism and barotrauma	Mastoiditis	Mastoiditis
			Trigeminal neuralgia	Trigeminal neuralgia	Trigeminal neuralgia
			Laryngeal cancer	Laryngeal cancer	Laryngeal cancer

Emergency Rule Out conditions shown in red. Entries in blue are for information only
Conditions are listed in approximate order of prevalence for this age range

257

Emergency Rule Out conditions shown in red. Entries in blue are for information only
Conditions are listed in approximate order of prevalence for this age range

Baby (0-1 yr)	Child (1-12 yr)	Adolescent (12-18 yr)	Adult (18-45 yr)	Middle Age Adult (45-65 yr)	Senior Adult (65+yr)
Non-traumatic tympanic membrane rupture	Non-traumatic tympanic membrane rupture	Non-traumatic tympanic membrane rupture	Non-traumatic tympanic membrane rupture	Non-traumatic tympanic membrane rupture	Non-traumatic tympanic membrane rupture
Acute ottis media	Ottis externa	Ottis externa	Ottis externa	Ottis externa	Ottis externa
Foreign body	Acute ottis media	Acute ottis media	Acute ottis media	Acute ottis media	Acute ottis media
Mastoiditis	Foreign body	Mastoiditis	Traumatic tympanic membrane rupture	Mastoiditis	Mastoiditis
Chronic ottis media	Mastoiditis	Traumatic tympanic membrane rupture	Mastoiditis	Chronic ottis media	Chronic ottis media
Cerebrospinal fluid leak	Chronic ottis media	Chronic ottis media	Chronic ottis media	Furunculosis	Furunculosis
	Cerebrospinal fluid leak	Foreign body	Furunculosis	Cholesteatoma	Cholesteatoma
		Cholesteatoma	Cholesteatoma	Foreign body	Foreign body
		Cerebrospinal fluid leak	Foreign body	Cerebrospinal fluid leak	Cerebrospinal fluid leak
			Cerebrospinal fluid leak		

Baby (0-1 yr)	Child (1-12 yr)	Adolescent (12-18 yr)	Adult (18-45 yr)	Middle Age Adult (45-65 yr)	Senior Adult (65+ yr)
Anemia due to acute blood loss	Anemia due to acute blood loss	Anemia due to acute blood loss	Anemia	Anemia	Anemia
Iron deficiency anemia	Iron deficiency anemia	Iron deficiency anemia	Aplastic anemia	Aplastic anemia	Aplastic anemia
Bronchiolitis	Bartonella infection (cat scratch disease)	Acute leukemia	Celiac disease	Acute leukemia	Celiac disease
Hemolytic disease of the newborn (erythroblastosis fetalis)	Celiac disease	Bartonella infection (cat scratch disease)	Acute leukemia	Celiac disease	Acute leukemia
Celiac disease	Bronchiolitis	Celiac disease	Bartonella infection (cat scratch disease)	Frostbite environmental hypothermia	Frostbite environmental hypothermia
Anemia	Acute leukemia	Anemia	Frostbite environmental hypothermia	Albinism	Albinism
Anemia of chronic disease	Anemia	Anemia of chronic disease	Albinism	Systemic lupus erythematosus	Systemic lupus erythematosus
Systemic lupus erythematosus	Anemia of chronic disease	Systemic lupus erythematosus	Systemic lupus erythematosus		
Albinism	Systemic lupus erythematosus	Albinism			
	Albinism				

Emergency Rule Out conditions shown in red. Entries in blue are for information only
Conditions are listed in approximate order of prevalence for this age range

Emergency Rule Out conditions shown in red. Entries in blue are for information only
Conditions are listed in approximate order of prevalence for this age range

Baby (0-1 yr)	Child (1-12 yr)	Adolescent (12-18 yr)	Adult (18-45 yr)	Middle Age Adult (45-65 yr)	Senior Adult (65+yr)
Orthostatic hypotension	Anxiety	Anxiety	Anxiety	Anxiety	Anxiety
Cardiomyopathy	Sinus tachycardia	Sinus tachycardia	Premature atrial contraction	Premature atrial contraction	Atrial fibrillation
Chronic fatigue syndrome	Aortic regurgitation	Premature atrial contraction	Atrial fibrillation	Atrial fibrillation	Orthostatic hypotension
Atrial septal defect	Chronic fatigue syndrome	Chronic fatigue syndrome	Atrial flutter	Atrial flutter	Chronic fatigue syndrome
	Cardiomyopathy	Orthostatic hypotension	Aortic regurgitation	Orthostatic hypotension	Atrial flutter
	Orthostatic hypotension	Cardiomyopathy	Chronic fatigue syndrome	Chronic fatigue syndrome	Paroxysmal atrial tachycardia
	Atrial septal defect	Atrial septal defect	Paroxysmal atrial tachycardia	Paroxysmal atrial tachycardia	Cardiomyopathy
	Wolff-Parkinson-White syndrome	Aortic regurgitation	Atrial septal defect	Caffeine abuse	Aortic regurgitation
	Recreational drug abuse	Premature ventricular contraction	Cardiomyopathy	Atrial septal defect	Ventricular tachycardia
		Wolff-Parkinson-White syndrome	Orthostatic hypotension	Cardiomyopathy	Atrial septal defect
		Recreational drug abuse	Caffeine abuse	Aortic regurgitation	Premature ventricular contraction
		Alcohol abuse	Recreational drug abuse	Recreational drug abuse	Sinus tachycardia
			Alcohol abuse	Alcohol abuse	Wolff-Parkinson-White syndrome
			Ventricular tachycardia	Ventricular tachycardia	
			Premature ventricular contraction	Premature ventricular contraction	
			Sinus tachycardia	Sinus tachycardia	
			Wolff-Parkinson-White syndrome	Wolff-Parkinson-White syndrome	

Baby (0-1 yr)	Child (1-12 yr)	Adolescent (12-18 yr)	Adult (18-45 yr)	Middle Age Adult (45-65 yr)	Senior Adult (65+ yr)
Parvovirus B19 infection	Parvovirus B19 infection	Parvovirus B19 infection	Aplastic anemia	Aplastic anemia	Aplastic anemia
Drug reaction	Drug reaction	Drug reaction	Systemic lupus erythematosus	Systemic lupus erythematosus	Myeloproliferative disorders
Acute leukemia	Intestinal parasites	Intestinal parasites	Myeloproliferative disorders	Myeloproliferative disorders	Megaloblastic anemias
Neuroblastoma	Acute leukemia	Babesiosis	Megaloblastic anemias	Megaloblastic anemias	Myelodysplastic syndromes
Myelodysplastic syndromes	Neuroblastoma	Acute leukemia	Babesiosis	Babesiosis	Drug reaction
Babesiosis	Myelodysplastic syndromes	Neuroblastoma	Intestinal parasites	Intestinal parasites	Babesiosis
Intestinal parasites	Babesiosis	Myelodysplastic syndromes	Myelodysplastic syndromes	Myelodysplastic syndromes	Acute leukemia
Fanconi's syndrome	Fanconi's syndrome	Fanconi's syndrome	Drug reaction	Drug reaction	Chronic lymphocytic leukemia
Primary HIV infection	Primary HIV infection	Primary HIV infection	Acute leukemia	Acute leukemia	Chronic myelogenous leukemia
Chronic lymphocytic leukemia	Chronic lymphocytic leukemia	Chronic lymphocytic leukemia	Chronic lymphocytic leukemia	Chronic lymphocytic leukemia	Intestinal parasites
Chronic myelogenous leukemia	Chronic myelogenous leukemia	Chronic myelogenous leukemia	Chronic myelogenous leukemia	Chronic myelogenous leukemia	

Emergency Rule Out conditions shown in red. Entries in blue are for information only
Conditions are listed in approximate order of prevalence for this age range

Emergency Rule Out conditions shown in red. Entries in blue are for information only
Conditions are listed in approximate order of prevalence for this age range

Baby (0-1 yr)	Child (1-12 yr)	Adolescent (12-18 yr)	Adult (18-45 yr)	Middle Age Adult (45-65 yr)	Senior Adult (65+ yr)
Raised intracranial pressure	Raised intracranial pressure	Raised intracranial pressure	Malignant hypertension	Malignant hypertension	Malignant hypertension
Hydrocephalus	Cerebral edema	Cerebral edema	Hydrocephalus	Hydrocephalus	Brain tumor
Brain tumor	Hydrocephalus	Hydrocephalus	Optic neuritis	Optic neuritis	Brain abscess
Cavernous sinus thrombosis	Trauma	Trauma	Brain tumor	Brain tumor	Hydrocephalus
Intracranial hemorrhage	Brain tumor	Cavernous sinus thrombosis	Brain abscess	Cavernous sinus thrombosis	Encephalitis
Trauma	Intracranial hemorrhage	Brain tumor	Encephalitis	Brain abscess	Cavernous sinus thrombosis
Encephalitis	Cavernous sinus thrombosis	Intracranial hemorrhage	Cavernous sinus thrombosis	Encephalitis	Benign intracranial hypertension
Encephalopathy	Brain abscess	Brain abscess	Benign intracranial hypertension	Benign intracranial hypertension	Cerebral edema
Cerebral edema	Encephalitis	Encephalitis	Cerebral edema	Cerebral edema	Encephalopathy
	Encephalopathy	Encephalopathy	Encephalopathy	Encephalopathy	Trauma
	Benign intracranial hypertension	Benign intracranial hypertension	Trauma	Trauma	Altitude sickness
	Malignant hypertension	Malignant hypertension	Altitude sickness	Altitude sickness	
	Altitude sickness	Altitude sickness			

Baby (0-1 yr)	Child (1-12 yr)	Adolescent (12-18 yr)	Adult (18-45 yr)	Middle Age Adult (45-65 yr)	Senior Adult (65+ yr)
Acute otitis media	Acute otitis media	Acute otitis media	Bell's palsy	Bell's palsy	Ischemic stroke
Chronic otitis media	Chronic otitis media	Chronic otitis media	Acute otitis media	Acute otitis media	Bell's palsy
Head injury	Bell's palsy	Acute sinusitis	Chronic otitis media	Chronic otitis media	Acute otitis media
Guillain-Barré syndrome (acute infective polyneuritis)	Head injury	Chronic sinusitis	Acute sinusitis	Acute sinusitis	Chronic otitis media
Herpes zoster, shingles	Guillain-Barré syndrome (acute infective polyneuritis)	Bell's palsy	Chronic sinusitis	Chronic sinusitis	Acute sinusitis
Myasthenia gravis	Herpes zoster, shingles	Head injury	Benign salivary gland tumor	Benign salivary gland tumor	Chronic sinusitis
	Myasthenia gravis	Guillain-Barré syndrome (acute infective polyneuritis)	Head injury	Head injury	Herpes zoster, shingles
		Herpes zoster, shingles	Ischemic stroke	Ischemic stroke	Benign salivary gland tumor
		Myasthenia gravis	Malignant salivary gland tumor	Malignant salivary gland tumor	Malignant salivary gland tumor
			Herpes zoster, shingles	Herpes zoster, shingles	Head injury
			Guillain-Barré syndrome (acute infective polyneuritis)	Guillain-Barré syndrome (acute infective polyneuritis)	Guillain-Barré syndrome (acute infective polyneuritis)
			Myasthenia gravis	Myasthenia gravis	Myasthenia gravis

Emergency Rule Out conditions shown in red. Entries in blue are for information only
Conditions are listed in approximate order of prevalence for this age range

Emergency Rule Out conditions shown in red. Entries in blue are for information only
Conditions are listed in approximate order of prevalence for this age range

Baby (0-1 yr)	Child (1-12 yr)	Adolescent (12-18 yr)	Adult (18-45 yr)	Middle Age Adult (45-65 yr)	Senior Adult (65+ yr)
Cerebral palsy	Cerebral palsy	Trauma	Trauma	Trauma	Trauma
Trauma	Trauma	Epidural abscess	Epidural abscess	Epidural abscess	Epidural abscess
Spinal cord compression	Spinal cord compression	Multiple sclerosis	Multiple sclerosis	Multiple sclerosis	Abdominal aortic dissection
Syringomyelia	Syringomyelia	Syringomyelia	Guillain-Barré syndrome (acute infective polyneuritis)	Guillain-Barré syndrome (acute infective polyneuritis)	Amyotrophic lateral sclerosis (motor neuron disease)
Hydrocephalus	Hydrocephalus	Cerebral palsy	Syringomyelia	Syringomyelia	Guillain-Barré syndrome (acute infective polyneuritis)
	Guillain-Barré syndrome (acute infective polyneuritis)	Spinal cord compression	Amyotrophic lateral sclerosis (motor neuron disease)	Amyotrophic lateral sclerosis (motor neuron disease)	Multiple sclerosis
		Hydrocephalus	Abdominal aortic dissection	Abdominal aortic aneurysm	Syringomyelia
		Guillain-Barré syndrome (acute infective polyneuritis)			

Baby (0-1 yr)	Child (1-12 yr)	Adolescent (12-18 yr)	Adult (18-45 yr)	Middle Age Adult (45-65 yr)	Senior Adult (65+ yr)
Not relevant to this age group	Not relevant to this age group	Not relevant to this age group	Brain tumor Ischemic stroke Brain abscess	Brain tumor Ischemic stroke Brain abscess	Brain tumor Ischemic stroke Brain abscess

Emergency Rule Out conditions shown in red. Entries in blue are for information only
Conditions are listed in approximate order of prevalence for this age range

Emergency Rule Out conditions shown in red. Entries in blue are for information only
Conditions are listed in approximate order of prevalence for this age range

Baby (0-1 yr)	Child (1-12 yr)	Adolescent (12-18 yr)	Adult (18-45 yr)	Middle Age Adult (45-65 yr)	Senior Adult (65+ yr)
Behçet's syndrome	Trauma	Trauma	Carpal tunnel syndrome	Diabetes mellitus type 1	Diabetes mellitus type 1
Creutzfeldt-Jakob disease	Nerve root compression	Nerve root compression	Diabetes mellitus type 1	Diabetes mellitus type 2	Diabetes mellitus type 2
Chronic fatigue syndrome	Hypocalcemia	Diabetes mellitus in children	Diabetes mellitus type 2	Carpal tunnel syndrome	Carpal tunnel syndrome
Herpes zoster, shingles	Chronic fatigue syndrome	Osteomalacia	Lumbar disc disorders	Lumbar disc disorders	Lumbar disc disorders
Herpes simplex	Herpes simplex	Charcot-Marie-Tooth disease	Herpes zoster, shingles	Herpes zoster, shingles	Bell's palsy
Hypocalcemia	Creutzfeldt-Jakob disease	Creutzfeldt-Jakob disease	Bell's palsy	Bell's palsy	Herpes simplex
Rickets in children	Herpes zoster, shingles	Chronic fatigue syndrome	Trigeminal neuralgia	Creutzfeldt-Jakob disease	Creutzfeldt-Jakob disease
	Diabetes mellitus in children	Herpes simplex	Charcot-Marie-Tooth disease	Herpes simplex	Herpes zoster, shingles
	Osteomalacia	Hypocalcemia	Hypocalcemia	Osteomalacia	Chronic fatigue syndrome
	Behçet's syndrome	Herpes zoster, shingles	Herpes simplex	Trigeminal neuralgia	Trigeminal neuralgia
	Reflex sympathetic dystrophy	Behçet's syndrome	Creutzfeldt-Jakob disease	Hypocalcemia	Osteomalacia
	Syringomyelia	Reflex sympathetic dystrophy	Osteomalacia	Charcot-Marie-Tooth disease	Hypocalcemia
	Cervical spine injury	Hereditary neuropathy of liability to pressure palsies	Behçet's syndrome	Chronic fatigue syndrome	Charcot-Marie-Tooth disease
	Rickets in children	Syringomyelia	Acoustic neuroma	Acoustic neuroma	Acoustic neuroma
		Cervical spine injury	Chronic fatigue syndrome	Thoracic outlet syndrome	Thoracic outlet syndrome
		Leprosy	Thoracic outlet syndrome	Behçet's syndrome	Multiple sclerosis
		Rickets in children	Multiple sclerosis	Multiple sclerosis	Behçet's syndrome
			Reflex sympathetic dystrophy	Reflex sympathetic dystrophy	Reflex sympathetic dystrophy
			Syringomyelia	Syringomyelia	Syringomyelia
			Brain tumor	Brain tumor	Brain tumor
			Hereditary neuropathy of liability to pressure palsies	Hereditary neuropathy of liability to pressure palsies	Hereditary neuropathy of liability to pressure palsies

Baby (0-1 yr)	Child (1-12 yr)	Adolescent (12-18 yr)	Adult (18-45 yr)	Middle Age Adult (45-65 yr)	Senior Adult (65+ yr)
			Nerve root compression	Nerve root compression	Nerve root compression
			Trauma	Trauma	Trauma
			Cervical spine injury	Cervical spine injury	Cervical spine injury
			Leprosy		

Emergency Rule Out conditions shown in red. Entries in blue are for information only
Conditions are listed in approximate order of prevalence for this age range

Baby (0-1 yr)	Child (1-12 yr)	Adolescent (12-18 yr)	Adult (18-45 yr)	Middle Age Adult (45-65 yr)	Senior Adult (65+ yr)
Not relevant to this age group	Allergic rhinitis Acute sinusitis Chronic sinusitis Trauma	Allergic rhinitis Acute sinusitis Chronic sinusitis Influenza Trauma	Allergic rhinitis Acute sinusitis Chronic sinusitis Influenza Trauma Brain tumor Malignancy Ischemic stroke Temporal lobe epilepsy	Allergic rhinitis Acute sinusitis Chronic sinusitis Influenza Trauma Brain tumor Malignancy Ischemic stroke Temporal lobe epilepsy	Influenza Allergic rhinitis Acute sinusitis Chronic sinusitis Trauma Brain tumor Malignancy Ischemic stroke Temporal lobe epilepsy

Baby (0-1 yr)	Child (1-12 yr)	Adolescent (12-18 yr)	Adult (18-45 yr)	Middle Age Adult (45-65 yr)	Senior Adult (65+ yr)
Mumps Sialadenitis Parotitis	Mumps Sialadenitis Parotitis	Mumps Sialadenitis Parotitis	Salivary gland calculi Parotitis Sialadenitis Benign salivary gland tumor Malignant salivary gland tumor Mumps	Salivary gland calculi Parotitis Sialadenitis Benign salivary gland tumor Malignant salivary gland tumor	Salivary gland calculi Parotitis Sialadenitis Benign salivary gland tumor Malignant salivary gland tumor

Emergency Rule Out conditions shown in red. Entries in blue are for information only
Conditions are listed in approximate order of prevalence for this age range

269

Emergency Rule Out conditions shown in red. Entries in blue are for information only
Conditions are listed in approximate order of prevalence for this age range

Baby (0-1 yr)	Child (1-12 yr)	Adolescent (12-18 yr)	Adult (18-45 yr)	Middle Age Adult (45-65 yr)	Senior Adult (65+ yr)
Mumps	Mumps	Mumps	Salivary gland calculi	Salivary gland calculi	Alcohol abuse
Sialadenitis	Parotitis	Parotitis	Alcohol abuse	Alcohol abuse	Benign salivary gland tumor
Parotitis	Sialadenitis	Parotid calculus	Anorexia nervosa	Benign salivary gland tumor	Malignant salivary gland tumor
Primary HIV infection	Parotid calculus	Sialadenitis	Benign salivary gland tumor	Parotitis	Salivary gland calculi
AIDS	Cystic fibrosis	Anorexia nervosa	Parotitis	Sialadenitis	Sjögren's syndrome
	Primary HIV infection	Bulimia nervosa	Bulimia nervosa	Anorexia nervosa	Parotitis
	AIDS	Cystic fibrosis	Malignant salivary gland tumor	Bulimia nervosa	Sialadenitis
		Primary HIV infection	Mumps	Malignant salivary gland tumor	Hodgkin's disease
		AIDS	Sialadenitis	Systemic lupus erythematosus	Non-Hodgkin's lymphoma
			Systemic lupus erythematosus	Sjögren's syndrome	Tuberculosis
			Hodgkin's disease	Mumps	Acute leukemia
			Sjögren's syndrome	Primary HIV infection	Anorexia nervosa
			Primary HIV infection	AIDS	Primary HIV infection
			AIDS	Tuberculosis	AIDS
			Tuberculosis	Hodgkin's disease	Mumps
			Cystic fibrosis	Non-Hodgkin's lymphoma	
			Non-Hodgkin's lymphoma	Acute leukemia	
			Acute leukemia		

Baby (0-1 yr)	Child (1-12 yr)	Adolescent (12-18 yr)	Adult (18-45 yr)	Middle Age Adult (45-65 yr)	Senior Adult (65+ yr)
Congenital heart disease **Aortic regurgitation** Cardiomyopathy	Congenital heart disease Cardiomyopathy Congestive heart failure **Aortic regurgitation**	Congestive heart failure Cardiomyopathy **Aortic regurgitation**	Congestive heart failure **Mitral stenosis** Aortic stenosis **Anxiety**	Congestive heart failure **Mitral stenosis** Aortic stenosis **Anxiety**	Congestive heart failure **Mitral stenosis** Aortic stenosis **Anxiety**

Paroxysmal nocturnal dyspnea

Emergency Rule Out conditions shown in red. Entries in blue are for information only
Conditions are listed in approximate order of prevalence for this age range

Emergency Rule Out conditions shown in red. Entries in blue are for information only
Conditions are listed in approximate order of prevalence for this age range

Baby (0-1 yr)	Child (1-12 yr)	Adolescent (12-18 yr)	Adult (18-45 yr)	Middle Age Adult (45-65 yr)	Senior Adult (65+yr)
Distended urinary bladder	Distended urinary bladder	Distended urinary bladder	Endometriosis	Pelvic inflammatory disease	Distended urinary bladder
Malignancy	Malignancy	Functional benign ovarian tumor	Pelvic inflammatory disease	Uterine myomas	Germ cell ovarian cancer
		Ruptured/hemorrhagic ovarian cyst	Ruptured/hemorrhagic ovarian cyst	Ruptured/hemorrhagic ovarian cyst	Sex cord/stromal ovarian cancer
		Pregnancy	Uterine myomas	Distended urinary bladder	Metastatic cancer
		Ectopic pregnancy	Functional benign ovarian tumor	Germ cell ovarian cancer	Endometrial cancer
		Endometriosis	Ectopic pregnancy	Sex cord/stromal ovarian cancer	Uterine myomas
		Polycystic ovarian disease	Distended urinary bladder	Functional benign ovarian tumor	Functional benign ovarian tumor
		Malignancy	Germ cell ovarian cancer	Endometrial cancer	Epithelial cell ovarian cancer
			Sex cord/stromal ovarian cancer	Metastatic cancer	Endometriosis
			Polycystic ovarian disease	Polycystic ovarian disease	Abdominal abscess
			Endometrial cancer	Epithelial cell ovarian cancer	
			Metastatic cancer	Endometriosis	
			Epithelial cell ovarian cancer	Abdominal abscess	
			Endometriosis		
			Abdominal abscess		

Baby (0-1 yr)	Child (1-12 yr)	Adolescent (12-18 yr)	Adult (18-45 yr)	Middle Age Adult (45-65 yr)	Senior Adult (65+ yr)
Not relevant to this age group	Urinary tract infection Phimosis and paraphimosis Polymyalgia rheumatica Benign ovarian tumor Dysmenorrhea Renal calculi Prepubescent vulvovaginitis	Dysmenorrhea Urinary tract infection Renal calculi Pregnancy Phimosis and paraphimosis Polymyalgia rheumatica Benign ovarian tumor Ruptured/hemorrhagic ovarian cyst Ectopic pregnancy Pelvic inflammatory disease Ovarian torsion Chlamydia trachomatis infection	Dysmenorrhea Premenstrual syndrome Urinary tract infection Ruptured/hemorrhagic ovarian cyst Phimosis and paraphimosis Pregnancy Ectopic pregnancy Polymyalgia rheumatica Pelvic inflammatory disease Chlamydia trachomatis infection Benign ovarian tumor Endometriosis Cervical malignancy Renal calculi Epithelial cell ovarian cancer Germ cell ovarian cancer Sex cord/stromal ovarian cancer Pelvic tumor	Dysmenorrhea Urinary tract infection Pelvic inflammatory disease Polymyalgia rheumatica Phimosis and paraphimosis Renal calculi Epithelial cell ovarian cancer Germ cell ovarian cancer Benign ovarian tumor Sex cord/stromal ovarian cancer Endometriosis Cervical malignancy Colon cancer Pelvic tumor Bladder tumor Ovarian torsion Ruptured/hemorrhagic ovarian cyst Chlamydia trachomatis infection	Urinary tract infection Cervical malignancy Pelvic tumor Epithelial cell ovarian cancer Phimosis and paraphimosis Polymyalgia rheumatica Germ cell ovarian cancer Benign ovarian tumor Sex cord/stromal ovarian cancer Colon cancer Renal calculi Bladder tumor Ovarian torsion Ruptured/hemorrhagic ovarian cyst

List continues on next page

Emergency Rule Out conditions shown in red. Entries in blue are for information only
Conditions are listed in approximate order of prevalence for this age range

List continued from previous page

Baby (0-1 yr)	Child (1-12 yr)	Adolescent (12-18 yr)	Adult (18-45 yr)	Middle Age Adult (45-65 yr)	Senior Adult (65+yr)
			Bladder tumor Colon cancer Ovarian torsion		

Baby (0-1 yr)	Child (1-12 yr)	Adolescent (12-18 yr)	Adult (18-45 yr)	Middle Age Adult (45-65 yr)	Senior Adult (65+ yr)
Drug reaction, peptic ulcer	Helicobacter pylori	Helicobacter pylori	Helicobacter pylori	Helicobacter pylori	Helicobacter pylori
Head injury	Drug reaction, peptic ulcer	Drug reaction, peptic ulcer	Alcohol abuse	Alcohol abuse	Alcohol abuse
Burns	Burns	Burns	Tobacco smoking	Tobacco smoking	Tobacco smoking
Poisoning	Head injury	Head injury	Drug reaction, peptic ulcer	Drug reaction, peptic ulcer	Drug reaction, peptic ulcer
Helicobacter pylori	Crohn's disease	Crohn's disease	Zollinger-Ellison syndrome	Zollinger-Ellison syndrome	Zollinger-Ellison syndrome
	Poisoning	Poisoning	Crohn's disease	Crohn's disease	Crohn's disease
		Alcohol abuse	Burns	Burns	Burns

Emergency Rule Out conditions shown in red. Entries in blue are for information only
Conditions are listed in approximate order of prevalence for this age range

275

Periarticular pain

Emergency Rule Out conditions shown in red. Entries in blue are for information only
Conditions are listed in approximate order of prevalence for this age range

Baby (0-1 yr)	Child (1-12 yr)	Adolescent (12-18 yr)	Adult (18-45 yr)	Middle Age Adult (45-65 yr)	Senior Adult (65+ yr)
Trauma	Trauma	Trauma Aseptic bursitis	Aseptic bursitis Nerve root compression Reflex sympathetic dystrophy Fibromyalgia Trauma	Aseptic bursitis Nerve root compression Reflex sympathetic dystrophy Polymyalgia rheumatica Fibromyalgia Trauma	Aseptic bursitis Nerve root compression Reflex sympathetic dystrophy Polymyalgia rheumatica Fibromyalgia Trauma

Baby (0-1 yr)	Child (1-12 yr)	Adolescent (12-18 yr)	Adult (18-45 yr)	Middle Age Adult (45-65 yr)	Senior Adult (65+yr)
Friedreich's ataxia	Guillain-Barré syndrome (acute infective polyneuritis)	Guillain-Barré syndrome (acute infective polyneuritis)	Carpal tunnel syndrome	Carpal tunnel syndrome	Diabetes mellitus type 2
Carbon monoxide poisoning	Chronic lead poisoning	Chemical/ pesticide poisoning	Diabetes mellitus type 2	Diabetes mellitus type 2	Chronic renal failure
	Friedreich's ataxia	Diabetes mellitus in children	Diabetes mellitus type 1	Chronic renal failure	Alcohol abuse
	Chemical/ pesticide poisoning	Friedreich's ataxia	Chronic renal failure	Alcohol abuse	Drug reaction
	Carbon monoxide poisoning	Chronic lead poisoning	Alcohol abuse	Drug reaction	Carpal tunnel syndrome
	Poisoning	Carbon monoxide poisoning	Drug reaction	Diabetes mellitus type 1	Vitamin B12 deficiency
	Diabetes mellitus in children	Chronic renal failure	Vitamin B12 deficiency	Vitamin B12 deficiency	Malignancy
	Chronic renal failure	Primary HIV infection	Malignancy	Friedreich's ataxia	Friedreich's ataxia
	Syringomyelia	AIDS	AIDS	Malignancy	Folate deficiency
	Charcot-Marie-Tooth disease	Syringomyelia	Friedreich's ataxia	Folate deficiency	Diabetes mellitus type 1
	Hereditary neuropathy of liability to pressure palsies	Charcot-Marie-Tooth disease	Folate deficiency	Myxedema	Myxedema
		Hereditary neuropathy of liability to pressure palsies	Myxedema	Sarcoidosis	Carbon monoxide poisoning
			Sarcoidosis	Pellagra	Sarcoidosis
			Pellagra	Carbon monoxide poisoning	Pellagra
			Carbon monoxide poisoning	Syphilis	Syphilis
			Syphilis	AIDS	Chronic lead poisoning
			Chronic lead poisoning	Chronic lead poisoning	Tabes dorsalis
			Tabes dorsalis	Tabes dorsalis	Polyarteritis nodosa
			Polyarteritis nodosa	Polyarteritis nodosa	Porphyria
			Porphyria	Porphyria	Amyloidosis
			Amyloidosis	Amyloidosis	Charcot-Marie-Tooth disease
			Charcot-Marie-Tooth disease	Charcot-Marie-Tooth disease	

List continues on next page

Emergency Rule Out conditions shown in red. Entries in blue are for information only
Conditions are listed in approximate order of prevalence for this age range

Peripheral neuropathy

List continued from previous page

Baby (0-1 yr)	Child (1-12 yr)	Adolescent (12-18 yr)	Adult (18-45 yr)	Middle Age Adult (45-65 yr)	Senior Adult (65+ yr)
			Hereditary neuropathy of liability to pressure palsies Syringomyelia Primary HIV infection	Hereditary neuropathy of liability to pressure palsies Syringomyelia Primary HIV infection	Hereditary neuropathy of liability to pressure palsies Syringomyelia Primary HIV infection AIDS

Baby (0-1 yr)	Child (1-12 yr)	Adolescent (12-18 yr)	Adult (18-45 yr)	Middle Age Adult (45-65 yr)	Senior Adult (65+ yr)
Not relevant to this age group	Head injury Depression Brain tumor	Depression Head injury Recreational drug abuse Alcohol abuse Brain tumor	Depression Head injury Recreational drug abuse Alcohol abuse Delirium Brain tumor Dementia	Depression Delirium Dementia Brain tumor Head injury	Dementia Drug reaction Depression Delirium Head injury Brain tumor

Emergency Rule Out conditions shown in red. Entries in blue are for information only
Conditions are listed in approximate order of prevalence for this age range

Personality change

Emergency Rule Out conditions shown in red. Entries in blue are for information only
Conditions are listed in approximate order of prevalence for this age range

Baby (0-1 yr)	Child (1-12 yr)	Adolescent (12-18 yr)	Adult (18-45 yr)	Middle Age Adult (45-65 yr)	Senior Adult (65+yr)
Viral infection	Idiopathic thrombocytopenic purpura	Idiopathic thrombocytopenic purpura	Sepsis	Sepsis	Sepsis
Sepsis	Viral infection	Viral infection	Idiopathic thrombocytopenic purpura	Idiopathic thrombocytopenic purpura	Drug reaction
Drug reaction	Sepsis	Sepsis	Drug reaction	Drug reaction	Idiopathic thrombocytopenic purpura
Meningococcemia	Meningococcemia	Meningococcemia	Idiopathic thrombocythemia	Idiopathic thrombocythemia	Idiopathic thrombocythemia
Idiopathic thrombocytopenic purpura	Bacterial meningitis	Dementia	Myelodysplastic syndromes	Myelodysplastic syndromes	Dementia
Bacterial meningitis	Viral meningitis	Bacterial meningitis	Bacteremia	Dementia	Myelodysplastic syndromes
Dementia	Dementia	Viral meningitis	Dementia	Bacteremia	Bacteremia
Viral meningitis	Drug reaction	Drug reaction	Aplastic anemia	Aplastic anemia	Aplastic anemia
Henoch-Schönlein purpura	Systemic lupus erythematosus	Systemic lupus erythematosus	Thrombotic thrombocytopenic purpura	Thrombotic thrombocytopenic purpura	Thrombotic thrombocytopenic purpura
Aplastic anemia	Acute leukemia	Acute leukemia	Meningococcemia	Meningococcemia	Meningococcemia
Thrombotic thrombocytopenic purpura	Myelodysplastic syndromes	Myelodysplastic syndromes	Henoch-Schönlein purpura	Henoch-Schönlein purpura	Henoch-Schönlein purpura
Idiopathic thrombocythemia	Henoch-Schönlein purpura	Henoch-Schönlein purpura	Connective tissue disease	Connective tissue disease	Connective tissue disease
Connective tissue disease	Aplastic anemia	Aplastic anemia	Systemic lupus erythematosus	Systemic lupus erythematosus	Systemic lupus erythematosus
Myelodysplastic syndromes	Thrombotic thrombocytopenic purpura	Thrombotic thrombocytopenic purpura	Acute leukemia	Acute leukemia	Acute leukemia
Disseminated intravascular coagulation	Idiopathic thrombocythemia	Idiopathic thrombocythemia	Viral infection	Viral infection	Viral infection
Acute leukemia	Connective tissue disease	Connective tissue disease			
Osteogenesis imperfecta					

Baby (0-1 yr)	Child (1-12 yr)	Adolescent (12-18 yr)	Adult (18-45 yr)	Middle Age Adult (45-65 yr)	Senior Adult (65+ yr)
Bacterial conjunctivitis	Retinal migraine	Retinal migraine	Migraine headache	Migraine headache	Glaucoma
Dry eye	Corneal abrasion	Corneal abrasion	Corneal abrasion	Corneal abrasion	Subarachnoid hemorrhage and cerebral aneurysm
Corneal abrasion	Uveitis	Uveitis	Uveitis	Uveitis	stroke
Glaucoma	Viral conjunctivitis	Viral conjunctivitis	Subarachnoid hemorrhage and cerebral aneurysm	Subarachnoid hemorrhage and cerebral aneurysm	Corneal abrasion
	Dry eye	Bacterial conjunctivitis	stroke	stroke	Uveitis
	Bacterial conjunctivitis	Dry eye	Bacterial meningitis	Bacterial meningitis	Bacterial meningitis
	Foreign body	Foreign body	Dry eye	Dry eye	Viral meningitis
	Viral meningitis	Bacterial meningitis	Glaucoma	Glaucoma	Dry eye
	Encephalitis	Viral meningitis	Viral meningitis	Viral meningitis	Migraine headache
	Bacterial meningitis	Encephalitis	Encephalitis	Encephalitis	Encephalitis
	Glaucoma	Glaucoma	Retinal migraine	Retinal migraine	Retinal migraine
			Bacterial conjunctivitis	Bacterial conjunctivitis	Bacterial conjunctivitis
			Viral conjunctivitis	Viral conjunctivitis	Viral conjunctivitis
			Foreign body	Foreign body	

Emergency Rule Out conditions shown in red. Entries in blue are for information only
Conditions are listed in approximate order of prevalence for this age range

281

Placental scan, abnormal

Emergency Rule Out conditions shown in red. Entries in blue are for information only
Conditions are listed in approximate order of prevalence for this age range

Baby (0-1 yr)	Child (1-12 yr)	Adolescent (12-18 yr)	Adult (18-45 yr)	Middle Age Adult (45-65 yr)	Senior Adult (65+yr)
Not relevant to this age group	Not relevant to this age group	Abruptio placentae Placenta previa Pregnancy-induced hypertension	Abruptio placentae Placenta previa Pregnancy-induced hypertension	Abruptio placentae Placenta previa Pregnancy-induced hypertension	Not relevant to this age group

Baby (0-1 yr)	Child (1-12 yr)	Adolescent (12-18 yr)	Adult (18-45 yr)	Middle Age Adult (45-65 yr)	Senior Adult (65+yr)
Bacterial pneumonia	Congestive heart failure	Congestive heart failure	Bacterial pneumonia	Bacterial pneumonia	Congestive heart failure
Pleurisy	Pleurisy	Pleurisy	Congestive heart failure	Congestive heart failure	Bacterial pneumonia
Congestive heart failure	Bacterial pneumonia	Bacterial pneumonia	Empyema	Empyema	Primary lung malignancy
Nephrotic syndrome	Nephrotic syndrome	Nephrotic syndrome	Tuberculosis	Tuberculosis	Liver failure
Pleural effusion	Pleural effusion	Liver failure	Nephrotic syndrome	Nephrotic syndrome	Tuberculosis
Liver failure	Liver failure	Pleural effusion	Liver failure	Liver failure	Empyema
Protein-losing enteropathy	Protein-losing enteropathy	Protein-losing enteropathy	Primary lung malignancy	Pleural effusion	Pleural effusion
Empyema	Empyema	Empyema	Pleural effusion	Primary lung malignancy	Acute pancreatitis
Tuberculosis	Tuberculosis	Tuberculosis	Acute pancreatitis	Acute pancreatitis	Nephrotic syndrome
	Fluid overload	Fluid overload	Hypothyroidism	Pleurisy	Chronic renal failure
	Malignancy	Malignancy	Pleurisy	Hypothyroidism	Pleurisy
			Systemic lupus erythematosus	Systemic lupus erythematosus	Rheumatoid arthritis
			Chronic renal failure	Chronic renal failure	Pericarditis
			Rheumatoid arthritis	Rheumatoid arthritis	Hypothyroidism
			Pericarditis	Pericarditis	Meig's syndrome
			Meig's syndrome	Meig's syndrome	Asbestosis
			Asbestosis	Asbestosis	Mesothelioma
			Mesothelioma	Mesothelioma	

Emergency Rule Out conditions shown in red. Entries in blue are for information only
Conditions are listed in approximate order of prevalence for this age range

P

Pleuritic chest pain

Emergency Rule Out conditions shown in red. Entries in blue are for information only
Conditions are listed in approximate order of prevalence for this age range

Baby (0-1 yr)	Child (1-12 yr)	Adolescent (12-18 yr)	Adult (18-45 yr)	Middle Age Adult (45-65 yr)	Senior Adult (65- yr)
Blastomycosis	Muscular strain	Muscular strain	Bacterial pneumonia	Bacterial pneumonia	Bacterial pneumonia
Chronic fatigue syndrome	Costochondritis	Costochondritis	Mycoplasmal pneumonia	Mycoplasmal pneumonia	Viral pneumonia
Acute allergic alveolitis	Pleurisy	Pleurisy	Viral pneumonia	Viral pneumonia	Mycoplasmal pneumonia
	Bacterial pneumonia	Bacterial pneumonia	Pleurisy	Pleurisy	Aspiration pneumonia
	Blastomycosis	Blastomycosis	Chlamydia pneumoniae	Chlamydia pneumoniae	Chronic fatigue syndrome
	Chronic fatigue syndrome	Acute allergic alveolitis	Mesothelioma	Chronic fatigue syndrome	Mesothelioma
	Acute allergic alveolitis	Chronic fatigue syndrome	Chronic fatigue syndrome	Mesothelioma	Pleurisy
	Tularemia	Mesothelioma	Acute allergic alveolitis	Acute allergic alveolitis	Acute allergic alveolitis
	Mesothelioma	Tularemia	Blastomycosis	Tularemia	Tularemia
	Viral pneumonia	Viral pneumonia	Rib fracture	Blastomycosis	Blastomycosis
	Rib fracture	Rib fracture	Tularemia	Rib fracture	Rib fracture
	Pericarditis	Pneumothorax	Pulmonary thromboembolism	Pulmonary thromboembolism	Primary lung malignancy
		Pericarditis	Pneumothorax	Pneumothorax	Pulmonary thromboembolism
			Eosinophilic pneumonias	Eosinophilic pneumonias	Pneumothorax
			Pericarditis	Pericarditis	Pericarditis
			Primary lung malignancy	Primary lung malignancy	Chlamydia pneumoniae
			Aspiration pneumonia	Aspiration pneumonia	Eosinophilic pneumonias

284

Baby (0-1 yr)	Child (1-12 yr)	Adolescent (12-18 yr)	Adult (18-45 yr)	Middle Age Adult (45-65 yr)	Senior Adult (65+ yr)
Intestinal fistula	Intestinal fistula Diabetes mellitus type 1 Diabetes mellitus type 2	Intestinal fistula Diabetes mellitus type 1 Diabetes mellitus type 2	Intestinal fistula Diabetes mellitus type 2 Diabetes mellitus type 1	Intestinal fistula Diabetes mellitus type 2 Diabetes mellitus type 1	Intestinal fistula Diabetes mellitus type 2 Diabetes mellitus type 1

Emergency Rule Out conditions shown in red. Entries in blue are for information only
Conditions are listed in approximate order of prevalence for this age range

Polyarticular arthritis

Emergency Rule Out conditions shown in red. Entries in blue are for information only
Conditions are listed in approximate order of prevalence for this age range

Baby (0-1 yr)	Child (1-12 yr)	Adolescent (12-18 yr)	Adult (18-45 yr)	Middle Age Adult (45-65 yr)	Senior Adult (65+ yr)
Chlamydia pneumoniae	Septic arthritis	Septic arthritis	Lyme disease	Osteoarthritis	Osteoarthritis
Fifth disease	Rheumatic fever	Fifth disease	Rheumatoid arthritis	Lyme disease	Rheumatoid arthritis
Kawasaki disease	Fifth disease	Rheumatic fever	Psoriatic arthritis	Rheumatoid arthritis	Lyme disease
	Juvenile idiopathic arthritis	Juvenile idiopathic arthritis	Ulcerative colitis	Psoriatic arthritis	Fifth disease
	Viral infection	Viral infection	Crohn's disease	Ulcerative colitis	Septic arthritis
	Henoch-Schönlein purpura	Cystic fibrosis	Pseudogout	Fifth disease	Ulcerative colitis
	Cystic fibrosis	Mycoplasmal pneumonia	Fifth disease	Crohn's disease	Amyloidosis
	Mycoplasmal pneumonia	Connective tissue disease	Chlamydia pneumoniae	Chlamydia pneumoniae	Chlamydia pneumoniae
	Chlamydia pneumoniae	Chlamydia pneumoniae	Amyloidosis	Amyloidosis	Crohn's disease
	Connective tissue disease	Lyme disease	Reiter's syndrome	Pseudogout	Pseudogout
	Lyme disease	Sickle cell anemia	Gonorrhea	Reiter's syndrome	Scleroderma
	Sickle cell anemia	Crohn's disease	Juvenile idiopathic arthritis	Septic arthritis	Gonorrhea
	Crohn's disease	Ulcerative colitis	Ankylosing spondylitis	Ankylosing spondylitis	Rheumatic fever
	Ulcerative colitis	Tuberculosis	Septic arthritis	Gonorrhea	Juvenile idiopathic arthritis
	Tuberculosis	Kawasaki disease	Rheumatic fever	Rheumatic fever	
	Kawasaki disease	Henoch-Schönlein purpura	Scleroderma	Scleroderma	
	Acute leukemia	Acute leukemia	Anicteric hepatitis	Juvenile idiopathic arthritis	
	Neuroblastoma	Neuroblastoma	Systemic lupus erythematosus	Anicteric hepatitis	
				Systemic lupus erythematosus	

Baby (0-1 yr)	Child (1-12 yr)	Adolescent (12-18 yr)	Adult (18-45 yr)	Middle Age Adult (45-65 yr)	Senior Adult (65+ yr)
Hypercalcemia	Diabetes mellitus in children	Diabetes mellitus in children	Diabetes mellitus type 1	Diabetes mellitus type 1	Diabetes mellitus type 2
Diabetic ketoacidosis	Hypercalcemia	Chronic renal failure	Diabetes mellitus type 2	Diabetes mellitus type 2	Diabetes mellitus type 1
	Diabetic ketoacidosis	Hypercalcemia	Drug reaction	Drug reaction	Diabetes insipidus
	Chronic renal failure	Diabetic ketoacidosis	Schizophrenia	Schizophrenia	Amyloidosis
	Fanconi's syndrome	Fanconi's syndrome	Hypercalcemia	Diabetic ketoacidosis	Diabetic ketoacidosis
	Diabetes insipidus	Diabetes insipidus	Diabetic ketoacidosis	Hypercalcemia	Hypercalcemia
	Psychosomatic	Psychosomatic	Sjögren's syndrome	Sjögren's syndrome	Schizophrenia
			Diabetes insipidus	Diabetes insipidus	Sjögren's syndrome
			Chronic renal failure	Chronic renal failure	Chronic renal failure
			Multiple myeloma	Multiple myeloma	Multiple myeloma
			Amyloidosis	Amyloidosis	Fanconi's syndrome
			Fanconi's syndrome	Fanconi's syndrome	Psychosomatic
			Psychosomatic	Psychosomatic	

Emergency Rule Out conditions shown in red. Entries in blue are for information only
Conditions are listed in approximate order of prevalence for this age range

Emergency Rule Out conditions shown in red. Entries in blue are for information only
Conditions are listed in approximate order of prevalence for this age range

Baby (0-1 yr)	Child (1-12 yr)	Adolescent (12-18 yr)	Adult (18-45 yr)	Middle Age Adult (45-65 yr)	Senior Adult (65+yr)
Not relevant to this age group	Nutritional deficiencies Guillain-Barré syndrome (acute infective polyneuritis) Chronic lead poisoning Systemic lupus erythematosus Malignancy	Nutritional deficiencies Guillain-Barré syndrome (acute infective polyneuritis) Hyperthyroidism Hypothyroidism Chronic lead poisoning Malignancy Systemic lupus erythematosus Porphyria	Diabetes mellitus in children Diabetes mellitus type 2 Alcohol abuse Malignancy Hyperthyroidism Hypothyroidism Multiple sclerosis Systemic lupus erythematosus Rheumatoid arthritis Guillain-Barré syndrome (acute infective polyneuritis) Nutritional deficiencies Amyloidosis Porphyria	Alcohol abuse Diabetes mellitus type 2 Diabetes mellitus type 1 Hyperthyroidism Multiple sclerosis Hypothyroidism Malignancy Rheumatoid arthritis Systemic lupus erythematosus Amyloidosis Guillain-Barré syndrome (acute infective polyneuritis) Nutritional deficiencies Porphyria	Malignancy Diabetes mellitus type 1 Diabetes mellitus type 2 Hyperthyroidism Multiple sclerosis Hypothyroidism Alcohol abuse Rheumatoid arthritis Amyloidosis Guillain-Barré syndrome (acute infective polyneuritis) Nutritional deficiencies Porphyria

Baby (0-1 yr)	Child (1-12 yr)	Adolescent (12-18 yr)	Adult (18-45 yr)	Middle Age Adult (45-65 yr)	Senior Adult (65+ yr)
Diabetic ketoacidosis	Prader-Willi syndrome Diabetic ketoacidosis Depression	Bulimia nervosa Pregnancy Diabetic ketoacidosis Prader-Willi syndrome Depression	Bulimia nervosa Diabetic ketoacidosis Depression Pregnancy	Bulimia nervosa Diabetic ketoacidosis Depression	Diabetic ketoacidosis Depression Bulimia nervosa

Emergency Rule Out conditions shown in red. Entries in blue are for information only
Conditions are listed in approximate order of prevalence for this age range

Emergency Rule Out conditions shown in red. Entries in blue are for information only
Conditions are listed in approximate order of prevalence for this age range

Baby (0-1 yr)	Child (1-12 yr)	Adolescent (12-18 yr)	Adult (18-45 yr)	Middle Age Adult (45-65 yr)	Senior Adult (65+ yr)
Not relevant to this age group	Diabetes mellitus in children	Diabetes mellitus in children	Diabetes mellitus type 1	Diabetes mellitus type 2	Diabetes mellitus type 2
	Fluid overload	Diabetes mellitus type 2	Diabetes mellitus type 2	Diabetes mellitus type 1	Diabetes mellitus type 1
	Sickle cell anemia	Fluid overload	Diabetic ketoacidosis	Diabetic ketoacidosis	Diabetic ketoacidosis
	Diabetic ketoacidosis	Diabetic ketoacidosis	Diuretic abuse	Hypercalcemia	Hypercalcemia
	Chronic renal failure	Sickle cell anemia	Hypercalcemia	Diabetes insipidus	Diabetes insipidus
	Fanconi's syndrome	Chronic renal failure	Diabetes insipidus	Diuretic abuse	Diuretic abuse
	Hypercalcemia	Hypercalcemia	Psychosomatic	Psychosomatic	Psychosomatic
	Diabetes insipidus	Diabetes insipidus			
	Diuretic abuse	Diuretic abuse			

Popliteal swelling

Baby (0-1 yr)	Child (1-12 yr)	Adolescent (12-18 yr)	Adult (18-45 yr)	Middle Age Adult (45-65 yr)	Senior Adult (65+ yr)
Septic arthritis	Trauma	Trauma	Deep vein thrombosis	Baker's cyst	Baker's cyst
Osteomyelitis	Septic arthritis	**Baker's cyst**	Cellulitis	Deep vein thrombosis	Deep vein thrombosis
Cellulitis	Osteomyelitis	Cellulitis	**Baker's cyst**	**Rheumatoid arthritis**	**Rheumatoid arthritis**
Trauma	Cellulitis	Septic arthritis	**Rheumatoid arthritis**	Cellulitis	**Osteoarthritis**
		Osteomyelitis	Septic arthritis	**Osteoarthritis**	Cellulitis
			Thrombophlebitis	Septic arthritis	Septic arthritis
			Trauma	Trauma	Trauma
			Osteomyelitis	**Thrombophlebitis**	**Thrombophlebitis**
				Osteomyelitis	Osteomyelitis

Emergency Rule Out conditions shown in red. Entries in blue are for information only
Conditions are listed in approximate order of prevalence for this age range

291

Emergency Rule Out conditions shown in red. Entries in blue are for information only
Conditions are listed in approximate order of prevalence for this age range

Baby (0-1 yr)	Child (1-12 yr)	Adolescent (12-18 yr)	Adult (18-45 yr)	Middle Age Adult (45-65 yr)	Senior Adult (65+ yr)
Tuberculosis	Tuberculosis	Tuberculosis BCG immunization	Tuberculosis BCG immunization	Tuberculosis BCG immunization	Tuberculosis BCG immunization

Baby (0-1 yr)	Child (1-12 yr)	Adolescent (12-18 yr)	Adult (18-45 yr)	Middle Age Adult (45-65 yr)	Senior Adult (65+ yr)
Not relevant to this age group	Vasovagal response	Vasovagal response	Vasovagal response	Vasovagal response	Vasovagal response
	Dehydration	Acute blood loss	Diabetes mellitus type 2	Diabetes mellitus type 2	Dehydration
	Acute blood loss	Dehydration	Parkinson's disease	Parkinson's disease	Parkinson's disease
	Orthostatic hypotension	Abruptio placentae	Dehydration	Dehydration	Diabetes mellitus type 2
	AV block, third degree	Orthostatic hypotension	Acute blood loss	Acute blood loss	Acute blood loss
	Nutritional deficiencies	AV block, third degree	Vitamin B12 deficiency	AV block, third degree	Vitamin B12 deficiency
	Anorexia nervosa	Anorexia nervosa	AV block, third degree	Orthostatic hypotension	Orthostatic hypotension
	Mucopolysaccharidosis	Nutritional deficiencies	Orthostatic hypotension	Vitamin B12 deficiency	AV block, third degree
		Pregnancy	Abruptio placentae	Abruptio placentae	Dementia
			Pregnancy	Venous insufficiency	Ischemic stroke
			Venous insufficiency	Amyotrophic lateral sclerosis (motor neuron disease)	Amyloidosis
			Wernicke's encephalopathy	Ischemic stroke	Wernicke's encephalopathy
			Amyloidosis	Dementia	Addison's disease
			Addison's disease	Wernicke's encephalopathy	Guillain-Barré syndrome (acute infective polyneuritis)
			Guillain-Barré syndrome (acute infective polyneuritis)	Amyloidosis	Venous insufficiency
			Amyotrophic lateral sclerosis (motor neuron disease)	Addison's disease	Shy-Drager syndrome
			Dementia	Guillain-Barré syndrome (acute infective polyneuritis)	
			Ischemic stroke		

Emergency Rule Out conditions shown in red. Entries in blue are for information only
Conditions are listed in approximate order of prevalence for this age range

293

Emergency Rule Out conditions shown in red. Entries in blue are for information only
Conditions are listed in approximate order of prevalence for this age range

Baby (0-1 yr)	Child (1-12 yr)	Adolescent (12-18 yr)	Adult (18-45 yr)	Middle Age Adult (45-65 yr)	Senior Adult (65+ yr)
Cerebral palsy	Kyphoscoliosis	Kyphoscoliosis	Ankylosing spondylitis	Osteoporosis	Osteoporosis
Kyphoscoliosis	Scoliosis	Scoliosis	Rheumatoid arthritis	Ankylosing spondylitis	Osteoarthritis
Scoliosis	Cerebral palsy	Friedreich's ataxia	Hepatic encephalopathy	Hepatic encephalopathy	Hepatic encephalopathy
Hepatic encephalopathy	Hepatic encephalopathy	Hepatic encephalopathy	Friedreich's ataxia	Rheumatoid arthritis	Rheumatoid arthritis
Muscular dystrophy	Friedreich's ataxia	Cerebral palsy	Osteoporosis	Osteoarthritis	Kyphoscoliosis
Spinal cord lesion	Spinal cord lesion	Spinal cord lesion	Kyphoscoliosis	Kyphoscoliosis	Scoliosis
Juvenile idiopathic arthritis	Muscular dystrophy	Muscular dystrophy	Scoliosis	Scoliosis	
	Juvenile idiopathic arthritis	Juvenile idiopathic arthritis		Friedreich's ataxia	

Baby (0-1 yr)	Child (1-12 yr)	Adolescent (12-18 yr)	Adult (18-45 yr)	Middle Age Adult (45-65 yr)	Senior Adult (65+ yr)
Periorbital cellulitis	Periorbital cellulitis	Periorbital cellulitis	Hyperthyroidism	Hyperthyroidism	Hyperthyroidism
Orbital cellulitis	Orbital cellulitis	Orbital cellulitis	Malignancy	Malignancy	Malignancy
Hyperthyroidism	Hyperthyroidism	Hyperthyroidism	Periorbital cellulitis	Periorbital cellulitis	Periorbital cellulitis
	Malignancy	Malignancy	Orbital cellulitis	Orbital cellulitis	Orbital cellulitis

Emergency Rule Out conditions shown in red. Entries in blue are for information only
Conditions are listed in approximate order of prevalence for this age range

Prostate abnormality

Emergency Rule Out conditions shown in red. Entries in blue are for information only
Conditions are listed in approximate order of prevalence for this age range

Baby (0-1 yr)	Child (1-12 yr)	Adolescent (12-18 yr)	Adult (18-45 yr)	Middle Age Adult (45-65 yr)	Senior Adult (65+ yr)
Blastomycosis	Blastomycosis	Blastomycosis	Prostatitis	Benign prostatic hyperplasia	Prostatic cancer
			Prostatic abscess	Prostatitis	Benign prostatic hyperplasia
			Benign prostatic hyperplasia	Blastomycosis	Blastomycosis
			Blastomycosis	Prostatic cancer	Prostatitis
			Prostate calculus	Prostatic abscess	Prostatic abscess
			Prostate cancer	Prostate calculus	Prostate calculus

Baby (0-1 yr)	Child (1-12 yr)	Adolescent (12-18 yr)	Adult (18-45 yr)	Middle Age Adult (45-65 yr)	Senior Adult (65+ yr)
Urinary tract infection	Urinary tract infection	Urinary tract infection	Urinary tract infection	Urinary tract infection	Urinary tract infection
Nephrotic syndrome	Orthostatic hypotension	Acute glomerulonephritis	Diabetes mellitus type 1	Diabetes mellitus type 1	Diabetes mellitus type 2
Henoch-Schönlein purpura	Nephrotic syndrome	Orthostatic hypotension	Diabetes mellitus type 2	Diabetes mellitus type 2	Diabetes mellitus type 1
Systemic lupus erythematosus	Henoch-Schönlein purpura	Henoch-Schönlein purpura	Pregnancy-induced hypertension	Nephrotic syndrome	Nephrotic syndrome
Nephrotic syndrome	Systemic lupus erythematosus	Systemic lupus erythematosus	Nephritic syndrome	Henoch-Schönlein purpura	Systemic lupus erythematosus
Diabetes mellitus in children	Acute glomerulonephritis	Nephrotic syndrome	Henoch-Schönlein purpura	Systemic lupus erythematosus	Henoch-Schönlein purpura
	Nephritic syndrome	Nephritic syndrome	Acute glomerulonephritis	Acute glomerulonephritis	Acute glomerulonephritis
	Diabetes mellitus in children	Diabetes mellitus in children	Systemic lupus erythematosus	Nephritic syndrome	Nephritic syndrome
		Pregnancy-induced hypertension	Nephrotic syndrome	Drug reaction	Drug reaction
			Drug reaction	Acute tubular necrosis	Amyloidosis
			Acute tubular necrosis	Amyloidosis	Acute tubular necrosis
			Amyloidosis	Renal vein thrombosis	Multiple myeloma
			Renal vein thrombosis	Polycystic kidney disease	Renal vein thrombosis
			Polycystic kidney disease	Multiple myeloma	
			Multiple myeloma		

Emergency Rule Out conditions shown in red. Entries in blue are for information only
Conditions are listed in approximate order of prevalence for this age range

Emergency Rule Out Conditions shown in red. Entries in blue are for information only
Conditions are listed in approximate order of prevalence for this age range

Baby (0-1 yr)	Child (1-12 yr)	Adolescent (12-18 yr)	Adult (18-45 yr)	Middle Age Adult (45-65 yr)	Senior Adult (65+ yr)
Atopic dermatitis	Atopic dermatitis	Atopic dermatitis	Contact dermatitis	Contact dermatitis	Contact dermatitis
Contact dermatitis	Contact dermatitis	Contact dermatitis	Atopic dermatitis	Atopic dermatitis	Atopic dermatitis
Insect and spider bites and stings	Insect and spider bites and stings	Insect and spider bites and stings	Sunburn	Seborrheic dermatitis	Seborrheic dermatitis
Allergic reactions and anaphylaxis	Herpes zoster, shingles	Allergic reactions and anaphylaxis	Seborrheic dermatitis	Lichen simplex chronicus	Lichen simplex chronicus
Herpes zoster, shingles	Allergic reactions and anaphylaxis	Chickenpox	Lichen simplex chronicus	Scabies	Folliculitis
Psoriasis	Chickenpox	Herpes zoster, shingles	Scabies	Herpes zoster, shingles	Herpes zoster, shingles
Bullous pemphigoid	Urticaria	Urticaria	Herpes zoster, shingles	Idiopathic myelofibrosis	Idiopathic myelofibrosis
Idiopathic myelofibrosis	Bullous pemphigoid	Psoriasis	Idiopathic myelofibrosis	Folliculitis	Bullous pemphigoid
Chickenpox	Psoriasis	Idiopathic myelofibrosis	Folliculitis	Sunburn	Sunburn
Urticaria	Idiopathic myelofibrosis	Fungal infection	Bullous pemphigoid	Bullous pemphigoid	Malignancy
Fungal infection	Fungal infection	Bullous pemphigoid	Psoriasis	Psoriasis	Psoriasis
Scabies	Scabies	Scabies	Non-Hodgkin's lymphoma	Non-Hodgkin's lymphoma	Chronic renal failure
Folliculitis	Pityriasis rosea	Pityriasis rosea	Hodgkin's disease	Hodgkin's disease	Hodgkin's disease
Liver failure	Folliculitis	Folliculitis	Chronic renal failure	Chronic renal failure	Non-Hodgkin's lymphoma
Enterobiasis	Dermatitis herpetiformis	Dermatitis herpetiformis	Liver failure	Liver failure	Scabies
Body lice	Enterobiasis	Enterobiasis	Primary biliary cirrhosis	Primary biliary cirrhosis	Polycythemia vera
Head lice	Liver failure	Liver failure	Malignancy	Polycythemia vera	Liver failure
Pubic lice	Body lice	Pregnancy	Pregnancy	Primary HIV infection	Primary biliary cirrhosis
Photodermatitis	Head lice	Primary HIV infection	Polycythemia vera	AIDS	Primary HIV infection
	Pubic lice	AIDS	Primary HIV infection	Body lice	AIDS
	Photodermatitis	Body lice	AIDS	Head lice	Body lice
			Body lice		Head lice
			Head lice		

Baby (0-1 yr)	Child (1-12 yr)	Adolescent (12-18 yr)	Adult (18-45 yr)	Middle Age Adult (45-65 yr)	Senior Adult (65+ yr)
		Head lice Pubic lice Photodermatitis	Pubic lice Photodermatitis	Pubic lice Photodermatitis	Pubic lice Photodermatitis

299

Emergency Rule Out conditions shown in red. Entries in blue are for information only
Conditions are listed in approximate order of prevalence for this age range

Baby (0-1 yr)	Child (1-12 yr)	Adolescent (12-18 yr)	Adult (18-45 yr)	Middle Age Adult (45-65 yr)	Senior Adult (65+ yr)
Trauma	Trauma	Trauma	Eyelid edema	Eyelid edema	Eyelid edema
Congenital facial palsy	Congenital facial palsy	Congenital facial palsy	Horner's syndrome	Horner's syndrome	Horner's syndrome
Cluster headache	Myasthenia gravis	Myasthenia gravis	Diabetic mononeuritis	Diabetic mononeuritis	Diabetic mononeuritis
Cavernous sinus thrombosis	Cavernous sinus thrombosis	Cluster headache	Cluster headache	Cluster headache	Cluster headache
Turner's syndrome	Cluster headache	Turner's syndrome	Turner's syndrome	Cavernous sinus thrombosis	Cavernous sinus thrombosis
Myasthenia gravis	Turner's syndrome	Cavernous sinus thrombosis	Cavernous sinus thrombosis	Turner's syndrome	Turner's syndrome
Botulism	Botulism	Botulism	Myasthenia gravis	Myasthenia gravis	Botulism
Horner's syndrome	Horner's syndrome	Horner's syndrome	Botulism	Botulism	Myasthenia gravis
Myotonic dystrophy	Myotonic dystrophy	Myotonic dystrophy	Posterior communicating artery aneurysm	Posterior communicating artery aneurysm	Posterior communicating artery aneurysm
			Myotonic dystrophy	Myotonic dystrophy	Myotonic dystrophy

Baby (0-1 yr)	Child (1-12 yr)	Adolescent (12-18 yr)	Adult (18-45 yr)	Middle Age Adult (45-65 yr)	Senior Adult (65+ yr)
Congenital heart disease	Adult respiratory distress syndrome	Adult respiratory distress syndrome	Congestive heart failure	Congestive heart failure	Congestive heart failure
Acute left ventricular failure	Drug reaction, allergic	Drug reaction, allergic	Acute left ventricular failure	Acute left ventricular failure	Acute left ventricular failure
Congestive heart failure	Aspiration pneumonia	Aspiration pneumonia	Drug reaction, allergic	Adult respiratory distress syndrome	Adult respiratory distress syndrome
Drug reaction, allergic	Near drowning	Cardiomyopathy	Adult respiratory distress syndrome	Aortic regurgitation	Drug reaction, allergic
Aspiration pneumonia	Cardiomyopathy	Acute left ventricular failure	syndrome	Primary intracerebral hemorrhage stroke	Primary intracerebral hemorrhage stroke
Cardiomyopathy	Aortic regurgitation	Congestive heart failure	Aortic regurgitation	Drug reaction, allergic	Aspiration pneumonia
Aortic regurgitation	Radiographic contrast media allergy	Smoke inhalation injury	Primary intracerebral hemorrhage stroke	Cardiomyopathy	Cardiomyopathy
Near drowning	Acute left ventricular failure	Aortic regurgitation	Cardiomyopathy	Gastroesophageal reflux disease	Aortic regurgitation
Smoke inhalation injury	Smoke inhalation injury	Near drowning	Aspiration pneumonia	Aspiration pneumonia	Near drowning
Salicylate poisoning	Salicylate poisoning	Salicylate poisoning	Aortic regurgitation	Near drowning	Radiographic contrast media allergy
Neonatal respiratory distress syndrome	Congestive heart failure	Radiographic contrast media allergy	Gastroesophageal reflux disease	Hypoxia	Gastroesophageal reflux disease
Radiographic contrast media allergy			Salicylate poisoning	Smoke inhalation injury	Hypoxia
			Hypoxia	Salicylate poisoning	Smoke inhalation injury
			Near drowning	Radiographic contrast media allergy	Salicylate poisoning
			Smoke inhalation injury	Altitude sickness	
			Radiographic contrast media allergy		
			Altitude sickness		

Emergency Rule Out conditions shown in red. Entries in blue are for information only
Conditions are listed in approximate order of prevalence for this age range

Pulmonary examination, crepitations

Emergency Rule Out conditions shown in red. Entries in blue are for information only
Conditions are listed in approximate order of prevalence for this age range

Baby (0-1 yr)	Child (1-12 yr)	Adolescent (12-18 yr)	Adult (18-45 yr)	Middle Age Adult (45-65 yr)	Senior Adult (65+yr)
Bronchiolitis	Bacterial pneumonia	Bacterial pneumonia	Congestive heart failure	Bronchiectasis	Bronchiectasis
Bacterial pneumonia	Bronchiectasis	Bronchiectasis	Bronchiectasis	Congestive heart failure	Bacterial pneumonia
Congestive heart failure	Cystic fibrosis	Cystic fibrosis	Bacterial pneumonia	Bacterial pneumonia	Congestive heart failure
	Congestive heart failure	Congestive heart failure	AIDS	AIDS	Idiopathic pulmonary interstitial fibrosis
		AIDS	Idiopathic pulmonary interstitial fibrosis	Idiopathic pulmonary interstitial fibrosis	AIDS

Baby (0-1 yr)	Child (1-12 yr)	Adolescent (12-18 yr)	Adult (18-45 yr)	Middle Age Adult (45-65 yr)	Senior Adult (65+ yr)
Pleural effusion Bacterial pneumonia	Pleural effusion Bacterial pneumonia	Pleural effusion Bacterial pneumonia	Pleural effusion Bacterial pneumonia Primary lung malignancy Hemothorax Metastatic neoplasm of the lung Mesothelioma	Pleural effusion Bacterial pneumonia Primary lung malignancy Hemothorax Metastatic neoplasm of the lung Mesothelioma	Pleural effusion Bacterial pneumonia Primary lung malignancy Hemothorax Metastatic neoplasm of the lung Mesothelioma

Pulmonary examination, dull to percussion

Emergency Rule Out conditions shown in red. Entries in blue are for information only
Conditions are listed in approximate order of prevalence for this age range

P

Pulmonary examination, reduced breath sounds

Emergency Rule Out conditions shown in red. Entries in blue are for information only
Conditions are listed in approximate order of prevalence for this age range

Baby (0-1 yr)	Child (1-12 yr)	Adolescent (12-18 yr)	Adult (18-45 yr)	Middle Age Adult (45-65 yr)	Senior Adult (65+ yr)
Bacterial pneumonia	Bacterial pneumonia	Bacterial pneumonia	Pleural effusion	Chronic obstructive pulmonary disease	Chronic obstructive pulmonary disease
Mycoplasmal pneumonia	Mycoplasmal pneumonia	Mycoplasmal pneumonia	Asthma	Asthma	Asthma
Viral pneumonia	Viral pneumonia	Viral pneumonia	Chronic obstructive pulmonary disease	Pleural effusion	Pleural effusion
Pleural effusion	Pleural effusion	Pleural effusion	Pneumothorax	Atelectasis	Atelectasis
Pneumothorax	Pneumothorax	Pneumothorax	Atelectasis	Pneumothorax	Mesothelioma
Foreign body	Foreign body	Foreign body	Mesothelioma	Mesothelioma	Pneumothorax
			Foreign body	Foreign body	Foreign body

304

Baby (0-1 yr)	Child (1-12 yr)	Adolescent (12-18 yr)	Adult (18-45 yr)	Middle Age Adult (45-65 yr)	Senior Adult (65+ yr)
Bacterial pneumonia	Bacterial pneumonia	Bacterial pneumonia	Chronic obstructive pulmonary disease	Chronic obstructive pulmonary disease	Chronic obstructive pulmonary disease
Pleural effusion	Pleural effusion	Pleural effusion	Asthma	Asthma	Asthma
Pneumothorax	Pneumothorax	Pneumothorax	Idiopathic pulmonary interstitial fibrosis	Idiopathic pulmonary interstitial fibrosis	Idiopathic pulmonary interstitial fibrosis
Asthma	Asthma	Asthma	Bacterial pneumonia	Bacterial pneumonia	Bacterial pneumonia
Pleurisy	Pleurisy	Pleurisy	Pleurisy	Pleurisy	Pleurisy
Atelectasis	Atelectasis	Atelectasis	Atelectasis	Atelectasis	Atelectasis
Kyphoscoliosis	Kyphoscoliosis	Kyphoscoliosis	Kyphoscoliosis	Kyphoscoliosis	Kyphoscoliosis
			Pleural effusion	Pleural effusion	Pleural effusion

Emergency Rule Out conditions shown in red. Entries in blue are for information only
Conditions are listed in approximate order of prevalence for this age range

Pulmonary examination, reduced expansion

Emergency Rule Out conditions shown in red. Entries in blue are for information only
Conditions are listed in approximate order of prevalence for this age range

Pulmonary nodule, solitary

Baby (0-1 yr)	Child (1-12 yr)	Adolescent (12-18 yr)	Adult (18-45 yr)	Middle Age Adult (45-65 yr)	Senior Adult (65-yr)
Tuberculosis	Tuberculosis	Tuberculosis	Primary lung malignancy	Primary lung malignancy	Primary lung malignancy
Lung abscess	Lung abscess	Lung abscess	Lung abscess	Lung abscess	Lung abscess
	Carcinoid syndrome	Carcinoid syndrome	Tuberculosis	Tuberculosis	Tuberculosis
	Pulmonary hamartoma	Pulmonary hamartoma	Carcinoid syndrome	Carcinoid syndrome	Carcinoid syndrome
	Metastatic neoplasm of the lung	Metastatic neoplasm of the lung	Pulmonary hamartoma	Pulmonary hamartoma	Pulmonary hamartoma

Pulsus paradoxus

Baby (0-1 yr)	Child (1-12 yr)	Adolescent (12-18 yr)	Adult (18-45 yr)	Middle Age Adult (45-65 yr)	Senior Adult (65+ yr)
Asthma Pericarditis Cardiac tamponade Cardiomyopathy Pericardial effusion	**Asthma** Pericarditis Cardiac tamponade Cardiomyopathy Pericardial effusion	**Asthma** Pericarditis Cardiac tamponade Cardiomyopathy Pericardial effusion	**Asthma** Pericarditis Cardiac tamponade Cardiomyopathy Pericardial effusion	**Asthma** Pericarditis Cardiac tamponade Cardiomyopathy Pericardial effusion	**Asthma** Pericarditis Cardiac tamponade Cardiomyopathy Pericardial effusion

Emergency Rule Out conditions shown in red. Entries in blue are for information only
Conditions are listed in approximate order of prevalence for this age range

Emergency Rule Out conditions shown in red. Entries in blue are for information only
Conditions are listed in approximate order of prevalence for this age range

Baby (0-1 yr)	Child (1-12 yr)	Adolescent (12-18 yr)	Adult (18-45 yr)	Middle Age Adult (45-65 yr)	Senior Adult (65+ yr)
Meningococcemia	Idiopathic thrombocytopenic purpura	Meningococcemia	Trauma	Trauma	Trauma
Child abuse	Henoch-Schönlein purpura	Vasculitis	Idiopathic thrombocytopenic purpura	Idiopathic thrombocytopenic purpura	Senile purpura
Trauma	Bacterial meningitis	Erythema multiforme	Vasculitis	Vasculitis	Idiopathic thrombocytopenic purpura
Vasculitis	Erythema multiforme	Bacterial meningitis	Vitamin K deficiency	Vitamin K deficiency	Amyloidosis
Erythema multiforme	Meningococcemia	Trauma	Erythema multiforme	Brucellosis	Erythema multiforme
Brucellosis	Brucellosis	Brucellosis	Thrombotic thrombocytopenic purpura	Erythema multiforme	Brucellosis
Bacterial meningitis	Trauma	Henoch-Schönlein purpura	Brucellosis	Bacterial meningitis	Vasculitis
Vitamin K deficiency	Child abuse	Idiopathic thrombocytopenic purpura	Henoch-Schönlein purpura	Thrombotic thrombocytopenic purpura	Bacterial meningitis
Childhood idiopathic immune thrombocytopenia	Vasculitis	Vitamin K deficiency	Bacterial meningitis	Senile purpura	Vitamin K deficiency
Idiopathic thrombocytopenic purpura	Vitamin K deficiency	Thrombotic thrombocytopenic purpura	Meningococcemia	Amyloidosis	Thrombotic thrombocytopenic purpura
Henoch-Schönlein purpura			Senile purpura	Henoch-Schönlein purpura	Henoch-Schönlein purpura
			Amyloidosis	Meningococcemia	Meningococcemia

Baby (0-1 yr)	Child (1-12 yr)	Adolescent (12-18 yr)	Adult (18-45 yr)	Middle Age Adult (45-65 yr)	Senior Adult (65+yr)
Urinary tract infection	Urinary tract infection	Urinary tract infection	Urinary tract infection	Urinary tract infection	Urinary tract infection
Polycystic kidney disease	Polycystic kidney disease	Polycystic kidney disease	Urethritis	Prostatitis	Urethritis
Urethritis	Renal calculi	Renal calculi	Prostatitis	Urethritis	Prostatitis
Tuberculosis	Urethritis	Acute appendicitis	Renal calculi	Renal calculi	Bladder tumor
	Acute appendicitis	Urethritis	Acute appendicitis	Acute appendicitis	Acute appendicitis
	Tuberculosis	Prostatitis	Tuberculosis	Tuberculosis	Renal calculi
		Tuberculosis	Bladder tumor	Bladder tumor	Tuberculosis
			Analgesic nephropathy	Analgesic nephropathy	Analgesic nephropathy
			Polycystic kidney disease	Polycystic kidney disease	

Emergency Rule Out conditions shown in red. Entries in blue are for information only
Conditions are listed in approximate order of prevalence for this age range

309

Raised intercranial pressure

Emergency Rule Out conditions shown in red. Entries in blue are for information only
Conditions are listed in approximate order of prevalence for this age range

Baby (0-1 yr)	Child (1-12 yr)	Adolescent (12-18 yr)	Adult (18-45 yr)	Middle Age Adult (45-65 yr)	Senior Adult (65+ yr)
Hydrocephalus	Brain tumor	Brain tumor	Brain tumor	Brain tumor	Brain tumor
Trauma	Trauma	Trauma	Subdural hematoma	Subdural hematoma	Subdural hematoma
Hypernatremia	Hypernatremia	Hypernatremia	Brain abscess	Hypernatremia	Hypernatremia
Brain tumor	Subdural hematoma	Subdural hematoma	Hypernatremia	Brain abscess	Brain abscess
Subdural hematoma	Hydrocephalus	Hydrocephalus	Hydrocephalus	Hydrocephalus	Hydrocephalus
Brain abscess	Brain abscess	Brain abscess	Meningioma	Meningioma	Meningioma
		Pseudotumor cerebri	Pseudotumor cerebri		

Baby (0-1 yr)	Child (1-12 yr)	Adolescent (12-18 yr)	Adult (18-45 yr)	Middle Age Adult (45-65 yr)	Senior Adult (65+ yr)
Bacterial pneumonia	Bacterial pneumonia	Bacterial pneumonia	Bacterial pneumonia	Bacterial pneumonia	Bacterial pneumonia
Viral pneumonia	Viral pneumonia	Viral pneumonia	Mycoplasmal pneumonia	Mycoplasmal pneumonia	Congestive heart failure
Tularemia	Tularemia	Tularemia	Viral pneumonia	Viral pneumonia	Viral pneumonia
Aortic regurgitation	Respiratory syncytial virus infection	Chlamydia pneumoniae	Congestive heart failure	Congestive heart failure	Atelectasis
Cardiomyopathy	Chlamydia pneumoniae	Respiratory syncytial virus infection	Tularemia	Tularemia	Respiratory syncytial virus infection
Respiratory syncytial virus infection	Cardiomyopathy	Cardiomyopathy	Chlamydia pneumoniae	Chlamydia pneumoniae	Aspiration pneumonia
Chlamydia pneumoniae	Mycoplasmal pneumonia	Aortic regurgitation	Respiratory syncytial virus infection	Respiratory syncytial virus infection	Aortic regurgitation
Atelectasis	Aortic regurgitation	Mycoplasmal pneumonia	Aortic regurgitation	Aortic regurgitation	Chlamydia pneumoniae
Congestive heart failure	Atelectasis	Atelectasis	Cardiomyopathy	Cardiomyopathy	Cardiomyopathy
Aspiration pneumonia	Congestive heart failure	Aspiration pneumonia	Atelectasis	Sarcoidosis	Mycoplasmal pneumonia
Poliomyelitis	Aspiration pneumonia	Congestive heart failure	Sarcoidosis	Aspiration pneumonia	Tularemia
Pulmonary thromboembolism	Poliomyelitis	Poliomyelitis	Aspiration pneumonia	Rheumatoid pneumoconiosis (Caplan's syndrome)	Idiopathic pulmonary interstitial fibrosis
	Pulmonary thromboembolism	Pulmonary thromboembolism	Rheumatoid pneumoconiosis (Caplan's syndrome)	Asbestosis	Sarcoidosis
			Asbestosis	Idiopathic pulmonary interstitial fibrosis	Rheumatoid pneumoconiosis (Caplan's syndrome)
			Idiopathic pulmonary interstitial fibrosis	Scleroderma	Asbestosis
			Scleroderma	Poliomyelitis	Scleroderma
			Poliomyelitis	Pulmonary thromboembolism	Poliomyelitis
			Pulmonary thromboembolism		Pulmonary thromboembolism

Emergency Rule Out conditions shown in red. Entries in blue are for information only
Conditions are listed in approximate order of prevalence for this age range

Emergency Rule Out conditions shown in red. Entries in blue are for information only
Conditions are listed in approximate order of prevalence for this age range

Baby (0-1 yr)	Child (1-12 yr)	Adolescent (12-18 yr)	Adult (18-45 yr)	Middle Age Adult (45-65 yr)	Senior Adult (65+ yr)
Idiopathic	Idiopathic	Idiopathic	Idiopathic	Idiopathic	Idiopathic
Drug reaction	Drug reaction	Drug reaction	Chronic vibration exposure	Chronic vibration exposure	Chronic vibration exposure
Cryoglobulinemia	Cryoglobulinemia	Cryoglobulinemia	Drug reaction	Drug reaction	Drug reaction
	Scleroderma	Scleroderma	Scleroderma	Scleroderma	Cryoglobulinemia
		Systemic lupus erythematosus	Cryoglobulinemia	Cryoglobulinemia	Scleroderma
			Zollinger-Ellison syndrome	Zollinger-Ellison syndrome	Zollinger-Ellison syndrome

Baby (0-1 yr)	Child (1-12 yr)	Adolescent (12-18 yr)	Adult (18-45 yr)	Middle Age Adult (45-65 yr)	Senior Adult (65+ yr)
Foreign body	Viral conjunctivitis	Viral conjunctivitis	Allergic conjunctivitis	Allergic conjunctivitis	Bacterial conjunctivitis
Bacterial conjunctivitis	Bacterial conjunctivitis	Bacterial conjunctivitis	Hordeolum, chalazion, blepharitis	Hordeolum, chalazion, blepharitis	Allergic conjunctivitis
Viral conjunctivitis	Allergic conjunctivitis	Allergic conjunctivitis	blepharitis	blepharitis	Hordeolum, chalazion,
Chlamydial conjunctivitis	Foreign body	Foreign body	Viral conjunctivitis	Measles	blepharitis
Corneal abrasion	Corneal abrasion	Cluster headache	Bacterial conjunctivitis	Bacterial conjunctivitis	Glaucoma
Cellulitis	Hordeolum, chalazion,	Corneal abrasion	Foreign body	Corneal abrasion	Corneal abrasion
Cluster headache	blepharitis	Hordeolum, chalazion,	Cluster headache	Cluster headache	Herpes simplex
Allergic conjunctivitis	Cluster headache	blepharitis	Cellulitis	Herpes simplex	Cluster headache
Hordeolum, chalazion,	Behçet's syndrome	Behçet's syndrome	Corneal abrasion	Uveitis	Uveitis
blepharitis	Herpes simplex	Herpes simplex	Behçet's syndrome	Cellulitis	Scleritis
Herpes simplex	Cellulitis	Measles	Herpes simplex	Behçet's syndrome	Cellulitis
Behçet's syndrome	Measles	Uveitis	Chlamydial conjunctivitis	Viral conjunctivitis	Behçet's syndrome
Measles	Uveitis	Cellulitis	Uveitis	Scleritis	Measles
Glaucoma	Glaucoma	Scleritis	Scleritis	Glaucoma	Chlamydial conjunctivitis
Uveitis	Scleritis	Glaucoma	Glaucoma	Chlamydial conjunctivitis	Viral conjunctivitis
Episcleritis	Episcleritis	Chlamydial conjunctivitis	Measles	Foreign body	Foreign body
	Chlamydial conjunctivitis	Episcleritis	Episcleritis	Episcleritis	Episcleritis

Emergency Rule Out conditions shown in red. Entries in blue are for information only
Conditions are listed in approximate order of prevalence for this age range

313

Emergency Rule Out conditions shown in red. Entries in blue are for information only
Conditions are listed in approximate order of prevalence for this age range

Baby (0-1 yr)	Child (1-12 yr)	Adolescent (12-18 yr)	Adult (18-45 yr)	Middle Age Adult (45-65 yr)	Senior Adult (65+ yr)
Myopia Hypermetropia Strabismus	Myopia Hypermetropia Strabismus	Myopia Hypermetropia Strabismus	Myopia Hypermetropia Strabismus	Myopia Hypermetropia Strabismus	Myopia Hypermetropia Strabismus

Baby (0-1 yr)	Child (1-12 yr)	Adolescent (12-18 yr)	Adult (18-45 yr)	Middle Age Adult (45-65 yr)	Senior Adult (65+ yr)
Asthma Bronchiolitis Viral pneumonia Bacterial pneumonia Congestive heart failure Atelectasis Pneumothorax	Asthma Viral pneumonia Bacterial pneumonia Congestive heart failure Atelectasis Pneumothorax	Asthma Viral pneumonia Bacterial pneumonia Congestive heart failure Atelectasis Pneumothorax	Asthma Chronic obstructive pulmonary disease Congestive heart failure Pulmonary thromboembolism Atelectasis Pneumothorax Bacterial pneumonia Idiopathic pulmonary interstitial fibrosis	Asthma Chronic obstructive pulmonary disease Congestive heart failure Pulmonary thromboembolism Atelectasis Pneumothorax Bacterial pneumonia Idiopathic pulmonary interstitial fibrosis	Asthma Chronic obstructive pulmonary disease Bacterial pneumonia Congestive heart failure Pulmonary thromboembolism Atelectasis Pneumothorax Idiopathic pulmonary interstitial fibrosis

Respiratory failure, type 1, CO2<6.5

Emergency Rule Out conditions shown in red. Entries in blue are for information only
Conditions are listed in approximate order of prevalence for this age range

Respiratory failure, type 2, CO2>6.5

Emergency Rule Out conditions shown in red. Entries in blue are for information only
Conditions are listed in approximate order of prevalence for this age range

Baby (0-1 yr)	Child (1-12 yr)	Adolescent (12-18 yr)	Adult (18-45 yr)	Middle Age Adult (45-65 yr)	Senior Adult (65+yr)
Neonatal respiratory distress syndrome	Asthma	Asthma	Chronic obstructive pulmonary disease	Chronic obstructive pulmonary disease	Chronic obstructive pulmonary disease
Viral pneumonia	Viral pneumonia	Pleural effusion	Asthma	Asthma	Asthma
Bacterial pneumonia	Bacterial pneumonia	Viral pneumonia	Pleural effusion	Pleural effusion	Pleural effusion
Raised intracranial pressure	Pleural effusion	Bacterial pneumonia	Pneumothorax	Foreign body	Bacterial pneumonia
Foreign body	Foreign body	Foreign body	Foreign body	Pneumothorax	Foreign body
Atelectasis	Atelectasis	Atelectasis	Atelectasis	Atelectasis	Atelectasis
Asthma	Pneumothorax	Pneumothorax	Bacterial pneumonia	Bacterial pneumonia	Raised intracranial pressure
Pleural effusion	Raised intracranial pressure	Muscular dystrophy	Raised intracranial pressure	Raised intracranial pressure	Pneumothorax
Pneumothorax	Muscular dystrophy	Myasthenia gravis	Myasthenia gravis	Myasthenia gravis	Myasthenia gravis
Congenital heart disease	Myasthenia gravis	Raised intracranial pressure	Amyotrophic lateral sclerosis (motor neuron disease)	Amyotrophic lateral sclerosis (motor neuron disease)	Amyotrophic lateral sclerosis (motor neuron disease)
Botulism	Botulism	Altitude sickness	Altitude sickness	Altitude sickness	Altitude sickness
Salicylate poisoning	Salicylate poisoning	Botulism	Botulism	Botulism	Botulism
		Salicylate poisoning	Salicylate poisoning	Salicylate poisoning	Salicylate poisoning

Baby (0-1 yr)	Child (1-12 yr)	Adolescent (12-18 yr)	Adult (18-45 yr)	Middle Age Adult (45-65 yr)	Senior Adult (65+ yr)
Glaucoma	Papilledema	Papilledema	Hypertensive retinopathy	Hypertensive retinopathy	Hypertensive retinopathy
Papilledema	Trauma	Trauma	Diabetic retinopathy	Diabetic retinopathy	Diabetic retinopathy
Optic atrophy	Chorioretinitis	Chorioretinitis	Glaucoma	Glaucoma	Glaucoma
Retinopathy of prematurity	Optic neuritis	Optic neuritis	Papilledema	Papilledema	Macular degeneration
Behçet's syndrome	Retinoblastoma	Retinoblastoma	Ocular trauma	Ocular trauma	Papilledema
Retinoblastoma	Glaucoma	Glaucoma	Lipemia retinalis	Lipemia retinalis	Cholesterol emboli
Retinitis pigmentosa	Retinitis pigmentosa	Retinitis pigmentosa	Macular degeneration	Macular degeneration	Behçet's syndrome
Tuberous sclerosis complex	Optic atrophy	Optic atrophy	Optic neuritis	Optic neuritis	Lipemia retinalis
Trauma	Mucopolysaccharidosis	Mucopolysaccharidosis	Retinal exudates	Behçet's syndrome	Optic atrophy
Infective endocarditis	Behçet's syndrome	Behçet's syndrome	Behçet's syndrome	Retinal exudates	Retinal exudates
Chorioretinitis	Infective endocarditis	Infective endocarditis	Optic atrophy	Optic atrophy	Retinal artery occlusion
Mucopolysaccharidosis	Hypertensive retinopathy	Hypertensive retinopathy	Retinal artery occlusion	Retinal artery occlusion	Retinal vein occlusion
	Tuberous sclerosis complex	Tuberous sclerosis complex	Retinal vein occlusion	Retinal vein occlusion	Angioid streaks
	Retinopathy of prematurity	Retinopathy of prematurity	Cholesterol emboli	Cholesterol emboli	Ocular trauma
			Angioid streaks	Angioid streaks	Hyperviscosity syndrome
			Hyperviscosity syndrome	Hyperviscosity syndrome	

Emergency Rule Out conditions shown in red. Entries in blue are for information only
Conditions are listed in approximate order of prevalence for this age range

Emergency Rule Out conditions shown in red. Entries in blue are for information only
Conditions are listed in approximate order of prevalence for this age range

Baby (0-1 yr)	Child (1-12 yr)	Adolescent (12-18 yr)	Adult (18-45 yr)	Middle Age Adult (45-65 yr)	Senior Adult (65+ yr)
Upper respiratory tract infections	Upper respiratory tract infections	Upper respiratory tract infections	Upper respiratory tract infections	Upper respiratory tract infections	Upper respiratory tract infections
Allergic rhinitis	Allergic rhinitis	Allergic rhinitis	Allergic rhinitis	Allergic rhinitis	Allergic rhinitis
Acute sinusitis	Acute sinusitis	Acute sinusitis	Chronic sinusitis	Chronic sinusitis	Chronic sinusitis
Pertussis	Pertussis	Pertussis	Vasomotor rhinitis	Vasomotor rhinitis	Pertussis
Bronchiolitis	Bronchiolitis	Vasomotor rhinitis	Pertussis	Pertussis	Acute bronchitis
Foreign body	Foreign body	Recreational drug abuse	Wegener's granulomatosis	Wegener's granulomatosis	Vasomotor rhinitis
Acute bronchitis	Acute bronchitis	Acute bronchitis	Acute bronchitis	Acute bronchitis	Wegener's granulomatosis
Vasomotor rhinitis	Vasomotor rhinitis	Foreign body	Foreign body	Foreign body	Foreign body
Cerebrospinal fluid leak	Cerebrospinal fluid leak	Cerebrospinal fluid leak	Cerebrospinal fluid leak	Cerebrospinal fluid leak	Cerebrospinal fluid leak

Baby (0-1 yr)	Child (1-12 yr)	Adolescent (12-18 yr)	Adult (18-45 yr)	Middle Age Adult (45-65 yr)	Senior Adult (65+ yr)
Bronchiolitis	Asthma	Asthma	Asthma	Asthma	Asthma
Acute bronchitis	Acute bronchitis	Acute bronchitis	Acute bronchitis	Acute bronchitis	Chronic obstructive pulmonary disease
Asthma	Bacterial pneumonia	Bacterial pneumonia	Bacterial pneumonia	Bacterial pneumonia	Acute bronchitis
Bacterial pneumonia	Bronchiolitis	Foreign body	Chronic obstructive pulmonary disease	Chronic obstructive pulmonary disease	Bacterial pneumonia
Foreign body	Foreign body	Congestive heart failure	Foreign body	Foreign body	Primary lung malignancy
Congestive heart failure	Congestive heart failure		Primary lung malignancy	Primary lung malignancy	Metastatic neoplasm of the lung
			Metastatic neoplasm of the lung	Metastatic neoplasm of the lung	Foreign body

Emergency Rule Out conditions shown in red. Entries in blue are for information only
Conditions are listed in approximate order of prevalence for this age range

319

Emergency Rule Out conditions shown in red. Entries in blue are for information only
Conditions are listed in approximate order of prevalence for this age range

Baby (0-1 yr)	Child (1-12 yr)	Adolescent (12-18 yr)	Adult (18-45 yr)	Middle Age Adult (45-65 yr)	Senior Adult (65+yr)
Glaucoma	Migraine headache	Migraine headache	Retinal detachment	Retinal detachment	Retinal detachment
Retinoblastoma	Acute retinitis	Retinal detachment	Glaucoma	Glaucoma	Glaucoma
Cataract	Retinal detachment	Acute retinitis	Vitreous opacities	Vitreous opacities	Vitreous opacities
Acute retinitis	Retinal tear	Retinal tear	Migraine headache	Amaurosis fugax	Amaurosis fugax
Retinal tear	Glaucoma	Retinoblastoma	Acute retinitis	Migraine headache	Cataract
Retinal detachment	Retinoblastoma	Glaucoma	Amaurosis fugax	Acute retinitis	Acute retinitis
Vitreous opacities	Vitreous opacities	Vitreous opacities	Retinal tear	Retinal tear	Retinal tear
Ocular trauma	Cataract	Cataract	Cataract	Cataract	Migraine headache
Retinal artery occlusion	Ocular trauma	Retinal artery occlusion	Retinal artery occlusion	Retinal artery occlusion	Retinal artery occlusion
Retinal and vitreous hemorrhage	Retinal artery occlusion	Retinal and vitreous hemorrhage	Retinal and vitreous hemorrhage	Retinal and vitreous hemorrhage	Retinal and vitreous hemorrhage
Retinal vein occlusion	Retinal and vitreous hemorrhage	Retinal vein occlusion	Retinal vein occlusion	Retinal vein occlusion	Retinal vein occlusion
Pituitary eosinophilic adenoma (prolactinoma)	Retinal vein occlusion	Pituitary eosinophilic adenoma (prolactinoma)	Pituitary eosinophilic adenoma (prolactinoma)	Pituitary eosinophilic adenoma (prolactinoma)	Pituitary eosinophilic adenoma (prolactinoma)
Pituitary basophilic adenoma (Cushing's disease, ACTH-producing adenoma)	Pituitary eosinophilic adenoma (prolactinoma)	Pituitary basophilic adenoma (Cushing's disease, ACTH-producing adenoma)	Pituitary basophilic adenoma (Cushing's disease, ACTH-producing adenoma)	Pituitary basophilic adenoma (Cushing's disease, ACTH-producing adenoma)	Pituitary basophilic adenoma (Cushing's disease, ACTH-producing adenoma)
Occipital cortex lesion	Pituitary basophilic adenoma (Cushing's disease, ACTH-producing adenoma)	Amaurosis fugax	Occipital cortex lesion	Occipital cortex lesion	Occipital cortex lesion
Solar retinopathy	Amaurosis fugax	Occipital cortex lesion	Ocular trauma	Ocular trauma	Ocular trauma
Optic neuritis	Occipital cortex lesion	Ocular trauma	Solar retinopathy	Solar retinopathy	Solar retinopathy
	Solar retinopathy	Solar retinopathy	Optic neuritis	Optic neuritis	Optic neuritis
	Optic neuritis	Optic neuritis			

Baby (0-1 yr)	Child (1-12 yr)	Adolescent (12-18 yr)	Adult (18-45 yr)	Middle Age Adult (45-65 yr)	Senior Adult (65+ yr)
Hydrocele	Inguinal hernia	Inguinal hernia	Epididymitis	Epididymitis	Orchitis
Inguinal hernia	Hydrocele	Hydrocele	Inguinal hernia	Inguinal hernia	Inguinal hernia
Trauma	Trauma	Trauma	Prostatitis	Genitofemoral neuralgia	Hydrocele
Behçet's syndrome	Testicular torsion	Testicular torsion	Hydrocele	Hydrocele	Epididymitis
Testicular torsion	Testicular malignancy	Testicular malignancy	Testicular malignancy	Testicular malignancy	Renal calculi
Testicular malignancy	Behçet's syndrome	Behçet's syndrome	Behçet's syndrome	Prostatitis	Genitofemoral neuralgia
	Orchitis	Orchitis	Genitofemoral neuralgia	Behçet's syndrome	Prostatitis
		Prostatitis	Orchitis	Orchitis	Behçet's syndrome
			Renal calculi	Renal calculi	Testicular malignancy

Scrotal pain

Emergency Rule Out conditions shown in red.   Entries in blue are for information only
Conditions are listed in approximate order of prevalence for this age range

Emergency Rule Out conditions shown in red. Entries in blue are for information only
Conditions are listed in approximate order of prevalence for this age range

Baby (0-1 yr)	Child (1-12 yr)	Adolescent (12-18 yr)	Adult (18-45 yr)	Middle Age Adult (45-65 yr)	Senior Adult (65+ yr)
Hydrocele	Inguinal hernia	Inguinal hernia	Inguinal hernia	Inguinal hernia	Inguinal hernia
Inguinal hernia	Hydrocele	Trauma	Epididymitis	Epididymitis	Sebaceous cyst
Testicular malignancy	Testicular torsion	Testicular torsion	Sebaceous cyst	Sebaceous cyst	Orchitis
Behçet's syndrome	Behçet's syndrome	Testicular malignancy	Testicular torsion	Varicocele	Testicular torsion
Testicular torsion	Testicular malignancy	Behçet's syndrome	Behçet's syndrome	Behçet's syndrome	Behçet's syndrome
Trauma	Trauma	Varicocele	Testicular malignancy	Testicular malignancy	Testicular malignancy
Orchitis	Orchitis	Orchitis	Varicocele	Testicular torsion	Varicocele
	Epididymitis	Epididymitis	Orchitis	Orchitis	Epididymitis
		Prostatitis	Prostatitis	Prostatitis	Genitofemoral neuralgia
			Genitofemoral neuralgia	Genitofemoral neuralgia	Prostatitis

Baby (0-1 yr)	Child (1-12 yr)	Adolescent (12-18 yr)	Adult (18-45 yr)	Middle Age Adult (45-65 yr)	Senior Adult (65+ yr)
Group B beta hemolytic streptococcus	Gram negative septicemia	Gram negative septicemia	Gram negative septicemia	Gram negative septicemia	Gram negative septicemia
Group A beta hemolytic streptococcus	Group A beta hemolytic streptococcus	Salmonella infection	Escherichia coli infection	Escherichia coli infection	Escherichia coli infection
Gram negative septicemia	Peritonitis	Peritonitis	Peritonitis	Peritonitis	Peritonitis
Peritonitis	Escherichia coli infection	Escherichia coli infection	Staphylococcal infection	Staphylococcal infection	Staphylococcal infection
Escherichia coli infection	Salmonella infection	Staphylococcal infection	Toxic shock syndrome	Toxic shock syndrome	Toxic shock syndrome
Necrotizing enterocolitis	Staphylococcal infection	Toxic shock syndrome	Campylobacter infection	Campylobacter infection	Campylobacter infection
Salmonella infection	Toxic shock syndrome	Campylobacter infection	Salmonella infection	Salmonella infection	Salmonella infection
Toxic shock syndrome	Campylobacter infection	Group A beta hemolytic streptococcus	Group A beta hemolytic streptococcus	Group A beta hemolytic streptococcus	Group A beta hemolytic streptococcus
Staphylococcal infection	Group B beta hemolytic streptococcus	Group B beta hemolytic streptococcus	Group B beta hemolytic streptococcus	Group B beta hemolytic streptococcus	Group B beta hemolytic streptococcus
Campylobacter infection	Necrotizing enterocolitis	Necrotizing enterocolitis	Necrotizing enterocolitis	Necrotizing enterocolitis	Necrotizing enterocolitis
Plague	Plague	Plague	Plague	Plague	Plague

Emergency Rule Out conditions shown in red. Entries in blue are for information only
Conditions are listed in approximate order of prevalence for this age range

Septic shock

Emergency Rule Out conditions shown in red. Entries in blue are for information only
Conditions are listed in approximate order of prevalence for this age range

Baby (0-1 yr)	Child (1-12 yr)	Adolescent (12-18 yr)	Adult (18-45 yr)	Middle Age Adult (45-65 yr)	Senior Adult (65+yr)
Sepsis	Trauma	Trauma	Myocardial infarction	Myocardial infarction	Myocardial infarction
Trauma	Sepsis	Sepsis	Sepsis	Sepsis	Sepsis
Dehydration	Dehydration	Dehydration	Allergic reactions and anaphylaxis	Allergic reactions and anaphylaxis	Allergic reactions and anaphylaxis
Ventricular tachycardia	Poisoning	Recreational drug abuse	Upper GI bleeding	Upper GI bleeding	Upper GI bleeding
Allergic reactions and anaphylaxis	Allergic reactions and anaphylaxis	Allergic reactions and anaphylaxis	Lower GI bleeding	Lower GI bleeding	Acute iron toxicity
Drug reaction	Upper GI bleeding	Adrenal insufficiency	Drug reaction	Dehydration	Lower GI bleeding
Cardiac tamponade	Lower GI bleeding	Mitral regurgitation	Dehydration	Drug reaction	Drug reaction
Intracranial hemorrhage	Adrenal insufficiency	Upper GI bleeding	Atrial fibrillation	Atrial fibrillation	Dehydration
Pericarditis	Mitral regurgitation	Lower GI bleeding	Pneumothorax	Pneumothorax	Atrial fibrillation
Sinoatrial arrest or block	Idiopathic hypertrophic subaortic stenosis	Drug reaction	Sinoatrial arrest or block	Sinoatrial arrest or block	Pneumothorax
AV block, third degree	AV block, third degree	Idiopathic hypertrophic subaortic stenosis	Mitral regurgitation	Mitral regurgitation	Sinoatrial arrest or block
Sinus bradycardia	Ventricular tachycardia	Aortic stenosis	Pulmonary thromboembolism	Pulmonary thromboembolism	Mitral regurgitation
Idiopathic hypertrophic subaortic stenosis	Acute iron toxicity	AV block, third degree	Aortic stenosis	Aortic stenosis	Pulmonary thromboembolism
Upper GI bleeding	Atrial fibrillation	Ventricular tachycardia	Ventricular tachycardia	Ventricular tachycardia	Aortic stenosis
Lower GI bleeding	Sinus bradycardia	Sinus bradycardia	AV block, third degree	AV block, third degree	Ventricular tachycardia
Adrenal insufficiency	Atrial flutter	Acute iron toxicity	Atrial flutter	Atrial flutter	AV block, third degree
Mitral regurgitation	Mitral regurgitation secondary to papillary muscle dysfunction	Atrial fibrillation	Idiopathic hypertrophic subaortic stenosis	Idiopathic hypertrophic subaortic stenosis	Atrial flutter
Cardiomyopathy	Cardiomyopathy	Atrial flutter	Mitral regurgitation secondary to papillary muscle dysfunction	Mitral regurgitation secondary to papillary muscle dysfunction	Idiopathic hypertrophic subaortic stenosis
Aortic stenosis	Cardiac tamponade	Mitral regurgitation secondary to papillary muscle dysfunction			
Atrial fibrillation					
Atrial flutter					

Baby (0-1 yr)	Child (1-12 yr)	Adolescent (12-18 yr)	Adult (18-45 yr)	Middle Age Adult (45-65 yr)	Senior Adult (65-yr)
Mitral regurgitation secondary to papillary muscle dysfunction	Pericarditis Sinoatrial arrest or block Intracranial hemorrhage Drug reaction Spinal cord lesion	Cardiomyopathy Pneumothorax Cardiac tamponade Pericarditis Sinoatrial arrest or block Intracranial hemorrhage Spinal cord lesion	Cardiomyopathy **Recreational drug abuse** Cardiac tamponade Intracranial hemorrhage Pericarditis Acute iron toxicity	Cardiomyopathy **Recreational drug abuse** Cardiac tamponade Intracranial hemorrhage Pericarditis Acute iron toxicity	Mitral regurgitation secondary to papillary muscle dysfunction Cardiomyopathy Cardiac tamponade Intracranial hemorrhage Pericarditis

Emergency Rule Out conditions shown in red. Entries in blue are for information only
Conditions are listed in approximate order of prevalence for this age range

Baby (0-1 yr)	Child (1-12 yr)	Adolescent (12-18 yr)	Adult (18-45 yr)	Middle Age Adult (45-65 yr)	Senior Adult (65+ yr)
Familial short stature	Familial short stature	Familial short stature	Familial short stature	Familial short stature	Familial short stature
Intrauterine growth retardation	Hypothyroidism	Hypothyroidism	Biliary tract disease	Biliary tract disease	Biliary tract disease
Failure to thrive	Congenital heart disease	Congenital heart disease	Nutritional deficiencies	Nutritional deficiencies	Nutritional deficiencies
Hypothyroidism	Nutritional deficiencies	Nutritional deficiencies	Diabetes mellitus type 1	Diabetes mellitus type 1	Diabetes mellitus type 1
Congenital heart disease	Diabetes mellitus in children	Diabetes mellitus in children	Diabetes insipidus	Diabetes insipidus	Diabetes insipidus
Nutritional deficiencies	Cystic fibrosis	Cystic fibrosis	Chronic renal failure	Chronic renal failure	Chronic renal failure
Cystic fibrosis	Celiac disease	Celiac disease	Congenital heart disease	Congenital heart disease	Congenital heart disease
Celiac disease	Crohn's disease	Crohn's disease	Hypothyroidism	Hypothyroidism	Hypothyroidism
Crohn's disease	Anemia of chronic disease	Anemia of chronic disease	Down syndrome	Down syndrome	Down syndrome
Anemia of chronic disease	Turner's syndrome	Turner's syndrome	Turner's syndrome	Turner's syndrome	Turner's syndrome
Turner's syndrome	Down syndrome	Down syndrome	Growth hormone deficiency	Growth hormone deficiency	Growth hormone deficiency
Down syndrome	Prader-Willi syndrome	Prader-Willi syndrome			
Prader-Willi syndrome	Noonan syndrome	Noonan syndrome			
Noonan syndrome	Growth hormone deficiency in children	Growth hormone deficiency in children			
Diabetes mellitus in children	Chronic renal failure	Chronic renal failure			
Growth hormone deficiency in children	Rickets in children	Rickets in children			
Chronic renal failure	Diabetes insipidus	Diabetes insipidus			
Rickets in children	Biliary tract disease	Biliary tract disease			
Diabetes insipidus					
Biliary tract disease					

326

Baby (0-1 yr)	Child (1-12 yr)	Adolescent (12-18 yr)	Adult (18-45 yr)	Middle Age Adult (45-65 yr)	Senior Adult (65+ yr)
Child abuse	Child abuse	Acromioclavicular joint separation	Rotator cuff syndrome	Rotator cuff syndrome	Rotator cuff syndrome
Trauma	Trauma	Tendinitis	Tendinitis	Tendinitis	Tendinitis
Acromioclavicular joint separation	Acromioclavicular joint separation	Rotator cuff syndrome	Impingement syndrome	Impingement syndrome	Impingement syndrome
Shoulder injury	Tendinitis	Impingement syndrome	Rotator cuff tear	Rotator cuff tear	Rotator cuff tear
Fracture	Fracture	Costochondritis	Acromioclavicular joint separation	Costochondritis	Frozen shoulder
Septic arthritis	Shoulder injury	Shoulder injury	Costochondritis	Acromioclavicular joint separation	Septic arthritis
Costochondritis	Costochondritis	Fracture	Septic arthritis	Cervical disk syndrome	Costochondritis
Cervical disk syndrome	Cervical disk syndrome	Septic arthritis	Cervical disk syndrome	Septic arthritis	Cervical disk syndrome
	Septic arthritis	Cervical disk syndrome	Shoulder injury	Shoulder injury	Polymyalgia rheumatica
	Primary lung malignancy	Glenohumeral joint instability	Fracture	Fracture	Adhesive capsulitis
	Rotator cuff syndrome	Rotator cuff tear	Adhesive capsulitis	Adhesive capsulitis	Shoulder injury
	Impingement syndrome	Adhesive capsulitis	Glenohumeral joint instability	Glenohumeral joint instability	Fracture
	Glenohumeral joint instability	Aseptic necrosis of the humeral head	Cervical spondylosis	Polymyalgia rheumatica	Aseptic necrosis of the humeral head
	Rotator cuff tear	Reflex sympathetic dystrophy	Reflex sympathetic dystrophy	Cervical spondylosis	Reflex sympathetic dystrophy
	Adhesive capsulitis	Cervical spondylosis	Aseptic necrosis of the humeral head	Reflex sympathetic dystrophy	Glenohumeral joint instability
	Aseptic necrosis of the humeral head	Primary lung malignancy	Frozen shoulder	Aseptic necrosis of the humeral head	Cervical spondylosis
	Reflex sympathetic dystrophy		Primary lung malignancy	Frozen shoulder	Acromioclavicular joint separation
	Cervical spondylosis			Primary lung malignancy	Primary lung malignancy

Emergency Rule Out conditions shown in red. Entries in blue are for information only
Conditions are listed in approximate order of prevalence for this age range

Emergency Rule Out conditions shown in red. Entries in blue are for information only
Conditions are listed in approximate order of prevalence for this age range

Baby (0-1 yr)	Child (1-12 yr)	Adolescent (12-18 yr)	Adult (18-45 yr)	Middle Age Adult (45-65 yr)	Senior Adult (65+ yr)
Autosomal recessive inherited	Autosomal recessive inherited	Autosomal recessive inherited	Aplastic anemia	Occult cancer	Occult cancer
Drug reaction	Drug reaction	Drug reaction	Occult cancer	Aplastic anemia	Aplastic anemia
Acute renal failure	Acute renal failure	Acute renal failure	Hypothyroidism	Idiopathic myelofibrosis	Idiopathic myelofibrosis
Hypothyroidism	Hypothyroidism	Hypothyroidism	Idiopathic myelofibrosis	Hypothyroidism	Hypothyroidism
Chronic renal failure	Chronic renal failure	Chronic renal failure	Acute renal failure	Acute renal failure	Acute renal failure
Inherited X-linked disorder	Inherited X-linked disorder	Inherited X-linked disorder	Chronic renal failure	Chronic renal failure	Chronic renal failure
			Autosomal recessive inherited	Rheumatoid arthritis	Rheumatoid arthritis
			Inherited X-linked disorder	Autosomal recessive inherited	Autosomal recessive inherited
			Rheumatoid arthritis	Inherited X-linked disorder	Inherited X-linked disorder

Baby (0-1 yr)	Child (1-12 yr)	Adolescent (12-18 yr)	Adult (18-45 yr)	Middle Age Adult (45-65 yr)	Senior Adult (65+ yr)
Not relevant to this age group	Acute sinusitis Chronic sinusitis	Acute sinusitis Chronic sinusitis	Acute sinusitis Chronic sinusitis Malignancy	Acute sinusitis Chronic sinusitis Malignancy	Acute sinusitis Chronic sinusitis Malignancy

Emergency Rule Out conditions shown in red. Entries in blue are for information only
Conditions are listed in approximate order of prevalence for this age range

Emergency Rule Out conditions shown in red. Entries in blue are for information only
Conditions are listed in approximate order of prevalence for this age range

Baby (0-1 yr)	Child (1-12 yr)	Adolescent (12-18 yr)	Adult (18-45 yr)	Middle Age Adult (45-65 yr)	Senior Adult (65+ yr)
Viral infection	Anxiety	Recreational drug abuse	Anxiety	Anemia	Anemia
Fright	Viral infection	Anxiety	Viral infection	Viral infection	Viral infection
Drug reaction	Fright	Viral infection	Hyperthyroidism	Anxiety	Anxiety
Sepsis	Dehydration	Drug reaction	Anemia	Hyperthyroidism	Hyperthyroidism
Dehydration	Sepsis	Dehydration	Recreational drug abuse	Congestive heart failure	Congestive heart failure
Anemia	Acute blood loss	Acute blood loss	Alcohol abuse	Alcohol abuse	Pulmonary thromboembolism
Congestive heart failure	Drug reaction	Sepsis	Pulmonary thromboembolism	Pulmonary thromboembolism	Alcohol abuse
Hyperthyroidism	Anemia	Hyperthyroidism	Congestive heart failure	Acute blood loss	Acute blood loss
Congenital heart disease	Hyperthyroidism	Anemia	Acute blood loss	Sepsis	Sepsis
Acute blood loss	Congestive heart failure	Congestive heart failure	Sepsis		
	Congenital heart disease	Alcohol abuse			
		Pulmonary thromboembolism			

330

Baby (0-1 yr)	Child (1-12 yr)	Adolescent (12-18 yr)	Adult (18-45 yr)	Middle Age Adult (45-65 yr)	Senior Adult (65+ yr)
Not relevant to this age group	Not relevant to this age group	Diabetic neuropathy	Nerve root compression	Nerve root compression	Nerve root compression
			Diabetic neuropathy	Diabetic neuropathy	Diabetic neuropathy
			Occult cancer	Occult cancer	Occult cancer
			Leprosy	Leprosy	Leprosy

Emergency Rule Out conditions shown in red. Entries in blue are for information only
Conditions are listed in approximate order of prevalence for this age range

Emergency Rule Out conditions shown in red. Entries in blue are for information only
Conditions are listed in approximate order of prevalence for this age range

Baby (0-1 yr)	Child (1-12 yr)	Adolescent (12-18 yr)	Adult (18-45 yr)	Middle Age Adult (45-65 yr)	Senior Adult (65+ yr)
Atopic dermatitis	Atopic dermatitis	Atopic dermatitis	Contact dermatitis	Contact dermatitis	Contact dermatitis
Seborrheic dermatitis	Contact dermatitis	Contact dermatitis	Atopic dermatitis	Acne rosacea	Tularemia
Neonatal acne	Seborrheic dermatitis	Acne vulgaris	Acne vulgaris	Drug reaction, skin	Toxic shock syndrome
Measles	Toxic shock syndrome	Toxic shock syndrome	Tularemia	Toxic shock syndrome	Acne rosacea
Viral infection	Drug reaction, skin	Drug reaction, skin	Toxic shock syndrome	Tularemia	Drug reaction, skin
Henoch-Schönlein purpura	Viral infection	Viral infection	Seborrheic dermatitis	Seborrheic dermatitis	Septic arthritis
Fifth disease	Scarlet fever	Scarlet fever	Scarlet fever	Scarlet fever	Scarlet fever
Kawasaki disease	Rocky Mountain spotted fever	Septic arthritis	Septic arthritis	Septic arthritis	Cellulitis
Tularemia	Ringworm	Rocky Mountain spotted fever	Rocky Mountain spotted fever	Rocky Mountain spotted fever	Rocky Mountain spotted fever
Rocky Mountain spotted fever	Septic arthritis	Ringworm	Drug reaction, skin	Cellulitis	Bartonella infection (cat scratch disease)
Chickenpox	Kawasaki disease	Measles	Measles	Ringworm	Measles
Bartonella infection (cat scratch disease)	Measles	Seborrheic dermatitis	Psoriasis	Kawasaki disease	Seborrheic dermatitis
Behçet's syndrome	Fifth disease	Kawasaki disease	Kawasaki disease	Measles	Henoch-Schönlein purpura
Scarlet fever	Henoch-Schönlein purpura	Henoch-Schönlein purpura	Henoch-Schönlein purpura	Henoch-Schönlein purpura	Kawasaki disease
Toxic shock syndrome	Chickenpox	Fifth disease	Fifth disease	Bartonella infection (cat scratch disease)	Ringworm
Septic arthritis	Behçet's syndrome	Acne rosacea	Bartonella infection (cat scratch disease)	Herpes zoster, shingles	Herpes zoster, shingles
Ringworm	Bartonella infection (cat scratch disease)	Bartonella infection (cat scratch disease)	Ringworm	Behçet's syndrome	Behçet's syndrome
Impetigo	Herpes zoster, shingles	Behçet's syndrome	Acne rosacea	Atopic dermatitis	Atopic dermatitis
Scabies	Tularemia	Chickenpox	Cellulitis	Vasculitis	Venous insufficiency
Fungal infection	Impetigo	Herpes zoster, shingles	Behçet's syndrome	Psoriasis	Vasculitis
Cellulitis	Fungal infection	Tularemia	Lichen planus	Fungal infection	Fungal infection

Baby (0-1 yr)	Child (1-12 yr)	Adolescent (12-18 yr)	Adult (18-45 yr)	Middle Age Adult (45-65 yr)	Senior Adult (65+ yr)
Drug reaction, skin	Acne vulgaris	Impetigo	Erythema nodosum	Scabies	Scabies
Hypothyroidism	Scabies	Cellulitis	Vasculitis	Diabetes mellitus type 2	Diabetes mellitus type 2
Vasculitis	Cellulitis	Scabies	Herpes zoster, shingles	Cutaneous T cell lymphoma	Psoriasis
Plague	Erythema nodosum	Fungal infection	Fungal infection	Erythema nodosum	Cutaneous T cell lymphoma
	Psoriasis	Erythema nodosum	Scabies	Acne vulgaris	Lichen planus
	Hypothyroidism	Psoriasis	Diabetes mellitus type 2	Lichen planus	Erythema nodosum
	Juvenile idiopathic arthritis	Juvenile idiopathic arthritis	Cutaneous T cell lymphoma	Venous insufficiency	Impetigo
	Lyme disease	Hypothyroidism	Venous insufficiency	Impetigo	Mumps
	Vasculitis	Lyme disease	Impetigo	Mumps	Fifth disease
	Plague	Vasculitis	Mumps	Fifth disease	Plague
		Plague	Plague	Plague	

Emergency Rule Out conditions shown in red. Entries in blue are for information only
Conditions are listed in approximate order of prevalence for this age range

Baby (0-1 yr)	Child (1-12 yr)	Adolescent (12-18 yr)	Adult (18-45 yr)	Middle Age Adult (45-65 yr)	Senior Adult (65+ yr)
Lichen sclerosis	Lichen sclerosis	Lichen sclerosis	Lichen sclerosis	Lichen sclerosis	Lichen sclerosis
Dupuytren's contracture	Dupuytren's contracture	Trauma	Trauma	Trauma	Dupuytren's contracture
Trauma	Trauma	Dupuytren's contracture	Dupuytren's contracture	Dupuytren's contracture	Trauma
Acromegaly (pituitary gigantism)	Acromegaly (pituitary gigantism)	Acromegaly (pituitary gigantism)	Acromegaly (pituitary gigantism)	Acromegaly (pituitary gigantism)	Acromegaly (pituitary gigantism)
	Scleroderma	Porphyria	Porphyria	Porphyria	Porphyria
		Scleroderma			

Skin thinning

Baby (0-1 yr)	Child (1-12 yr)	Adolescent (12-18 yr)	Adult (18-45 yr)	Middle Age Adult (45-65 yr)	Senior Adult (65+ yr)
Cushing's syndrome	Cushing's syndrome	Cushing's syndrome	Cushing's syndrome	Reflex sympathetic dystrophy	Cushing's syndrome
Reflex sympathetic dystrophy	Drug reaction, skin	Reflex sympathetic dystrophy	Reflex sympathetic dystrophy	Menopause	Menopause
Drug reaction, skin	Reflex sympathetic dystrophy	Menopause	Menopause	Cushing's syndrome	Reflex sympathetic dystrophy
Ehlers-Danlos syndrome	Ehlers-Danlos syndrome	Drug reaction, skin	Drug reaction, skin	Drug reaction, skin	Drug reaction, skin
		Ehlers-Danlos syndrome			

Emergency Rule Out conditions shown in red. Entries in blue are for information only
Conditions are listed in approximate order of prevalence for this age range

Emergency Rule Out conditions shown in red. Entries in blue are for information only
Conditions are listed in approximate order of prevalence for this age range

Baby (0-1 yr)	Child (1-12 yr)	Adolescent (12-18 yr)	Adult (18-45 yr)	Middle Age Adult (45-65 yr)	Senior Adult (65+yr)
Insomnia	Insomnia	Depression	Depression	Depression	Depression
Hypersomnia	Nightmares	Insomnia	Insomnia	Insomnia	Insomnia
Teething	Night terrors	Anxiety	Anxiety	Anxiety	Anxiety
Sexual assault	Obstructive sleep apnea	Sexual assault	Obstructive sleep apnea	Hypersomnia	Hypersomnia
Chronic fatigue syndrome	Sleep walking	Chronic fatigue syndrome	Hypersomnia	Chronic fatigue syndrome	Dementia
Hepatic encephalopathy	Sexual assault	Autism	Narcolepsy	Obstructive sleep apnea	Sexual assault
Post-traumatic stress disorder	Chronic fatigue syndrome	Nightmares	Chronic fatigue syndrome	Post-traumatic stress disorder	Obstructive sleep apnea
Autism	Hepatic encephalopathy	Post-traumatic stress disorder	Post-traumatic stress disorder	Hepatic encephalopathy	Menopause
Narcolepsy	Autism	Sleep walking	Sexual assault	Menopause	Sleep walking
Obstructive sleep apnea	Post-traumatic stress disorder	Obstructive sleep apnea	Autism	Autism	Chronic fatigue syndrome
	Hypersomnia	Hypersomnia	Hepatic encephalopathy	Narcolepsy	Hepatic encephalopathy
	Anxiety	Narcolepsy	Menopause	Sexual assault	Autism
	Narcolepsy		Nightmares	Nightmares	Post-traumatic stress disorder
	Depression		Sleep walking	Sleep walking	Narcolepsy
					Nightmares
					Night terrors

Baby (0-1 yr)	Child (1-12 yr)	Adolescent (12-18 yr)	Adult (18-45 yr)	Middle Age Adult (45-65 yr)	Senior Adult (65+ yr)
Not relevant to this age group	Hearing loss	Hearing loss	Alcohol abuse	Alcohol abuse	Alcohol abuse
	Head injury	Head injury	Ischemic stroke	Ischemic stroke	Ischemic stroke
	Poisoning	Recreational drug abuse	Multiple sclerosis	Multiple sclerosis	Drug reaction
	Guillain-Barré syndrome (acute infective polyneuritis)	Poisoning	Parkinson's disease	Drug reaction	Parkinson's disease
	Poliomyelitis	Guillain-Barré syndrome (acute infective polyneuritis)	Guillain-Barré syndrome (acute infective polyneuritis)	Parkinson's disease	Myasthenia gravis
	Myasthenia gravis	Poliomyelitis	Poliomyelitis	Guillain-Barré syndrome (acute infective polyneuritis)	Multiple sclerosis
	Hepatic encephalopathy	Myasthenia gravis	Hepatic encephalopathy	Hepatic encephalopathy	Guillain-Barré syndrome (acute infective polyneuritis)
	Friedreich's ataxia	Hepatic encephalopathy	Myasthenia gravis	Myasthenia gravis	Hepatic encephalopathy
	Narcolepsy	Friedreich's ataxia	Poisoning	Poisoning	Poliomyelitis
		Narcolepsy	Recreational drug abuse	Recreational drug abuse	Poisoning
				Poliomyelitis	

Slurred speech

Emergency Rule Out conditions shown in red. Entries in blue are for information only
Conditions are listed in approximate order of prevalence for this age range

337

Emergency Rule Out conditions shown in red. Entries in blue are for information only
Conditions are listed in approximate order of prevalence for this age range

Baby (0-1 yr)	Child (1-12 yr)	Adolescent (12-18 yr)	Adult (18-45 yr)	Middle Age Adult (45-65 yr)	Senior Adult (65+ yr)
Upper respiratory tract infections	Upper respiratory tract infections	Upper respiratory tract infections	Upper respiratory tract infections	Upper respiratory tract infections	Upper respiratory tract infections
Allergic rhinitis	Allergic rhinitis	Allergic rhinitis	Allergic rhinitis	Allergic rhinitis	Allergic rhinitis
Influenza	Influenza	Influenza	Influenza	Influenza	Influenza
Foreign body	Foreign body				

Baby (0-1 yr)	Child (1-12 yr)	Adolescent (12-18 yr)	Adult (18-45 yr)	Middle Age Adult (45-65 yr)	Senior Adult (65+ yr)
Upper respiratory tract infections	Upper respiratory tract infections	Upper respiratory tract infections	Upper respiratory tract infections	Upper respiratory tract infections	Upper respiratory tract infections
Pharyngitis	Streptococcal throat infection	Streptococcal throat infection	Streptococcal throat infection	Streptococcal throat infection	Mucocutaneous candidiasis
Mucocutaneous candidiasis	Tonsillitis	Tonsillitis	Tonsillitis	Mucocutaneous candidiasis	Streptococcal throat infection
Laryngitis	Mononucleosis	Mononucleosis	Mononucleosis	Tonsillitis	Tonsillitis
Acute bronchitis	Laryngitis	Peritonsillar abscess	Peritonsillar abscess	Laryngitis	Laryngitis
Scarlet fever	Scarlet fever	Influenza	Influenza	Peritonsillar abscess	Influenza
Epiglottitis	Peritonsillar abscess	Laryngitis	Laryngitis	Acute bronchitis	Poliomyelitis
Tonsillitis	Epiglottitis	Acute bronchitis	Acute bronchitis	Chronic fatigue syndrome	Chronic fatigue syndrome
Peritonsillar abscess	Acute bronchitis	Chronic fatigue syndrome	Chronic fatigue syndrome	Laryngeal cancer	Laryngeal cancer
Poliomyelitis	Herpes simplex	Laryngeal cancer	Laryngeal cancer	Gonorrhea	Xerostomia
Gonorrhea	Poliomyelitis	Gonorrhea	Oral cavity cancer	Influenza	Gonorrhea
Chronic fatigue syndrome	Atypical mycobacterial infection	Scarlet fever	Gonorrhea	Oral cavity cancer	Herpes simplex
Oral cavity cancer	Influenza	Poliomyelitis	Chlamydia pneumoniae	Chlamydia pneumoniae	Oral cavity cancer
Influenza	Chronic fatigue syndrome	Chlamydia pneumoniae	Poliomyelitis	Poliomyelitis	Chlamydia pneumoniae
Chlamydia pneumoniae	Laryngeal cancer	Oral cavity cancer	Mucocutaneous candidiasis	Scarlet fever	Scarlet fever
Laryngeal cancer	Gonorrhea	Herpes simplex	Scarlet fever	Mononucleosis	Chronic lymphocytic leukemia
Herpes simplex	Oral cavity cancer	Trauma	Herpes simplex	Herpes simplex	Mononucleosis
Primary HIV infection	Chlamydia pneumoniae	Mucocutaneous candidiasis	Chronic lymphocytic leukemia	Primary HIV infection	Epiglottitis
Diphtheria	Trauma	Epiglottitis	Epiglottitis	AIDS	
Lymphogranuloma venereum		Atypical mycobacterial infection		Epiglottitis	
Tularemia					

List continues on next page

Emergency Rule Out conditions shown in red. Entries in blue are for information only
Conditions are listed in approximate order of prevalence for this age range

List continued from previous page

Baby (0-1 yr)	Child (1-12 yr)	Adolescent (12-18 yr)	Adult (18-45 yr)	Middle Age Adult (45-65 yr)	Senior Adult (65+ yr)
	Mucocutaneous candidiasis	Primary HIV infection	Primary HIV infection	Chronic lymphocytic leukemia	Primary HIV infection
	Primary HIV infection	AIDS	AIDS	Diphtheria	AIDS
	AIDS	Diphtheria	Diphtheria	Lymphogranuloma venereum	Diphtheria
	Diphtheria	Lymphogranuloma venereum	Lymphogranuloma venereum	Tularemia	Lymphogranuloma venereum
	Lymphogranuloma venereum	Tularemia	Tularemia		Tularemia
	Tularemia				

Baby (0-1 yr)	Child (1-12 yr)	Adolescent (12-18 yr)	Adult (18-45 yr)	Middle Age Adult (45-65 yr)	Senior Adult (65+ yr)
Hemolysis Hereditary spherocytosis	Hemolysis Hereditary spherocytosis	Hemolysis Hereditary spherocytosis	Hemolysis Hereditary spherocytosis	Hemolysis Hereditary spherocytosis	Hemolysis Hereditary spherocytosis

Emergency Rule Out conditions shown in red. Entries in blue are for information only
Conditions are listed in approximate order of prevalence for this age range

Emergency Rule Out conditions shown in red. Entries in blue are for information only
Conditions are listed in approximate order of prevalence for this age range

Baby (0-1 yr)	Child (1-12 yr)	Adolescent (12-18 yr)	Adult (18-45 yr)	Middle Age Adult (45-65 yr)	Senior Adult (65+yr)
Liver failure	Liver failure	Oral contraception Liver failure Alcoholic hepatitis	Alcoholic hepatitis Oral contraception Liver failure	Alcoholic hepatitis Liver failure	Alcoholic hepatitis Liver failure

Baby (0-1 yr)	Child (1-12 yr)	Adolescent (12-18 yr)	Adult (18-45 yr)	Middle Age Adult (45-65 yr)	Senior Adult (65+ yr)
Not relevant to this age group	Adenoid hypertrophy Obstructive sleep apnea Peritonsillar abscess	Adenoid hypertrophy Obstructive sleep apnea Peritonsillar abscess	Peritonsillar abscess Obstructive sleep apnea Brain tumor Primary intracerebral hemorrhage stroke	Obstructive sleep apnea Brain tumor Primary intracerebral hemorrhage stroke	Obstructive sleep apnea Brain tumor Primary intracerebral hemorrhage stroke

Emergency Rule Out conditions shown in red. Entries in blue are for information only
Conditions are listed in approximate order of prevalence for this age range

Stool color abnormality

Emergency Rule Out conditions shown in red. Entries in blue are for information only
Conditions are listed in approximate order of prevalence for this age range

Baby (0-1 yr)	Child (1-12 yr)	Adolescent (12-18 yr)	Adult (18-45 yr)	Middle Age Adult (45-65 yr)	Senior Adult (65+yr)
Campylobacter infection	Campylobacter infection	Campylobacter infection	Upper GI bleeding	Upper GI bleeding	Upper GI bleeding
Intussusception	Salmonella infection	Salmonella infection	Lower GI bleeding	Lower GI bleeding	Lower GI bleeding
Salmonella infection	Malabsorption	Celiac disease	Campylobacter infection	Campylobacter infection	Biliary tract disease
Malabsorption	Intussusception	Upper GI bleeding	Salmonella infection	Salmonella infection	Campylobacter infection
Cystic fibrosis	Cystic fibrosis	Lower GI bleeding	Malabsorption	Malabsorption	Malabsorption
Upper GI bleeding	Celiac disease	Malabsorption	Intussusception	Intussusception	Salmonella infection
Celiac disease	Upper GI bleeding	Intussusception	Celiac disease	Biliary tract disease	Intussusception
Lower GI bleeding	Lower GI bleeding	Cystic fibrosis	Biliary tract disease	Celiac disease	Celiac disease
Indirect neonatal hyperbilirubinemia	Direct hyperbilirubinemia	Direct hyperbilirubinemia	Cystic fibrosis	Cystic fibrosis	

Baby (0-1 yr)	Child (1-12 yr)	Adolescent (12-18 yr)	Adult (18-45 yr)	Middle Age Adult (45-65 yr)	Senior Adult (65+ yr)
Malabsorption Abetalipoproteinemia Celiac disease	Malabsorption Abetalipoproteinemia Celiac disease	Malabsorption Abetalipoproteinemia Celiac disease	Malabsorption Abetalipoproteinemia Celiac disease	Malabsorption Celiac disease	Malabsorption Celiac disease

Emergency Rule Out conditions shown in red. Entries in blue are for information only
Conditions are listed in approximate order of prevalence for this age range

Emergency Rule Out conditions shown in red. Entries in blue are for information only
Conditions are listed in approximate order of prevalence for this age range

Baby (0-1 yr)	Child (1-12 yr)	Adolescent (12-18 yr)	Adult (18-45 yr)	Middle Age Adult (45-65 yr)	Senior Adult (65+ yr)
Crohn's disease	Crohn's disease	Irritable bowel syndrome	Irritable bowel syndrome	Irritable bowel syndrome	Colon cancer
Intussusception	Irritable bowel syndrome	Crohn's disease	Crohn's disease	Crohn's disease	Irritable bowel syndrome
Amebic dysentery	Intussusception	Amebic dysentery	Intussusception	Ulcerative colitis	Intussusception
Behçet's syndrome	Amebic dysentery	Intussusception	Behçet's syndrome	Intussusception	Behçet's syndrome
	Behçet's syndrome	Behçet's syndrome	Amebic dysentery	Colon cancer	Ulcerative colitis
	Ulcerative colitis	Ulcerative colitis	Ulcerative colitis	Amebic dysentery	Crohn's disease
			Colon cancer	Behçet's syndrome	Amebic dysentery

346

Baby (0-1 yr)	Child (1-12 yr)	Adolescent (12-18 yr)	Adult (18-45 yr)	Middle Age Adult (45-65 yr)	Senior Adult (65+ yr)
Ischiorectal abscess Salmonella infection Campylobacter infection	Ischiorectal abscess Salmonella infection Campylobacter infection	Ischiorectal abscess Salmonella infection Campylobacter infection	Ischiorectal abscess Salmonella infection Campylobacter infection	Ischiorectal abscess Salmonella infection Campylobacter infection	Ischiorectal abscess Salmonella infection Campylobacter infection

Emergency Rule Out conditions shown in red. Entries in blue are for information only
Conditions are listed in approximate order of prevalence for this age range

Stool pus abnormality

Emergency Rule Out conditions shown in red. Entries in blue are for information only
Conditions are listed in approximate order of prevalence for this age range

Baby (0-1 yr)	Child (1-12 yr)	Adolescent (12-18 yr)	Adult (18-45 yr)	Middle Age Adult (45-65 yr)	Senior Adult (65+ yr)
Cushing's syndrome	Cushing's syndrome	Rapid weight gain	Pregnancy	Obesity	Obesity
Drug reaction, skin	Drug reaction, skin	Pregnancy	Obesity	Cushing's syndrome	Cushing's syndrome
	Rapid weight gain	Cushing's syndrome	Cushing's syndrome		
		Drug reaction, skin			

Baby (0-1 yr)	Child (1-12 yr)	Adolescent (12-18 yr)	Adult (18-45 yr)	Middle Age Adult (45-65 yr)	Senior Adult (65+ yr)
Upper respiratory tract infections	Upper respiratory tract infections	Upper respiratory tract infections	Angioedema	Angioedema	Angioedema
Croup	Croup	Peritonsillar abscess	Peritonsillar abscess	Peritonsillar abscess	Epiglottitis
Foreign body	Foreign body	Epiglottitis	Epiglottitis	Epiglottitis	Laryngeal cancer
Epiglottitis	Peritonsillar abscess	Angioedema	Laryngeal cancer	Laryngeal cancer	
Angioedema	Epiglottitis				
	Angioedema				

Emergency Rule Out conditions shown in red. Entries in blue are for information only
Conditions are listed in approximate order of prevalence for this age range

349

Subcutaneous nodules

Emergency Rule Out conditions shown in red. Entries in blue are for information only
Conditions are listed in approximate order of prevalence for this age range

Baby (0-1 yr)	Child (1-12 yr)	Adolescent (12-18 yr)	Adult (18-45 yr)	Middle Age Adult (45-65 yr)	Senior Adult (65+ yr)
Not relevant to this age group	Juvenile idiopathic arthritis Granuloma annulare Rheumatic fever Tuberous sclerosis complex Neurofibromatosis	Juvenile idiopathic arthritis Rheumatic fever Granuloma annulare Neurofibromatosis Tuberous sclerosis complex	Rheumatoid arthritis Chronic tophaceous gout Polyarteritis nodosa Tuberous sclerosis complex Granuloma annulare Neurofibromatosis Rheumatic fever	Rheumatoid arthritis Chronic tophaceous gout Polyarteritis nodosa Tuberous sclerosis complex Granuloma annulare Neurofibromatosis Rheumatic fever	Rheumatoid arthritis Chronic tophaceous gout Tuberous sclerosis complex Granuloma annulare Neurofibromatosis Rheumatic fever

Baby (0-1 yr)	Child (1-12 yr)	Adolescent (12-18 yr)	Adult (18-45 yr)	Middle Age Adult (45-65 yr)	Senior Adult (65+ yr)
Breath-holding	Vasovagal response	Vasovagal response	Vasovagal response	Vasovagal response	Vasovagal response
Febrile seizure	Hyperventilation	Hyperventilation	Orthostatic hypotension	Orthostatic hypotension	Orthostatic hypotension
Epilepsy	Conversion disorder	Conversion disorder	Stokes-Adams attacks	Stokes-Adams attacks	Stokes-Adams attacks
Vasovagal response	Febrile seizure	Orthostatic hypotension	Sinoatrial arrest or block	Sinoatrial arrest or block	Sinoatrial arrest or block
Congenital heart disease	Orthostatic hypotension	Non-diabetic hypoglycemia	Myocardial infarction	Myocardial infarction	Myocardial infarction
Aortic stenosis	Non-diabetic hypoglycemia	Epilepsy	Pulmonary thromboembolism	Pulmonary thromboembolism	Pulmonary thromboembolism
Carbon monoxide poisoning	Epilepsy	Marfan's syndrome	Aortic stenosis	Aortic stenosis	Carbon monoxide poisoning
Paroxysmal atrial tachycardia	Congenital heart disease	Carbon monoxide poisoning	Carbon monoxide poisoning	Carbon monoxide poisoning	Aortic stenosis
Cardiomyopathy	Marfan's syndrome	Aortic stenosis	Epilepsy	Epilepsy	Epilepsy
Ventricular tachycardia	Carbon monoxide poisoning	Cardiomyopathy	Ventricular tachycardia	Ventricular tachycardia	Ventricular tachycardia
AV block, third degree	Aortic stenosis	Paroxysmal atrial tachycardia	Subclavian steal syndrome	Subclavian steal syndrome	Subclavian steal syndrome
Cardiac tamponade	Cardiomyopathy	Ventricular tachycardia	Ischemic stroke	Ischemic stroke	Ischemic stroke
	Paroxysmal atrial tachycardia	AV block, third degree	Cardiac tamponade	Cardiac tamponade	Cardiac tamponade
	Ventricular tachycardia	Cardiac tamponade	Thoracic aortic dissection	Thoracic aortic dissection	Thoracic aortic dissection
	AV block, third degree		Abdominal aortic dissection	Abdominal aortic dissection	Abdominal aortic dissection
	Cardiac tamponade				

Emergency Rule Out conditions shown in red. Entries in blue are for information only
Conditions are listed in approximate order of prevalence for this age range

Emergency Rule Out conditions shown in red. Entries in blue are for information only
Conditions are listed in approximate order of prevalence for this age range

Baby (0-1 yr)	Child (1-12 yr)	Adolescent (12-18 yr)	Adult (18-45 yr)	Middle Age Adult (45-65 yr)	Senior Adult (65+ yr)
Viral infection	Viral infection	Viral infection	Viral infection	Hypoxia	Hypoxia
Fever	Fever	Fever	Fever	Asthma	Viral infection
Bronchiolitis	Asthma	Asthma	Asthma	Viral infection	Fever
Croup	Viral pneumonia	Anxiety	Anxiety	Fever	Congestive heart failure
Viral pneumonia	Bacterial pneumonia	Viral pneumonia	Viral pneumonia	Viral pneumonia	Pulmonary thromboembolism
Neonatal respiratory distress syndrome	Croup	Hypoxia	Hypoxia	Bacterial pneumonia	Chronic obstructive pulmonary disease
Bacterial pneumonia	Anxiety	Mycoplasmal pneumonia	Mycoplasmal pneumonia	Anxiety	Asthma
Sepsis	Sepsis	Bacterial pneumonia	Pulmonary thromboembolism	Mycoplasmal pneumonia	Viral pneumonia
Salicylate poisoning	Salicylate poisoning	Salicylate poisoning	Intracranial hemorrhage	Chronic obstructive pulmonary disease	Bacterial pneumonia
Adult respiratory distress syndrome	Adult respiratory distress syndrome	Adult respiratory distress syndrome	Metabolic acidosis	Pulmonary thromboembolism	Intracranial hemorrhage
Aortic regurgitation	Aortic regurgitation	Aortic regurgitation	Salicylate poisoning	Congestive heart failure	Metabolic acidosis
Cardiac tamponade	Cardiac tamponade	Pneumothorax	Aortic regurgitation	Salicylate poisoning	Cardiac tamponade
Pneumothorax	Mycoplasmal pneumonia	Congestive heart failure	Acute blood loss	Intracranial hemorrhage	Croup
Intracranial hemorrhage	Pneumothorax	Cardiac tamponade	Adult respiratory distress syndrome	Metabolic acidosis	Salicylate poisoning
Congestive heart failure	Congestive heart failure	Bronchiectasis	Cardiac tamponade	Adult respiratory distress syndrome	Adult respiratory distress syndrome
Acute blood loss	Bronchiectasis	Intracranial hemorrhage	Chronic obstructive pulmonary disease	Cardiac tamponade	Acute blood loss
	Intracranial hemorrhage	Acute blood loss	Bronchiectasis	Aortic regurgitation	Aortic regurgitation
	Acute blood loss	Pulmonary thromboembolism	Bacterial pneumonia	Acute blood loss	Bronchiectasis
	Pulmonary thromboembolism		Pneumothorax	Bronchiectasis	Pneumothorax
			Congestive heart failure	Pneumothorax	

Baby (0-1 yr)	Child (1-12 yr)	Adolescent (12-18 yr)	Adult (18-45 yr)	Middle Age Adult (45-65 yr)	Senior Adult (65+yr)
					Anxiety Mycoplasmal pneumonia

Emergency Rule Out conditions shown in red. Entries in blue are for information only
Conditions are listed in approximate order of prevalence for this age range

Baby (0-1 yr)	Child (1-12 yr)	Adolescent (12-18 yr)	Adult (18-45 yr)	Middle Age Adult (45-65 yr)	Senior Adult (65+ yr)
Klinefelter's syndrome	Growth hormone excess Hyperthyroidism Klinefelter's syndrome Precocious puberty Marfan's syndrome	Growth hormone excess Klinefelter's syndrome Hyperthyroidism Marfan's syndrome	Hyperthyroidism Klinefelter's syndrome Marfan's syndrome	Hyperthyroidism Klinefelter's syndrome Marfan's syndrome	Hyperthyroidism Klinefelter's syndrome Marfan's syndrome

Baby (0-1 yr)	Child (1-12 yr)	Adolescent (12-18 yr)	Adult (18-45 yr)	Middle Age Adult (45-65 yr)	Senior Adult (65+ yr)
Sun damage Spider angioma Liver failure Hereditary hemorrhagic telangectasia Ataxia-telangiectasia Systemic lupus erythematosus Osler-Weber-Rendu syndrome	Sun damage Spider angioma Hereditary hemorrhagic telangectasia Ataxia-telangiectasia Essential hypertension Scleroderma Liver failure Juvenile idiopathic arthritis Osler-Weber-Rendu syndrome Polymyositis/ dermatomyositis	Sun damage Spider angioma Hereditary hemorrhagic telangectasia Ataxia-telangiectasia Essential hypertension Systemic lupus erythematosus Scleroderma Liver failure Juvenile idiopathic arthritis Polymyositis/ dermatomyositis Osler-Weber-Rendu syndrome	Sun damage Acne rosacea Essential hypertension Liver failure Polymyositis/ dermatomyositis Hereditary hemorrhagic telangectasia Scleroderma Systemic lupus erythematosus Carcinoid syndrome	Sun damage Acne rosacea Essential hypertension Liver failure Hereditary hemorrhagic telangectasia Scleroderma Systemic lupus erythematosus Polymyositis/ dermatomyositis Carcinoid syndrome	Sun damage Acne rosacea Essential hypertension Liver failure Scleroderma Hereditary hemorrhagic telangectasia Carcinoid syndrome

Emergency Rule Out conditions shown in red. Entries in blue are for information only
Conditions are listed in approximate order of prevalence for this age range

355

Emergency Rule Out conditions shown in red. Entries in blue are for information only
Conditions are listed in approximate order of prevalence for this age range

Baby (0-1 yr)	Child (1-12 yr)	Adolescent (12-18 yr)	Adult (18-45 yr)	Middle Age Adult (45-65 yr)	Senior Adult (65+ yr)
Campylobacter infection	Campylobacter infection	Irritable bowel syndrome	Irritable bowel syndrome	Irritable bowel syndrome	Irritable bowel syndrome
	Proctitis	Proctitis	Proctitis	Proctitis	Campylobacter infection
	Irritable bowel syndrome	Campylobacter infection	Campylobacter infection	Campylobacter infection	Colon cancer
	Ulcerative colitis	Ulcerative colitis	Ulcerative colitis	Colon cancer	Proctitis
	Crohn's disease	Crohn's disease	Crohn's disease	Ulcerative colitis	Ulcerative colitis
			Colon cancer	Crohn's disease	Crohn's disease

Tenosynovitis

Baby (0-1 yr)	Child (1-12 yr)	Adolescent (12-18 yr)	Adult (18-45 yr)	Middle Age Adult (45-65 yr)	Senior Adult (65+ yr)
Not relevant to this age group	Repetitive strain injury Septic arthritis Gonorrhea	Septic arthritis Repetitive strain injury Gonorrhea	Repetitive strain injury Septic arthritis Gonorrhea	Septic arthritis Repetitive strain injury Gonorrhea	Septic arthritis Repetitive strain injury Gonorrhea

Emergency Rule Out conditions shown in red. Entries in blue are for information only
Conditions are listed in approximate order of prevalence for this age range

Emergency Rule Out conditions shown in red. Entries in blue are for information only
Conditions are listed in approximate order of prevalence for this age range

Baby (0-1 yr)	Child (1-12 yr)	Adolescent (12-18 yr)	Adult (18-45 yr)	Middle Age Adult (45-65 yr)	Senior Adult (65+yr)
Sepsis	Sepsis	Sepsis	Disseminated intravascular coagulation	Disseminated intravascular coagulation	Disseminated intravascular coagulation
Birth asphyxia	Idiopathic thrombocytopenic purpura	Idiopathic thrombocytopenic purpura	Alcohol abuse	Alcohol abuse	Alcohol abuse
Idiopathic thrombocytopenic purpura	Drug reaction	Drug reaction	Drug reaction	Myeloproliferative disorders	Myeloproliferative disorders
Drug reaction	Aplastic anemia	Aplastic anemia	Myeloproliferative disorders	Drug reaction	Drug reaction
Malaria	Systemic lupus erythematosus	Disseminated intravascular coagulation	Aplastic anemia	Aplastic anemia	Aplastic anemia
Aplastic anemia	Disseminated intravascular coagulation	Hodgkin's disease	Systemic lupus erythematosus	Systemic lupus erythematosus	Systemic lupus erythematosus
Disseminated intravascular coagulation	Babesiosis	Malaria	Megaloblastic anemias	Megaloblastic anemias	Megaloblastic anemias
Babesiosis	Hodgkin's disease	Non-Hodgkin's lymphoma	Malaria	Brucellosis	Malaria
Systemic lupus erythematosus	Brucellosis	Brucellosis	Brucellosis	Thrombotic thrombocytopenic purpura	Brucellosis
Hodgkin's disease	Malaria	Babesiosis	Thrombotic thrombocytopenic purpura	Babesiosis	Thrombotic thrombocytopenic purpura
Non-Hodgkin's lymphoma	Babesiosis	Myeloproliferative disorders	Myelodysplastic syndromes	Malaria	Myelodysplastic syndromes
Megaloblastic anemias	Non-Hodgkin's lymphoma	Megaloblastic anemias	Babesiosis	Myelodysplastic syndromes	Babesiosis
Brucellosis	Megaloblastic anemias	Systemic lupus erythematosus	Sepsis	Sepsis	Sepsis
Thrombotic thrombocytopenic purpura	Thrombotic thrombocytopenic purpura	Thrombotic thrombocytopenic purpura	Acute leukemia	Acute leukemia	Acute leukemia
Liver failure	Liver failure	Liver failure	Chronic lymphocytic leukemia	Chronic lymphocytic leukemia	Chronic lymphocytic leukemia
Paroxysmal nocturnal hemoglobinuria	Paroxysmal nocturnal hemoglobinuria	Paroxysmal nocturnal hemoglobinuria	Chronic myelogenous leukemia	Chronic myelogenous leukemia	Chronic myelogenous leukemia
Acute leukemia	Acute leukemia		Hodgkin's disease	Hodgkin's disease	Hodgkin's disease
Hemolytic uremic syndrome			Non-Hodgkin's lymphoma	Non-Hodgkin's lymphoma	Non-Hodgkin's lymphoma

Baby (0-1 yr)	Child (1-12 yr)	Adolescent (12-18 yr)	Adult (18-45 yr)	Middle Age Adult (45-65 yr)	Senior Adult (65+ yr)
Fanconi's anemia	Hemolytic uremic syndrome	Acute leukemia	Liver failure	Liver failure	Liver failure
Thrombocytopenia absent radius syndrome	Fanconi's anemia	Fanconi's anemia	Paroxysmal nocturnal hemoglobinuria	Paroxysmal nocturnal hemoglobinuria	Paroxysmal nocturnal hemoglobinuria
Congenital rubella syndrome	Myelodysplastic syndromes	Myelodysplastic syndromes			
Myelodysplastic syndromes					

Thrombocytopenia (continued)

359

Emergency Rule Out conditions shown in red. Entries in blue are for information only
Conditions are listed in approximate order of prevalence for this age range

Baby (0-1 yr)	Child (1-12 yr)	Adolescent (12-18 yr)	Adult (18-45 yr)	Middle Age Adult (45-65 yr)	Senior Adult (65+ yr)
Acute blood loss	Acute blood loss	Acute blood loss	Asplenia syndromes	Myeloproliferative disorders	Myeloproliferative disorders
Malignancy	Malignancy	Asplenia syndromes	Acute blood loss	Asplenia syndromes	Acute blood loss
Asplenia syndromes	Asplenia syndromes	Malignancy	Myeloproliferative disorders	Acute blood loss	Asplenia syndromes
Kawasaki disease	Kawasaki disease	Myeloproliferative disorders	Malignancy	Malignancy	Malignancy
Iron deficiency anemia	Juvenile idiopathic arthritis	Kawasaki disease	Kawasaki disease	Kawasaki disease	Kawasaki disease
Viral meningitis	Iron deficiency anemia	Juvenile idiopathic arthritis	Chronic lymphocytic leukemia	Chronic lymphocytic leukemia	Chronic lymphocytic leukemia
Bacterial meningitis	Bacterial meningitis	Iron deficiency anemia	Chronic myelogenous leukemia	Chronic myelogenous leukemia	Chronic myelogenous leukemia
Hereditary spherocytosis	Viral meningitis	Bacterial meningitis	Acute leukemia	Acute leukemia	Acute leukemia
Thalassemia	Hereditary spherocytosis	Viral meningitis	Multiple myeloma	Multiple myeloma	Multiple myeloma
Sickle cell anemia	Thalassemia	Hereditary spherocytosis	Iron deficiency anemia	Iron deficiency anemia	Iron deficiency anemia
Idiopathic thrombocythemia	Sickle cell anemia	Thalassemia	Viral meningitis	Viral meningitis	Viral meningitis
Acute leukemia	Idiopathic thrombocythemia	Sickle cell anemia	Bacterial meningitis	Bacterial meningitis	Bacterial meningitis
	Acute leukemia	Idiopathic thrombocythemia	Hereditary spherocytosis	Hereditary spherocytosis	Hereditary spherocytosis
		Acute leukemia	Thalassemia	Sickle cell anemia	Thalassemia
		Chronic myelogenous leukemia	Sickle cell anemia	Idiopathic thrombocythemia	Sickle cell anemia
			Idiopathic thrombocythemia		Idiopathic thrombocythemia

Baby (0-1 yr)	Child (1-12 yr)	Adolescent (12-18 yr)	Adult (18-45 yr)	Middle Age Adult (45-65 yr)	Senior Adult (65+ yr)
Thyroid cyst	Thyroid cyst	Thyroid cyst	Follicular adenoma	Follicular adenoma	Follicular adenoma
Thyroglossal duct cyst	Thyroglossal duct cyst	Thyroglossal duct cyst	Multinodular goiter	Multinodular goiter	Multinodular goiter
Multinodular goiter	Multinodular goiter	Multinodular goiter	Thyroid cyst	Thyroid cyst	Thyroid cyst
Follicular adenoma	Follicular adenoma	Follicular adenoma	Thyroid carcinoma	Thyroid carcinoma	Thyroid carcinoma
Thyroiditis	Thyroiditis	Thyroiditis			
Thyroid carcinoma	Thyroid carcinoma	Thyroid carcinoma			

Emergency Rule Out conditions shown in red. Entries in blue are for information only
Conditions are listed in approximate order of prevalence for this age range

Emergency Rule Out conditions shown in red. Entries in blue are for information only
Conditions are listed in approximate order of prevalence for this age range

Baby (0-1 yr)	Child (1-12 yr)	Adolescent (12-18 yr)	Adult (18-45 yr)	Middle Age Adult (45-65 yr)	Senior Adult (65+ yr)
Thyroiditis	Thyroiditis	Adolescence	Hypothyroidism	Hypothyroidism	Hypothyroidism
Thyroid carcinoma	Thyroid carcinoma	Thyroiditis	Graves' disease	Graves' disease	Graves' disease
Iodine deficiency	Iodine deficiency	Pregnancy	Thyroiditis	Thyroiditis	Amyloidosis
Hodgkin's disease	Hodgkin's disease	Iodine deficiency	Pregnancy	Thyroid carcinoma	Thyroiditis
Non-Hodgkin's lymphoma	Non-Hodgkin's lymphoma	Thyroid carcinoma	Multinodular goiter	Pregnancy	Thyroid carcinoma
		Hodgkin's disease	Thyroid carcinoma	Multinodular goiter	Multinodular goiter
		Non-Hodgkin's lymphoma	Amyloidosis	Amyloidosis	Iodine deficiency
			Iodine deficiency	Iodine deficiency	

Baby (0-1 yr)	Child (1-12 yr)	Adolescent (12-18 yr)	Adult (18-45 yr)	Middle Age Adult (45-65 yr)	Senior Adult (65+ yr)
Not relevant to this age group	Impacted cerumen	Impacted cerumen	Impacted cerumen	Impacted cerumen	Impacted cerumen
	Acute otitis media	Eustachian tube dysfunction	Eustachian tube dysfunction	Acute otitis media	Acute otitis media
	Chronic otitis media	Acute otitis media	Acute otitis media	Chronic otitis media	Chronic otitis media
	Hearing loss	Chronic otitis media	Chronic otitis media	Eustachian tube dysfunction	Ménière's disease
	Tinnitus	Tinnitus	Tinnitus	Tinnitus	Salicylate poisoning
	Salicylate poisoning	Salicylate poisoning	Temporomandibular joint syndrome	Presbycusis	Eustachian tube dysfunction
	Migraine headache	Migraine headache	Drug reaction, tinnitus	Ménière's disease	Tinnitus
	Temporomandibular joint syndrome	Temporomandibular joint syndrome	Salicylate poisoning	Drug reaction, tinnitus	Temporomandibular joint syndrome
	Acoustic neuroma	Hearing loss	Presbycusis	Temporomandibular joint syndrome	Drug reaction, tinnitus
	Eustachian tube dysfunction	Vascular aneurysm	Ménière's disease	Salicylate poisoning	Presbycusis
	Vascular aneurysm	Arteriovenous malformation	Vascular aneurysm	Vascular aneurysm	Vascular aneurysm
	Arteriovenous malformation	Glomus tumor (paraganglioma)	Acoustic neuroma	Acoustic neuroma	Acoustic neuroma
	Glomus tumor (paraganglioma)		Glomus tumor (paraganglioma)	Glomus tumor (paraganglioma)	Glomus tumor (paraganglioma)
			Migraine headache	Migraine headache	Migraine headache

Emergency Rule Out conditions shown in red. Entries in blue are for information only
Conditions are listed in approximate order of prevalence for this age range

Emergency Rule Out conditions shown in red. Entries in blue are for information only
Conditions are listed in approximate order of prevalence for this age range

Baby (0-1 yr)	Child (1-12 yr)	Adolescent (12-18 yr)	Adult (18-45 yr)	Middle Age Adult (45-65 yr)	Senior Adult (65+yr)
Tongue tie	Tongue tie	Scarlet fever	Mucocutaneous candidiasis	Mucocutaneous candidiasis	Mucocutaneous candidiasis
Mucocutaneous candidiasis	Geographic tongue	Geographic tongue	Vitamin B12 deficiency	Vitamin B12 deficiency	Vitamin B12 deficiency
Herpes simplex	Scarlet fever	Trauma	Hyperthyroidism	Hyperthyroidism	Hyperthyroidism
Trauma	Trauma	Macroglossia	Herpes simplex	Oral cavity cancer	Oral leukoplakia
Down syndrome	Oral cavity cancer	Down syndrome	Oral cavity cancer	Herpes simplex	Oral cavity cancer
Macroglossia	Down syndrome	Mucocutaneous candidiasis	Down syndrome	Down syndrome	Down syndrome
Geographic tongue	Macroglossia	Herpes simplex	Malignancy	Malignancy	Malignancy
Oral cavity cancer	Mucocutaneous candidiasis	Vitamin B12 deficiency	Angioedema	Polyarteritis nodosa	Herpes simplex
Beckwith-Wiedemann syndrome	Herpes simplex	Hyperthyroidism	Acromegaly (pituitary gigantism)	Angioedema	Acromegaly (pituitary gigantism)
Acromegaly (pituitary gigantism)	Hyperthyroidism	Oral cavity cancer	Syphilis	Oral leukoplakia	Scarlet fever
Angioedema	Vitamin B12 deficiency	Angioedema	Oral leukoplakia	Acromegaly (pituitary gigantism)	Angioedema
Vitamin B12 deficiency	Angioedema	Oral leukoplakia	Scarlet fever	Scarlet fever	Syphilis
Hyperthyroidism	Acromegaly (pituitary gigantism)	Acromegaly (pituitary gigantism)	Polyarteritis nodosa	Syphilis	Amyloidosis
Congenital syphilis	Beckwith-Wiedemann syndrome	Syphilis	Amyloidosis	Amyloidosis	Geographic tongue
		Beckwith-Wiedemann syndrome	Geographic tongue	Geographic tongue	

Tongue swelling

Baby (0-1 yr)	Child (1-12 yr)	Adolescent (12-18 yr)	Adult (18-45 yr)	Middle Age Adult (45-65 yr)	Senior Adult (65+ yr)
Scarlet fever	Scarlet fever	Scarlet fever	Stomatitis	Stomatitis	Stomatitis
Stomatitis	Stomatitis	Stomatitis	Angioedema	Angioedema	Angioedema
Macroglossia	Angioedema	Angioedema	Oral leukoplakia	Oral leukoplakia	Oral leukoplakia
Glossitis	Glossitis	Glossitis	Scarlet fever	Glossitis	Glossitis
Hypothyroidism	Down syndrome	Hypothyroidism	Glossitis	Scarlet fever	Malignancy
Angioedema	Oral cavity cancer	Oral cavity cancer	Oral cavity cancer	Hyperthyroidism	Hypothyroidism
Oral cavity cancer	Hypothyroidism	Hyperthyroidism	Hypothyroidism	Hypothyroidism	Oral cavity cancer
Down syndrome	Hyperthyroidism	Malignancy	Hyperthyroidism	Oral cavity cancer	Vitamin B12 deficiency
Hyperthyroidism	Malignancy	Down syndrome	Vitamin B12 deficiency	Vitamin B12 deficiency	Amyloidosis
Acromegaly (pituitary gigantism)	Acromegaly (pituitary gigantism)	Acromegaly (pituitary gigantism)	Malignancy	Malignancy	Hyperthyroidism
Beckwith-Wiedemann syndrome	Beckwith-Wiedemann syndrome	Beckwith-Wiedemann syndrome	Amyloidosis	Amyloidosis	Scarlet fever
Vitamin B12 deficiency	Vitamin B12 deficiency	Vitamin B12 deficiency	Down syndrome	Acromegaly (pituitary gigantism)	Acromegaly (pituitary gigantism)
			Acromegaly (pituitary gigantism)	Down syndrome	

Emergency Rule Out conditions shown in red. Entries in blue are for information only
Conditions are listed in approximate order of prevalence for this age range

Emergency Rule Out conditions shown in red. Entries in blue are for information only
Conditions are listed in approximate order of prevalence for this age range

Baby (0-1 yr)	Child (1-12 yr)	Adolescent (12-18 yr)	Adult (18-45 yr)	Middle Age Adult (45-65 yr)	Senior Adult (65+yr)
Hepatic encephalopathy	Anxiety	Anxiety	Anxiety	Anxiety	Anxiety
Cerebral palsy	Hepatic encephalopathy	Benign essential/familial tremor syndrome	Alcohol abuse	Alcohol abuse	Alcohol abuse
Charcot-Marie-Tooth disease	Charcot-Marie-Tooth disease	Hyperthyroidism	Benign essential/familial tremor syndrome	Benign essential/familial tremor syndrome	Charcot-Marie-Tooth disease
Diabetic hypoglycemia	Diabetic hypoglycemia	Hepatic encephalopathy	Hyperthyroidism	Hepatic encephalopathy	Hyperthyroidism
Non-diabetic hypoglycemia	Cerebral palsy	Charcot-Marie-Tooth disease	Parkinson's disease	Charcot-Marie-Tooth disease	Parkinson's disease
Dementia	Hyperthyroidism	Cerebral palsy	Charcot-Marie-Tooth disease	Cerebral palsy	Hepatic encephalopathy
	Wilson's disease	Dementia	Hepatic encephalopathy	Hyperthyroidism	Cerebral palsy
	Dementia	Brain tumor	Brain tumor	Dementia	Dementia
		Alcohol abuse	Encephalopathy	Brain tumor	Brain tumor
		Diabetic hypoglycemia	Dementia	Parkinson's disease	Benign essential/familial tremor syndrome
		Wilson's disease	Cerebral palsy	Encephalopathy	Encephalopathy
			Multiple sclerosis	Multiple sclerosis	Multiple sclerosis
			Amyotrophic lateral sclerosis (motor neuron disease)	Diabetic hypoglycemia	Amyotrophic lateral sclerosis (motor neuron disease)
			Diabetic hypoglycemia	Amyotrophic lateral sclerosis (motor neuron disease)	Diabetic hypoglycemia
				Diabetic hypoglycemia	

Baby (0-1 yr)	Child (1-12 yr)	Adolescent (12-18 yr)	Adult (18-45 yr)	Middle Age Adult (45-65 yr)	Senior Adult (65+ yr)
Trauma	Trauma	Trauma	Candida	Candida	Candida
Staphylococcal infection	Staphylococcal infection	Candida	Endometriosis	Trauma	Trauma
Sepsis	Candida	Staphylococcal infection	Trauma	Endometriosis	Staphylococcal infection
Candida			Staphylococcal infection	Staphylococcal infection	
Hemorrhagic disease of newborn					

Emergency Rule Out conditions shown in red. Entries in blue are for information only
Conditions are listed in approximate order of prevalence for this age range

Emergency Rule Out conditions shown in red. Entries in blue are for information only
Conditions are listed in approximate order of prevalence for this age range

Baby (0-1 yr)	Child (1-12 yr)	Adolescent (12-18 yr)	Adult (18-45 yr)	Middle Age Adult (45-65 yr)	Senior Adult (65+ yr)
Diabetes mellitus in children	Diabetes mellitus in children	Diabetes mellitus in children	Drug reaction, uremia	Drug reaction, uremia	Drug reaction, uremia
Essential hypertension	Essential hypertension	Essential hypertension	Congestive heart failure	Congestive heart failure	Amyloidosis
Pyelonephritis	Pyelonephritis	Pyelonephritis	Amyloidosis	Amyloidosis	Congestive heart failure
Obstruction of ureter	Obstruction of ureter	Obstruction of ureter	Pyelonephritis	Pyelonephritis	Pyelonephritis
Membranous glomerulonephritis	Membranous glomerulonephritis	Membranous glomerulonephritis	Obstruction of ureter	Obstruction of ureter	Essential hypertension
Polycystic kidney disease	Polycystic kidney disease	Liver failure	Essential hypertension	Essential hypertension	Obstruction of ureter
Liver failure	Liver failure	Polycystic kidney disease	Membranous glomerulonephritis	Membranous glomerulonephritis	Membranous glomerulonephritis
Hemolytic uremic syndrome	Systemic lupus erythematosus	Systemic lupus erythematosus	Essential hypertension	Multiple myeloma	Multiple myeloma
Inborn errors of metabolism	Hemolytic uremic syndrome	Inborn errors of metabolism	Multiple myeloma	Urate nephropathy	Urate nephropathy
Acute renal failure	Inborn errors of metabolism	Acute renal failure	Polycystic kidney disease	Polyarteritis nodosa	Renal artery stenosis
Reye's syndrome	Acute renal failure	Chronic renal failure	Urate nephropathy	Urate nephropathy	Liver failure
Poisoning	Chronic renal failure	Reye's syndrome	Polyarteritis nodosa	Systemic lupus erythematosus	Acute renal failure
Renal artery stenosis	Reye's syndrome	Poisoning	Systemic lupus erythematosus	Renal artery stenosis	Chronic renal failure
	Poisoning	Renal artery stenosis	Renal artery stenosis	Liver failure	Poisoning
	Renal artery stenosis		Liver failure	Acute renal failure	Renal vein thrombosis
			Acute renal failure	Chronic renal failure	Hypothyroidism
			Chronic renal failure	Poisoning	
			Poisoning	Renal vein thrombosis	
			Renal vein thrombosis	Hypothyroidism	
			Hypothyroidism		

368

Baby (0-1 yr)	Child (1-12 yr)	Adolescent (12-18 yr)	Adult (18-45 yr)	Middle Age Adult (45-65 yr)	Senior Adult (65+ yr)
Foreign body	Urethritis	Urethritis	Urethritis	Urethritis	Urethritis
Cystitis	Foreign body	Foreign body	Cystitis	Cystitis	Gonorrhea
Urethral prolapse	Urethral prolapse	Cystitis	Gonorrhea	Gonorrhea	Mucocutaneous candidiasis
Sexual abuse	Sexual abuse	Urethral prolapse	Chlamydia trachomatis infection	Balanitis and balanoposthitis	Cystitis
	Cystitis	Sexual abuse	Balanitis and balanoposthitis	Chlamydia trachomatis infection	Balanitis and balanoposthitis
	Balanitis and balanoposthitis	Balanitis and balanoposthitis	Trichomoniasis	Trichomoniasis	Trichomoniasis
	Gonorrhea	Gonorrhea	Mucocutaneous candidiasis	Mucocutaneous candidiasis	Chlamydia trachomatis infection
	Chlamydia trachomatis infection	Chlamydia trachomatis infection			
	Syphilis	Syphilis			
	Reiter's syndrome	Reiter's syndrome			

Emergency Rule Out conditions shown in red. Entries in blue are for information only
Conditions are listed in approximate order of prevalence for this age range

Urethral discharge

Urge incontinence

Emergency Rule Out conditions shown in red. Entries in blue are for information only
Conditions are listed in approximate order of prevalence for this age range

Baby (0-1 yr)	Child (1-12 yr)	Adolescent (12-18 yr)	Adult (18-45 yr)	Middle Age Adult (45-65 yr)	Senior Adult (65+ yr)
Not relevant to this age group	Cystitis	Cystitis	Cystitis	Cystitis	Weakness of pelvic floor muscles
	Neurogenic bladder	Neurogenic bladder	Prostatitis	Weakness of pelvic floor muscles	Cystitis
	Bladder outlet obstruction	Bladder outlet obstruction	Weakness of pelvic floor muscles	Prostatitis	Benign prostatic hyperplasia
	Spinal cord lesion	Brain tumor	Benign prostatic hyperplasia	Benign prostatic hyperplasia	Prostatic cancer
	Brain tumor	Spinal cord lesion	Bladder outlet obstruction	Bladder outlet obstruction	Prostatitis
		Prostatitis	Prostatic cancer	Menopause	Menopause
			Spinal cord lesion	Prostatic cancer	Alzheimer's disease
			Multiple sclerosis	Parkinson's disease	Parkinson's disease
			Parkinson's disease	Multiple sclerosis	Brain tumor
			Brain tumor	Alzheimer's disease	Spinal cord lesion
			Alzheimer's disease	Brain tumor	Bladder outlet obstruction
				Spinal cord lesion	Multiple sclerosis

Baby (0-1 yr)	Child (1-12 yr)	Adolescent (12-18 yr)	Adult (18-45 yr)	Middle Age Adult (45-65 yr)	Senior Adult (65+ yr)
Meatal stenosis	Urethral stricture	Urethral stricture	Urethral stricture	Benign prostatic hyperplasia	Benign prostatic hyperplasia
Posterior urethral valves	Meatal stenosis	Meatal stenosis	Meatal stenosis	Prostatic cancer	Prostatic cancer
Neurogenic bladder	Bladder outlet obstruction	Ectopic ureter	Bladder outlet obstruction	Urethral stricture	Urethral stricture
Megaureter	Ectopic ureter	Neurogenic bladder	Ectopic ureter	Meatal stenosis	Meatal stenosis
Ectopic ureter	Neurogenic bladder	Ureterocele	Benign prostatic hyperplasia	Bladder outlet obstruction	Bladder outlet obstruction
Bladder diverticula	Ureterocele	Megaureter	Neurogenic bladder	Ectopic ureter	Ectopic ureter
Ureterocele	Megaureter	Bladder diverticula	Prostatic cancer	Neurogenic bladder	Neurogenic bladder
Bladder outlet obstruction	Bladder diverticula	Posterior urethral valves	Ureterocele	Ureterocele	Ureterocele
	Posterior urethral valves		Megaureter	Megaureter	Megaureter
			Bladder diverticula	Bladder diverticula	Bladder diverticula

Emergency Rule Out conditions shown in red. Entries in blue are for information only
Conditions are listed in approximate order of prevalence for this age range

Urinary stream, weak

Emergency Rule Out conditions shown in red. Entries in blue are for information only
Conditions are listed in approximate order of prevalence for this age range

Baby (0-1 yr)	Child (1-12 yr)	Adolescent (12-18 yr)	Adult (18-45 yr)	Middle Age Adult (45-65 yr)	Senior Adult (65+ yr)
Allergic reactions and anaphylaxis	Allergic reactions and anaphylaxis	Allergic reactions and anaphylaxis	Allergic reactions and anaphylaxis	Allergic reactions and anaphylaxis	Allergic reactions and anaphylaxis
Drug reaction, skin	Drug reaction, skin	Drug reaction, skin	Drug reaction, skin	Drug reaction, skin	Drug reaction, skin
Insect and spider bites and stings	Insect and spider bites and stings	Insect and spider bites and stings	Insect and spider bites and stings	Insect and spider bites and stings	Insect and spider bites and stings
Mononucleosis	Mononucleosis	Mononucleosis	Sunburn	Viral hepatitis	Viral hepatitis
Chemical/ pesticide poisoning	Chemical/ pesticide poisoning	Chemical/ pesticide poisoning	Mononucleosis	Sunburn	Sunburn
Viral hepatitis	Sunburn	Sunburn	Viral hepatitis	Mononucleosis	Malignancy
Sunburn	Viral hepatitis	Viral hepatitis	Hyperthyroidism	Hyperthyroidism	Hyperthyroidism
Hyperthyroidism	Discoid lupus erythematosus	Discoid lupus erythematosus	Discoid lupus erythematosus	Malignancy	Discoid lupus erythematosus
Malignancy	Hyperthyroidism	Hyperthyroidism	Chemical/ pesticide poisoning	Discoid lupus erythematosus	Chemical/ pesticide poisoning
Collagen vascular disease	Malignancy	Malignancy	Malignancy	Chemical/ pesticide poisoning	Mononucleosis
Serum sickness	Collagen vascular disease	Collagen vascular disease	Collagen vascular disease	Collagen vascular disease	Collagen vascular disease
	Serum sickness	Serum sickness	Serum sickness	Serum sickness	Serum sickness

Baby (0-1 yr)	Child (1-12 yr)	Adolescent (12-18 yr)	Adult (18-45 yr)	Middle Age Adult (45-65 yr)	Senior Adult (65+ yr)
Maternal estrogen	Trauma	Oral contraception	Dysfunctional uterine bleeding	Menopause	Cervical malignancy
Trauma	Foreign body	Dysfunctional uterine bleeding	Ovulatory bleeding	Ovulatory bleeding	Endometrial cancer
Bacterial vulvovaginitis	Cystitis	Ovulatory bleeding	Polycystic ovarian disease	Dysfunctional uterine bleeding	Estrogen deficient vulvovaginitis
Chlamydia trachomatis infection	Cervicitis	Cystitis	Ectopic pregnancy	Polycystic ovarian disease	Chlamydia trachomatis infection
Uterine myomas	Uterine myomas	Genital warts	Vaginal bleeding during pregnancy	Drug reaction	Excessive anticoagulation
Foreign body	Chlamydia trachomatis infection	Trauma	Chlamydia trachomatis infection	Chlamydia trachomatis infection	Uterine myomas
Idiopathic thrombocytopenic purpura	Urethral prolapse	Cervicitis	Miscarriage	Miscarriage	Drug reaction
Urethral prolapse	Polycystic ovarian disease	Polycystic ovarian disease	Pelvic inflammatory disease	Vaginal bleeding during pregnancy	Vaginal malignancy
Vaginal malignancy	Vaginal malignancy	Bacterial vulvovaginitis	Estrogen deficient vulvovaginitis	Estrogen deficient vulvovaginitis	Cervical ectropion
	Bacterial vulvovaginitis	Hypothyroidism	Uterine myomas	Ectopic pregnancy	Idiopathic thrombocytopenic purpura
	Precocious puberty	Vaginal bleeding during pregnancy	Oral contraception	Uterine myomas	
	Genital warts	Chlamydia trachomatis infection	Vaginal malignancy	Oral contraception	
	Idiopathic thrombocytopenic purpura	Cervical ectropion	Drug reaction	Vaginal malignancy	
	Ruptured/hemorrhagic ovarian cyst	Cervical polyp	Retained products of gestation	Cervical malignancy	
		Uterine myomas	Endometriosis	Pelvic inflammatory disease	
		Urethral prolapse	Menopause	Endometriosis	
		Vaginal malignancy	Cervical ectropion	Excessive anticoagulation	
		Pelvic inflammatory disease		Cervical ectropion	
		Foreign body			

List continues on next page

Emergency Rule Out conditions shown in red. Entries in blue are for information only
Conditions are listed in approximate order of prevalence for this age range

Vaginal bleeding, abnormal

List continued from previous page

Baby (0-1 yr)	Child (1-12 yr)	Adolescent (12-18 yr)	Adult (18-45 yr)	Middle Age Adult (45-65 yr)	Senior Adult (65+ yr)
		Miscarriage	Cervical polyp	Retained products of gestation	
		Ectopic pregnancy	Excessive anticoagulation	Cervical polyp	
		Placenta previa	Cervical malignancy	Endometrial cancer	
		Ruptured/hemorrhagic ovarian cyst	Endometrial cancer	Idiopathic thrombocythemia	
		Abruptio placentae	Idiopathic thrombocythemia		
		Retained products of gestation			
		Idiopathic thrombocytopenic purpura			

Baby (0-1 yr)	Child (1-12 yr)	Adolescent (12-18 yr)	Adult (18-45 yr)	Middle Age Adult (45-65 yr)	Senior Adult (65+ yr)
Physiological	Physiological	Physiological	Physiological	Physiological	Estrogen deficient vulvovaginitis
Bacterial vulvovaginitis	Bacterial vulvovaginitis	Bacterial vulvovaginitis	Mucocutaneous candidiasis	Mucocutaneous candidiasis	Mucocutaneous candidiasis
Prepubescent vulvovaginitis	Prepubescent vulvovaginitis	Mucocutaneous candidiasis	Bacterial vulvovaginitis	Bacterial vulvovaginitis	Bacterial vulvovaginitis
Mucocutaneous candidiasis	Mucocutaneous candidiasis	Contact dermatitis	Cervical ectropion	Estrogen deficient vulvovaginitis	Contact dermatitis
Contact dermatitis	Contact dermatitis	Cystitis	Cervicitis	Cervical ectropion	Cervicitis
Foreign body	Cystitis	Foreign body	Puerperal infection (endometritis)	Cervicitis	Urethritis
Urethritis	Foreign body	Sexual abuse	Chlamydia trachomatis infection	Trichomoniasis	Trichomoniasis
Sexual abuse	Sexual abuse	Urethritis	Trichomoniasis	Urethritis	Chlamydia trachomatis infection
Ectopic ureter	Herpes simplex	Cervical ectropion	Urethritis	Chlamydia trachomatis infection	Chancroid
Trichomoniasis	Gonorrhea	Gonorrhea	Chancroid	Chancroid	Vaginal malignancy
Vaginal malignancy	Ectopic ureter	Chlamydia trachomatis infection	Genital warts	Cervical malignancy	Genital warts
Chancroid	Urethritis	Chancroid	Gonorrhea	Genital warts	Cervical malignancy
Chlamydia trachomatis infection	Trichomoniasis	Puerperal infection (endometritis)	Herpes simplex	Gonorrhea	Gonorrhea
Herpes simplex	Vaginal malignancy	Vaginal malignancy	Contact dermatitis	Herpes simplex	Herpes simplex
Genital warts	Chancroid	Trichomoniasis	Cervical malignancy	Contact dermatitis	Foreign body
Gonorrhea	Chlamydia trachomatis infection	Genital warts	Foreign body	Foreign body	
	Genital warts	Herpes simplex	Vaginal malignancy	Vaginal malignancy	
	Vulval lichen sclerosis	Ectopic ureter		Puerperal infection (endometritis)	
	Cervical malignancy	Cervical malignancy			

Emergency Rule Out conditions shown in red. Entries in blue are for information only
Conditions are listed in approximate order of prevalence for this age range

375

Emergency Rule Out conditions shown in red. Entries in blue are for information only
Conditions are listed in approximate order of prevalence for this age range

Baby (0-1 yr)	Child (1-12 yr)	Adolescent (12-18 yr)	Adult (18-45 yr)	Middle Age Adult (45-65 yr)	Senior Adult (65+ yr)
Physiological	Physiological	Physiological	Mucocutaneous candidiasis	Mucocutaneous candidiasis	Estrogen deficient vulvovaginitis
Prepubescent vulvovaginitis	Prepubescent vulvovaginitis	Bacterial vulvovaginitis	Bacterial vulvovaginitis	Estrogen deficient vulvovaginitis	Mucocutaneous candidiasis
Bacterial vulvovaginitis	Bacterial vulvovaginitis	Mucocutaneous candidiasis	Trichomoniasis	Bacterial vulvovaginitis	Bacterial vulvovaginitis
Mucocutaneous candidiasis	Mucocutaneous candidiasis	Gonorrhea	Gonorrhea	Herpes simplex	Vaginal malignancy
Trichomoniasis	Foreign body	Chlamydia trachomatis infection	Chlamydia trachomatis infection	Genital warts	Vulvar malignancy
Foreign body	Contact dermatitis	Trichomoniasis	Herpes simplex	Trichomoniasis	Contact dermatitis
Contact dermatitis	Sexual abuse	Herpes simplex	Genital warts	Contact dermatitis	Trichomoniasis
Sexual abuse	Trichomoniasis	Genital warts	Contact dermatitis	Vaginal malignancy	Herpes simplex
Giardiasis	Diabetes mellitus in children	Foreign body	Foreign body	Vulvar malignancy	Genital warts
Enterobiasis	Congenital chlamydia	Oral contraception	Cervical polyp	Foreign body	Foreign body
Congenital chlamydia	Congenital gonorrhea	Cervical polyp	Vaginal malignancy	Cervical polyp	
Congenital gonorrhea	Trauma	Contact dermatitis	Vulvar malignancy		
Trauma	Herpes simplex	Giardiasis	Diabetes mellitus type 1		
Herpes simplex	Genital warts	Enterobiasis			
Genital warts	Giardiasis	Sexual abuse			
	Enterobiasis	Trauma			
		Diabetes mellitus in children			

Baby (0-1 yr)	Child (1-12 yr)	Adolescent (12-18 yr)	Adult (18-45 yr)	Middle Age Adult (45-65 yr)	Senior Adult (65+ yr)
Labyrinthitis	Benign paroxysmal positional vertigo	Benign paroxysmal positional vertigo	Labyrinthitis	Labyrinthitis	Labyrinthitis
Temporal lobe epilepsy	Labyrinthitis	Labyrinthitis	Acute otitis media	Acute otitis media	Acute otitis media
Trauma	Migraine headache	Hyperventilation	Benign paroxysmal positional vertigo	Benign paroxysmal positional vertigo	Benign paroxysmal positional vertigo
Transient ischemic attack	Hyperventilation	Drug reaction	Infectious myringitis	Infectious myringitis	Infectious myringitis
Brain tumor	Drug reaction	Transient ischemic attack	Otosclerosis	Otosclerosis	Otosclerosis
Migraine headache	Trauma	Migraine headache	Migraine headache	Migraine headache	Migraine headache
Drug reaction	Brain tumor	Trauma	Ménière's disease	Ménière's disease	Ménière's disease
Posterior fossa tumor	Temporal lobe epilepsy	Brain tumor	Alcohol abuse	Alcohol abuse	Alcohol abuse
Cholesteatoma	Transient ischemic attack	Temporal lobe epilepsy	Drug reaction	Drug reaction	Drug reaction
Arnold-Chiari malformation	Acoustic neuroma	Acoustic neuroma	Transient ischemic attack	Brain tumor	Vertebrobasilar insufficiency
Ramsay Hunt syndrome	Cholesteatoma	Cholesteatoma	Brain tumor	Transient ischemic attack	Brain tumor
	Posterior fossa tumor	Posterior fossa tumor	Multiple sclerosis	Ramsay Hunt syndrome	Transient ischemic attack
	Arnold-Chiari malformation	Arnold-Chiari malformation	Ramsay Hunt syndrome	Multiple sclerosis	Ramsay Hunt syndrome
	Ramsay Hunt syndrome	Ramsay Hunt syndrome	Acoustic neuroma	Acoustic neuroma	Multiple sclerosis
		Multiple sclerosis	Herpes zoster, shingles	Herpes zoster, shingles	Acoustic neuroma
					Herpes zoster, shingles

Emergency Rule Out conditions shown in red. Entries in blue are for information only
Conditions are listed in approximate order of prevalence for this age range

Emergency Rule Out conditions shown in red. Entries in blue are for information only
Conditions are listed in approximate order of prevalence for this age range

Baby (0-1 yr)	Child (1-12 yr)	Adolescent (12-18 yr)	Adult (18-45 yr)	Middle Age Adult (45-65 yr)	Senior Adult (65+yr)
Insect and spider bites and stings	Insect and spider bites and stings	Insect and spider bites and stings	Stomatitis	Contact dermatitis	Contact dermatitis
Atopic dermatitis	Atopic dermatitis	Atopic dermatitis	Atopic dermatitis	Atopic dermatitis	Atopic dermatitis
Stomatitis	Stomatitis	Stomatitis	Folliculitis	Folliculitis	Folliculitis
Contact dermatitis	Contact dermatitis	Folliculitis	Contact dermatitis	Burns	Burns
Hand-foot-and-mouth disease	Hand-foot-and-mouth disease	Contact dermatitis	Chickenpox	Herpes simplex	Herpes zoster, shingles
Folliculitis	Folliculitis	Bartonella infection (cat scratch disease)	Burns	Impetigo	Erythema multiforme
Scabies	Scabies	Hand-foot-and-mouth disease	Herpes simplex	Herpes zoster, shingles	Herpes simplex
Herpes simplex	Herpes simplex	Scabies	Impetigo	Dermatitis herpetiformis	Stomatitis
Impetigo	Impetigo	Herpes simplex	Bartonella infection (cat scratch disease)	Bartonella infection (cat scratch disease)	Bartonella infection (cat scratch disease)
Bartonella infection (cat scratch disease)	Burns	Impetigo	Herpes zoster, shingles	Stomatitis	Impetigo
Burns	Trauma	Burns	Dermatitis herpetiformis	Erythema multiforme	Dermatitis herpetiformis
Trauma	Bartonella infection (cat scratch disease)	Trauma	Erythema multiforme	Bullous pemphigoid	Bullous pemphigoid
Erythema multiforme	Erythema multiforme	Erythema multiforme	Bullous pemphigoid	Pemphigus vulgaris	Pemphigus vulgaris
Diabetes mellitus in children	Diabetes mellitus in children	Diabetes mellitus in children	Pemphigus vulgaris	Hand-foot-and-mouth disease	Hand-foot-and-mouth disease
Herpes zoster, shingles	Herpes zoster, shingles	Herpes zoster, shingles	Hand-foot-and-mouth disease	Chickenpox	Congenital syphilis
Dermatitis herpetiformis	Dermatitis herpetiformis	Dermatitis herpetiformis	Congenital syphilis	Congenital syphilis	Epidermolysis bullosa
Pemphigus vulgaris	Pemphigus vulgaris	Pemphigus vulgaris	Epidermolysis bullosa	Epidermolysis bullosa	Toxic epidermal necrolysis
Epidermolysis bullosa	Bullous pemphigoid	Bullous pemphigoid	Toxic epidermal necrolysis	Toxic epidermal necrolysis	
Erythema toxicum	Epidermolysis bullosa	Epidermolysis bullosa			
Toxic epidermal necrolysis	Chronic bullous dermatosis				

Baby (0-1 yr)	Child (1-12 yr)	Adolescent (12-18 yr)	Adult (18-45 yr)	Middle Age Adult (45-65 yr)	Senior Adult (65+ yr)
Transient neonatal pustular melanosis Congenital syphilis	Toxic epidermal necrolysis Congenital syphilis	Toxic epidermal necrolysis Congenital syphilis			

Emergency Rule Out conditions shown in red. Entries in blue are for information only
Conditions are listed in approximate order of prevalence for this age range

Baby (0-1 yr)	Child (1-12 yr)	Adolescent (12-18 yr)	Adult (18-45 yr)	Middle Age Adult (45-65 yr)	Senior Adult (65+ yr)
Scleritis	Brain tumor	Brain tumor	Retinal and vitreous hemorrhage	Macular degeneration	Macular degeneration
Down syndrome	Retinal and vitreous hemorrhage	Retinal and vitreous hemorrhage	Ischemic stroke	Ischemic stroke	Giant cell arteritis
Diabetes insipidus	Brain abscess	Brain abscess	Ischemic stroke	Giant cell arteritis	Ischemic stroke
	Scleritis	Retinal artery occlusion	Macular degeneration	Retinal artery occlusion	Retinal artery occlusion
	Down syndrome	Scleritis	Transient ischemic attack	Scleritis	Scleritis
	Retinal artery occlusion	Down syndrome	Down syndrome	Retinal vein occlusion	Transient ischemic attack
	Transient ischemic attack	Transient ischemic attack	Scleritis	Transient ischemic attack	Retinal vein occlusion
	Retinal vein occlusion	Retinal vein occlusion	Pituitary basophilic adenoma (Cushing's disease, ACTH-producing adenoma)	Retinal and vitreous hemorrhage	Glaucoma
	Glaucoma	Glaucoma	Pituitary eosinophilic adenoma (prolactinoma)	Glaucoma	Retinal and vitreous hemorrhage
	Pituitary basophilic adenoma (Cushing's disease, ACTH-producing adenoma)	Pituitary basophilic adenoma (Cushing's disease, ACTH-producing adenoma)	Retinal artery occlusion	Down syndrome	Down syndrome
	Pituitary eosinophilic adenoma (prolactinoma)	Pituitary eosinophilic adenoma (prolactinoma)	Retinal vein occlusion	Brain tumor	Brain tumor
	Coloboma	Coloboma	Brain tumor	Brain abscess	Brain abscess
	Diabetes insipidus	Diabetes insipidus	Glaucoma	Pituitary basophilic adenoma (Cushing's disease, ACTH-producing adenoma)	Pituitary basophilic adenoma (Cushing's disease, ACTH-producing adenoma)
			Brain abscess	Pituitary eosinophilic adenoma (prolactinoma)	Pituitary eosinophilic adenoma (prolactinoma)
			Diabetes insipidus	Diabetes insipidus	Diabetes insipidus

380

Baby (0-1 yr)	Child (1-12 yr)	Adolescent (12-18 yr)	Adult (18-45 yr)	Middle Age Adult (45-65 yr)	Senior Adult (65+ yr)
Viral conjunctivitis	Viral conjunctivitis	Myopia	Amaurosis fugax	Amaurosis fugax	Amaurosis fugax
Strabismus	Strabismus	Hypermetropia	Hypermetropia	Hypermetropia	Hypermetropia
Retinopathy of prematurity	Myopia	Strabismus	Cataract	Cataract	Cataract
Retinoblastoma	Psychosomatic	Ocular trauma	Viral conjunctivitis	Macular degeneration	Giant cell arteritis
Cataract	Ocular trauma	Viral conjunctivitis	Retinal migraine	Viral conjunctivitis	Viral conjunctivitis
Glaucoma	Hypermetropia	Cataract	Retinal detachment	Hyperprolactinemia	Macular degeneration
Scleritis	Cataract	Glaucoma	Macular degeneration	Retinal migraine	Diabetic retinopathy
Optic atrophy	Scleritis	Retinal migraine	Scleritis	Scleritis	Scleritis
Cellulitis	Glaucoma	Optic atrophy	Retinal and vitreous hemorrhage	Diabetic retinopathy	Hyperprolactinemia
Cavernous sinus thrombosis	Retinal migraine	Retinitis pigmentosa	Hyperprolactinemia	Retinal and vitreous hemorrhage	Retinal migraine
Hyperprolactinemia	Hyperprolactinemia	Scleritis	Diabetic retinopathy	Optic atrophy	Retinal artery occlusion
Retinitis pigmentosa	Cavernous sinus thrombosis	Retinoblastoma	Cavernous sinus thrombosis	Orbital cellulitis	Cavernous sinus thrombosis
Myopia	Optic atrophy	Cavernous sinus thrombosis	Optic atrophy	Retinal detachment	Retinal vein occlusion
Hypermetropia	Retinitis pigmentosa	Retinal and vitreous hemorrhage	Ocular trauma	Cavernous sinus thrombosis	Cellulitis
Retinal and vitreous hemorrhage	Retinoblastoma	Hyperprolactinemia	Orbital cellulitis	Hypertensive retinopathy	Glaucoma
Retinal detachment	Retinal and vitreous hemorrhage	Retinal vein occlusion	Melanoma	Cellulitis	Hypertensive retinopathy
Amaurosis fugax	Cellulitis	Retinal artery occlusion	Cellulitis	Retinal artery occlusion	Retinal and vitreous hemorrhage
Ocular trauma	Retinal vein occlusion	Retinal detachment	Hypertensive retinopathy	Retinal vein occlusion	Optic atrophy
Uveitis	Retinal artery occlusion	Amaurosis fugax	Retinitis pigmentosa	Ocular trauma	Retinal detachment
Orbital cellulitis	Retinal detachment	Orbital cellulitis	Glaucoma	Glaucoma	Orbital cellulitis
	Amaurosis fugax	Cellulitis	Optic neuritis	Giant cell arteritis	Ocular trauma

List continues on next page

Emergency Rule Out conditions shown in red. Entries in blue are for information only
Conditions are listed in approximate order of prevalence for this age range

381

List continued from previous page

Baby (0-1 yr)	Child (1-12 yr)	Adolescent (12-18 yr)	Adult (18-45 yr)	Middle Age Adult (45-65 yr)	Senior Adult (65+yr)
	Orbital cellulitis	Uveitis	Retinal artery occlusion	Melanoma	Melanoma
	Uveitis	Optic neuritis	Retinal vein occlusion	Optic neuritis	Retinitis pigmentosa
	Optic neuritis	**Melanoma**	Giant cell arteritis	**Retinitis pigmentosa**	Psychosomatic
		Psychosomatic	Psychosomatic	Psychosomatic	
		Diabetic retinopathy			

Baby (0-1 yr)	Child (1-12 yr)	Adolescent (12-18 yr)	Adult (18-45 yr)	Middle Age Adult (45-65 yr)	Senior Adult (65+ yr)
Retinitis pigmentosa	Retinal migraine	Retinal migraine	Retinal migraine	Retinal migraine	Retinal migraine
Retinal detachment	Retinitis pigmentosa	Retinal detachment	Retinal detachment	Retinal detachment	Diabetic retinopathy
Uveitis	Infective endocarditis	Retinitis pigmentosa	Essential hypertension	Essential hypertension	Essential hypertension
Infective endocarditis	Diabetic retinopathy	Infective endocarditis	Diabetic retinopathy	Diabetic retinopathy	Retinal detachment
Tuberculosis	Essential hypertension	Essential hypertension	Uveitis	Uveitis	Uveitis
Acute leukemia	Uveitis	Uveitis	Retinal artery occlusion	Retinal artery occlusion	Retinal artery occlusion
	Acute leukemia	Diabetic retinopathy	Retinal vein occlusion	Retinal vein occlusion	Retinal vein occlusion
	Tuberculosis	Retinal artery occlusion	Infective endocarditis	Infective endocarditis	Infective endocarditis
	Retinal artery occlusion	Retinal vein occlusion	Tuberculosis	Tuberculosis	Tuberculosis
	Retinal vein occlusion	Acute leukemia	Systemic lupus erythematosus	Systemic lupus erythematosus	Acute leukemia
	Retinal detachment	Systemic lupus erythematosus	Acute leukemia	Acute leukemia	
		Tuberculosis			

Emergency Rule Out conditions shown in red. Entries in blue are for information only
Conditions are listed in approximate order of prevalence for this age range

Vitreous floaters and flashes

Emergency Rule Out conditions shown in red. Entries in blue are for information only
Conditions are listed in approximate order of prevalence for this age range

Baby (0-1 yr)	Child (1-12 yr)	Adolescent (12-18 yr)	Adult (18-45 yr)	Middle Age Adult (45-65 yr)	Senior Adult (65+yr)
Overuse	Overuse	Overuse	Angioedema	Angioedema	Angioedema
Croup	Croup	Vocal cord nodules	Multiple sclerosis	Multiple sclerosis	Ischemic stroke
Epiglottitis	Vocal cord nodules	Vocal cord polyp	Oral cavity cancer	Oral cavity cancer	Oral cavity cancer
Foreign body	Vocal cord polyp	Glossitis	Parkinson's disease	Parkinson's disease	Parkinson's disease
Glossitis	Glossitis	Angioedema	Myasthenia gravis	Myasthenia gravis	Myasthenia gravis
Angioedema	Epiglottitis	Epiglottitis	Bacterial meningitis	Bacterial meningitis	Brainstem disorders
Recurrent laryngeal nerve palsy	Recurrent laryngeal nerve palsy	Viral meningitis	Glossitis	Glossitis	Glossitis
Botulism	Botulism	Recurrent laryngeal nerve palsy	Viral meningitis	Recurrent laryngeal nerve palsy	Amyloidosis
Viral meningitis	Angioedema	Laryngeal cancer	Recurrent laryngeal nerve palsy	Laryngeal cancer	Recurrent laryngeal nerve palsy
Bacterial meningitis	Foreign body	Bacterial meningitis	Laryngeal cancer	Viral meningitis	Laryngeal cancer
Poliomyelitis	Viral meningitis	Guillain-Barré syndrome (acute infective polyneuritis)	Ischemic stroke	Ischemic stroke	Bacterial meningitis
Vocal cord nodules	Bacterial meningitis	Poliomyelitis	Guillain-Barré syndrome (acute infective polyneuritis)	Arteriosclerosis	Arteriosclerosis
Vocal cord polyp	Pseudobulbar palsy	Brainstem disorders	Arteriosclerosis	Guillain-Barré syndrome (acute infective polyneuritis)	Viral meningitis
Pseudobulbar palsy	Guillain-Barré syndrome (acute infective polyneuritis)	Pseudobulbar palsy	Brainstem disorders	Amyloidosis	Multiple sclerosis
Guillain-Barré syndrome (acute infective polyneuritis)	Poliomyelitis	Multiple sclerosis	Poliomyelitis	Brainstem disorders	Amyotrophic lateral sclerosis (motor neuron disease)
Brainstem disorders	Brainstem disorders	Amyloidosis	Pseudobulbar palsy	Pseudobulbar palsy	Pseudobulbar palsy
Post-tracheostomy	Post-tracheostomy	Post-tracheostomy	Amyotrophic lateral sclerosis (motor neuron disease)	Poliomyelitis	Guillain-Barré syndrome (acute infective polyneuritis)
Trauma	Trauma	Trauma	Post-tracheostomy	Amyotrophic lateral sclerosis (motor neuron disease)	Poliomyelitis
Laryngeal cancer	Laryngeal cancer	Botulism			
Cleft lip and palate					

Baby (0-1 yr)	Child (1-12 yr)	Adolescent (12-18 yr)	Adult (18-45 yr)	Middle Age Adult (45-65 yr)	Senior Adult (65+ yr)
			Trauma **Amyloidosis** Botulism	Post-tracheostomy Trauma Botulism	Post-tracheostomy Trauma Botulism

Emergency Rule Out conditions shown in red. Entries in blue are for information only
Conditions are listed in approximate order of prevalence for this age range

Baby (0-1 yr)	Child (1-12 yr)	Adolescent (12-18 yr)	Adult (18-45 yr)	Middle Age Adult (45-65 yr)	Senior Adult (65+ yr)
Posseting	Gastroenteritis	Food poisoning	Food poisoning	Food poisoning	Food poisoning
Gastroenteritis	Cough	Gastroenteritis	Gastroenteritis	Gastroenteritis	Gastroenteritis
Gastroesophageal reflux disease	Acute appendicitis	Migraine headache	Pregnancy	Migraine headache	Gastroesophageal reflux disease
Malaria	Acute pancreatitis	Gastroesophageal reflux disease	Migraine headache	Gastroesophageal reflux disease	Intestinal obstruction
Ménière's disease	Gastroesophageal reflux disease	Acute pancreatitis	Alcohol abuse	Alcohol abuse	Brain injury
Intussusception	Head injury	Acute iron toxicity	Motion sickness	Acute appendicitis	Labyrinthitis
Intracranial hemorrhage	Malaria	Rocky Mountain spotted fever	Labyrinthitis	Labyrinthitis	Toxic shock syndrome
Hyponatremia	Renal calculi	Malaria	Acoustic neuroma	Intestinal obstruction	Alcohol abuse
Heat stroke and heat exhaustion	Rocky Mountain spotted fever	Tonsillitis	Acute appendicitis	Brain injury	Scarlet fever
Hypercalcemia	Intussusception	Intussusception	Toxic shock syndrome	Toxic shock syndrome	Salicylate poisoning
Renal calculi	Intracranial hemorrhage	Renal calculi	Addison's disease	Head injury	Head injury
Glaucoma	Hyponatremia	Intracranial hemorrhage	Scarlet fever	Salicylate poisoning	Rocky Mountain spotted fever
Pyloric stenosis	Heat stroke and heat exhaustion	Hyponatremia	Diabetic ketoacidosis	Rocky Mountain spotted fever	Acute pancreatitis
Diabetes mellitus in children	Hypercalcemia	Hypercalcemia	Salicylate poisoning	Acute pancreatitis	Poliomyelitis
Campylobacter infection	Glaucoma	Heat stroke and heat exhaustion	Acute pancreatitis	Poliomyelitis	Acoustic neuroma
Rocky Mountain spotted fever	Scarlet fever	Glaucoma	Poliomyelitis	Scarlet fever	Babesiosis
Cholera	Ménière's disease	Ménière's disease	Acute iron toxicity	Babesiosis	Malaria
Congenital megacolon	Campylobacter infection	Campylobacter infection	Babesiosis	Acute iron toxicity	Ménière's disease
Tonsillitis	Congenital megacolon	Poliomyelitis	Rocky Mountain spotted fever	Malaria	Intussusception
Poliomyelitis	Diabetes mellitus in children	Diabetes mellitus in children	Malaria	Renal calculi	Hyponatremia
			Intussusception	Intussusception	Intracranial hemorrhage
			Intracranial hemorrhage		

Baby (0-1 yr)	Child (1-12 yr)	Adolescent (12-18 yr)	Adult (18-45 yr)	Middle Age Adult (45-65 yr)	Senior Adult (65+yr)
Babesiosis	Cholera	Congenital megacolon	Renal calculi	Hyponatremia	Hypercalcemia
Carbon monoxide poisoning	Poliomyelitis	Cholera	Hyponatremia	Hypercalcemia	Heat stroke and heat exhaustion
Carcinoid syndrome	Salicylate poisoning	Chlamydia pneumoniae	Heat stroke and heat exhaustion	Intracranial hemorrhage	Renal calculi
Chlamydia pneumoniae	Carbon monoxide poisoning	Babesiosis	Hypercalcemia	Heat stroke and heat exhaustion	Glaucoma
Acute pancreatitis	Tonsillitis	Brain injury	Glaucoma	Glaucoma	Raised intracranial pressure
Salicylate poisoning	Carcinoid syndrome	Carcinoid syndrome	Ménière's disease	Campylobacter infection	Diabetes mellitus in children
Scarlet fever	Babesiosis	Carbon monoxide poisoning	Chlamydia pneumoniae	Ménière's disease	Carbon monoxide poisoning
Toxic shock syndrome	Toxic shock syndrome	Salicylate poisoning	Diabetes mellitus in children	Diabetes mellitus in children	Congenital megacolon
Brain injury	Chlamydia pneumoniae	Scarlet fever	Congenital megacolon	Chlamydia pneumoniae	Cholera
Intestinal obstruction	Brain injury	Toxic shock syndrome	Intestinal obstruction	Congenital megacolon	Campylobacter infection
Raised intracranial pressure	Addison's disease	Acute appendicitis	Cholera	Cholera	Tonsillitis
Bacterial meningitis	Acute iron toxicity	Addison's disease	Carbon monoxide poisoning	Carbon monoxide poisoning	Chlamydia pneumoniae
Viral meningitis	Migraine headache	Intestinal obstruction	Campylobacter infection	Diabetic ketoacidosis	Carcinoid syndrome
Sarcoidosis	Raised intracranial pressure	Head injury	Head injury	Acoustic neuroma	Acute iron toxicity
Volvulus	Bacterial meningitis	Alcohol abuse	Carcinoid syndrome	Carcinoid syndrome	Addison's disease
	Viral meningitis	Pyelonephritis	Brain injury	Addison's disease	Benign paroxysmal positional vertigo
	Reye's syndrome	Bacterial meningitis	Pyelonephritis	Raised intracranial pressure	Acute renal failure
	Sarcoidosis	Viral meningitis	Drug reaction	Benign paroxysmal positional vertigo	Metabolic acidosis
	Volvulus	Sarcoidosis	Bacterial meningitis	Pyelonephritis	Diabetic ketoacidosis
		Volvulus	Benign paroxysmal positional vertigo	Drug reaction	Drug reaction
				Metabolic acidosis	Severe pain

List continues on next page

Vomiting (continued)

List continued from previous page

Baby (0-1 yr)	Child (1-12 yr)	Adolescent (12-18 yr)	Adult (18-45 yr)	Middle Age Adult (45-65 yr)	Senior Adult (65+ yr)
			Metabolic acidosis	Severe pain	Anxiety
			Severe pain	Anxiety	Brain tumor
			Anxiety	Ocular trauma	Ocular trauma
			Brain tumor	Brain tumor	Sarcoidosis
			Ocular trauma	Sarcoidosis	Volvulus
			Sarcoidosis	Volvulus	
			Volvulus		

Baby (0-1 yr)	Child (1-12 yr)	Adolescent (12-18 yr)	Adult (18-45 yr)	Middle Age Adult (45-65 yr)	Senior Adult (65+ yr)
Hyperthyroidism	Hyperthyroidism	Hyperthyroidism	Hypothyroidism	Hypothyroidism	Hypothyroidism
Hypothyroidism	Hypothyroidism	Hypothyroidism	Primary intracerebral hemorrhage stroke	Primary intracerebral hemorrhage stroke	Primary intracerebral hemorrhage stroke
Hyperkalemia	Hyperkalemia	Hyperkalemia	Hyperthyroidism	Hyperthyroidism	Dehydration
Hypokalemia	Hypokalemia	Hypokalemia	Nerve root compression	Dehydration	Hyperthyroidism
Hyperparathyroidism	Hyperparathyroidism	Hyperparathyroidism	Dehydration	Nerve root compression	Nerve root compression
Hyperaldosteronism	Hyperaldosteronism	Hyperaldosteronism	Cushing's syndrome	Cushing's syndrome	Cushing's syndrome
Cushing's syndrome	Cushing's syndrome	Cushing's syndrome	Hypokalemia	Hypokalemia	Hypokalemia
Nutritional deficiencies	Diabetes mellitus in children	Diabetes mellitus in children	Guillain-Barré syndrome (acute infective polyneuritis)	Hyperparathyroidism	Guillain-Barré syndrome (acute infective polyneuritis)
Osteomalacia	Nutritional deficiencies	Nutritional deficiencies	Hyperparathyroidism	Guillain-Barré syndrome (acute infective polyneuritis)	Hyperparathyroidism
Tuberculosis	Osteomalacia	Osteomalacia	Hyperaldosteronism	Hyperaldosteronism	Hyperaldosteronism
Dehydration	Tuberculosis	Tuberculosis	Polymyositis/ dermatomyositis	Polymyositis/ dermatomyositis	Amyotrophic lateral sclerosis (motor neuron disease)
Transient ischemic attack	Dehydration	Transient ischemic attack	Amyotrophic lateral sclerosis (motor neuron disease)	Amyotrophic lateral sclerosis (motor neuron disease)	Malignancy
Down syndrome	Tuberculosis	Ischemic stroke	Malignancy	Malignancy	Osteomalacia
Poliomyelitis	Transient ischemic attack	Poliomyelitis	Osteomalacia	Osteomalacia	Myasthenia gravis
Ischemic stroke	Hydrocephalus	Dehydration	Myasthenia gravis	Myasthenia gravis	Muscular dystrophy
Myocardial infarction	Ischemic stroke	Myocardial infarction	Tuberculosis	Muscular dystrophy	Transient ischemic attack
Multiple sclerosis	Poliomyelitis	Multiple sclerosis			Ischemic stroke
Insect and spider bites and stings	Orthostatic hypotension	Hydrocephalus			
Influenza	Myocardial infarction	Influenza			
Intracranial hemorrhage	Intracranial hemorrhage	Insect and spider bites and stings			
Brucellosis	Multiple sclerosis	Hypercalcemia			
	Influenza				

List continues on next page

Emergency Rule Out conditions shown in red. Entries in blue are for information only
Conditions are listed in approximate order of prevalence for this age range

389

Baby (0-1 yr)	Child (1-12 yr)	Adolescent (12-18 yr)	Adult (18-45 yr)	Middle Age Adult (45-65 yr)	Senior Adult (65+ yr)
Hypercalemia	Insect and spider bites and stings	Brucellosis	Muscular dystrophy	Tuberculosis	Poliomyelitis
Heat stroke and heat exhaustion	Brucellosis	Friedreich's ataxia	Ischemic stroke	Ischemic stroke	Tuberculosis
Friedreich's ataxia	Hypercalemia	Heat stroke and heat exhaustion	Poliomyelitis	Diabetes mellitus type 2	Diabetes mellitus type 2
Cardiomyopathy	Heat stroke and heat exhaustion	Celiac disease	Transient ischemic attack	Poliomyelitis	Multiple sclerosis
Orthostatic hypotension	Cardiomyopathy	Cardiomyopathy	Myocardial infarction	Orthostatic hypotension	Intracranial hemorrhage
Chronic lymphocytic leukemia	Friedreich's ataxia	Congestive heart failure	Multiple sclerosis	Myocardial infarction	Porphyria
Addison's disease	Congestive heart failure	Addison's disease	Intracranial hemorrhage	Multiple sclerosis	Influenza
Congestive heart failure	Chronic lymphocytic leukemia	Chronic lymphocytic leukemia	Orthostatic hypotension	Intracranial hemorrhage	Insect and spider bites and stings
Hydrocephalus	Addison's disease	Intracranial hemorrhage	Influenza	Influenza	Brucellosis
Celiac disease	Mucopolysaccharidosis	Orthostatic hypotension	Insect and spider bites and stings	Insect and spider bites and stings	Myocardial infarction
Mucopolysaccharidosis	Myasthenia gravis	Muscular dystrophy	Brucellosis	Brucellosis	Hypercalemia
Muscular dystrophy	Muscular dystrophy	Myasthenia gravis	Hypercalemia	Transient ischemic attack	Friedreich's ataxia
Myasthenia gravis	Nerve root compression	Nerve root compression	Heat stroke and heat exhaustion	Friedreich's ataxia	Heat stroke and heat exhaustion
Nerve root compression	Brain abscess	Brain abscess	Friedreich's ataxia	Cardiomyopathy	Orthostatic hypotension
Brain abscess	Celiac disease	Brain tumor	Congestive heart failure	Heat stroke and heat exhaustion	Congestive heart failure
Brain tumor	Brain tumor	Malignancy	Cardiomyopathy	Congestive heart failure	Chronic lymphocytic leukemia
Primary intracerebral hemorrhage stroke	Malignancy	Guillain-Barré syndrome (acute infective polyneuritis)	Addison's disease	Addison's disease	Addison's disease
Malignancy	Guillain-Barré syndrome (acute infective polyneuritis)	Diphtheria	Chronic lymphocytic leukemia	Chronic lymphocytic leukemia	Cardiomyopathy
Chronic lead poisoning		Lyme disease	Diabetes mellitus type 2	Celiac disease	Hyperkalemia
Poisoning			Porphyria	Porphyria	Celiac disease

List continues on next page

390

Baby (0-1 yr)	Child (1-12 yr)	Adolescent (12-18 yr)	Adult (18-45 yr)	Middle Age Adult (45-65 yr)	Senior Adult (65+yr)
Diphtheria	Diphtheria	Botulism	Hyperkalemia	Hyperkalemia	Polymyalgia rheumatica
Lyme disease	Lyme disease	Chronic lead poisoning	Celiac disease	Polymyalgia rheumatica	Nutritional deficiencies
Botulism	Botulism	Poisoning	Polymyalgia rheumatica	Nutritional deficiencies	Diabetes mellitus type 1
Trauma	Poisoning	Polymyositis/ dermatomyositis	Nutritional deficiencies	Hypercalcemia	Hydrocephalus
	Chronic lead poisoning	Porphyria	Diabetes mellitus type 1	Diabetes mellitus type 1	Brain abscess
	Polymyositis/ dermatomyositis		Hydrocephalus	Hydrocephalus	Brain tumor
	Porphyria		Brain abscess	Brain abscess	Diphtheria
			Brain tumor	Brain tumor	Lyme disease
			Diphtheria	Diphtheria	Botulism
			Lyme disease	Lyme disease	Chronic lead poisoning
			Botulism	Botulism	Poisoning
			Chronic lead poisoning	Chronic lead poisoning	Polymyositis/ dermatomyositis
			Poisoning	Poisoning	Charcot-Marie-Tooth disease
			Charcot-Marie-Tooth disease	Charcot-Marie-Tooth disease	

Weakness (continued)

391

Emergency Rule Out conditions shown in red. Entries in blue are for information only
Conditions are listed in approximate order of prevalence for this age range

Baby (0-1 yr)	Child (1-12 yr)	Adolescent (12-18 yr)	Adult (18-45 yr)	Middle Age Adult (45-65 yr)	Senior Adult (65+ yr)
Overfeeding	Overfeeding	Depression	Pregnancy	Depression	Hypothyroidism
Hypothyroidism	Hypothyroidism	Overfeeding	Depression	Hypothyroidism	Depression
Cushing's syndrome	Depression	Bulimia nervosa	Hypothyroidism	Menopause	Congestive heart failure
Hypopituitarism	Cushing's syndrome	Hypothyroidism	Polycystic ovarian disease	Alcohol abuse	Alcohol abuse
Prader-Willi syndrome	Hypopituitarism	Polycystic ovarian disease	Alcohol abuse	Congestive heart failure	Cushing's syndrome
Insulinoma	Prader-Willi syndrome	Pregnancy	Menopause	Cushing's syndrome	Hypopituitarism
	Polycystic ovarian disease	Alcohol abuse	Bulimia nervosa	Hypopituitarism	Insulinoma
	Insulinoma	Cushing's syndrome	Cushing's syndrome	Bulimia nervosa	Bulimia nervosa
		Hypopituitarism	Hypopituitarism	Insulinoma	Insulin resistance
		Insulinoma	Insulinoma	Insulin resistance	
		Prader-Willi syndrome	Insulin resistance		
		Insulin resistance			

392

Baby (0-1 yr)	Child (1-12 yr)	Adolescent (12-18 yr)	Adult (18-45 yr)	Middle Age Adult (45-65 yr)	Senior Adult (65+ yr)
Gastroenteritis	Anxiety	Anemia	Anxiety	Anxiety	Anxiety
Lactose intolerance	Gastroenteritis	Anxiety	Depression	Depression	Depression
Anemia	Tularemia	Gastroenteritis	Gastroenteritis	Tularemia	Gastroenteritis
Chronic allergic alveolitis	Chronic allergic alveolitis	Bulimia nervosa	Bulimia nervosa	Gastroenteritis	Malignancy
Giardiasis	Tuberculosis	Tularemia	Diabetes mellitus type 1	Tuberculosis	Ulcerative colitis
Tularemia	Diabetes mellitus in children	Manic depression	Tularemia	Chronic infection	Tuberculosis
Diabetes mellitus in children	Giardiasis	Chronic allergic alveolitis	Anorexia nervosa	Celiac disease	Polyarteritis nodosa
Chronic fatigue syndrome	Chronic fatigue syndrome	Myelodysplastic syndromes	Tuberculosis	Ulcerative colitis	Systemic lupus erythematosus
Myelodysplastic syndromes	Idiopathic myelofibrosis	Giardiasis	Chronic infection	Polyarteritis nodosa	Idiopathic myelofibrosis
Amebic dysentery	Myelodysplastic syndromes	Idiopathic myelofibrosis	Ulcerative colitis	Malabsorption	Myelodysplastic syndromes
Manic depression	Systemic lupus erythematosus	Chronic fatigue syndrome	Crohn's disease	Idiopathic myelofibrosis	Chronic obstructive pulmonary disease
Idiopathic myelofibrosis	Polyarteritis nodosa	Diabetes mellitus in children	Systemic lupus erythematosus	Myelodysplastic syndromes	Chronic infection
Polyarteritis nodosa	Manic depression	Tuberculosis	Polyarteritis nodosa	Amebic dysentery	Chronic allergic alveolitis
Blastomycosis	Blastomycosis	Polyarteritis nodosa	Amebic dysentery	Manic depression	Manic depression
Reiter's syndrome	Reiter's syndrome	Blastomycosis	Blastomycosis	Chronic allergic alveolitis	Giardiasis
Systemic lupus erythematosus	Amebic dysentery	Reiter's syndrome	Idiopathic myelofibrosis	Blastomycosis	Chronic fatigue syndrome
Tuberculosis	Malabsorption	Systemic lupus erythematosus	Manic depression	Giardiasis	Malabsorption
Celiac disease	Bulimia nervosa	Amebic dysentery	Chronic allergic alveolitis	Chronic fatigue syndrome	Blastomycosis
Pyloric stenosis	Anorexia nervosa	Anorexia nervosa	Myelodysplastic syndromes	Diabetes mellitus type 1	Reiter's syndrome
Inborn errors of metabolism	Celiac disease	Celiac disease	Giardiasis	Malignancy	Tularemia
Malignancy	Malignancy	Chronic infection	Chronic fatigue syndrome	Reiter's syndrome	

List continues on next page

Emergency Rule Out conditions shown in red. Entries in blue are for information only
Conditions are listed in approximate order of prevalence for this age range

393

List continued from previous page

Baby (0-1 yr)	Child (1-12 yr)	Adolescent (12-18 yr)	Adult (18-45 yr)	Middle Age Adult (45-65 yr)	Senior Adult (65+ yr)
Pancreatic cancer	Pancreatic cancer	Crohn's disease	Malabsorption	Systemic lupus erythematosus	Amebic dysentery
Proctitis	Proctitis	Malabsorption	Reiter's syndrome	Hyperthyroidism	Hyperthyroidism
		Malignancy	Malignancy	Malnutrition	Malnutrition
		Pancreatic cancer	Hyperthyroidism	Chronic obstructive pulmonary disease	Peptic ulcer
		Proctitis	Malnutrition	Intestinal parasites	Intestinal parasites
			AIDS	Addison's disease	Liver failure
			Peptic ulcer	AIDS	Carcinoid syndrome
			Intestinal parasites	Liver failure	Diabetes mellitus type 1
			Addison's disease	Gastric cancer	Addison's disease
			Liver failure	Carcinoid syndrome	Pancreatic cancer
			Chronic obstructive pulmonary disease	Pancreatic cancer	Proctitis
			Carcinoid syndrome	Proctitis	
			Pancreatic cancer		
			Proctitis		

Baby (0-1 yr)	Child (1-12 yr)	Adolescent (12-18 yr)	Adult (18-45 yr)	Middle Age Adult (45-65 yr)	Senior Adult (65+ yr)
Asthma	Asthma	Asthma	Asthma	Asthma	Chronic obstructive pulmonary disease
Bronchiolitis	Bronchiolitis	Cystic fibrosis	Chronic obstructive pulmonary disease	Chronic obstructive pulmonary disease	Asthma
Cystic fibrosis	Cystic fibrosis	Foreign body	Gastroesophageal reflux disease	Acute bronchitis	Acute bronchitis
Gastroesophageal reflux disease	Gastroesophageal reflux disease	Gastroesophageal reflux disease	Acute bronchitis	Gastroesophageal reflux disease	Gastroesophageal reflux disease
Foreign body	Foreign body	Acute bronchitis	Aspiration pneumonia	Aspiration pneumonia	Aspiration pneumonia
Congenital heart disease	Congenital heart disease	Respiratory syncytial virus infection	Bacterial pneumonia	Bacterial pneumonia	Bacterial pneumonia
Respiratory syncytial virus infection	Acute bronchitis	Congenital heart disease	Allergic reactions and anaphylaxis	Mycoplasmal pneumonia	Mycoplasmal pneumonia
Bronchiectasis	Bronchiectasis	Bronchiectasis	Respiratory syncytial virus infection	Respiratory syncytial virus infection	Viral pneumonia
Acute bronchitis	Respiratory syncytial virus infection	Bacterial pneumonia	Mycoplasmal pneumonia	Primary lung malignancy	Bronchiectasis
Bacterial pneumonia	Bacterial pneumonia	Viral pneumonia	Viral pneumonia	Viral pneumonia	Primary lung malignancy
Viral pneumonia	Viral pneumonia	Mycoplasmal pneumonia	Bronchiectasis	Bronchiectasis	Behçet's syndrome
Allergic reactions and anaphylaxis	Mycoplasmal pneumonia	Allergic reactions and anaphylaxis	Primary lung malignancy	Carcinoid syndrome	Respiratory syncytial virus infection
Angioedema	Allergic reactions and anaphylaxis	Angioedema	Carcinoid syndrome	Congestive heart failure	Congestive heart failure
Drug reaction	Angioedema	Drug reaction	Bronchiolitis	Allergic reactions and anaphylaxis	Carcinoid syndrome
Behçet's syndrome	Drug reaction	Behçet's syndrome	Congestive heart failure	Drug reaction	Allergic reactions and anaphylaxis
Primary lung malignancy	Behçet's syndrome	Primary lung malignancy	Drug reaction	Behçet's syndrome	Drug reaction
Carcinoid syndrome	Primary lung malignancy	Carcinoid syndrome	Behçet's syndrome	Pulmonary thromboembolism	Pulmonary thromboembolism
	Carcinoid syndrome				

List continues on next page

Emergency Rule Out conditions shown in red. Entries in blue are for information only
Conditions are listed in approximate order of prevalence for this age range

395

List continued from previous page

Baby (0-1 yr)	Child (1-12 yr)	Adolescent (12-18 yr)	Adult (18-45 yr)	Middle Age Adult (45-65 yr)	Senior Adult (65+yr)
			Pulmonary thromboembolism Idiopathic pulmonary interstitial fibrosis Vocal cord dysfunction Angioedema Foreign body	Idiopathic pulmonary interstitial fibrosis Vocal cord dysfunction Angioedema Foreign body	Idiopathic pulmonary interstitial fibrosis Vocal cord dysfunction Angioedema Foreign body

Baby (0-1 yr)	Child (1-12 yr)	Adolescent (12-18 yr)	Adult (18-45 yr)	Middle Age Adult (45-65 yr)	Senior Adult (65+ yr)
Trauma	Trauma	Trauma	Trauma	Trauma	Trauma
Wrist injury	Overuse	Muscular strain	Muscular strain	Muscular strain	Muscular strain
Muscular strain	Wrist injury	Overuse	Overuse	Overuse	Overuse
	Muscular strain	Wrist injury	Acute gout	Acute gout	Osteoarthritis
	Juvenile idiopathic arthritis	Carpal tunnel syndrome	Wrist injury	Wrist injury	Wrist injury
		Juvenile idiopathic arthritis	Osteoarthritis	Rheumatoid arthritis	Acute gout
		Systemic lupus erythematosus	Rheumatoid arthritis	Osteoarthritis	Rheumatoid arthritis
		Scleroderma	Gonorrhea	Psoriatic arthritis	Scleroderma
			Psoriatic arthritis	Gonorrhea	Systemic lupus erythematosus
			Systemic lupus erythematosus	Systemic lupus erythematosus	Gonorrhea
			Scleroderma	Scleroderma	

Emergency Rule Out conditions shown in red. Entries in blue are for information only
Conditions are listed in approximate order of prevalence for this age range

Wrist pain

Part Two

Clinical Benchmarks

- Clinical Benchmarks are listed by diagnosis in alphabetical order.

- Based on your clinical judgment or your use of the tables in Part One, find the Clinical Benchmarks for the diagnoses under consideration and compare and contrast them to the patient.

- As necessary, compare Clinical Benchmarks between diagnoses to help further define the patient's profile.

Clinical Benchmarks can facilitate your thinking regarding the evaluation and workup necessary to confirm your patient's condition or status.

Abdominal abscess ●*Onset:* Subacute ●*Male:female ratio:* M=F ●*Ethnicity:* All ●*Character:* Fever, anorexia, malaise, usually with abdominal pain, but may be relatively painless; if persistent, there is often weight loss ●*Location:* Abdomen ●*Pattern:* Nonspecific ●*Precipitating factors:* None relevant ●*Relieving factors:* Both antibiotic therapy and drainage of the abscess are required; drainage may be via percutaneous catheter or surgery ●*Clinical course:* Usually progresses over days to weeks; not self-limited ●*Co-morbidities:* Abdominal trauma, diverticulitis, appendicitis, inflammatory bowel disease, postoperative complication ●*Procedure results:* Abdominal CT scan usually reveals the abscess; diagnosis is confirmed by sampling of the abscess contents (Gram stain and culture) ●*Test findings:* WBC, ESR usually elevated

Abdominal aortic aneurysm ●*Onset:* Subacute/insidious ●*Male:female ratio:* M(4):F(1) ●*Ethnicity:* All ●*Character:* Asymptomatic or constant pain ●*Location:* Lower abdomen and/or lower back ●*Pattern:* Steady ●*Precipitating factors:* Age, smoking, family history, atherosclerosis ●*Relieving factors:* Beta-blockers ●*Clinical course:* Progressive: rupture; risk of rupture increased with size >5.0cm and rate of growth >0.5cm/year ●*Co-morbidities:* Hypertension, hyperlipidemia, atherosclerosis ●*Procedure results:* No relevant procedures ●*Test findings:* U/S, CT, MRI, aortogram with dilation of aorta 1.5x normal

Abdominal aortic dissection ●*Onset:* Acute ●*Male:female ratio:* M(2):F(1) ●*Ethnicity:* All ●*Character:* Severe, sudden, sharp, tearing or ripping pain ●*Location:* Abdominal ●*Pattern:* Hypertension, pulse deficit, renal insufficiency ●*Precipitating factors:* Trauma, connective tissue disease ●*Relieving factors:* Surgery, nitroprusside, beta-blockers ●*Clinical course:* Progressive: vascular compromise or rupture, death ●*Co-morbidities:* Hypertension, atherosclerosis, aortic aneurysm, Marfan's, Noonan's, giant cell arteritis, trauma ●*Procedure results:* CT or MRI: two lumens and/or intimal flap ●*Test findings:* Hypertension, pulse deficit, renal insufficiency

Abdominal hernias ●*Onset:* Acute/subacute/chronic ●*Male:female ratio:* M=F ●*Ethnicity:* All ●*Character:* Swelling (protrusion) at involved site with tenderness; may develop vomiting, diffuse abdominal pain, decreased bowel sounds; usually reducible ●*Location:* Most common are inguinal (direct and indirect), femoral, umbilical, incisional ●*Pattern:* Nonspecific ●*Precipitating factors:* Often congenital, may follow repetitive contraction/relaxation of abdominal musculature; may be more obvious with increasing intra-abdominal pressure (standing position, valsalva maneuver) ●*Relieving factors:* Reducing hernia relieves pain, wearing an elastic wrap or girdle, surgical repair is definitive treatment ●*Clinical course:* Hernias may become incarcerated (not reducible) or strangulated (vascular compromise of herniated contents) requiring immediate surgery ●*Co-morbidities:* Advancing age (direct inguinal hernias), prior surgery (incisional hernias) ●*Procedure results:* Abdominal radiographs may show obstruction ●*Test findings:* No relevant tests

Abdominal migraine ●*Onset:* Acute ●*Male:female ratio:* M=F ●*Ethnicity:* All ●*Character:* Nausea, abdominal pain, recurrent vomiting, diarrhea, headache ●*Location:* Abdomen ●*Pattern:* Repetitious pattern ●*Precipitating factors:* Family history ●*Relieving factors:* Sleeping, propanolol ●*Clinical course:* Lasting minutes to hours ●*Co-morbidities:* Migraines ●*Procedure results:* No relevant procedures ●*Test findings:* Family history

Abetalipoproteinemia ●*Onset:* Age: 2 to 6 years ●*Male:female ratio:* M=F ●*Ethnicity:* All ●*Character:* Mutation in gene encoding microsomal triglyceride transfer protein (MTP) ●*Location:* Defective assembly and secretion of apolipoprotein B resulting in defective absorption of lipids in intestine ●*Pattern:* Retinitis pigmentosa, sensory motor neuropathy, ataxia, mental retardation in one third of patients, distal muscle atrophy, absent deep tendon reflexes ●*Precipitating factors:* Clinical spectrum dependent on severity of metabolic derangement: homozygous inheritance most severe ●*Relieving factors:* No treatment for primary defect; supplemental vitamin E and other fat soluble vitamins may improve retinopathy and neuropathy ●*Clinical course:* Progressive deterioration ●*Co-morbidities:* Fat-soluble vitamin deficiencies ●*Procedure results:* Peripheral nerve biopsy shows loss of large myelinated fibers; nerve conduction studies show low sensory amplitude; visual and somatosensory evoked potentials abnormal ●*Test findings:* Serum cholesterol, very low density lipoprotein (VLDL) and beta lipoprotein absent; acanthocytes; MRI shows posterior column degeneration

Abruptio placentae ●*Onset:* Acute ●*Male:female ratio:* F ●*Ethnicity:* All ●*Character:* Sharp pain, cramping, contractions, vaginal bleeding ●*Location:* Uterine ●*Pattern:* Vaginal bleeding and onset of cramping possibly accompanied by sharp pain ●*Precipitating factors:* May be related to trauma, hypertension, preterm premature rupture of membranes or idiopathic ●*Relieving factors:* None relevant ●*Clinical course:* Variable ●*Co-morbidities:* Disseminated intravascular coagulopathy, fetal hypoxia ●*Procedure results:* Hematoma on U/S, nonreassuring fetal heart rate pattern ●*Test findings:* No relevant tests

Achalasia ●*Onset:* Insidious ●*Male:female ratio:* M=F ●*Ethnicity:* All ●*Character:* Progressive dysphagia to liquids and solids; retrosternal pain with swallowing in one-thrid to one-half of patients; regurgitation of food; progressive weight loss ●*Location:* Pain is retrosternal ●*Pattern:* Nonspecific ●*Precipitating factors:* Swallowing solids or liquids ●*Relieving factors:* Regurgitation of swallowed material; slow deliberate swallowing with an erect posture may help; balloon dilation of the lower esohageal sphincter, myotomy, or injection of botulinum toxin ●*Clinical course:* Slowly progressive over months; not self-limited ●*Co-morbidities:* Squamous cell carcinoma of the esophagus is more common in patients with achalasia ●*Procedure results:* Definitve test: esophageal manometry showing lower esophageal sphincter hypertension and aperistalsis; esophagogastroduodenoscopy to rule out other structural diseases of the esophagus ●*Test findings:* Barium swallow may show dilated esophagus with poor motility and a tapering stricture at the gastroesophageal junction

Acne rosacea ●*Onset:* Subacute ●*Male:female ratio:* M<F ●*Ethnicity:* Fair skin ❶ *Character:* Flushing ❷ *Location:* Midforehead, cheeks, nose, chin ❸ *Pattern:* Papules, pustules, telangiectasias ●*Precipitating factors:* Alcohol, caffeine, spicy foods, sun exposure ●*Relieving factors:* Tetracyclines, topical metronidazole ●*Clinical course:* Persistent ●*Co-morbidities:* None relevant ●*Procedure results:* No relevant procedures ●*Test findings:* No relevant tests

Images of ❶ *Character,* ❷ *Location,* ❸ *Pattern on page 402*

Acne vulgaris ●*Onset:* Subacute ●*Male:female ratio:* M=F ●*Ethnicity:* Caucasians more commonly affected ❶ *Character:* Skin lesions ❷ *Location:* Face, back, chest, upper arms ❸ *Pattern:* Comedones, papules, pustules, cysts ●*Precipitating factors:* Oral contraceptive pill, topical oils ●*Relieving factors:* Benzoyl peroxides, antibiotics, topical and oral retinoids ●*Clinical course:* Persistent ●*Co-morbidities:* None relevant ●*Procedure results:* No relevant procedures ●*Test findings:* No relevant tests

Images of ❶ *Character,* ❷ *Location,* ❸ *Pattern on page 402*

Acoustic neuroma ●*Onset:* Acute to insidious ●*Male:female ratio:* M<F ●*Ethnicity:* All ●*Character:* Hearing loss, tinnitus, facial paresthesias, if progression; ataxia, dysphagia ●*Location:* Nonspecific ●*Pattern:* Nonspecific ●*Precipitating factors:* Acoustic trauma (exposure to loud noise), neurofibromatosis ●*Relieving factors:* Surgical resection, radiation ●*Clinical course:* If tumor is small and completely excised the prognosis is good ●*Co-morbidities:* None relevant ●*Procedure results:* Abnormal audiometry (asymmetric sensorineural hearing loss), lesion in auditory canal on MRI (preferred imaging) or CT ●*Test findings:* No relevant tests

Acne rosacea: Images *see text page 401*

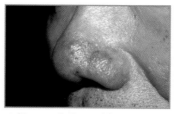

❶ *Character* Erythema of the nose

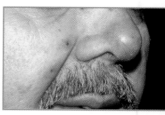

❷ *Location* Papules on the cheeks and erythema of the nose

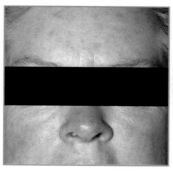

❷ *Location* Red nose and patchy erythema of cheeks and forehead

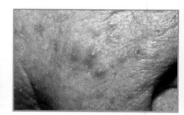

❸ *Pattern* Close up of papules and pustules on cheek

Acne vulgaris: Images *see text page 401*

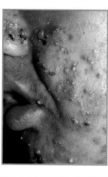

❶ *Character* Multiple papules and pustules of severe acne

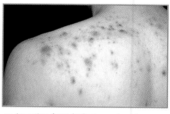

❷ *Location* Acne lesions on shoulders are multiple and in different stages

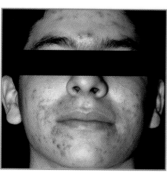

❸ *Pattern* Moderate acne of the face

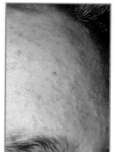

❸ *Pattern* Multiple comedones - both open (white) and closed (black)

Acromegaly (pituitary gigantism) ●*Onset:* Insidious except in the setting of pituitary apoplexy ●*Male:female ratio:* M=F ●*Ethnicity:* All ●*Character:* Increase in hat, shoe, and/or ring size; coarsening of facial features, increase in spacing between teeth in adults ●*Location:* Pituitary adenoma most common; also recorded in lung, pancreas, other locations ●*Pattern:* Nonspecific ●*Precipitating factors:* Pituitary adenoma/ectopic production of growth hormone releasing hormone (GHRH) (bronchial carcinoid or islet cell tumor); overadministration of growth hormone (GH) ●*Relieving factors:* Surgery/radiotherapy to remove tumor; somatostatin analog to lower GH levels ●*Clinical course:* Progressive ●*Co-morbidities:* Accelerated atherosclerosis, hypertension, diabetes mellitus ●*Procedure results:* Pituitary tumor on CT or MRI ●*Test findings:* GH does not suppress in response to an oral glucose load; elevated somatomedin C; ectopic may have elevated plasma GHRH; imaging procedures may reveal nonpituitary tumor

Acromioclavicular joint separation ●*Onset:* Acute ●*Male:female ratio:* M=F ●*Ethnicity:* All ●*Character:* Dull ache ●*Location:* Shoulders ●*Pattern:* Worse with movement of affected shoulder ●*Precipitating factors:* Trauma, usually downward over outer shoulder ●*Relieving factors:* Sling, NSAIDs, open reduction and internal fixation (rarely) ●*Clinical course:* Types IV-VI must be surgically corrected; early degenerative acromioclavicular arthritis not uncommon ●**Co-morbidities:** None relevant ●*Procedure results:* Confirmed by standing anterior-posterior shoulder films with an axillary lateral view ●*Test findings:* No relevant tests

Acute allergic alveolitis ●*Onset:* Abrupt within 4-6 hours ●*Male:female ratio:* M=F ●*Ethnicity:* All ●*Character:* Fever, chills, malaise, nausea, cough, chest tightness, dyspnea ●*Location:* Pulmonary symptoms and signs include cough dyspnea, tachypnea, diffuse fine rales, wheezing (rare) ●*Pattern:* Intensity of symptoms variable depending on inciting antigen ●*Precipitating factors:* Exposure to inciting agents including agricultural dusts, bioaerosols, micro-organisms including fungal, bacterial or protozoal, certain reaction chemicals ●*Relieving factors:* Symptoms resolve within 12 hours-to-days after removal from exposure to inciting antigen ●*Clinical course:* Symptoms recur with re-exposure ●*Co-morbidities:* Increased incidence of chronic bronchitis in agricultural workers with past history of farmer's lung ●*Procedure results:* Bronchoalveolar lavage lymphocytosis usually present. Pulmonary function tests show restrictive defect. Lung biopsy positive for non-caseating interstitial granulomas or peribronchial mononuclear cell infiltration ●*Test findings:* Nonspecific: elevated ESR, lactate dehydrogenase, C-reactive protein. Positive IgG serum antibodies to common causative antigens. Chest X-ray frequently normal, CT may show interstitial pneumonitis

Acute appendicitis ●*Onset:* Subacute ●*Male:female ratio:* M=F ●*Ethnicity:* All ●*Character:* Vague generalized abdominal pain, anorexia, nausea, followed by migration of pain to right lower quadrant (RLQ) with increased severity and peritoneal signs ●*Location:* Early: epigastic and periumbillical pain; later: localized RLQ pain ●*Pattern:* Generalized abdominal pain is first, then anorexia and nausea, then localized RLQ pain ●*Precipitating factors:* Thigh extension increases pain; in later stages, any movement aggravates pain ●*Relieving factors:* Lying still relieves pain ●*Clinical course:* Most patients seek medical attention in 12-48 hours after onset; requires surgical intervention ●*Co-morbidities:* None relevant ●*Procedure results:* CT or U/S may aid in the diagnosis, but it is generally suspected clinically and confirmed at operation ●*Test findings:* WBC usually elevated >10,000

Acute blood loss ●*Onset:* Acute ●*Male:female ratio:* M=F ●*Ethnicity:* All ●*Character:* Lightheadedness ●*Location:* Nonspecific ●*Pattern:* Nonspecific ●*Precipitating factors:* Anticoagulation, thrombolysis, trauma ●*Relieving factors:* None relevant ●*Clinical course:* Variable ●*Co-morbidities:* None relevant ●*Procedure results:* No relevant procedures ●*Test findings:* Low hematocrit

Acute bronchitis ● *Onset:* Acute ● *Male:female ratio:* M=F ● *Ethnicity:* All ● *Character:* Cough with phlegm, fever is unusual (except with influenza) ● *Location:* Chest ● *Pattern:* Bilateral expiratory rhonchi ● *Precipitating factors:* Upper respiratory infection ● *Relieving factors:* Reassurance and symptomatic treatment; antibiotics and bronchodilators if obstructive lung disease ● *Clinical course:* Recovery over days to weeks, c.75% improved by day 14 ● *Co-morbidities:* Pneumonitis, asthma, chronic obstructive pulmonary disease, sinusitis, rhinitis ● *Procedure results:* Chest X-ray not indicated unless focal abnormality on lung examination or patient is febrile ● *Test findings:* Purulent sputum

Acute glomerulonephritis ● *Onset:* Subacute over days-to-weeks ● *Male:female ratio:* M(6):F(4) ● *Ethnicity:* All ● *Character:* Glomerular disease leading to hematuria, RBC casts, lipiduria, proteinuria ● *Location:* Peripheral edema, hypertension, renal insufficiency ● *Pattern:* Focal nephritic involves < half glomeruli; diffuse nephritic affects most or all glomeruli ● *Precipitating factors:* Immune complex deposition, e.g. systemic lupus erythematosus (SLE), hepatitis C, drug-induced (e.g. penicillamine), postinfectious ● *Relieving factors:* Dependent on underlying etiology. Postinfectious: antibiotic and supportive therapy; SLE: glucocorticoids and cytotoxics; Goodpasture's: may require plasma exchange, IV glucocorticoids ● *Clinical course:* Dependent on underlying etiology; some forms (e.g. poststreptococcal) are self-limited ● *Co-morbidities:* SLE, postviral (hepatitis B and C, EBV, varicella, coxsackie); poststreptococcal; other postinfection including parasitic; endocarditis, malignancy, Henoch-Schönlein purpura, vasculitis, cryoglobulinemia, Goodpasture's ● *Procedure results:* Renal biopsy distinguishes focal from diffuse glomerulonephritis ● *Test findings:* Urine sediment positive for RBCs and RBC casts; serum elevated creatinine, reduced complement, positive antistrepsolysin titer, antiglomerular basement membrane (GBM) antibodies

Acute gout ● *Onset:* Acute ● *Male:female ratio:* M(5):F(1) ● *Ethnicity:* All ● *Character:* Severe, constant joint pain, joint swelling and redness ● *Location:* First metatarsophalangeal joint, ankle, knee, wrist, other joints less common ● *Pattern:* 80% monoarticular ● *Precipitating factors:* Alcohol, diuretics, low-dose aspirin, renal disease, obesity, treatment of myeloproliferative disorders ● *Relieving factors:* NSAIDs, glucocorticoids, colchicine, aspiration ● *Clinical course:* If untreated, attack lasts days-to-weeks; usually recurs ● *Co-morbidities:* Hypertension, renal failure, hypothyroidism, hyperparathyroidism, hyperlipidemia, alcoholism, high cell turnover states (e.g. psoriasis, polycythemia) ● *Procedure results:* No relevant procedures ● *Test findings:* Negatively birefringent crystals (monosodium urate) on polarized microscopy of synovial fluid

Acute iron toxicity ● *Onset:* Acute ● *Male:female ratio:* M=F ● *Ethnicity:* All ● *Character:* Nausea, vomiting, diarrhea, hematemesis ● *Location:* Abdomen ● *Pattern:* Acute GI distress within 30 min-6 h after ingestion; >6 h can have hypotension, coma, hepatitis ● *Precipitating factors:* Iron, a gastric corrosive that causes direct injury and mitochondrial damage to cells ● *Relieving factors:* Ipecac-induced vomiting, bowel irrigation, deferoxamine chelation ● *Clinical course:* Mild ingestion causes self-limited GI symptoms; moderate-to-severe causes hematemesis and hypotension, coma in 6-12 hours; gastric scarring and pyloric stenosis can develop in 2-4 weeks ● *Co-morbidities:* Hepatitis, coma, pyloric stenosis ● *Procedure results:* Abdominal film reveals radiopaque pills ● *Test findings:* Metabolic acidosis by electrolytes and blood gas, iron level, elevated liver function tests, coagulation studies

Acute left ventricular failure ● *Onset:* Acute ● *Male:female ratio:* M=F ● *Ethnicity:* All ● *Character:* Sudden onset of chest pain, shortness of breath, hypotension with or without syncope ● *Location:* Chest pain may be present in the substernal area with radiation to the jaw and left arm; may radiate to the back as in aortic dissection; examination may reveal diffuse pulmonary crackles, new murmur, elevated neck veins, S3 or S4 heart sounds ● *Pattern:* Worsening shortness of breath; progression of symptoms; usually occurs due to acute myocardial infarction, myocarditis, acute valvular insufficiency ● *Precipitating factors:* Acute myocardial infarction, myocarditis, acute valvular insufficiency ● *Relieving factors:* Acute therapy is to protect airway, breathing, circulation; etiology of acute left ventricular dysfunction should be determined promptly ● *Clinical course:* If left untreated, acute left ventricular dysfunction is associated with high morbidity/mortality ●*Co-morbidities:* Often coronary artery disease, diabetes, hyperlipidemia, hypertension, cocaine use; acute myocarditis may be idiopathic or result from viral infection ●*Procedure results:* Hemodynamic instability may be present; shortness of breath is always present ●*Test findings:* Chest X-ray reveals heart failure; ECG may show ischemic/infarct pattern; blood work may reveal elevated creatine kinase/myocardial band fraction or troponin/lactase dehydrogenase levels; Echo reveals left ventricular dysfunction with or without valvular insufficiency; cardiac catheterization reveals elevated right/left ventricular pressures with or without coronary artery disease

Acute leukemia ●*Onset:* Usually subacute but can be acute ●*Male:female ratio:* M>F ●*Ethnicity:* All ●*Character:* Bleeding, infection, fatigue, gum hypertrophy, headache, change in mental status, bone pain, rash ●*Location:* Bleeding is usually mucosal, infection commonly in lung, skin, and perirectal areas ●*Pattern:* Nonspecific ●*Precipitating factors:* Radiation, toxins (benzene), alkylating chemotherapy agents ●*Relieving factors:* Intensive chemotherapy, bone marrow transplant, supportive care, retinoic acid (M3 AML) ●*Clinical course:* Adults <60 years, 30-40% cure with aggressive treatment; children: 60-70% cure ●*Co-morbidities:* None relevant ●*Procedure results:* Bone marrow biopsy: hypercellular, >30% blasts; spinal tap: blasts (AML); chest X-ray: mediastinal mass (ALL) ●*Test findings:* Blood smear: blasts, Auer rods (AML), elevated prothrombin time, fibrin split products; monoclonal antibody tests positive for specific B/T cell antigens

Acute mesenteric adenitis ●*Onset:* Subacute ●*Male:female ratio:* M=F ●*Ethnicity:* All ●*Character:* Low-grade fever, abdominal tenderness, nausea/vomiting, rash (uncommon), arthritis, diarrhea (fairly uncommon) ●*Location:* Pain in right lower quadrant, rash is generalized, arthritis: multiple joints and asymmetric ●*Pattern:* Nonspecific ●*Precipitating factors:* Infection with Yersinia enterocolitica ●*Relieving factors:* Supportive care; if septicemia, then antibiotics ●*Clinical course:* Usually self-limited, but if septicemic, mortality is 10-50% ●*Co-morbidities:* None relevant ●*Procedure results:* Abdominal CT finding enlarged mesenteric lymph nodes and terminal ileal thickening ●*Test findings:* Stool culture positive for Y. enterocolitica or pseudotuberculosis, positive serologic test for Yersinia, mild leukocytosis with left shift

Acute mesenteric ischemia ●*Onset:* Acute ●*Male:female ratio:* M=F ●*Ethnicity:* All ●*Character:* Sudden onset of abdominal pain, forceful bowel evacuation following onset of pain, blood per rectum ●*Location:* Nonspecific ●*Pattern:* Nonspecific ●*Precipitating factors:* Poorly controlled congestive heart failure (CHF), atrial fibrillation ●*Relieving factors:* Usually requires surgery/embolectomy, supportive care, broad spectrum antibiotics, infusion of papaverine via angiography ●*Clinical course:* Mortality 70-90% without early intervention ●*Co-morbidities:* Atrial fibrillation, CHF, vascular disease ●*Procedure results:* Angiography: spasm or occlusion; endoscopy: ulceration, edema; CT: bowel wall thickening and dilation, vascular thrombosis ●*Test findings:* Leukocytosis, acidemia, elevated lactate

Acute otitis media ●*Onset:* Acute ●*Male:female ratio:* M>F ●*Ethnicity:* All ●*Character:* Otalgia, decreased hearing, fever ●*Location:* Affected ear ●*Pattern:* Persistent otalgia ●*Precipitating factors:* Upper respiratory infection: viruses, Streptococcus pneumoniae, Hemophilus influenzae, Moraxella catarrhalis; dysfunctional eustachian tube, enlarged adenoids, immature immune system, day care attendance, smoke exposure in the home ●*Relieving factors:* Topical anesthetic ear drops, cold compress ●*Clinical course:* Acute phase may be self-limited, 3-7 days; fluid may persist for weeks ●*Co-morbidities:* Cleft palates, eustachian tube dysfunction; adenoid hypertrophy ●*Procedure results:* Fluid behind red, bulging, inflamed tympanic membrane on otoscopy ●*Test findings:* Flat tympanogram

Acute pancreatitis ●*Onset:* Acute ●*Male:female ratio:* M=F ●*Ethnicity:* All ●*Character:* Epigastric/diffuse abdominal pain, nausea, vomiting that is worse after food intake; pain worse lying supine, improved with sitting forward; may have low-grade fever ●*Location:* Upper abdomen ●*Pattern:* Pain exacerbated by eating ●*Precipitating factors:* Food intake, alcohol ingestion ●*Relieving factors:* Patients should be given nothing by mouth, with IV hydration; narcotic analgesics are often required ●*Clinical course:* Usually self-limited; average: 2-7 days but may be longer ●*Co-morbidities:* Alcohol use, gallstones, hypercalcemia, severe hypertriglyceridemia ●*Procedure results:* CT scan shows pancreatic edema with peripancreatic fat stranding ●*Test findings:* Amylase and lipase are usually elevated

Acute renal failure ●*Onset:* Acute ●*Male:female ratio:* M=F ●*Ethnicity:* All ●*Character:* Abrupt reduction/cessation of renal function leading to reduced glomerular filtration ●*Location:* Prerenal: reduced glomerular perfusion; obstructive uropathy: must be bilateral to produce acute renal failure; vascular: usually vasculitis; glomerular disease; tubular and interstitial ●*Pattern:* Variable depending on underlying etiology; decreased urine output or anuria, flank pain, edema, hematuria, anorexia, vomiting, hypertension, mental status changes ●*Precipitating factors:* Drugs including acetaminophen, NSAIDs, IV contrast, cyclosporine, amphotericin B, pentamidine, acyclovir; obstruction due to intra-abdominal malignancy or prostatic enlargement; pregnancy ●*Relieving factors:* Treatment primarily supportive; dialysis for uremic patient or patient with severe fluid and electrolyte abnormalities ●*Clinical course:* Variable depending on underlying etiology; most causes resolve over weeks-to-months with supportive therapy ●*Co-morbidities:* Thrombotic thrombocytopenic purpura-hemolytic/uremic syndrome, HIV/AIDS, multiple myeloma, systemic lupus erythematosus, cryoglobulinemia, hepatitis C, Wegener's polyarteritis nodosa, Henoch-Schönlein purpura ●*Procedure results:* Renal biopsy distinguishes cause of glomerulonephritis, vasculitis, nephrotic syndrome; abdominal radiograph (kidneys and upper bladder), renal U/S is key diagnostic imaging tool; CT, MRI, intravenous pyelogram secondary ●*Test findings:* Plasma creatinine, blood urea nitrogen, electrolytes; urinalysis including sediment examination; urine sodium excretion

Acute retinitis ●*Onset:* Acute ●*Male:female ratio:* M=F ●*Ethnicity:* All ●*Character:* Blurred distance and near vision ●*Location:* One or both eyes involved, depending on the cause ●*Pattern:* Usually progressive visual loss ●*Precipitating factors:* Patient may be immunocompromised, but not necessarily so ●*Relieving factors:* Only specific treatments directed against the cause of the retinitis relieve symptoms ●*Clinical course:* Progresses over a period of days, not self-limited ●*Co-morbidities:* AIDS or other conditions that produce an immunocompromised state ●*Procedure results:* Fundus examination; sometimes vitreous or retinal biopsy is necessary ●*Test findings:* No relevant tests

Acute sinusitis ●*Onset:* Acute ●*Male:female ratio:* M=F ●*Ethnicity:* All ●*Character:* Dull pain, pressure over affected sinuses; purulent rhinorrhea; nasal congestion ●*Location:* Periorbital or facial ●*Pattern:* May be worse with bending over ●*Precipitating factors:* Antecedent upper respiratory tract infection ●*Relieving factors:* Oral or topical decongestants; manual counter pressure; hot pack over eyes ●*Clinical course:* Usually self-limited for 7-10 days ●*Co-morbidities:* None relevant ●*Procedure results:* Plain film sinus X-rays (relatively insensitive) may reveal air fluid level; rhinoscopy may reveal pus, erythema, edema ●*Test findings:* No relevant tests

Acute tubular necrosis ●*Onset:* Acute ●*Male:female ratio:* M=F ●*Ethnicity:* All ●*Character:* Acute renal failure due to ischemia or administration of a nephrotoxin ●*Location:* Renal tubules ●*Pattern:* Oliguric vs nonoliguric ●*Precipitating factors:* Hypotension, prolonged prerenal azotemia, postoperative sepsis, rhabdomyolysis, hemolysis, drugs (IV contrast, aminoglycosides, cisplatin) ●*Relieving factors:* Treatment of underlying infection and correction of hypotension and hypercatabolic state; may require dialysis ●*Clinical course:* Generally 7-21 days; mortality rate 40-60% ●*Co-morbidities:* Patients at risk include: postsurgical, postmyocardial infarction and postseizure; cardiovascular accident, chronic immunosuppression and mechanical ventilation are also risks ●*Procedure results:* Failure to respond to IV saline distinguishes from prerenal azotemia ●*Test findings:* Normal blood urea nitrogen:plasma creatinine ratio; urinalysis positive for muddy brown granular and epithelial cell casts; elevated urine sodium; fractional excretion of sodium >2mmol/L; urine osmolality <450mOsm/kg water, due to loss of concentrating ability

Addison's disease ●*Onset:* Insidious but may be present acutely with adrenal crisis ●*Male:female ratio:* M(1):F(2) ●*Ethnicity:* All ●*Character:* Weakness, fatigue, nausea, abdominal pain, hyperpigmentation, salt craving, hypotension, may have fever ●*Location:* Pigmentation in palmar creases and buccal mucosa ●*Pattern:* Nonspecific ●*Precipitating factors:* Anticoagulation or hypotension leading to adrenal hemorrhage, HIV infection, disseminated tuberculosis ●*Relieving factors:* Cortisol and mineralocorticoid replacement ●*Clinical course:* Progressive ●*Co-morbidities:* Other autoimmune disease (type 1 diabetes, hypothyroidism, or Graves' disease, premature ovarian failure, vitamin B12 deficiency) ●*Procedure results:* None relevant ●*Test findings:* Low cortisol (check in the morning), blunted Cortrosyn stimulation test, hyperkalemia

Adenoid hypertrophy ●*Onset:* Chronic ●*Male:female ratio:* M=F ●*Ethnicity:* All ●*Character:* Nasal obstruction, nasal congestion, recurrent ear infections ●*Location:* Nasal cavity, ears ●*Pattern:* Nonspecific ●*Precipitating factors:* Symptoms much worse in the setting of an upper respiratory tract infection ●*Relieving factors:* None relevant ●*Clinical course:* Persistent symptomatology; child may outgrow ●*Co-morbidities:* Tonsillar hypertrophy, chronic otitis media with effusion ●*Procedure results:* Adenoid enlargement on nasal endoscopy ●*Test findings:* Enlarged adenoid pad on lateral neck plain film

Adhesions ●*Onset:* Acute if becomes symptomatic ●*Male:female ratio:* M=F ●*Ethnicity:* All ●*Character:* Crampy abdominal pain, vomiting, constipation, absence of flatus, abdominal distention, possibly fever ●*Location:* Pain is usually periumbilical or hypogastric ●*Pattern:* Acute onset, then paroxysms of pain ●*Precipitating factors:* Abdominal surgery (especially colectomy, appendectomy, gynecologic procedures); intra-abdominal infection, ischemia, foreign bodies such as sutures ●*Relieving factors:* Nasogastric suction, surgery ●*Clinical course:* If complete obstruction usually does not resolve spontaneously; without surgery, bowel ischemia and infarction ensue ●*Co-morbidities:* Previous surgery ●*Procedure results:* Exploratory laparotomy finding: dilated, possibly ischemic bowel ●*Test findings:* Electrolyte disorders, acidosis, leukocytosis; air-fluid levels and dilated small bowel on imaging studies

Adhesive capsulitis ●*Onset:* Insidious ●*Male:female ratio:* M=F ●*Ethnicity:* All ●*Character:* Dull ache ●*Location:* Shoulders ●*Pattern:* Worse with immobility ●*Precipitating factors:* Immobility ●*Relieving factors:* NSAIDs, intra-articular corticosteroids, physical therapy ●*Clinical course:* Chronic if not treated ●*Co-morbidities:* Diabetes, inflammatory arthritis, hypothyroidism, trauma to the shoulder ●*Procedure results:* Arthrography shows a decrease in shoulder volume ●*Test findings:* No relevant tests

Adrenal insufficiency ●*Onset:* Acute: infants; subacute: older children ●*Male:female ratio:* M<F ●*Ethnicity:* All ●*Character:* Infant: failure to thrive, vomiting, lethargy, dehydration; older children: muscle weakness, weight loss, abdominal pain ●*Location:* Increased skin pigment, muscle wasting ●*Pattern:* Worsening symptoms, increased thirst ●*Precipitating factors:* Depends on cause: congenital adrenal hypoplasia, pituitary hypoplasia, aldosterone deficient (autosomal recessive), Addison's disease, adrenoleukodystrophy (X-linked), adrenal gland hemorrhage; certain drugs: ketoconazole ●*Relieving factors:* Acute treatment: hydrocortisone, fluids, glucose; chronic treatment: cortisol ●*Clinical course:* Progressive unless treated ●*Co-morbidities:* Addison's disease with Type I autoimmune polyendocrinopathy, adrenoleukodystrophy, mitochondrial disorder, congenital adrenal hypoplasia, cryptorchidism, adrenocorticotropic hormone (ACTH) resistance associated with Allgrove's syndrome (achalasia/alacrima), Duchenne's muscular dystrophy ●*Procedure results:* No relevant procedures ●*Test findings:* Low serum sodium, high potassium, increased plasma renin, increased urinary sodium/chloride, decreased urinary potassium, acidosis, hypoglycemia, abnormal ACTH challenge, low aldosterone, abnormal cortisol precursors

Adrenocortical carcinoma/ adenoma ●*Onset:* Insidious ●*Male:female ratio:* M<F ●*Ethnicity:* All ●*Character:* Cushing's syndrome (weight gain, truncal obesity, striae, hirsutism, plethoric complexion); aldosteronism (hypertension, weakness, thirst, muscle cramps); sex hormone excess (virilization or feminization) ●*Location:* Nonspecific ●*Pattern:* Nonspecific ●*Precipitating factors:* Nonspecific ●*Relieving factors:* Surgical removal of the tumor/adrenal gland with replacement glucocorticoids; mitotane, other chemotherapeutic agents, adrenal enzyme inhibitors (e.g. ketoconazole) ●*Clinical course:* Most adenomas are cured with surgery; carcinomas have a poor prognosis even in early stage, no efficacious therapy for metastatic disease which is often present at diagnosis ●*Co-morbidities:* None relevant ●*Procedure results:* Adrenal mass biopsy showing adenoma or adenocarcinoma ●*Test findings:* Lack of suppression on dexamethasone test, elevated free urine cortisol, hypokalemia, elevated aldosterone/renin ratio, lack of aldosterone suppression with captopril, elevated urinary sex hormones, imaging study localizing adrenal mass

Adult respiratory distress syndrome ●*Onset:* Acute, 4-48 hours ●*Male:female ratio:* M=F ●*Ethnicity:* All ●*Character:* Dyspnea with or without cough ●*Location:* Chest: rapid shallow breathing ●*Pattern:* Bilateral, diffuse inspiratory rales ●*Precipitating factors:* Sepsis, aspiration, pneumonia, trauma, massive blood transfusion, drugs, others ●*Relieving factors:* Supplemental oxygen, assisted ventilation, consider diuresis ●*Clinical course:* Days-to-weeks, self-limiting ●*Co-morbidities:* Multiorgan system failure ●*Procedure results:* Pulmonary arterial occlusion pressure <18mmHg ●*Test findings:* Bilateral diffuse alveolar infiltrates on chest X-ray, hypoxemia

Agoraphobia ●*Onset:* Often in early adulthood ●*Male:female ratio:* M(1):F(3) ●*Ethnicity:* All ●*Character:* Anxiety about places/situations from which escape would be difficult ●*Location:* Nonspecific ●*Pattern:* Nonspecific ●*Precipitating factors:* Psychosocial stress may precede development of agoraphobia ●*Relieving factors:* Avoidance of feared places/situations ●*Clinical course:* Often lifelong; may be associated with significant impairment ●*Co-morbidities:* Panic attacks, depression, obsessive compulsive disorders, eating disorders ●*Procedure results:* No relevant procedures ●*Test findings:* No relevant tests

AIDS ●*Onset:* Insidious ●*Male:female ratio:* M>F ●*Ethnicity:* All ●*Character:* Progressive weight loss, wasting, constitutional symptoms, dementia, recurrent opportunistic infections, malignancies ●*Location:* Systemic (with constitutional symptoms), skin, oral mucosa, lymphoid organs, CNS (HIV encephalopathy, myelopathy, dementia complex, progressive multifocal leukoencephalopathy [PML]), peripheral nerves, dorsal nerve roots, psychiatric, GI tract (mouth to anus), liver and biliary tree (cholangiopathy), genitals, kidneys (HIV nephropathy), lungs (opportunistic infections, lymphocytic interstitial pneumonia [LIP], malignancies), joints (polyarthropathy, psoriatic arthritis), endocrine glands (adrenal, ovaries, other), any other organ ●*Pattern:* Progressive wasting, progressive dementia, persistent skin rashes, persistent constitutional symptoms, persistent generalized adenopathy, opportunistic infection ●*Precipitating factors:* Men who have sex with men, individuals who have injected drugs, had multiple sex partners, had unprotected vaginal, anal, or oral sex; received blood products before the 1980s, been exposed to blood or contaminated body fluids, born to HIV-infected mother, residence in highly endemic/epidemic areas ●*Relieving factors:* None relevant ●*Clinical course:* Chronic progressive wasting, dementia, myopathy, neuropathy, immunosuppression, leading to opportunistic infections, malignancies, death ●*Co-morbidities:* Pneumocystis carinii pneumonia, CNS toxoplasmosis, cytomegalovirus [CMV] retinitis, disseminated mycobacterium avium intracellulare [MAI], extrapulmonary cryptococcosis (especially meningitis), recurrent bacterial pneumoniae, invasive cervical cancer, tuberculosis, esophageal candidiasis, extrapulmonary coccidioidomycosis or histoplasmosis, persistent or disseminated herpes simplex virus [HSV], dementia, isosporosis, prolonged cryptosporidiosis, non-Hodgkin's lymphoma, Kaposi's sarcoma, nocardiosis, PML, recurrent salmonella bacteremia, extraintestinal strongyloidosis, bacillary angiomatosis, nephropathy, psoriatic arthropathy ●*Procedure results:* Diffuse, nonenhancing, deep white matter disease on brain MRI ●*Test findings:* Leukopenia, anemia, thrombocytopenia, low CD4+ cell count and %, high globulins, low albumin, low cholesterol

Airway irritants ●*Onset:* Episodic, acute ●*Male:female ratio:* M=F ●*Ethnicity:* All ●*Character:* Cough, dyspnea, chest tightness ●*Location:* Chest ●*Pattern:* Expiratory rhonchi and wheeze ●*Precipitating factors:* Cigarette smoke, cold air, irritant gases, fumes and chemicals ●*Relieving factors:* Inhaled corticosteroids, albuterol ●*Clinical course:* With avoidance, c.50% resolve within 6 months ●*Co-morbidities:* Asthma ●*Procedure results:* No relevant procedures ●*Test findings:* Airway hyperreactivity to methacholine or decreased FEV1

Albinism ●*Onset:* Congenital ●*Male:female ratio:* M=F ●*Ethnicity:* All ●*Character:* Skin and eye involvement ●*Location:* Generalized ●*Pattern:* Light skin/hair, nystagmus, photophobia ●*Precipitating factors:* Light precipitates visual symptoms ●*Relieving factors:* None relevant ●*Clinical course:* Chronic progressive ●*Co-morbidities:* Decreased visual acuity, skin cancer ●*Procedure results:* No relevant procedures ●*Test findings:* No relevant tests

Alcohol abuse ●*Onset:* Acute, subacute ●*Male:female ratio:* M>F ●*Ethnicity:* All ●*Character:* Intoxication: slurred speech, disinhibited behavior, CNS depression, decreased coordination; withdrawal: tremor, anxiety, agitation, seizures ●*Location:* Nonspecific ●*Pattern:* Nonspecific ●*Precipitating factors:* None relevant ●*Relieving factors:* Treatment mainly supportive; protect airway in severe intoxication; withdrawal treated with benzodiazepines or phenobarbital ●*Clinical course:* Withdrawal may progress to delerium tremens with hallucinations, severe agitation, seizures ●*Co-morbidities:* Assess patients carefully for physical trauma, hypothermia, hypoglycemia ●*Procedure results:* No relevant procedures ●*Test findings:* Check glucose, electrolytes, liver function tests

Alcoholic hepatitis ●*Onset:* Subacute ●*Male:female ratio:* M=F ●*Ethnicity:* All ●*Character:* Fever, jaundice, right upper quadrant (RUQ) pain and tenderness in a patient with a history of alcohol use; patients become encephalopathic in severe cases, and may have onset or worsening of ascites or pedal edema; bleeding common due to coagulopathy that is usually present ●*Location:* Pain is usually in RUQ of abdomen ●*Pattern:* Gradually worsens over days, with no pattern to symptoms ●*Precipitating factors:* Alcohol use ●*Relieving factors:* Abstinence from alcohol is essential, but the disorder runs its course with variable severity; in severe cases, steroids are used to decrease the hepatic inflammation, and may improve survival ●*Clinical course:* Progresses over days-to-weeks after cessation of alcohol; inhospital mortality in severe cases is >50%, but even severe cases may resolve in time ●*Co-morbidities:* Alcohol abuse, hepatic cirrhosis ●*Procedure results:* Liver biopsy is diagnostic, showing steatosis and hepatic inflammation with a predominance of PMN leukocytes; usually, however, the diagnosis is made on clinical grounds ●*Test findings:* WBC usually elevated, bilirubin often markedly elevated; aspartate transaminase (APT) and alanine transaminase (ALT) elevated to varying degrees, with AST/ALT ratio usually 2:1 or greater; prothrombin time usually high

Allergic conjunctivitis ●*Onset:* Acute ●*Male:female ratio:* M=F ●*Ethnicity:* All ●*Character:* Ocular itching ●*Location:* Both eyes ●*Pattern:* Worse in spring and fall, can be perennial ●*Precipitating factors:* Exposure to inciting antigens ●*Relieving factors:* Cool compresses, topical or oral antihistamines, artificial tears ●*Clinical course:* Self-limited ●*Co-morbidities:* Allergic rhinitis, asthma ●*Procedure results:* Conjunctival hyperemia, chemosis, lid edema, mucous discharge ●*Test findings:* No relevant tests

Allergic reactions and anaphylaxis ●*Onset:* Acute/subacute ●*Male:female ratio:* M=F ●*Ethnicity:* All ●*Character:* Rapid onset of itching, urticaria, flushing, shortness of breath and/or wheezing; may develop edema of tongue or larynx, hypotension or pulmonary edema ●*Location:* Nonspecific ●*Pattern:* Nonspecific ●*Precipitating factors:* Exposure to drugs (most common), foods, vaccines, pollens, and insect venoms ●*Relieving factors:* Supportive measures: oxygen, IV fluids; epinephrine (subcutaneous or intravenous), diphenhydramine, H2-blockers, corticosteroids ●*Clinical course:* Usually responds quickly to medical management; hospital admission required for more refractory or severe reactions ●*Co-morbidities:* None relevant ●*Procedure results:* No relevant procedures ●*Test findings:* No relevant tests

Allergic rhinitis ●*Onset:* Subacute ●*Male:female ratio:* M=F ●*Ethnicity:* All ●*Character:* Itching nose, sneezing, thin and colorless nasal discharge, nasal obstruction, facial pressure and pain ●*Location:* Nasal symptoms accompanied by itchy, watery eyes, loss of smell and taste, sleep disturbance ●*Pattern:* Seasonal or perennial, depending on trigger ●*Precipitating factors:* 5-20 micron particulate antigens causing IgE production after initial allergen exposure ●*Relieving factors:* Identification and avoidance of triggers; nasal corticosteroids, oral anithistamines, sympathomimetic agents, nasal cromolyn, allergy desensitization ●*Clinical course:* Symptoms peak in childhood and 30-40 years old; varying severity throughout life, including periods of remission ●*Co-morbidities:* Increased incidence with family or personal history of atopy, rhinitis, asthma ●*Procedure results:* Skin testing to identify allergens ●*Test findings:* Nasal cytology positive for eosinophils can distinguish allergic from nonallergic etiology

Alopecia areata ●*Onset:* Subacute/acute ●*Male:female ratio:* M=F ●*Ethnicity:* All ❶ *Character:* Hair loss ❷ *Location:* Scalp; all body hair possible ❸ *Pattern:* Circumscribed hair loss without inflammation ●*Precipitating factors:* Stress ●*Relieving factors:* Intralesional steroids ●*Clinical course:* Usually resolves in months, can recur ●*Co-morbidities:* Vitiligo, thyroid ●*Procedure results:* No relevant procedures ●*Test findings:* No relevant tests

Images of ❶ *Character,* ❷ *Location,* ❸ *Pattern on page 411*

Alpha-1-antitrypsin deficiency ●*Onset:* 15% of newborns have cholestasis; otherwise onset usually insidious ●*Male:female ratio:* M=F ●*Ethnicity:* Increased prevalence in Caucasians (northern European); rare in African-Americans, Hispanics, Asians ●*Character:*

Alopecia areata: Images *see text page 410*

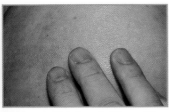

❶ *Character* Note the nail pitting and the complete alopecia of the scalp

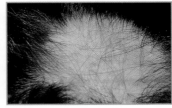

❷ *Location* Nonscarring alopecic patch. Look for exclamation point hairs at edges

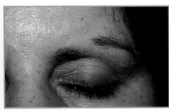

❷ *Location* Occasionally, the eyebrows may be affected

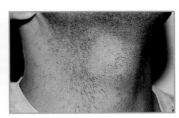

❸ *Pattern* A typical lesion on the beard

Infant: jaundice, slow weight gain, irritability, lethargy, bleeding tendency; adult: abdominal distension, hepatosplenomegaly, ascites, upper GI hemorrhage ●*Location:* Multiple organ systems involved ●*Pattern:* Often presents with abnormal liver function tests without symptoms; can progress to emphysema/lung disease and liver disease ●*Precipitating factors:* None relevant ●*Relieving factors:* Symptomatic care, prolonged breast-feeding for infants, fat-soluble vitamins, avoidance of smoking, perhaps alpha-antitrypsin replacement therapy, liver transplant for end-stage disease ●*Clinical course:* Variable; some patients progress to cirrhosis and others remain asymptomatic ●*Co-morbidities:* Lung disease ●*Procedure results:* Liver biopsy: findings change with age; infant: decreased ducts, cholestasis; adult: resolution or progression to cirrhosis ●*Test findings:* Phenotype analysis revealing alpha-antitrypsin; alpha antitrypsin level is not diagnostic

Altitude sickness ●*Onset:* Subacute ●*Male:female ratio:* M=F ●*Ethnicity:* All ●*Character:* Headache, nausea, fatigue, insomnia ●*Location:* Nonspecific ●*Pattern:* Nonspecific ●*Precipitating factors:* Ascent to altitude ●*Relieving factors:* Stop ascent, administer acetazolamide, oxygen, steroids; descend ●*Clinical course:* Ranges from self-limited to fatal ●*Co-morbidities:* Pulmonary edema, cerebral edema ●*Procedure results:* No relevant procedures ●*Test findings:* Chest X-ray may show pulmonary edema; ECG may show right heart strain

411

Alzheimer's disease ●*Onset:* Insidious ●*Male:female ratio:* M=F ●*Ethnicity:* All ●*Character:* Early loss of operational judgment followed by the failure of recent memory; patient resorts to keeping written notes to circumvent the failure of recent memory; loss of insight, inappropriate behavior, uncritical statements, irratability, grandiosity may occur ●*Location:* Nonspecific ●*Pattern:* Dominant system often reflects the premorbid personality of the patient; focal signs including dysphagia, syscalculia, dyslexia, dysgraphia, and dyspraxia can develop at any time ●*Precipitating factors:* None relevant ●*Relieving factors:* Certain anticholinergic medications slow progression but there is no cure ●*Clinical course:* Progressive; mean survival time 5-10 years after diagnosis; death usually from intercurrent infection ●*Co-morbidities:* None relevant ●*Procedure results:* MRI of brain: atrophy of medial temporal lobes; single photon emission computerized tomography (SPECT) imaging: hypoperfusion of temporal parietal regions ●*Test findings:* General physical examination and biochemical tests for infection normal; sustained deterioration in memory in alert patient; impairment in 3 of following: orientation, judgment and problem solving, function in community affairs, function in home and hobbies, function in personal care, duration of 6 months or longer

Amaurosis fugax ●*Onset:* Acute ●*Male:female ratio:* M=F ●*Ethnicity:* All ●*Character:* Monocular visual loss lasting <10 min ●*Location:* Eye ●*Pattern:* Usually painless loss of both central and peripheral vision ●*Precipitating factors:* Usually none relevant ●*Relieving factors:* Attacks generally transient and resolve spontaneously ●*Clinical course:* Symptoms develop rapidly, resolve quickly and last 2-10 min ●*Co-morbidities:* Most commonly carotid artery disease ●*Procedure results:* Atherosclerosis of the carotid vasculature, or thrombotic lesions on cardiac Echo may reveal embolic source ●*Test findings:* Often fundus examination is normal; rarely embolus seen in retinal vasculature; ECG may reveal atrial fibrillation if the atrium is the embolic source

Ambiguous genitalia ●*Onset:* Acute ●*Male:female ratio:* M=F ●*Ethnicity:* All ●*Character:* Hypospadias/unilateral cryptorchidism, abnormal urethral opening, fusion of labioscrotal folds ●*Location:* Genitalia ●*Pattern:* Nonspecific ●*Precipitating factors:* Chromosomal: hermaphroditism mosaic; gonadal dysgenesis; hereditary: testosterone enzyme synthesis defect, incomplete testicular feminization syndrome, androgenital syndrome; maternal drug ingestion: phenytoin, progesterone ●*Relieving factors:* Sex assignment, removal of intra-abdominal testes, surgery and hormone replacement as needed ●*Clinical course:* Progressive unless treated ●*Co-morbidities:* XX newborn: congenital adrenocortical hypoplasia, female pseudohermaphroditism due to drugs/maternal virilizing tumor, true pseudohermaphrodite; XY newborn: defects of testicular differentiation or testosterone synthesis, deficient placental luteinizing hormone (LH), Leydig cell agenesis, Kallmans' syndrome ●*Procedure results:* Abnormal pelvic U/S, MRI, genitogram/urethrogram ●*Test findings:* Abnormal buccal smear cytogenetics/karyotype, elevated 17-OH-progesterone, androstenedione, low cortisol, abnormal follicle-stimulating hormone (FSH), LH, testosterone, dehydroepiandrosterone (DHA), 17-OH-pregnenolone, urinary 17-ketosteroids, abnormal serum/urine sodium, potassium

Amebic dysentery ●*Onset:* Subacute ●*Male:female ratio:* M=F ●*Ethnicity:* All ●*Character:* Crampy abdominal pain, flatulence, small-volume bloody diarrhea, no fever; fulminant: profuse diarrhea, fever, more common in children, pregnant women, steroid recipients ●*Location:* Colon (colitis); complications: amebic liver abscess, ameboma, other less common ●*Pattern:* Small amount of fecal material with blood and mucus; onset more gradual than bacterial dysentery ●*Precipitating factors:* Contaminated food/water, travel to/residence in tropical and subtropical areas, institutionalized individuals, men who have sex with men; severe disease: steroid use, malnutrition, pregnancy, young age ●*Relieving factors:* Hydration, metronidazole/tinidazole followed by luminal agent (paromomycin, iodoquinol) ●*Clinical course:* Incubation 1-6 weeks or longer, symptoms in <10%, asymptomatic eliminate parasites within 12 months, symptomatic require therapy; complications: fulminant colitis, bowel perforation, liver abscess ●*Co-morbidities:* Malnutrition, amebic liver abscess ●*Procedure results:* Heme-positive stool, small mucosal ulcers on sigmoidoscopy, flask-shaped ulcers on histopathology ●*Test findings:* Trophozoites in fresh stool, heme-positive stool with no WBC, positive serology for 6-12 months

Amino acidurea ●*Onset:* Infancy/childhood ●*Male:female ratio:* M=F ●*Ethnicity:* All ●*Character:* Lethargy, vomiting, hypotonia, seizures, neurologic abnormalities: mental retardation ●*Location:* Multisystem: neurologic, ophthalmalogic, respiratory, cardiovascular, liver, kidney, spleen ●*Pattern:* Worsening symptoms without treatment, some life-threatening ●*Precipitating factors:* Abnormal metabolic pathways of amino acids due to enzyme defect; possible gene mutation ●*Relieving factors:* Depending on diagnosis: altered diet (low protein), coenzyme replacement (riboflavin, pyridoxine, carnitine), some syndromes without treatment ●*Clinical course:* Worsening symptoms without treatment, some life-threatening ●*Co-morbidities:* Depend on syndrome ●*Procedure results:* Depend on diagnosis: abnormal MRIs, enzyme activity ●*Test findings:* Metabolic acidosis, hypoglycemia with/without ketosis, elevated ammonia, abnormal liver enzymes, abnormal levels of amino acid in blood, urine and/or CSF

Amyloidosis ●*Onset:* Gradual ●*Male:female ratio:* M>F ●*Ethnicity:* All ●*Character:* Extracellular tissue deposition of fibrils of normal serum protein formed into antiparallel beta-pleated sheets; codeposition of serum amyloid P (SAP), glycoaminoglycans, E and J apolipoproteins ●*Location:* Heart: congestive heart failure; kidney: nephrotic range proteinuria, edema; nervous system: neuropathy especially carpal tunnel syndrome; liver: hepatomegaly, liver failure; GI: perforation, bleeding ●*Pattern:* Primary amyloidosis due to deposition of monoclonal light chains; secondary amyloidosis due to increased hepatic production of serum amyloid A protein, an acute phase reactant; dialysis-related amyloidosis due to beta-2 microglobulin ●*Precipitating factors:* Secondary amyloidosis due to chronic inflammatory states; dialysis-related amyloidosis linked to duration of treatment; occurs with both hemo- and peritoneal dialysis ●*Relieving factors:* Primary amyloidosis treated with alkylating agents, corticosteroids; bone marrow stem cell transplantation rarely; secondary: treatment directed at underlying disease ●*Clinical course:* Primary: poor prognosis: 15% 5-year survival, death due to cardiac, hepatic, or renal failure; secondary: poor prognosis 50-60% 4-year survival, prognosis worse with high levels of circulating SAP ●*Co-morbidities:* Primary: monoclonal gammopathy of uncertain significance (MGUS), multiple myeloma; secondary: rheumatoid arthritis, bronchiectasis, osteomyelitis, familial Mediterranean fever, anklyosing spondylitis, juvenile chronic polyarthritis ●*Procedure results:* Biopsy of abdominal fat pad, rectum, bone marrrow, kidney, or liver positive for presence of antiparallel beta pleated sheets and binding of Congo red leading to birefringence in polarized light ●*Test findings:* Scintigraphy following intravenous injection of technetium-labeled SAP; highly sensitive except in cardiac amyloid

Amyotrophic lateral sclerosis (motor neuron disease) ●*Onset:* Insidious ●*Male:female ratio:* M>F ●*Ethnicity:* All ●*Character:* Progressive weakness in a limb or palate/throat ●*Location:* If speech and swallowing is affected more, the term bulbar motor neuron disease is used; if the weakness in the limbs predominate, generalized motor neuron disease is used ●*Pattern:* Motor weakness and no sensory change ●*Precipitating factors:* None relevant ●*Relieving factors:* Supportive ●*Clinical course:* Progressive and eventually patient succumbs to respiratory distress or infections; 30 to 50% die in the first 3-5 years ●*Co-morbidities:* Systemic lymphoma ●*Procedure results:* No relevant procedures ●*Test findings:* Electomyogram showing fibrillations, fasciculations and large motor units; nerve conduction is normal and sensory nerve action potentials are normal

Anal carcinoma ●*Onset:* Insidious ●*Male:female ratio:* M=F ●*Ethnicity:* All ●*Character:* Rectal bleeding, pain, pruritis, drainage, change in bowel habits, mass ●*Location:* Anus ●*Pattern:* Nonspecific ●*Precipitating factors:* Human papilloma virus (HPV), immunosuppression (e.g. HIV or organ transplant) ●*Relieving factors:* Surgery, radiation, chemotherapy ●*Clinical course:* Complete regression in 75-100%; poor prognosis if refractory to initial therapy ●*Co-morbidities:* HIV, organ transplant recipient ●*Procedure results:* Endoscopy: anal mass; biopsy: cells typical of anal carcinoma, presence of HPV ●*Test findings:* Anemia

Anal fissure ●*Onset:* Acute ●*Male:female ratio:* M>F ●*Ethnicity:* All ●*Character:* Sharp anal pain with defecation; sometimes with gnawing perianal discomfort between bowel movements, lasting hours; occasional bright red blood per rectum ●*Location:* Anal canal ●*Pattern:* Pain worst with defecation, but may occur at other times ●*Precipitating factors:* Defecation ●*Relieving factors:* Warm water bath; bulk agents for stool; glycerin suppositories; nitropaste applied to anal canal; surgical repair if the fissure is a chronic problem ●*Clinical course:* Often self-limited, but a minority of cases become chronic and unremitting ●*Co-morbidities:* Constipation ●*Procedure results:* Anoscopy or flexible sigmoidoscopy shows fissure; chronic cases have a sentinel skin tag and hypertrophied anal papilla ●*Test findings:* No relevant tests

Analgesic nephropathy ●*Onset:* Insidious ●*Male:female ratio:* M>F ●*Ethnicity:* All ●*Character:* Prolonged use of analgesic medication, leading to renal injury ●*Location:* Renal papillary necrosis and chronic interstitial nephritis; early injury most prominent in renal medulla ●*Pattern:* Can present with hematuria and flank pain; combination analgesics especially phenacetin/acetaminophen are most toxic; toxicity is dose-dependent ●*Precipitating factors:* Phenacetin, acetaminophen, NSAIDs ●*Relieving factors:* Early diagnosis and discontinuing drug can stop progressive renal injury ●*Clinical course:* Progression to chronic renal failure and end-stage renal disease; late course may be complicated by atherosclerosis and malignancy ●*Co-morbidities:* Chronic pain syndromes, e.g. low back pain and headache; somatic complaints; peptic ulcer disease associated with prolonged NSAID use ●*Procedure results:* CT more sensitive than U/S; avoid contrast if renal insufficiency present ●*Test findings:* Urinanalysis may be normal or positive for sterile pyuria and/or proteinuria

Anemia ●*Onset:* Acute if due to rapid blood loss, subacute when loss of red cells is moderately fast, most often insidious with slow blood loss or hypoproduction ●*Male:female ratio:* M(1):F(1-7) ●*Ethnicity:* All ●*Character:* Fatigue, weakness, shortness of breath, pallor, headache ●*Location:* Nonspecific ●*Pattern:* Nonspecific ●*Precipitating factors:* Symptoms worse with exertion; precipitants are numerous and depend on type/source of anemia ●*Relieving factors:* Iron, vitamin B12, folate supplementation depending on deficiency, treatment of bleeding source, blood transfusions if anemia is severe, treatment of underlying disease if related to anemia ●*Clinical course:* Depends on cause: many self-limited (e.g. anemia due to blood loss); anemia of chronic disease tends to follow related disease; hereditary anemias are lifelong ●*Co-morbidities:* Depends on type of anemia ●*Procedure results:* Bone marrow biopsy varies with type of anemia ●*Test findings:* Low hematocrit and hemoglobin; red blood cells vary according to cause of anemia

Anemia due to acute blood loss ●*Onset:* Acute ●*Male:female ratio:* M=F ●*Ethnicity:* All ●*Character:* Upper GI bleeding: melena; lower GI bleeding: hematochezia; bleeding from any source: dizziness, fatigue ●*Location:* Nonspecific ●*Pattern:* Nonspecific ●*Precipitating factors:* Aspirin or NSAID usage (peptic ulcers); alcoholism (esophageal varices); trauma (internal bleeding) ●*Relieving factors:* Blood transfusions, iron supplementation, treatment of bleeding source ●*Clinical course:* Often requires emergent treatment and if untreated can be progressive and life-threatening ●*Co-morbidities:* Chronic liver disease ●*Procedure results:* Depends on source of blood loss; esophagogastroduodenoscopy (EGD): ulcers, varices; colonoscopy: diverticulosis; angiography: localization of bleeding source ●*Test findings:* Drop in hematocrit (though if bleeding very acute may not reflect volume loss); blood in stools (melena or hematochezia)

Anemia of chronic disease ●*Onset:* Insidious ●*Male:female ratio:* M=F ●*Ethnicity:* All ●*Character:* Fatigue, dyspnea on exertion, headache ●*Location:* Nonspecific ●*Pattern:* Nonspecific ●*Precipitating factors:* None relevant ●*Relieving factors:* Blood transfusions, erythropoietin, treatment of the underlying disease ●*Clinical course:* Indolent without treatment, follows course of underlying disease ●*Co-morbidities:* Chronic infection or inflammation, cancer, liver disease, renal insufficiency ●*Procedure results:* Bone marrow biopsy: increased iron stores, hypoproliferative ● *Test findings:* Mild-to-moderate normocytic, normochromic anemia, often reduced reticulocyte count, decreased iron, total iron binding capacity and transferrin saturation, increased ferritin and ESR

Angina ● *Onset:* Acute/subacute ● *Male:female ratio:* M>F ● *Ethnicity:* All ● *Character:* Chest discomfort described as pressure, heaviness, squeezing; sometimes nausea ● *Location:* Typically located in midsternum with radiation to jaw, left shoulder and both arms; can present atypically with no associated chest pain and only with arm pain with or without shortness of breath ● *Pattern:* In stable angina, symptoms usually improve at rest. If unstable angina, pattern may be progressive and can even occur at rest ● *Precipitating factors:* Exertion, emotion (anger/stress) ● *Relieving factors:* Stable angina usually relieved by rest or sublingual nitroglycerin; unstable angina is an emergency and requires referral to a cardiologist for complete assessment ● *Clinical course:* Clinical course very variable depending on the severity of coronary artery disease; can lead to unstable angina or myocardial infarction ● *Co-morbidities:* Diabetes mellitus, hypertension, hyperlipidemia, smoking, cocaine use, positive family history of coronary artery disease ● *Procedure results:* Positive cardiac stress test indicating ischemia ● *Test findings:* ECG changes, including ST- or T-wave changes; coronary angiography reveals epicardial coronary artery disease

Angiodysplasia ● *Onset:* Insidious; generally after fifth decade of life ● *Male:female ratio:* M=F ● *Ethnicity:* All ● *Character:* Painless rectal bleeding, ranging from bright blood to melena ● *Location:* Mostly in cecum or ascending colon; less frequently, in small bowel ● *Pattern:* Bleeding can be either chronic and intermittent or acute and massive ● *Precipitating factors:* None relevant ● *Relieving factors:* None relevant ● *Clinical course:* Most episodes stop spontaneously; some require nonoperative management; a few require endoscopic ablation or right hemicolectomy ● *Co-morbidities:* None relevant ● *Procedure results:* Radionuclide scan may show presence of localized hemorrhage; colonoscopy or angiography may show evidence of vascular ectasia ● *Test findings:* No relevant tests

Angioedema ● *Onset:* Acute ● *Male:female ratio:* M=F ● *Ethnicity:* All ● *Character:* Itching, swelling ● *Location:* Any area, particularly lips, eyelids, genitals, tongue, larynx possible ● *Pattern:* Transitory, light-colored, edematous plaques ● *Precipitating factors:* Medication, foods ● *Relieving factors:* Antihistamines ● *Clinical course:* Self-limited ● *Co-morbidities:* None relevant ● *Procedure results:* No relevant procedures ● *Test findings:* No relevant tests

Angioid streaks ● *Onset:* Acute if leakage; otherwise no symptoms ● *Male:female ratio:* M=F ● *Ethnicity:* Depends on the underlying disorder ● *Character:* Blurred vision, metamorphopsia ● *Location:* Eye ● *Pattern:* Central vision ● *Precipitating factors:* None relevant ● *Relieving factors:* None relevant ● *Clinical course:* When leaking, rapidly progressive; lesions rarely resolve spontaneously ● *Co-morbidities:* Pseudoxanthoma elasticum, Paget's disease, sickle cell anemia and other hematologic conditions, lead poisoning, Ehlers-Danlos, and others ● *Procedure results:* Typical railroad track with leakage on fluorescein angiography ● *Test findings:* Slightly irregular linear lesions centered around the disc and deep to the retina

Angular cheilitis ● *Onset:* Insidious ● *Male:female ratio:* M=F ● *Ethnicity:* All ● *Character:* Skin eruption ● *Location:* Angle of mouth ● *Pattern:* Redness, scaling and crusting ● *Precipitating factors:* Denture problems, hypersalivation ● *Relieving factors:* Steroid, nystatin, antibiotic cream ● *Clinical course:* Controlled with medication, may resolve ● *Co-morbidities:* None relevant ● *Procedure results:* No relevant procedures ● *Test findings:* No relevant tests

Anicteric hepatitis ●*Onset:* Toddler/adolescence/adulthood ●*Male:female ratio:* M=F ●*Ethnicity:* All ●*Character:* Minor flu-like illness, fatigue, nausea, fever, decreased appetite, no jaundice ●*Location:* Liver ●*Pattern:* Worsening symptoms, with resolution as illness resolves ●*Precipitating factors:* Viral illness ●*Relieving factors:* Resolution of illness ●*Clinical course:* Self-limited ●*Co-morbidities:* None relevant ●*Procedure results:* Liver inflammation on biopsy ●*Test findings:* Increased liver function tests: aspartate aminotransferase (AST), alanine transaminase (ALT)

Ankle injury ●*Onset:* Acute ●*Male:female ratio:* M=F ●*Ethnicity:* All ●*Character:* Pain, swelling in ankle after injury; inability to bear weight indicates more significant sprain/possible fracture ●*Location:* Lateral ligament sprains most common ●*Pattern:* Nonspecific ●*Precipitating factors:* Inversion or eversion type injuries most common ●*Relieving factors:* Anti-inflammatories, ice, elevation, splinting, rest ●*Clinical course:* Some fractures may require operative repair ●*Co-morbidities:* None relevant ●*Procedure results:* Radiographs rule out fractures ●*Test findings:* Check Achilles tendon for possible injury or rupture

Ankylosing spondylitis ●*Onset:* Insidious ●*Male:female ratio:* M(10):F(1) ●*Ethnicity:* Rare in African-Americans ●*Character:* Dull ache with stiffness ●*Location:* Low back symptoms often starting in sacroiliac joint, hip and shoulder joints, peripheral joints less common ●*Pattern:* Bilateral ●*Precipitating factors:* Inactivity ●*Relieving factors:* NSAIDs, sulfasalazine, exercise ●*Clinical course:* Often mild and remitting, but hip or peripheral joint involvement predicts a progressive course ●*Co-morbidities:* Secondary ankylosing spondylitis occurs in patients with Reiter's syndrome, psoriasis, inflammatory bowel disease ●*Procedure results:* Symmetric sacroiliitis on plain radiographs ●*Test findings:* HLA-B27 positive, elevated ESR

Ankylosis of hip ●*Onset:* Insidious ●*Male:female ratio:* M=F ●*Ethnicity:* All ●*Character:* Dull ache ●*Location:* Hips ●*Pattern:* Worse in the morning and improves with activity ●*Precipitating factors:* Immobility and weightbearing ●*Relieving factors:* Physical therapy, NSAIDs, sulfasalazine ●*Clinical course:* Progressive ●*Co-morbidities:* Ankylosing spondylitis, Reiter's syndrome, psoriatic arthritis, inflammatory bowel disease ●*Procedure results:* Plain radiographs show ankylosis ●*Test findings:* No relevant tests

Anorectal problems ●*Onset:* Depends on disorder; often insidious or subacute ●*Male:female ratio:* M=F ●*Ethnicity:* All ●*Character:* Rectal or anal pain/discomfort, rectal bleeding, constipation, change in bowel movements, incontinence, rectal mass ●*Location:* Nonspecific ●*Pattern:* Nonspecific ●*Precipitating factors:* Constipation, Crohn's disease, ulcerative colitis and others depending on abnormality ●*Relieving factors:* Mass lesions: surgical excision; prolapse: often surgical repair; hemorrhoids, pruritus: often treated supportively ●*Clinical course:* Depends on disorder; hemorrhoids, prolapse: tend to be chronic; early cancers: can be cured; pruritis: usually self-limited; abscess/fistula due to Crohn's: self-limited but recurs ●*Co-morbidities:* Chronic constipation, Crohn's disease, ulcerative colitis, STDs ●*Procedure results:* Endoscopy: anal abnormality; anal manometry: abnormal sphincter/motility; defecography: prolapse, rectocele, other abnormality ●*Test findings:* CBC for quantifying anemia if bleeding; anal swab for detection of human papilloma virus in cancer and dysplasia

Anorexia nervosa ●*Onset:* Mean age onset middle teens, may occur late in life ●*Male:female ratio:* M(1):F(9) ●*Ethnicity:* All ●*Character:* Subtypes include restricting (starvation) and binge-eating/purging (self-induced vomiting, misuse of laxatives); often anorectics exhibit limited insight and considerable denial about their illness; frequently poor historians ●*Location:* Nonspecific ●*Pattern:* Nonspecific ●*Precipitating factors:* Onset often associated with life stressor, such as leaving home for college ●*Relieving factors:* Psychotherapy, family therapy may be more effective for younger patients ●*Clinical course:* Highly variable; some recover after single episode, others have chronic deteriorating course ●*Co-morbidities:* Depression, obsessive-compulsive disorder, physiologic sequelae of malnutrition and starvation ●*Procedure results:* Emaciation, amenorrhea, bradycardia, findings related to starvation and/or purging behaviors (e.g. dental problems), diffusely abnormal EEG ●*Test findings:* Related to starvation, vomiting, use of laxatives: low serum estrogen, leukopenia and anemia common, electrolyte abnormalities, evidence of dehydration

Anterior cruciate ligament tear ●*Onset:* Acute ●*Male:female ratio:* M=F ●*Ethnicity:* All ●*Character:* Intermittent pain with 'giving way' of the knee ●*Location:* Knee ●*Pattern:* Pain worse with activity ●*Precipitating factors:* Sudden trauma to lower leg with a foot planted ●*Relieving factors:* Quadriceps and hamstring strengthening or anterior cruciate ligament repair ●*Clinical course:* Pain and swelling may be short-lived; can also lead to instability ●*Co-morbidities:* None relevant ●*Procedure results:* MRI shows disruption of anterior cruciate ligament ●*Test findings:* No relevant tests

Antidepressant overdose ●*Onset:* Acute/subacute ●*Male:female ratio:* M=F ●*Ethnicity:* All ●*Character:* Tricyclic antidepressants cause anticholinergic effects (dry mouth, sedation, agitation) and cardiovascular effects (hypotension, ECG changes, dysrhythmias). Selective serotonin reuptake inhibitors (SSRIs) may cause adverse effects in larger doses: tachycardia, agitation, hypertension, diaphoresis ●*Location:* Nonspecific ●*Pattern:* Nonspecific ●*Precipitating factors:* Overdosage of medications. Multiple drug interactions are recognized ●*Relieving factors:* Sodium bicarbonate and antiarrhythmics for tricyclic overdose ●*Clinical course:* Overdoses are lifethreatening ●*Co-morbidities:* Depression ●*Procedure results:* No relevant procedures ●*Test findings:* Dysrhythmias, acidosis

Anxiety ●*Onset:* Acute/subacute/chronic ●*Male:female ratio:* M(1):F(2) ●*Ethnicity:* All ●*Character:* Restlessness, difficulty concentrating, irritability, muscle tension, sleep difficulty, easily fatigued ●*Location:* May report palpitations, sweating, moist palms, shortness of breath, chest pain, 'butterflies' or GI complaints ●*Pattern:* Anxiety occurs more days than not for at least six months and patient cannot control the worry ●*Precipitating factors:* May follow stressful life event(s) but some have strong genetic component ●*Relieving factors:* Progressive relaxation/meditation, short-term benzodiazepines, buspirone, selective serotonin reuptake inhibitors ●*Clinical course:* Often responds fairly quickly to reassurance and benzodiazepenes; may become chronic, recurring, relapsing and disabling if not treated; anxiety common symptom in other conditions such as psychosis, mood disorders, organic disorders ●*Co-morbidities:* Panic disorder, social anxiety disorder, obsessive compulsive disorders, mood disorders, substance abuse; probably comorbid with some suicides ●*Procedure results:* Based on history and mental status examination; patient appears anxious, may have moist palms, dry mouth, appear shaky or trembling ●*Test findings:* Tests are generally normal; check thyroid

Aortic regurgitation ●*Onset:* Acute, insidious ●*Male:female ratio:* M=F ●*Ethnicity:* All ●*Character:* Acute: severe shortness of breath, hemodynamic collapse; chronic: asymptomatic-to-severe shortness of breath ●*Location:* Soft S2, with or without S3, early diastolic murmur, Austin-Flint murmur; if chronic also get wide pulse pressure and peripheral pulse signs, e.g. de Musset's, Corrigan's, Traube's, Muller's, Duroziez's, Quincke's, Hill's signs ●*Pattern:* Worse with exertion, when lying flat ●*Precipitating factors:* Aortic valve disease (bicuspid, myxomatous), aortic root dilatation, infection, connective tissue disease, rheumatologic disease, trauma ●*Relieving factors:* Vasodilators, diuretics ●*Clinical course:* Acute can lead to death within days; chronic: progressive ●*Co-morbidities:* Rheumatic fever, infective endocarditis, trauma, Marfan's, aortic dissection, systemic lupus erythematosus, rheumatoid arthritis, ankylosing spondylitis, Jacoud's arthropathy, Whipple's disease, Crohn's disease ●*Procedure results:* Echo, catheterization with diastolic flow from aorta to left ventricle ●*Test findings:* No relevant tests

Aortic sclerosis ●*Onset:* Insidious ●*Male:female ratio:* M=F ●*Ethnicity:* All ●*Character:* Asymptomatic ●*Location:* Nonspecific ●*Pattern:* Nonspecific ●*Precipitating factors:* Age ●*Relieving factors:* None relevant ●*Clinical course:* May rarely progress to give aortic stenosis ●*Co-morbidities:* Fibrocalcific conduction system disease ●*Procedure results:* Echo with fibrocalcific thickening at bases of previously normal trileaflet aortic valve cusps at the level of insertion into the sinuses of Valsalva, without stenosis ●*Test findings:* Examination with crescendo-decrescendo systolic murmur heard best in the right second intercostal space

Aortic stenosis ●*Onset:* Insidious ●*Male:female ratio:* M=F ●*Ethnicity:* All ●*Character:* Chest pain, lightheadedness, shortness of breath. Normal: soft S1, single or paradoxically split S2, with or without S4 ●*Location:* Anterior chest, left arm, jaw, neck pain. Crescendo-decrescendo systolic murmur heard loudest at the base, radiating to the neck. Carotid pulsus parvus et tardus ●*Pattern:* All symptoms worse with exertion. Shortness of breath worse with lying down ●*Precipitating factors:* Congenital aortic valve disease (uni-, bi- tricuspid), rheumatic fever, degeneration, calcification. Symptoms worse with nitrates, beta-blockers, diuretics in critical aortic stenosis (AS) ●*Relieving factors:* Balloon valvuloplasty for infants and adolescents with congenital AS. Surgery if critical AS ●*Clinical course:* Progressive. Average survival: 5 years after angina, 3 years after syncope, 2 years after congestive heart failure ●*Co-morbidities:* Aortic insufficiency, mitral valve disease, rheumatoid arthritis, Paget's disease, atrioventricular malformations ●*Procedure results:* Echo with decreased aortic leaflet mobility and increased transaortic gradient in systole ●*Test findings:* ECG: left ventricular hypertrophy

Aphthous ulcers ●*Onset:* Insidious to subacute ●*Male:female ratio:* M=F ●*Ethnicity:* All ●*Character:* Pain with contact, pain with citrus beverages ●*Location:* Localized pain at the site of the ulcer ●*Pattern:* Varies widely, ranging from solitary ulcers to multiple ulcers of different sizes ●*Precipitating factors:* Burn injury, recent dental work, recent viral illness ●*Relieving factors:* Ice cubes, over-the-counter anesthetic preparations ●*Clinical course:* Variable: ulcers may cycle in the 5-7 day range ●*Co-morbidities:* Behçet's disease, autoimmune disease, Crohn's disease ●*Procedure results:* Biopsy reveals fibrin, lymphocytic cellular infiltrate ●*Test findings:* No relevant tests

Aplastic anemia ●*Onset:* Usually insidious ●*Male:female ratio:* M=F ●*Ethnicity:* All ●*Character:* Fatigue, weakness, bleeding. Less common: fever and signs of infection ●*Location:* Bleeding is from skin, nose, gums, vagina or GI tract ●*Pattern:* Nonspecific ●*Precipitating factors:* Usually none. Other causes: drugs, radiation, chemicals, viruses, paroxysmal nocturnal hemoglobinuria, pregnancy, hereditary syndromes ●*Relieving factors:* Withdrawal of etiologic agent if possible. Bone marrow transplantation is curative. Immunosuppressive agents. Hematopoietic growth factors ●*Clinical course:* Progressive and lifethreatening without treatment (50% 1-year mortality), bone marrow transplant cures 60-90% of patients ●*Co-morbidities:* None relevant ●*Procedure results:* Bone marrow aspirate: empty fatty spaces and few cells. Bone marrow biopsy: hypocellular, positive cytogenetic studies ●*Test findings:* Pancytopenia, normochromic/normocytic anemia, decreased reticulocyte count, normal-sized platelets, normal white cell differential

Arnold-Chiari malformation ●*Onset:* Chiari I = adolescence, Chiari II = at birth ●*Male:female ratio:* M=F ●*Ethnicity:* All ●*Character:* Chiari I: cerebromedullary malformation without meningocele/dysraphism, presenting with headaches, progressive ataxia and spastic quadriplegia or syringomyelia (segmental amyotrophy and sensory loss); Chiari II, with meningomyelocele, presenting with progressive hydrocephalus resulting in lower cranial nerve involvement with laryngeal stridor, deafness ●*Location:* Variety of presentations with lower cranial nerve involvement, ataxia and occipital headaches; location of all lesions in cerebellum and medulla with some changes in the pons as well ●*Pattern:* Disease is progressive: Chiari I with headaches becoming worse, progressive ataxia and spastic quadriparesis; Chiari II with lower cranial nerve changes first, then ataxia as child gets older ●*Precipitating factors:* Chiari type I malformation: cerebellar tonsils protrude through the foramen magnum and into the cervical spinal canal; when this abnormality is associated with protrusion of meninges (meningocele) or meninges and cord (meningomyelocele) through a spinal canal that has incompletely closed, it is designated a Chiari type II (or Arnold-Chiari) malformation; any space-occupying lesion in the cerebellum or brainstem area can exacerbate the condition ●*Relieving factors:* Treatment is generally unsatisfactory; surgery can cause death: aim is to decompress the hydrocephalus ●*Clinical course:* Progressive worsening especially if hydrocephalus worsens ●*Co-morbidities:* Basilar compression, developmental abnormalities of cerebellum (polymicrogyria), lower end of spinal cord (filum terminale) may extend longer, as low as sacrum; posterior fossa is smaller, foramen magnum is enlarged, basilar impression (base of the skull is flattened or infolded) ●*Procedure results:* Decompression of hydrocephalus may help halt disease progression ●*Test findings:* MRI and myelography show obstruction of CSF flow; CSF may show elevated protein and increased pressure

Arterial embolus and thrombosis ●*Onset:* Acute ●*Male:female ratio:* M=F ●*Ethnicity:* All ●*Character:* Ischemic symptoms in affected organ (typically lower extremity); pain, paresthesia, numbness, coolness, cyanosis/pallor, weakness/possible paralysis ●*Location:* Symptoms are in the affected limb or organ, distal to the location of arterial occlusion ●*Pattern:* Sudden onset with rapid progression over minutes-to-hours ●*Precipitating factors:* Usually consequence of underlying cardiac/vascular abnormality, but can be precipitated by local trauma to artery ●*Relieving factors:* Relieved only by restoration of blood supply through occluded artery; either spontaneous (unusual), or with anticoagulation (heparin) and prompt surgical intervention (thrombectomy or arterial bypass) ●*Clinical course:* Depends on presence of collateral blood supply and degree of arterial occlusion; with complete arterial occlusion, rapidly progressive until surgical intervention; if blood supply not restored rapidly, irreversible ischemia with gangrene/loss of organ or limb ●*Co-morbidities:* Emboli can originate in atrial fibrillation/flutter, acute myocardial infarction, cardiomyopathy, ventricular aneurysm, endocarditis, atrial myxoma, atherosclerosis of great vessels, aortic aneurysm, rarely from venous system via patent foramen ovale or atrial septal defect; insitu thrombosis in hypercoagulable states (e.g. antiphospholipid antibody syndrome) ●*Procedure results:* Arteriography reveals location and extent of arterial occlusion; Doppler evaluation of artery beyond occlusion: diminished/absent waveform; CT/MRI: may show intraluminal thrombus/embolus in affected artery ●*Test findings:* Diagnosis should be made clinically from history and physical examination to expedite treatment

Arterial insufficiency ●*Onset:* Acute/chronic ●*Male:female ratio:* M=F ●*Ethnicity:* All ●*Character:* Acute: pain, paresthesias, numbness, coldness, cyanosis, pallor in involved extremity; chronic: pain or numbness with exercise that resolves with rest (claudication), diminished pulses, bruits ●*Location:* Most common in lower extremities ●*Pattern:* Nonspecific ●*Precipitating factors:* Symptoms worse with exertion; may occur at rest with severe insufficiency ●*Relieving factors:* Rest may relieve symptoms; platelet inhibitors, revascularization (angioplasty or surgery) ●*Clinical course:* Symptoms stabilize in most non-diabetic patients; may worsen and lead to amputation ●*Co-morbidities:* Atherosclerosis, diabetes, hypercholesterolemia, smoking, hypertension, coronary artery and cerebral vascular disease ●*Procedure results:* Low flow in Doppler studies, arterial blockage in angiography ●*Test findings:* None relevant

Arterial-intestinal fistula ●*Onset:* Subacute to acute; often a small, herald gastrointestinal bleed prior to a massive one ●*Male:female ratio:* M=F ●*Ethnicity:* All ●*Character:* Intermittent melena followed by massive bleeding; fever, abdominal pain are less common ●*Location:* Nonspecific ●*Pattern:* Recurrent, minor bleeding followed by massive bleeding; interval can be hours-to-months ●*Precipitating factors:* Abdominal aortic aneurysm or abdominal vascular graft replacement (usually years or more in the past) ●*Relieving factors:* Surgical correction, supportive care: blood products, intravenous fluids ●*Clinical course:* If diagnosed and treated promptly, prognosis is good, though bleeding is often life-threatening ●*Co-morbidities:* Vascular disease, salmonella infection ●*Procedure results:* Upper endoscopy: may locate source of bleeding in third portion of duodenum; arteriography: extravasation of blood; radionuclide scanning: bleeding source in small bowel; CT: aortic aneurysm ●*Test findings:* Anemia

Arteriosclerosis ●*Onset:* Insidious ●*Male:female ratio:* M>F ●*Ethnicity:* More common in Western countries ●*Character:* Gradual progression of ischemic symptoms in organs fed by atherosclerotic arteries (heart, legs, brain, viscera) ●*Location:* Symptoms depend on affected target organ: angina with heart, claudication with legs, transient ischemic attacks/stroke with brain, abdominal pain with viscera ●*Pattern:* Worse symptoms when oxygen demand in target organ is increased: angina with exertion, leg claudication with walking, visceral pain after eating ●*Precipitating factors:* Activities/situations that require more oxygen supply in target organ precipitate symptoms: angina with exertion, leg claudication with walking, visceral pain after eating ●*Relieving factors:* Cessation of provoking activity, decreasing oxygen demand; medications to decrease oxygen demand in target organ (mainly with heart: nitrates, beta-blockers relieving angina) ●*Clinical course:* Gradually progressive over a lifetime; course slowed with smoking cessation, blood pressure control, LDL cholesterol lowering, diabetes control ●*Co-morbidities:* Tobacco use, hypertension, diabetes, hypercholesterolemia (LDL) ●*Procedure results:* Arteriography of affected vessel reveals narrowed, irregular lumen, sometimes with occlusion and development of collaterals ●*Test findings:* Depending on artery affected, may use U/S or Doppler to see increased blood velocity/turbulence (e.g. in carotid arteries)

Arteriovenous fistula ●*Onset:* Congenital or acute ●*Male:female ratio:* M=F ●*Ethnicity:* All ●*Character:* Frequently asymptomatic; may have ischemic symptoms, edema, tortuous varicose veins associated with chronic arteriovenous (AV) fistula; if high flow across fistula, may see high-output heart failure over time ●*Location:* If symptoms are present, seen locally in affected extremity ●*Pattern:* If fistula large enough to cause symptoms, gradual progression of symptoms over months-to-years ●*Precipitating factors:* May be purposefully created for dialysis access; otherwise, most frequently seen with vascular trauma, including complication after arterial catheterization/surgical dissection ●*Relieving factors:* Decreasing/eliminating AV communication; acquired fistulas typically repaired surgically; congenital AV fistulas harder to treat (combination of ligation, embolization, elastic support hose on affected limb) ●*Clinical course:* Typically does not spontaneously resolve, and may cause stable or gradually progressive symptoms over time ●*Co-morbidities:* Mainly seen in renal failure patients on dialysis (purposeful creation of AV fistula), and after percutaneous/surgical procedures involving invasion of an artery ●*Procedure results:* Arteriography shows communication between artery and vein; Doppler study reveals communication between artery and vein, with arterialized waveform in vein ●*Test findings:* Physical examination reveals bruit heard through both systole and diastole sometimes with a palpable thrill and possibly a pulsatile mass

Arteriovenous malformation ●*Onset:* Often bleeding is acute but can be insidious if small in volume ●*Male:female ratio:* M=F ●*Ethnicity:* All ●*Character:* Most commonly rectal bleeding or hematochezia; hematemesis, melena also common; fatigue, weakness secondary to anemia ●*Location:* Commonly in the colon and small intestine ●*Pattern:* Nonspecific ●*Precipitating factors:* Antiplatelet agents precipitate bleeding; hereditary syndromes ●*Relieving factors:* Endoscopy with electrocautery, supportive care with iron or blood products, estrogen therapy ●*Clinical course:* Often recurrent; if localized and treated, prognosis excellent; bleeding can be life-threatening ●*Co-morbidities:* Endstage renal disease, aortic stenosis ●*Procedure results:* Arteriography: extravasation; endoscopy: bleeding tuft of vessels; radionuclide scanning: positive for bleeding source ●*Test findings:* Anemia

Arteriovenous malformation of the colon ●*Onset:* Acute ●*Male:female ratio:* M=F ●*Ethnicity:* All ●*Character:* Painless rectal bleeding - usually bright red or maroon stools ●*Location:* Colon ●*Pattern:* Episodes of bleeding are acute, and occur sporadically, without pattern ●*Precipitating factors:* None relevant ●*Relieving factors:* Colonoscopy with cautery of the vascular lesions; estrogen therapy may decrease incidence of bleeding from arteriovenous malformations ●*Clinical course:* Intermittent lower GI bleeding; may be frequent or rare ●*Co-morbidities:* Osler-Weber-Rendu syndrome ●*Procedure results:* Colonoscopy reveals vascular lesions ●*Test findings:* Anemia is often present after hemorrhage

Asbestosis ●*Onset:* Insidious ●*Male:female ratio:* M>F ●*Ethnicity:* All ●*Character:* Dyspnea on exertion ●*Location:* Chest: inspiratory crackles; extremities: clubbing ●*Pattern:* Bibasilar inspiratory crackles ●*Precipitating factors:* Exposure to asbestos fibers ●*Relieving factors:* No specific treatment, supplemental oxygen ●*Clinical course:* 20-30 year latency period between exposure and symptoms ●*Co-morbidities:* Asbestos-related pleural disease, lung cancer ●*Procedure results:* No relevant procedures ●*Test findings:* Pulmonary function tests: restrictive lung disease; chest X-ray: bilateral lower lobe interstitial infiltrates

Aseptic bursitis ●*Onset:* Acute or subacute ●*Male:female ratio:* M>F ●*Ethnicity:* All ●*Character:* Constant pain with exacerbations brought on by pressure or overuse ●*Location:* Single extra-articular area including greater trochanter, pes anserine, subdeltoid, and subacromial, olecranon, or prepatellar ●*Pattern:* Worse with pressure over bursa; therefore often worse while lying down ●*Precipitating factors:* Overuse phenomenon or imbalance of normal kinematics ●*Relieving factors:* NSAIDs, cortisone injection, ice ●*Clinical course:* Acute or subacute attacks that are usually self-limited ●*Co-morbidities:* Gout, rheumatoid arthritis, osteoarthritis ●*Procedure results:* Aspiration of bursa reveals WBC <1000 with negative Gram stain and culture ●*Test findings:* MRI shows inflammation in characteristic regions

Aseptic necrosis of the humeral head ●*Onset:* Subacute ●*Male:female ratio:* M=F ●*Ethnicity:* African-American ●*Character:* Dull ache ●*Location:* Shoulder ●*Pattern:* Worse with shoulder rotation ●*Precipitating factors:* Lifting using the affected shoulder ●*Relieving factors:* Core decompression or total shoulder arthroplasty ●*Clinical course:* Frequently self-limited ●*Co-morbidities:* Steroid use, alcohol abuse, systemic lupus erythematosus, sickle cell disease ●*Procedure results:* MRI shows bone infarcts ●*Test findings:* Synovial fluid analysis with WBC <500

Aspergillosis ●*Onset:* Acute/subacute/chronic ●*Male:female ratio:* M=F ●*Ethnicity:* All ●*Character:* Airway colonization, aspergilloma: asymptomatic, chronic productive cough, hemoptysis; allergic bronchopulmonary aspergillosis (ABPA): asthma; invasive aspergillosis: rapidly progressive fever, cough, dyspnea; aspergillus sinusitis: chronic nasal obstruction, proptosis (less common) ●*Location:* Upper/lower airway, lung, sinuses most common; dissemination to CNS, skin, bone, heart, other, in immunocompromised hosts; eye (endophthalmitis) after penetrating trauma ●*Pattern:* Invasive disease rapidly progressive; others chronic-to-stable or progressive ●*Precipitating factors:* Invasive: neutropenia (<500), neutrophil dysfunction, lymphoproliferative disorders (leukemia), transplantation, AIDS, prolonged steroid/cytotoxic drug therapy, chronic granulomatous diseases, massive exposure in normal host (rare); noninvasive: chronic lung disease, old cavity, asthma, allergic rhinitis ●*Relieving factors:* Invasive: IV amphotericin-B/lipid-amphotericin; noninvasive: no therapy, oral itraconazole, IV amphotericin ●*Clinical course:* Invasive/immunocompromised: rapidly fatal without therapy; noninvasive: chronic stable or progressive, hemoptysis may be fatal ●*Co-morbidities:* Chronic pulmonary disease, lung cavities, asthma, allergic rhinitis, chronic immunosuppression, prolonged neutropenia, steroid therapy, chronic granulomatous diseases ●*Procedure results:* Colonization or infection: branching hyphae on smear, isolation from clinical specimen (usually sputum); biopsy to confirm invasive disease; aspergilloma: fungal ball on chest X-ray ●*Test findings:* Invasive disease: histopathology shows invasion of blood vessels, thrombosis, infarction; blood, CSF cultures are rarely positive; eosinophilia, high IgE, anti-Aspergillus IgE, IgG in ABPA

Aspiration pneumonia ●*Onset:* Acute ●*Male:female ratio:* M=F ●*Ethnicity:* All ●*Character:* Cough with purulent and often fetid sputum, fever and chills, dyspnea, chest discomfort, nausea and vomiting (less common) ●*Location:* Chest ●*Pattern:* Bronchial breath sounds, inspiratory rales, egophony ●*Precipitating factors:* Poor dentition with gingivitis; loss of consciousness; abnormal swallowing, esophageal dysmotility, laryngeal or vocal cord dysfunction; pregnancy, labor, delivery ●*Relieving factors:* Antibiotics ●*Clinical course:* Illness lasts days-to-weeks, longer if a lung abscess is present ●*Co-morbidities:* Seizures, stroke with residual dysphagia, esophageal motility disorders, substance abuse, alcoholism, pregnancy, gingivitis ●*Procedure results:* No relevant procedures ●*Test findings:* Leukocytosis, focal infiltrate on chest X-ray, sputum with neutrophils yet no definitive organism

Asplenia syndromes ●*Onset:* Can be acute if surgically-removed spleen; is insidious if due to sickle cell disease ●*Male:female ratio:* M=F ●*Ethnicity:* All ●*Character:* Nonspecific ●*Location:* Nonspecific ●*Pattern:* Nonspecific ●*Precipitating factors:* Bacterial infections, particularly encapsulated (Streptococcus pneumoniae, Hemophilus influenzae) ●*Relieving factors:* Antibiotics ●*Clinical course:* Lifetime risk of infection is 25% ●*Co-morbidities:* Sickle cell disease, Hodgkin's disease, and certain leukemias for which splenectomy is therapeutic ●*Procedure results:* No relevant procedures ●*Test findings:* Post-spleen removal, mild leukocytosis and thrombocytosis

Asthma ●*Onset:* Acute ●*Male:female ratio:* M=F ●*Ethnicity:* All ●*Character:* Intermittent cough, dyspnea, wheezing ●*Location:* Chest ●*Pattern:* Prolonged expiratory phase of respiration, evidence of hyperinflation by chest percussion, expiratory wheezing or rhonchi; if lung function <25% of normal, pulsus paradoxus, use of accessory respiratory muscles, diaphoresis and difficulty lying supine may be present ●*Precipitating factors:* Exposure to specific antigens (e.g. environmental allergens, occupational sensitizing agents), respiratory viral infections, nonspecific stimuli (e.g. strong odors, cigarette smoke, cold air, exercise) ●*Relieving factors:* Bronchodilators (e.g. albuterol, metaproterenol, salmeterol), glucocorticoids (e.g. beclomethasone, triamcinolone, budesonide, fluticasone), antileukotrienes (e.g. zileuton, zafirlukast, montelulkast), allergen avoidance ●*Clinical course:* Episodic, but symptoms and airflow obstruction may be persistent with increased disease severity or chronicity; exacerbations usually last 1 day-5 weeks ●*Co-morbidities:* Eczema, allergic rhinosinusitus, gastroesophageal reflux disease ●*Procedure results:* Pulmonary function test: airfllow obstruction; positive metacholine, cold air, exercise challenge test ●*Test findings:* FEV1/FVC <95% predicted plus FEV1 <100% predicted

Asymptomatic carotid stenosis ●*Onset:* Insidious ●*Male:female ratio:* M>F ●*Ethnicity:* All ethnicities but more in Caucasians ●*Character:* Asymptomatic ●*Location:* Carotid area ●*Pattern:* Bruit heard on auscultation ●*Precipitating factors:* Hypertension, elevated cholesterol, homocysteinemia, diabetes, peripheral atherosclerosis ●*Relieving factors:* Surgical carotid endarectomy if the stenosis is greater than 60% ●*Clinical course:* Progressive to stroke or carotid occlusion ●*Co-morbidities:* None relevant ●*Procedure results:* No relevant procedures ●*Test findings:* Stenosis on carotid ultrasound, MR angiogram, or CT angiogram of the neck

Ataxia-telangiectasia ●*Onset:* Subacute ●*Male:female ratio:* M=F ●*Ethnicity:* All ●*Character:* Telangiectasia and progressive cerebellar ataxia (clumsiness) ●*Location:* Ataxia in all four extremities and telangiectasia first appear in the conjunctiva and later on the cheeks and across the bridge of the nose; eyelids and pinnae may be involved ●*Pattern:* Facial appearance described as 'sad' ●*Precipitating factors:* Autosomal recessive ●*Relieving factors:* Supportive ●*Clinical course:* Chronic progressive and non-limiting ●*Co-morbidities:* Repeated attacks of sinusitis, chronic bronchiitis, bronchiectasis, pneumonia due to altered immune resistance ●*Procedure results:* No relevant procedures ●*Test findings:* Depression of IgA and IgE; serum alpha fetoprotein levels are elevated; skull X-rays show chronic sinusitis; MRI of the brain shows presence of cerebellar atrophy in older children

Atelectasis ●*Onset:* Acute, subacute, postoperative ●*Male:female ratio:* M=F ●*Ethnicity:* All ●*Character:* Dyspnea, hypoxemia ●*Location:* Dependent portions of the lungs or distal to airway obstruction ●*Pattern:* Postoperative hypoxemia ●*Precipitating factors:* Low lung volumes or airway obstruction (e.g. foreign body aspiration) ●*Relieving factors:* Deep respirations, cough, chest physical therapy; if severe, consider bronchoscopy to exclude airway lesion and eliminate retained secretions ●*Clinical course:* Resolves over days unless fixed airway obstruction or associated with pleural fibrosis ('round' atelectasis) ●*Co-morbidities:* Respiratory muscle weakness, structural lung disease ●*Procedure results:* No relevant procedures ●*Test findings:* Atelectasis evident by chest X-ray, CT scan

Athetosis ●*Onset:* Depends on cause: acute/subacute/chronic/progressive ●*Male:female ratio:* M=F ●*Ethnicity:* All ●*Character:* Slow, continuous, involuntary writhing movements ●*Location:* Most commonly, distal arms and hands; also head, neck, trunk ●*Pattern:* Nonspecific ●*Precipitating factors:* Exercise, stress ●*Relieving factors:* None relevant ●*Clinical course:* Depends on underlying cause ●*Co-morbidities:* Cerebral palsy, encephalitis, medications, hepatic encephalopathy, Huntington's disease ●*Procedure results:* No relevant procedures ●*Test findings:* No relevant tests

Atlantoaxial subluxation ●*Onset:* Insidious if related to rheumatoid arthritis; acute if traumatic ●*Male:female ratio:* M=F ●*Ethnicity:* All ●*Character:* Pain and paresthesias ●*Location:* Neck, occiput, arms ●*Pattern:* Nonspecific ●*Precipitating factors:* Trauma if not related to rheumatoid arthritis ●*Relieving factors:* Halo traction ●*Clinical course:* Progressive ●*Co-morbidities:* Rheumatoid arthritis ●*Procedure results:* Plain radiographs show abnormal alignment of C1 and C2 ●*Test findings:* No relevant tests

Atopic dermatitis ●*Onset:* Chronic ●*Male:female ratio:* M=F ●*Ethnicity:* All ❶ *Character:* Inflammatory skin disorder characterized by thickened skin, lichenification, excoriated fibrotic papules ❷ *Location:* Adults: flexural surfaces (antecubital and popliteal fossae) neck, face, wrists, and forearms; head, face, and neck in children ❸ *Pattern:* Dry skin and itching papulovesicular eruptions ●*Precipitating factors:* Chronic scratching contributes to activity and chronicity ●*Relieving factors:* Controlled with topical steroids ●*Clinical course:* Chronic nonprogressive ●*Co-morbidities:* Allergic rhinitis, asthma ●*Procedure results:* Positive skin tests for IgE antibodies against many environmental and food allergens ●*Test findings:* Increased serum IgE and eosinophilia

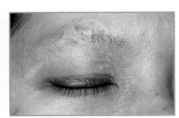

❶ *Character Red, scaly plaques often occur in atopic dermatitis*

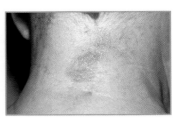

❷ *Location Typically affected are the flexures of the neck, arms and legs*

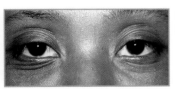

❸ *Pattern Multiple erosions are scattered around the eyes*

Atrial fibrillation ●*Onset:* Acute ●*Male:female ratio:* M>F ●*Ethnicity:* All ●*Character:* Palpitations, chest pain, shortness of breath, lightheadedness ●*Location:* Anterior chest, jaw, neck, left arm ●*Pattern:* Worse with rapid ventricular rates ●*Precipitating factors:* Age, valvular heart disease, hypertension, cardiomyopathy, coronary artery disease, left atrial enlargement, thyrotoxicosis, pulmonary embolus, pericarditis, atrial septal defect, alcohol ●*Relieving factors:* Ventricular rate control with beta-blockers, calcium channel blockers, digoxin, amiodarone, sotalol; direct-current cardioversion if unstable or direct-current/chemical cardioversion ●*Clinical course:* Intermittent or chronic; stroke if unanticoagulated ●*Co-morbidities:* Valvular heart disease, hypertension, cardiomyopathy, pericarditis, pulmonary embolus, thyrotoxicosis, stroke ●*Procedure results:* Echo with evidence of structural heart disease (except in lone atrial fibrillation), left atrial enlargement ●*Test findings:* ECG with no detectable P waves and irregularly, irregular rhythm

Atrial flutter ●*Onset:* Acute ●*Male:female ratio:* M=F ●*Ethnicity:* All ●*Character:* Palpitations, chest pain, shortness of breath, lightheadedness ●*Location:* Anterior chest, jaw, neck, left arm pain ●*Pattern:* Worse with rapid ventricular rates ●*Precipitating factors:* Age, valvular heart disease, hypertension, cardiomyopathy, coronary artery disease, left atrial enlargement, thyrotoxicosis, pulmonary embolus, pericarditis, atrial septal defect, alcohol ●*Relieving factors:* Ventricular rate control with beta-blockers, calcium channel blockers, digoxin, amiodarone, sotalol; direct current-cardioversion if unstable or direct current/chemical cardioversion ●*Clinical course:* Intermittent or chronic; stroke if unanticoagulated ●*Co-morbidities:* Valvular heart disease, hypertension, cardiomyopathy, pericarditis, pulmonary embolus, thyrotoxicosis, stroke ●*Procedure results:* Echo with evidence of structural heart disease, left atrial enlargement ●*Test findings:* EKG with 'sawtooth' flutter waves, atrial rate of 300 and ventricular rate usually an integer ratio of atrial rate; ventricular rate can be irregular with concomitant Mobitz type I AV block

Atrial myxoma ●*Onset:* Insidious ●*Male:female ratio:* M=F ●*Ethnicity:* All ●*Character:* A number of conditions may be confused with atrial myxoma (e.g. rheumatic heart disease, mitral stenosis, pulmonary hypertension) ●*Location:* Nonspecific for symptoms; most myxomas occur in the left atrium ●*Pattern:* Patients may have chest pain, shortness of breath, constitutional symptoms such as fever, weight loss ●*Precipitating factors:* There are sporadic myxomas and syndrome myxomas; 27% of the syndrome myxomas can be familial ●*Relieving factors:* Surgical excision is the treatment of choice ●*Clinical course:* Clinical course and the development of symptoms depend on whether the myxoma is in the right or left atria; after excision of the myxoma about 1-5% of cases recur ●*Co-morbidities:* Embolization can occur; also, sudden death, dizziness, and hemoptysis have been reported ●*Procedure results:* Examination may reveal murmur (systolic/diastolic), third heart sound, pulmonary hypertension, right heart failure, anemia, elevated ESR, clubbing, atrial fibrillation, Raynaud's phenomenon ●*Test findings:* Atrial mass on cardiac Echo (transthoracic with or without transesophageal); CT or MRI may be helpful in some cases; pathology should be reviewed to rule out other malignancies

Atrial septal defect ●*Onset:* Congenital ●*Male:female ratio:* M(1):F(2) ●*Ethnicity:* All ●*Character:* Usually asymptomatic in early life; gradual development of fatigue, shortness of breath, palpitations, chest pain, lightheadedness ●*Location:* Congenital cardiac anomaly; markedly wide and fixed split S2, accentuated P2, pulmonic, tricuspid, tricuspid insufficiency murmurs, prominent right ventricular cardiac impulse ●*Pattern:* Worse with exertion; shortness of breath worse with lying down ●*Precipitating factors:* Genetic defects, e.g. Holt-Oram syndrome, Noonan syndrome; teratogens, e.g. ethanol, hydantoin; infections, e.g. rubella; trauma/iatrogenic ●*Relieving factors:* IV filters to prevent paradoxical embolus; anticoagulation if history of transient ischemic attacks, stroke, or atrial fibrillation; operative or percutaneous closure ●*Clinical course:* Depending on size on atrial septal defect (ASD): progressive worsening of symptoms leading to pulmonary hypertension/Eisenmenger's syndrome if untreated ●*Co-morbidities:* Cleft in anterior mitral valve leaflet with ostium primum ASDs, mitral valve prolapse with secundum ASDs, partial anomolous pulmonary venous return with sinus venosus ASDs, atrial fibrillation, congestive heart failure, pulmonary hypertension/Eisenmenger's syndrome ●*Procedure results:* Echo shows interatrial septal defect, quantitation of shunt fraction using Echo or nuclear imaging ●*Test findings:* ECG with prolonged PR interval, a rSR' pattern in the right-sided chest leads, right atrial enlargement, left axis deviation, counterclockwise rotation of the QRS loop in the frontal plane in ostium primum ASDs; ECG with right axis deviation, right ventricular hypertrophy, rSR' pattern in right precordial leads in secundum ASDs; left axis deviation of the P wave in the frontal plane suggests a sinus venosus ASD rather than a secundum ASD

Attention deficit hyperactivity disorder ●*Onset:* Subacute ●*Male:female ratio:* M=F ●*Ethnicity:* All ●*Character:* Inattentiveness, hyperactivity ●*Location:* Nonspecific ●*Pattern:* Child cannot sit still in class, talks when teacher is talking, fidgets ●*Precipitating factors:* Structured setting usually school ●*Relieving factors:* One-on-one attention, medication ●*Clinical course:* Usually controlled with behavior modification by adolescence ●*Co-morbidities:* Tic disorders ●*Procedure results:* No relevant procedures ●*Test findings:* High scores on behavioral rating scales, e.g. Connor's

Atypical mycobacterial infection ●*Onset:* Insidious in non-AIDS, acute/subacute in AIDS ●*Male:female ratio:* M=F ●*Ethnicity:* All ●*Character:* Progressive cough, often productive, less often hemoptysis, fever, and weight loss (M. avium intracellulare, others); cavitary lung disease (M. avium intracellulare, M. kansasii); lymphadenitis (M. scrofulaceum); draining skin nodules (M. marinum). AIDS (M. avium intracellulare, fever, night sweats, weight loss, anorexia, diarrhea, widespread organ involvement ●*Location:* Lung (interstitial, nodular, cavitary), skin and soft tissue (bone and joint less common), regional lymph nodes, other; AIDS: bacteremia, bone marrow involvement, gastroenteritis, liver, spleen, lymph nodes, any organ ●*Pattern:* In AIDS patients, fever may be very high ●*Precipitating factors:* Advanced AIDS, steroid and cytotoxic therapy, transplantation, chronic pulmonary disease, cystic fibrosis, elderly, water exposure for M. marinum ●*Relieving factors:* Organ-specific multidrug therapy, debridement of severe soft tissue infections ●*Clinical course:* Progressive illnesses; prolonged multidrug therapy is required; disseminated M. avium intracellulare, in AIDS is associated with decreased survival ●*Co-morbidities:* Chronic pulmonary conditions, immunosuppression, AIDS ●*Procedure results:* Acid-fast bacilli in sputum, bronchoalveolar lavage, lymph node aspirate, bone marrow, blood culture, other biopsy material, granulomata on histopathology, lymphocytic pleocytosis, increased protein in CSF ●*Test findings:* Isolation of acid-fast bacilli from sterile clinical specimen (lymph node, bone marrow, blood, biopsy) is diagnostic; isolation from sputum or bronchoalveolar lavage may represent colonization; anemia, leukopenia, elevated alkaline phosphatase in AIDS

Aural atresia ●*Onset:* Congenital ●*Male:female ratio:* M=F ●*Ethnicity:* All ●*Character:* Absent ear canal ●*Location:* Ear ●*Pattern:* Nonspecific ●*Precipitating factors:* None relevant ●*Relieving factors:* None relevant ●*Clinical course:* Permanent unless surgically corrected ●*Co-morbidities:* May be associated with deformities of the auricular pinna ●*Procedure results:* Otoscopy reveals a blind or absent external auditory canal ●*Test findings:* No relevant tests

Autism ●*Onset:* Insidious ●*Male:female ratio:* M(4):F(1) ●*Ethnicity:* All ●*Character:* Failure of language development, severe impairment of interpersonal relationships, restricted repertoire of activities ●*Location:* Nonspecific ●*Pattern:* Onset of symptoms before 3 years of age ●*Precipitating factors:* None relevant ●*Relieving factors:* Behavioral modification ●*Clinical course:* Static ●*Co-morbidities:* None relevant ●*Procedure results:* No relevant procedures ●*Test findings:* Mental retardation

Autoimmune hemolytic anemia ●*Onset:* Depends on underlying cause and severity. Can be acute, subacute, insidious ●*Male:female ratio:* M<F ●*Ethnicity:* All ●*Character:* Fatigue, dyspnea, pallor, mild icterus, hemoglobinuria ●*Location:* Nonspecific ●*Pattern:* Nonspecific ●*Precipitating factors:* Certain medications (methyldopa, penicillin, quinine), certain infections (mycoplasma, mononucleosis), exposure to cold ●*Relieving factors:* Transfusions, corticosteroids, other immunosuppressive drugs, splenectomy (if refractory) ●*Clinical course:* Self-limited in most though durative varies from several weeks to several years (with relapses) ●*Co-morbidities:* Lymphomas, collagen vascular diseases, postviral syndromes, drugs, other tumors (rare) ●*Procedure results:* No relevant procedures ●*Test findings:* Positive direct Coombs' test, anemia (normomacrocytic), reticulocytosis, nucleated red blood cells, spherocytosis

Autonomic dysfunction ●*Onset:* Insidious ●*Male:female ratio:* M=F ●*Ethnicity:* All ●*Character:* Depends whether secondary to CNS degenerative disease or severe peripheral neuropathy ●*Location:* Nonspecific ●*Pattern:* Urinary hesitancy, xerostomia, constipation, male impotence, anhydrosis with heat intolerance and postural hypotension manifested by lightheadedness and ataxia on change of posture and occasional syncope ●*Precipitating factors:* None relevant ●*Relieving factors:* Thigh high stockings and fludrocortisone help prevent orthostasis ●*Clinical course:* Progressive ●*Co-morbidities:* None relevant ●*Procedure results:* No relevant procedures ●*Test findings:* No relevant tests

AV block, first degree ●*Onset:* Acute ●*Male:female ratio:* M=F ●*Ethnicity:* All ●*Character:* Asymptomatic. Rarely shortness of breath secondary to presystolic mitral regurgitation ●*Location:* Prolonged PR interval ●*Pattern:* Nonspecific ●*Precipitating factors:* Coronary ischemia/infarction, increased vagal tone, AV nodal blocking agents, hyperkalemia ●*Relieving factors:* Vagotonic agents, e.g. atropine ●*Clinical course:* Intermittent or chronic ●*Co-morbidities:* Lev's disease, Lenegre's disease, coronay artery disease (CAD), hyperkalemia, aortic endocarditis, Lyme disease, sarcoidosis, ankylosing spondylitis, Reiter's disease, rheumatoid arthritis ●*Procedure results:* Electrophysiology testing with conduction delay in the AV node (AH interval) and less commonly intra-atrially (PA interval) ●*Test findings:* ECG with PR prolongation (PR >0.2s) but all impulses are conducted

AV block, second degree ●*Onset:* Acute ●*Male:female ratio:* M=F ●*Ethnicity:* All ●*Character:* Asymptomatic, lightheadedness, syncope, chest pain, shortness of breath ●*Location:* Anterior chest, left arm, jaw, neck ●*Pattern:* Nonspecific ●*Precipitating factors:* Age, congenital, increased vagal tone, Lev's disease, AV nodal blocking agents, valvular heart disease ●*Relieving factors:* Vagotonic agents, e.g. atropine for Mobitz type I, cardiac pacing for Mobitz type II ●*Clinical course:* Intermittent or chronic. Mobitz type II may progress to complete heart block ●*Co-morbidities:* Lev's disease, Lenegre's disease, coronary artery disease (CAD), valvular heart disease, Lyme disease, sarcoidosis, ankylosing spondylitis, Reiter's syndrome, rheumatoid arthritis ●*Procedure results:* Electrophysiology testing with conduction delay in the AV node (AH interval) for Mobitz type I and with conduction delay in the His-Purkinje system (HV interval) for Mobitz type II ●*Test findings:* Mobitz type I (Wenckebach): ECG with PR prolongation, culminating in a nonconducted P wave; Mobitz type II: ECG with occasional or repetitive nonconducted P waves, without measurable PR prolongation

AV block, third degree ●*Onset:* Typically acute ●*Male:female ratio:* M=F ●*Ethnicity:* All ●*Character:* Symptoms variably present, depending on ventricular escape rate and resultant BP. Primarily symptoms of hypotension (lightheadedness, syncope). May also present as fatigue ●*Location:* Nonspecific ●*Pattern:* Symptoms persistent if third-degree AV block is persistent (intermittent block results in intermittent symptoms of unpredictable onset and duration) ●*Precipitating factors:* Symptoms typically spontaneous and unpredictable in onset/duration; lightheadedness may be exacerbated by dehydration, fatigue may be noted with activity (exercise intolerance) ●*Relieving factors:* Resting, lying supine; atropine (temporary); electrical pacing (definitive) ●*Clinical course:* Depends on etiology: mostly is persistent problem requiring pacemaker implantation. In Lyme disease, antibiotic treatment can be curative. After valve surgery, may resolve spontaneously within days. Drug toxicity resolves with discontinuation of offending agent(s) ●*Co-morbidities:* Commonly age-related degeneration of electrical conduction system. Also drug toxicity, myocardial infarction, Lyme disease, aortic or mitral valve surgery, amyloidosis, sarcoidosis, electrolyte disturbance, Chagas' disease, hypothyroidism ●*Procedure results:* ECG reveals AV dissociation with ventricular rate slower than atrial rate and no association whatsoever between P waves and QRS complexes ●*Test findings:* No relevant tests

Avascular necrosis ●*Onset:* Subacute ●*Male:female ratio:* M=F ●*Ethnicity:* African-American ●*Character:* Dull ache ●*Location:* Hip, knee, shoulder, foot, wrist ●*Pattern:* Pain worse with weight bearing ●*Precipitating factors:* Trauma, scaphoid fracture, peripheral vascular disease, trauma, diabetes ●*Relieving factors:* Unloading joint with assistive device, core decompressive surgery, total joint replacement ●*Clinical course:* Progressive in weight-bearing joints, e.g. hips or knees, frequently self-limiting in shoulders ●*Co-morbidities:* Steroid use, alcohol abuse, systemic lupus erythematosus (SLE), sickle cell disease ●*Procedure results:* MRI with bone infarcts ●*Test findings:* Synovial fluid analysis with WBC <500

Babesiosis ●*Onset:* Acute, subacute ●*Male:female ratio:* M>F ●*Ethnicity:* All ●*Character:* Gradual onset of fever, chills, myalgia, malaise, fatigue. Less common: headache, arthralgia, abdominal pain, anorexia. Uncommon: photophobia, conjunctivitis, pulmonary involvement ●*Location:* Initial symptoms are nonspecific, flu-like illness is most common ●*Pattern:* Fever sustained or intermittent, severe hemolysis may predominate, hepatosplenomegaly ●*Precipitating factors:* Tick exposure (not all recalled); endemic areas (New England, upper Midwest; more recently: northeast) ●*Relieving factors:* Oral clindamycin and quinine, exchange blood transfusions if life-threatening. Other agents: experimental ●*Clinical course:* Incubation: 1-4 weeks, usually subclinical and self-limited, untreated symptomatic infection lasts weeks-to-months, more severe in immunosuppressed, splenectomized, elderly ●*Co-morbidities:* Coinfection with Lyme and Ehrlichia organisms (same tick vector) ●*Procedure results:* Intraerythrocytic parasite in Giemsa- or Wright-stained thin or thick blood smears ●*Test findings:* Parasitized red blood cells (RBC), hemolytic anemia (low hemoglobin, low haptoglobin), normal-low white blood cells (WBC), mildly elevated aspartate transaminase (AST), alanine transaminase (ALT), lactate dehydrogenase (LDH), proteinuria, hemoglobinuria

Bacteremia ●*Onset:* Acute or subacute ●*Male:female ratio:* M=F ●*Ethnicity:* All ●*Character:* The presence of bacteria in the blood stream ●*Location:* Blood stream, may seed any organ system ●*Pattern:* Nonspecific ●*Precipitating factors:* Vascular catheters, indwelling devices, focal infection, chronic illness, IV drug abuse, neutropenia, skin or mucosal disruption, AIDS, splenectomy, many other factors ●*Relieving factors:* None relevant ●*Clinical course:* May evolve into sepsis ●*Co-morbidities:* Diabetes, cancer, injection drug use, AIDS, splenectomy, surgery, hospitalization, neutropenia, cirrhosis, burn, trauma, vascular catheters, indwelling devices, foreign bodies, other ●*Procedure results:* No relevant procedures ●*Test findings:* Finding of bacteria from blood culture, leukocytosis or leukopenia, left shift (bandemia)

Bacterial conjunctivitis ●*Onset:* Most forms acute; gonococcal hyperacute; chlamydial subacute ●*Male:female ratio:* M=F ●*Ethnicity:* All ❶ *Character:* Mucopurulent discharge from eye ❷ *Location:* Conjunctiva ❸ *Pattern:* Unilateral, bilateral ●*Precipitating factors:* Exposure to person with bacterial conjunctivitis; preceding upper respiratory illness (URI) ●*Relieving factors:* Topical antibiotic shortens the course of condition ●*Clinical course:* Usually lasts up to 10 days and is usually self-limiting ●*Co-morbidities:* None relevant ●*Procedure results:* Small conjunctival papillae and turbid tear film noted on slit lamp examination ●*Test findings:* Gram stain and culture/sensitivity if gonococcal infection suspected

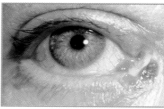

❶ *Character Normal pupil, peripheral conjunctival injection, and purulent discharge (especially nasally)*

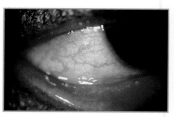

❷ *Location Peripheral conjunctival injection, mild discharge, and inclusion cysts*

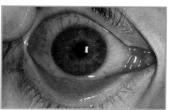

❸ *Pattern Normal pupil and conjunctival injection, most marked peripherally away from cornea*

Bacterial meningitis ●*Onset:* Acute ●*Male:female ratio:* M=F ●*Ethnicity:* All ●*Character:* Acute onset of severe headache, meningismus, fever, with neutrophilic pleocytosis of CSF ●*Location:* Meninges, CSF ●*Pattern:* Worst headache of life with photophobia, meningismus and fever, occasional confusion, delirium, or severely altered consciousness; less common: cranial nerve palsies ●*Precipitating factors:* Causative organisms vary with age ●*Relieving factors:* Avoidance of light ●*Clinical course:* Rapidly progressive, may lead to coma, severe neurologic sequelae, death ●*Co-morbidities:* None relevant ●*Procedure results:* Elevated opening spinal pressure, CSF: neutrophilic pleocytosis (usually thousands), elevated protein, low glucose, organisms on Gram stain, positive rapid assay for specific bacteria; contrast MRI or CT of head: meningeal enhancement ●*Test findings:* Blood: leukocytosis with a left shift (rarely leukopenia)

Bacterial pneumonia ●*Onset:* Acute ●*Male:female ratio:* M>F ●*Ethnicity:* All ●*Character:* Cough, fevers, sputum, chest discomfort, malaise ●*Location:* Chest ●*Pattern:* Bronchial breath sounds, inspiratory rales, egophony ●*Precipitating factors:* Risk factors: immunodeficiency, structural lung disease, postoperative state, aspiration ●*Relieving factors:* Antibiotics ●*Clinical course:* Overall mortality 13.7% (5.1% for ambulatory patients, 36.5% for critically ill); clinical improvement within days, radiographic resolution within weeks (usually <4 weeks). Be aware for peripneumonic effusions and the development of empyemas ●*Co-morbidities:* None relevant ●*Procedure results:* No relevant procedures ●*Test findings:* Leukocytosis, focal infiltrate(s) on chest X-ray, sputum with neutrophils and a prominent bacterial organism

Bacterial vulvovaginitis ●*Onset:* Acute ●*Male:female ratio:* F ●*Ethnicity:* All ●*Character:* Vaginal burning, discharge, dysuria ●*Location:* Vagina, vulva, periurethral ●*Pattern:* Discharge is malodorous ●*Precipitating factors:* Oral contraceptives, douches, stress, prior antibiotic usage ●*Relieving factors:* Treatment with metronidazole orally or vaginally, sexual partner not treated ●*Clinical course:* Persistent unless treated, may be recurrent ●*Co-morbidities:* Assess for presence of STDs, may be associated with preterm deliveries, premature rupture of membranes, postpartum endometritis ●*Procedure results:* No relevant procedures ●*Test findings:* Sodium chloride wet mount positive for clue cells, potassium hydroxide negative, culture positive for Gardnerella vaginalis

Baker's cyst ●*Onset:* Subacute, rupture is acute ●*Male:female ratio:* M<F ●*Ethnicity:* All ●*Character:* Dull ache ●*Location:* Behind knee joint, ruptures cause pain into calf ●*Pattern:* Pain worsens as the day proceeds ●*Precipitating factors:* Worse with activity ●*Relieving factors:* Aspiration of knee joint, cortisone injection in knee, elevation of calf ●*Clinical course:* Baker's cyst remains as long as knee pathology continues, ruptured cysts are self-limited ●*Co-morbidities:* Osteoarthritis, rheumatoid arthritis ●*Procedure results:* Able to aspirate moderate amounts of fluid from knee joint ●*Test findings:* Ultrasound demonstrating the cyst

Balanitis and balanoposthitis ●*Onset:* Subacute ●*Male:female ratio:* M ●*Ethnicity:* All ●*Character:* Itching and burning pain ●*Location:* Penis ●*Pattern:* Progressive ulceration and inflammation ●*Precipitating factors:* Phimosis, uncircumcised males, poor genital hygiene ●*Relieving factors:* Antifungals for candida; improve hygiene, circumcision ●*Clinical course:* May progress to cause phimosis. Consider biopsy for squamous cell carcinoma if not responding to treatment ●*Co-morbidities:* Phimosis, diabetes ●*Procedure results:* No relevant procedures ●*Test findings:* Bright red inflammation suggests candida. Potassium hydroxide preparation of scraping confirms Candida. Ulcer or solid lesion needs referral

Barotitis media ●*Onset:* Acute ●*Male:female ratio:* M=F ●*Ethnicity:* All ●*Character:* Ranges from sudden severe ear pain to dull ache with associated hearing loss and possibly vertigo ●*Location:* Affected ear (may be bilateral) ●*Pattern:* Pain may be initially severe, then subsides ●*Precipitating factors:* Airplane flight, scuba diving ●*Relieving factors:* 'Ear popping', valsalva, oral decongestants ●*Clinical course:* Initial pain generally subsides to manifest as a blockage over several hours to days; disease is often self-limited to within 2 weeks ●*Co-morbidities:* Chronic sinusitis, allergic rhinitis, eustachian dysfunction, ear surgery ●*Procedure results:* Otoscopic visualization of fluid or hemorrhage within the middle ear space or tympanic membrane ●*Test findings:* Conductive hearing loss on audiometry, flat tympanogram

Bartholin cyst ●*Onset:* Asympomatic, subacute. Can become acutely enlarged and painful if infected ●*Male:female ratio:* F ●*Ethnicity:* All ●*Character:* Pain at introitus worsened by penile insertion; usually painless lump discovered by patient ●*Location:* Swelling postlaterally at introitus ●*Pattern:* 2cm rubbery lystic nodular density. Can increase up to 8cm ●*Precipitating factors:* Worsened by intercourse or insertion of tampon, diaphragm ●*Relieving factors:* Frequent warm soaks can produce spontaneous drainage ●*Clinical course:* Small asymptomatic cysts may persist indefinitely, spontaneously resolve or progress to infection requiring surgical drainage ●*Co-morbidities:* Gonococcal infection of cervix and vagina can lead to gonococcal Bartholin cyst ●*Procedure results:* Contains sterile mucus when punctured ●*Test findings:* No relevant tests

Bartonella infection (cat scratch disease) ●*Onset:* Acute, subacute ●*Male:female ratio:* M>F ●*Ethnicity:* All ●*Character:* Skin papule to crusted-over pustule at site of cat scratch, tender regional lymphadenopathy ●*Location:* Scratch sites: hands and face most common, any other site. Adenopathy: axillary, cervical, epitrochlear, pectoral most common, any other site. Systemic: fever, malaise. Severe complications: encephalitis, seizure, coma, meningitis, transverse myelitis, hepatitis, splenic lesions, conjunctivitis, osteomyelitis, other ●*Pattern:* Adenopathy is tender, and localized, more common in upper limbs, axillae, neck, other ●*Precipitating factors:* Cat scratch, exposure to cat fleas/young cats ●*Relieving factors:* Needle aspiration of lymph node relieves pain, antibiotics shorten course ●*Clinical course:* Untreated resolves in 1-6 months ●*Co-morbidities:* None relevant ●*Procedure results:* Lymph node biopsy (Warthin-Starry silver stain), granulomata with central necrosis and clustered bacilli; positive polymerase chain reaction (PCR) of biopsy material ●*Test findings:* Positive Bartonella henselae serology, positive PCR of infected material

Bartter's syndrome ●*Onset:* Gradual ●*Male:female ratio:* M=F ●*Ethnicity:* All ●*Character:* Weakness, polydipsia, salt craving, failure to thrive in childhood ●*Location:* Nonspecific ●*Pattern:* Nonspecific ●*Precipitating factors:* Familial, cystinosis may predispose to acquired form ●*Relieving factors:* Potassium chloride and/or magnesium supplementation, occasionally amiloride or triamterene ●*Clinical course:* Chronic ●*Co-morbidities:* Cystinosis ●*Procedure results:* No relevant procedures ●*Test findings:* Hypokalemic alkalosis, hypomagnesemia, high urine potassium/magnesium/chloride excretion

Basal cell carcinoma ●*Onset:* Subacute ●*Male:female ratio:* M>F ●*Ethnicity:* Fair skin ❶ *Character:* Nonhealing lesion ❷ *Location:* Sun-exposed skin ❸ *Pattern:* Shiny papule/plaque with telangiectasias ●*Precipitating factors:* Years of sun exposure ●*Relieving factors:* Surgical excision, curettage and electrodessication, cryotherapy ●*Clinical course:* Progressive ●*Co-morbidities:* Other skin cancers ●*Procedure results:* Positive skin biopsy ●*Test findings:* No relevant tests

Images of ❶ *Character,* ❷ *Location,* ❸ *Pattern on page 431*

Beckwith-Wiedemann syndrome ●*Onset:* Congenital ●*Male:female ratio:* M=F ●*Ethnicity:* All ●*Character:* Macroglossia, omphalocele, gigantism ●*Location:* Nonspecific ●*Pattern:* Hypoglycemia in neonatal period ●*Precipitating factors:* Patient fasts ●*Relieving factors:* Food ●*Clinical course:* Chronic ●*Co-morbidities:* Wilm's tumor, congenital heart defects ●*Procedure results:* Increased insulin ●*Test findings:* Hypoglycemia

Behavioral problem in children ●*Onset:* Late infancy/toddlers/children ●*Male:female ratio:* M=F ●*Ethnicity:* All ●*Character:* Inappropriate behavior ●*Location:* Mood/behavior/temperament ●*Pattern:* Persistent inappropriate behavior with/without modification ●*Precipitating factors:* Fatigue, environmental stress, frustration, inadequate behavior modification ●*Relieving factors:* Behavior modification, maturation ●*Clinical course:* Usual improvement with behavior modiification/intervention ●*Co-morbidities:* Delayed developmental milestones (i.e. speech), sensory integration disorders, ADHD, unstable home environment or other social stressor ●*Procedure results:* No relevant procedures ●*Test findings:* Abnormal behavior observation

Basal cell carcinoma: Images *see text page 430*

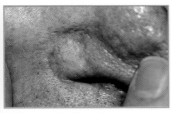

❶ *Character A solitary, slow-growing, yellowish plaque is a typical presentation*

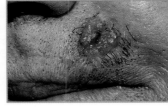

❶ *Character A larger, eroded nodule with a rolled border*

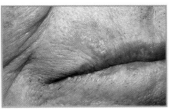

❷ *Location A pearly papule in a sun-exposed location is typical*

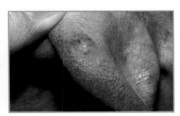

❷ *Location A pearly papule with a slight blood tinge*

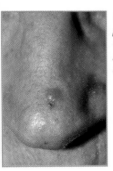

❸ *Pattern A pearly papule, with a focal area of crusting*

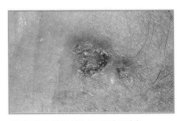

❸ *Pattern Note the crusted nodule*

Behçet's syndrome ●*Onset:* Subacute, episodic ●*Male:female ratio:* M>F ●*Ethnicity:* Japanese and Middle Eastern ❶ *Character:* Painful oral and genital ulcers, uveitis, large joint arthritis ●*Location:* Mouth, genitals, large joints ●*Pattern:* Joints involved: ankles and knees most common. Cutaneous lesions such as erythema nodosum, photosensitivity also common ●*Precipitating factors:* None relevant ●*Relieving factors:* Corticosteroids, colchicine, chlorambucil for CNS disease ●*Clinical course:* Episodic disease that is generally chronic ●*Co-morbidities:* None relevant ●*Procedure results:* No relevant procedures ●*Test findings:* No relevant tests

Image of ❶ *Character on page 432*

Bell's palsy ●*Onset:* Acute, subacute ●*Male:female ratio:* M=F ●*Ethnicity:* All ●*Character:* Unilateral facial weakness with difficulty closing the affected eye. Associated with retroricular pain ●*Location:* Upper and lower face involved ●*Pattern:* Nonspecific ●*Precipitating factors:* None relevant ●*Relieving factors:* None relevant ●*Clinical course:* Full recovery in 85% ●*Co-morbidities:* Lyme disease and varicella zoster ●*Procedure results:* No relevant procedures ●*Test findings:* Normal MRI or CT of the brain

Behçet's syndrome: Image *see text page 431*

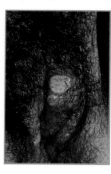

❶ *Character* Two moist, painful, ulcers in the vulva of a young woman

Benign essential myoclonus ●*Onset:* Prior to age 20 ●*Male:female ratio:* M=F ●*Ethnicity:* All ●*Character:* Simple jerklike movement not coordinated or suppressible; often activated by volitional movement ●*Location:* May involve a single motor unit or simultaneously involve groups of muscles ●*Pattern:* Inherited as simple autosomal dominant pattern ●*Precipitating factors:* None relevant ●*Relieving factors:* Drugs: clonazepam, piracetam, levetiracetam, valproic acid, 5-OH tryptophan, tetrabenazine, reserpine, levodopa, trohexyphenidyl, lisuride ●*Clinical course:* Variable ●*Co-morbidities:* Essential tremor, seizures ●*Procedure results:* No relevant procedures ●*Test findings:* Neurological examination and testing negative for other associated deficits

Benign essential/familial tremor syndrome ●*Onset:* Insidious ●*Male:female ratio:* M=F ●*Ethnicity:* All ●*Character:* Bilateral symmetric tremor but can be asymmetric ●*Location:* Beginning in fingers and hands ●*Pattern:* Nonspecific ●*Precipitating factors:* Autosomal dominate. Worse with anger, excitement, extreme emotions ●*Relieving factors:* Beta blockers, primidone, alcohol ●*Clinical course:* Symptoms progress but do plateau ●*Co-morbidities:* None relevant ●*Procedure results:* No relevant procedures ●*Test findings:* Non-Parkinsonian patient

Benign intracranial hypertension ●*Onset:* Subacute/insidious ●*Male:female ratio:* M<F ●*Ethnicity:* All ●*Character:* Headache, nausea and vomiting, visual difficulties ●*Location:* Head ●*Pattern:* Diurnal variation of headache: worse in the morning ●*Precipitating factors:* Obesity, idiopathic, lateral sinous thrombosis, hypovitaminosis, hypervitaminosis A, carbon dioxide retention, endocrine disorders, tetracyclines, head trauma ●*Relieving factors:* Lowering of intracranial pressure with acetazolamide or prednisone, which decreases amount of CSF produced; lumbar puncture ●*Clinical course:* Most cases resolve spontaneously in 6-18 months ●*Co-morbidities:* None relevant ●*Procedure results:* CT/MRI of brain: normal or slit-like lateral ventricles. Opening pressure of the lumbar puncture is >20cm/H2O ●*Test findings:* CSF: normal

Benign ovarian tumor ●*Onset:* Insidious over weeks-to-months ●*Male:female ratio:* F ●*Ethnicity:* All ●*Character:* Asymptomatic or vague bloating, distension, pressure. Severe acute pain with torsion/rupture ●*Location:* Increased abdominal girth, pressure on intra-abdominal organs. Rupture produces peritoneal irritation radiating to inguinal area, external genitalia and upper thigh ●*Pattern:* Mild intermittent pelvic pain ●*Precipitating factors:* None relevant ●*Relieving factors:* Surgical resection required for large symptomatic tumors ●*Clinical course:* 5-10% potential for malignancy. May grow extremely large and fill entire pelvis ●*Co-morbidities:* Functioning ovarian tumors produce feminizing or virilizing effects ●*Procedure results:* Transvaginal ultrasound, CT or MRI: >8cm, multiocular or solid ovarian lesion, can be bilateral. Cell type origin determined by surgical resection: stromal, germ cell, epithelial ●*Test findings:* CA-125 elevated in 20% of cases

Benign paroxysmal positional vertigo ●*Onset:* Acute ●*Male:female ratio:* M=F ●*Ethnicity:* All ●*Character:* Severe vertigo induced by rapid change in head position ●*Location:* Nonspecific ●*Pattern:* Nonspecific ●*Precipitating factors:* Idiopathic, head trauma, viral labyrinthitis, vertebral basilar insufficiency ●*Relieving factors:* Repositioning of the calcium otolith, anticholinergics, benzodiazepines ●*Clinical course:* Usually resolves spontaneously but attacks may last more than one year ●*Co-morbidities:* None relevant ●*Procedure results:* Normal MRI/MRA of the brainstem ●*Test findings:* With Barany's maneuver, symptoms and nystagmus are exacerbated when appropriate ear is towards the floor

Benign prostatic hyperplasia ●*Onset:* Insidious ●*Male:female ratio:* M ●*Ethnicity:* All ●*Character:* Pain. Obstructive and irritative voiding symptoms ●*Location:* Suprapubic area/bladder ●*Pattern:* Nonspecific ●*Precipitating factors:* Cold medicine (alpha-adrenergics), urinary tract infeciton (UTI), prostatitis ●*Relieving factors:* Medications: alpha-blockers, finasteride; surgery ●*Clinical course:* Slowly progressive over years or decades ●*Co-morbidities:* UTI, retention, hematuria, prostatitis ●*Procedure results:* No relevant procedures ●*Test findings:* Enlarged prostate without nodule or fixation; normal prostate-specific antigen (PSA)

Benign salivary gland tumor ●*Onset:* Insidious ●*Male:female ratio:* M=F ●*Ethnicity:* All ●*Character:* Asymptomatic enlargement of salivary gland ●*Location:* Affected salivary gland ●*Pattern:* Nonspecific ●*Precipitating factors:* None relevant ●*Relieving factors:* None relevant ●*Clinical course:* Slow progressive enlargement ●*Co-morbidities:* Radiation therapy to head and neck ●*Procedure results:* CT or MRI with contrast demonstrates mass or tumor ●*Test findings:* No relevant tests

Bennet's fracture ●*Onset:* Acute ●*Male:female ratio:* M=F ●*Ethnicity:* All ●*Character:* Sharp or dull pain, swelling ●*Location:* Base of thumb metacarpal ●*Pattern:* Persistent pain or swelling despite conservative therapy ●*Precipitating factors:* May occur during fist fights, axial blow to partially flexed metacarpal ●*Relieving factors:* Ice, elevation, splint, analgesia ●*Clinical course:* Needs reduction and internal fixation of volar ulnar fragment ●*Co-morbidities:* Trapezium fracture, rupture of MP joint collateral ligaments ●*Procedure results:* No relevant procedures ●*Test findings:* X-ray showing volnar ulnar fragment dislocation and fractured metacarpal shaft

Biliary atresia ●*Onset:* Subacute ●*Male:female ratio:* M>F ●*Ethnicity:* All ●*Character:* Neonatal jaundice, acholic stools, hepatomegaly, sometimes splenomegaly ●*Location:* Biliary tree ●*Pattern:* Nonspecific ●*Precipitating factors:* None relevant ●*Relieving factors:* Surgical decompression of the extrahepatic biliary tree ●*Clinical course:* Fatal within 2 years if not surgically treated; with treatment 20% survive >10 years ●*Co-morbidities:* Cardiovascular defects, polyspenia, malrotation, situs inversus and bowel atresias ●*Procedure results:* Exploratory laparotomy finding obstructed extrahepatic biliary tree ●*Test findings:* Elevated bilirubin (6-12mg/dL), moderately elevated alkaline phosphatase and aminotransferases

Biliary tract disease ●*Onset:* Insidious if slow growth of a lesion; gallstones present acutely though often preceding biliary colic ●*Male:female ratio:* M=F ●*Ethnicity:* All ●*Character:* Right upper quadrant pain, jaundice, fevers, weight loss, bloating, clay-colored stools, dark urine ●*Location:* Nonspecific ●*Pattern:* Biliary colic often occurs at night and/or postprandially and lasts for 30 min to hours ●*Precipitating factors:* Gallstones: obesity, high cholesterol, rapid weight loss, parenteral nutrition ●*Relieving factors:* Usually surgical (gallstones, tumor); endoscopic stent replacement or stone removal. Antibiotics for infection. Oral bile salts or lithotripsy for stones ●*Clinical course:* Depends on disorder: good prognosis for gallstones unless accompanied by pancreatitis which can be life-threatening; biliary tumors have poor prognosis ●*Co-morbidities:* Obesity, inflammatory bowel disease, disorders of hemoglobin synthesis/hemolysis ●*Procedure results:* Endoscopic retrograde choleopancreatoscopy or radiographic studies can identify gallstones, mass ●*Test findings:* Elevated bilirubin/liver function tests/amylase and lipase

Birth asphyxia ●*Onset:* Acute ●*Male:female ratio:* M=F ●*Ethnicity:* All ●*Character:* Depressed respiration, hypo/hypertonia, cyanosis, apnea, bradycardia ●*Location:* Respiratory/cardiac/neurologic symptoms ●*Pattern:* Nonspecific ●*Precipitating factors:* Fetal: inadequate maternal blood oxygenation, placental insufficiency, premature placental separation, compression of umbilical cord. After birth: severe anemia, hemorrhage, inadequate oxygenation ●*Relieving factors:* Adequate oxygenation, corrective hypotension, fluid balance, electrolyte abnormalities ●*Clinical course:* Severity dictates outcome and long-term effects ●*Co-morbidities:* Cerebral palsy, mental retardation, encephalopathy, seizures ●*Procedure results:* No relevant procedures ●*Test findings:* Low fetal scalp pH, acidosis, hypoxemia

Black widow spider bite ●*Onset:* Acute ●*Male:female ratio:* M=F ●*Ethnicity:* All ●*Character:* Local pain, muscle cramping or rigidity, dizziness, diaphoresis, hypertension and tachycardia; abdominal muscle pain may simulate an acute abdomen ●*Location:* Extremities, genitalia most common ●*Pattern:* Nonspecific ●*Precipitating factors:* None relevant ●*Relieving factors:* Ice to bite, narcotics for pain, benzodiazepines for cramps, antivenin in severe cases ●*Clinical course:* Effects self-limited, mortality about 5% ●*Co-morbidities:* None relevant ●*Procedure results:* No relevant procedures ●*Test findings:* No relevant tests

Bladder diverticula ●*Onset:* Chronic ●*Male:female ratio:* M(5):F(1) ●*Ethnicity:* All ●*Character:* Mostly asymptomatic ●*Location:* Bladder ●*Pattern:* Nonspecific ●*Precipitating factors:* Bladder outlet obstruction (benign prostatic hypertrophy [BPH], stricture, posterior urethral valves); neurogenic bladder ●*Relieving factors:* Surgical repair ●*Clinical course:* Slowly progressive in adults ●*Co-morbidities:* Bladder outlet obstruction (BPH, stricture) and neurogenic bladder in adults; vesivoureteral reflux and posterior urethral valves in children ●*Procedure results:* No relevant procedures ●*Test findings:* Intravenous pyelogram, ultrasound, voiding cystouretogram all diagnostic

Bladder outlet obstruction ●*Onset:* Acute, subacute, or chronic ●*Male:female ratio:* M>F ●*Ethnicity:* All ●*Character:* Difficulty in voiding with obstructive voiding symptoms; pain and discomfort when in retention ●*Location:* Bladder and suprapubic area ●*Pattern:* Nonspecific ●*Precipitating factors:* Urinary tract infection (UTI), prostatitis, pelvic mass ●*Relieving factors:* Bladder drainage: catheter or surgical; alpha blockers in patients with benign prostatic hyperplasia (BPH); surgery (transurethral prostatectomy [TURP], prostatectomy, bladder neck incision) will resolve symptoms ●*Clinical course:* Progressive when not treated; may lead to azotemia with chronic urine retention ●*Co-morbidities:* Urinary tract infection (UTI), prostatitis, congenital abnormalities in newborns ●*Procedure results:* CT/ultrasound: distended bladder, pelvic mass; cystoscopy: BPH, strictures and/or stenosis ●*Test findings:* Urine analysis: possible hematuria and pyuria; urine culture and sensitivity: possible bacterial growth

Bladder trauma ●*Onset:* Acute ●*Male:female ratio:* M=F ●*Ethnicity:* All ●*Character:* Severe pain with hematuria ●*Location:* Suprapubic area/bladder ●*Pattern:* Nonspecific ●*Precipitating factors:* Distended bladder at time of trauma ●*Relieving factors:* Drainage with catheter for extraperitoneal rupture; surgical repair for intraperitoneal rupture ●*Clinical course:* Progressive if not treated ●*Co-morbidities:* Congenital malformation of bladder; prior pelvic or bladder surgery ●*Procedure results:* Cystogram best in making correct diagnosis ●*Test findings:* Hematuria

Bladder tumor ●*Onset:* Subacute ●*Male:female ratio:* M>F ●*Ethnicity:* Caucasians at higher risk than African-Americans ●*Character:* Painless gross hematuria ●*Location:* Bladder ●*Pattern:* Possibly multifocal ●*Precipitating factors:* Long history of smoking and/or exposure to carcinogens ●*Relieving factors:* Surgery, radiation therapy, chemotherapy ●*Clinical course:* Rapidly progressive and fatal if not treated ●*Co-morbidities:* Chronic bladder inflammation and urinary tract infections (UTIs) ●*Procedure results:* Tumor possibly seen as a filling defect on intravenous pyelogram (IVP), CT or ultrasound; transurethral resection of bladder tumor (TURBT) or biopsy are diagnostic ●*Test findings:* Urine analysis: positive red blood cells (RBC)

Blastomycosis ●*Onset:* Acute, insidious (most) ●*Male:female ratio:* M>F ●*Ethnicity:* Mostly seen in US ●*Character:* Progressive fever, cough, hemoptysis, fatigue, weight loss, skin lesions, dissemination ●*Location:* Lungs: lobar/segmental alveolar consolidation, nodules, cavities, hilar adenopathy; skin: verrucae, ulcers, subcutaneous nodules; dissemination: skeleton, prostate, epididymis, meninges, other ●*Pattern:* Chronic progressive lung and skin infection, dissemination ●*Precipitating factors:* Most cases in southeastern, central, mid-Atlantic US, Canada, Africa, India ●*Relieving factors:* Amphotericin-B if severe, oral itraconazole if mild-to-moderate ●*Clinical course:* Acute infection often asymptomatic/unrecognized, diagnosed cases are chronic-to-progressive and if left untreated mortality exceeds 60% ●*Co-morbidities:* None relevant ●*Procedure results:* Segmental alveolar-consolidation, nodules, cavitation, hilar adenopathy on chest X-ray; yeast forms in wet/stained sputum, pus, CSF, urine, other preparations ●*Test findings:* Thick-walled, broad-based, budding yeast forms in clinical preparations or histopathology, growth of Blastomycosis dermatitidis in culture; identification with DNA probe, positive serology

Blepharitis ●*Onset:* Insidious ●*Male:female ratio:* M=F ●*Ethnicity:* All ●*Character:* Itching, ocular burning usually worse in the morning ●*Location:* Both eyes ●*Pattern:* Erythematous eyelid margins; worse in the morning ●*Precipitating factors:* Frequent hand-to-eye contact sometimes precipitates symptoms ●*Relieving factors:* Improved lid hygiene ●*Clinical course:* Not progressive, chronic but not self-limiting ●*Co-morbidities:* Conjunctivitis, keratoconjunctivitis, rosacea, phlyctenulosis ●*Procedure results:* High magnification of the eyelid margins helps identify problem ●*Test findings:* Edema and erythema of eyelid

Body lice ●*Onset:* Acute/subacute/chronic ●*Male:female ratio:* M=F ●*Ethnicity:* All ●*Character:* Pruritic tiny macules and papules with secondary excoriations ●*Location:* Trunk, limbs (common), face (less common) ●*Pattern:* Nits (eggs) and lice are in clothing not on skin. Macules and papules are tiny, extremely pruritic. Longstanding disease results in hyperpigmentation ●*Precipitating factors:* Poor hygiene, overcrowding, poor sanitation, sharing bed linens, clothing ●*Relieving factors:* Hot-cycle (130°F) machine washing of all clothing, bed linens; carefully ironing seams of clothing; improving hygiene ●*Clinical course:* Chronic persistent unless hygiene improved; nits are viable in clothing for 1 month, lice survive without blood source for 10 days ●*Co-morbidities:* Epidemic typhus, trench fever, relapsing fever ●*Procedure results:* No relevant tests ●*Test findings:* Finding nits in seams of clothing or live nymphs/adult lice in clothing

Botulism ●*Onset:* Acute ●*Male:female ratio:* M=F ●*Ethnicity:* All ●*Character:* Symmetric, descending, flaccid paralysis, progressive bowel and urinary retention, no fever ●*Location:* Bilateral cranial nerves (diplopia, dysarthria, dysphagia, other), symmetric descending weakness, blurry vision, dry mouth, dry sore throat, diffuse abdominal pain, constipation, nausea, urinary retention, respiratory failure ●*Pattern:* Symmetric descending weakness, patient responsive, normal or low heart rate (unless hypotensive), no sensory loss, no fever ●*Precipitating factors:* Toxin ingestion (home-canned food, restaurant outbreaks); infected wounds; ingestion of Clostridia spores in foods such as honey: infant botulism ●*Relieving factors:* Botulism antitoxin, supportive care ●*Clinical course:* Food-borne: 12-36 hours incubation, rapidly progressive, respiratory failure within 24 hours, prolonged mechanical ventilation, recovery takes months; infant: progression over 1-2 weeks, stabilization for 2-3 weeks, slow recovery; wound: 4-14 days incubation, progressive, then slow recovery ●*Co-morbidities:* None relevant ●*Procedure results:* Nerve stimulation, electromyogram (EMG), and the Tensilon test helpful but nonspecific, paralysis induced in mice inoculated with patient's serum or stool ●*Test findings:* Clostridium botulinum in anaerobic culture of wound or stool, positive toxin assay of serum, stool, implicated food (ELISA or mouse bioassay), normal white blood cells (WBC), normal erythrocyte sedimentation rate (ESR), abnormal EMG

Brain abscess ●*Onset:* Acute, subacute ●*Male:female ratio:* M(2):F(1) ●*Ethnicity:* All ●*Character:* Weakness, numbness, confusion, headache, seizure, fevers ●*Location:* Nonspecific ●*Pattern:* Nonspecific ●*Precipitating factors:* Poor dentition, immunocompromised, trauma, severe sinusitis ●*Relieving factors:* Neurosurgical intervention and antibiotics ●*Clinical course:* Fatal if untreated ●*Co-morbidities:* None relevant ●*Procedure results:* MRI or CT of brain with contrast showing lesion ●*Test findings:* No relevant tests

Brain tumor ●*Onset:* Insidious, subacute, acute ●*Male:female ratio:* M=F ●*Ethnicity:* All ●*Character:* Weakness, confusion, numbness, mental status change, seizures, headache ●*Location:* Nonspecific ●*Pattern:* Nonspecific ●*Precipitating factors:* None relevant ●*Relieving factors:* Steroids, brain surgery ●*Clinical course:* Usually not self-limited and depends on the pathology ●*Co-morbidities:* None relevant ●*Procedure results:* CT/MRI of the brain showing the lesion. Positive brain biopsy ●*Test findings:* No relevant tests

Brainstem disorders ●*Onset:* Acute/subacute/insidious ●*Male:female ratio:* M=F ●*Ethnicity:* All ●*Character:* Diplopia, dysarthria, crossed sensory or motor findings, nausea, vomiting, vertigo, tongue heaviness ●*Location:* Nonspecific ●*Pattern:* Variable ●*Precipitating factors:* Depends on the etiology ●*Relieving factors:* Variable ●*Clinical course:* Variable ●*Co-morbidities:* None relevant ●*Procedure results:* No relevant procedures ●*Test findings:* No relevant tests

Branchial cyst ●*Onset:* Subacute (may be acute if appears during acute infection) ●*Male:female ratio:* M=F ●*Ethnicity:* All ●*Character:* Usually asymptomatic spontaneous swelling of lateral neck; may be painful if infected ●*Location:* Lateral neck, anterior to sternocleidomastoid muscle ●*Pattern:* Persistent swelling; may cycle with upper respiratory tract infection ●*Precipitating factors:* Upper respiratory tract infection or trauma ●*Relieving factors:* None relevant ●*Clinical course:* Swelling usually persists until surgically excised ●*Co-morbidities:* None relevant ●*Procedure results:* Needle biopsy yields proteinaceous fluid ●*Test findings:* CT scan delineates cystic mass in lateral neck

Breast abscess ●*Onset:* Acute to subacute ●*Male:female ratio:* M(1):F(10) ●*Ethnicity:* All ●*Character:* Purulent nipple discharge, usually due to Staphylococcus aureus or Streptococcus. Systemic symptoms include fever, chills ●*Location:* Local erythema tenderness and induration of affected breast ●*Pattern:* Nonspecific ●*Precipitating factors:* Lactating women, recent breast surgery, including biopsy ●*Relieving factors:* Incision and drainage required for abscess formation, cessation of nursing, oral antibiotics ●*Clinical course:* Improvement rapid following definitive surgical incision and drainage ●*Co-morbidities:* Hydradenitis suppurativa ●*Procedure results:* Culture of abscess fluid from incision and drainage reveals organism and antibiotic sensitivities ●*Test findings:* Blood cultures to assess for sepsis; leukocytosis common

Breast cancer ●*Onset:* Insidious ●*Male:female ratio:* M(1):F(100) ●*Ethnicity:* Caucasian>African-American>Asian ●*Character:* Breast lump, nipple discharge, nipple changes, skin changes, breast pain (inflammatory carcinoma), itching, erosion (Paget's) ●*Location:* Breast (most prevalent in upper outer quadrant) ●*Pattern:* Nonspecific ●*Precipitating factors:* None relevant ●*Relieving factors:* Surgery (lumpectomy vs mastectomy), hormonal treatment, radiation, chemotherapy ●*Clinical course:* Depends on stage and type; inflammatory carcinoma: poor prognosis; low stage/favorable type: good prognosis with treatment ●*Co-morbidities:* None relevant ●*Procedure results:* Breast biopsy: positive for malignant cells ●*Test findings:* Ultrasound: solid mass; mammogram: suspicious abnormality; in metastatic disease - elevated erythrocyte sedimentation rate (ESR) and alkaline phosphatase

Breast cyst ●*Onset:* Subacute ●*Male:female ratio:* M<F ●*Ethnicity:* All ●*Character:* Firm, mobile, tender ●*Location:* Usually well-demarcated from surrounding breast tissue ●*Pattern:* Fluctuates with menstrual cycle ●*Precipitating factors:* Hormonal irregularity, hormone replacement therapy ●*Relieving factors:* Warm compress, NSAIDs, aspiration ●*Clinical course:* Self limited, resolve on own or by aspiration, can recur ●*Co-morbidities:* If aspirated fluid is bloody or there is associated mass, consider breast cancer ●*Procedure results:* If no

associated solid mass and mammogram normal, aspiration for treatment only ●*Test findings:* Ultrasound shows cystic mass

Breast fibroadenoma ●*Onset:* Insidious ●*Male:female ratio:* M<F ●*Ethnicity:* Nonspecific ●*Character:* Usually asymptomatic breast mass ●*Location:* Breast ●*Pattern:* Usually asymptomatic ●*Precipitating factors:* None relevant ●*Relieving factors:* Surgical excision ●*Clinical course:* Benign ●*Co-morbidities:* None relevant ●*Procedure results:* Fibroadenoma on biopsy ●*Test findings:* Homogeneous well-defined mass on mammogram

Bronchiectasis ●*Onset:* Episodic, subacute ●*Male:female ratio:* M=F ●*Ethnicity:* All ●*Character:* Cough, daily sputum production, dyspnea ●*Location:* Chest: inspiratory crackles, expiratory rhonchi ●*Pattern:* Worse in morning ●*Precipitating factors:* Infection; impaired drainage, airflow obstruction, defect in host defense ●*Relieving factors:* Antibiotics, bronchodilators, chest physical therapy, postural drainage and exercise ●*Clinical course:* Episodic cough, phlegm with or without hemoptysis for years ●*Co-morbidities:* Cystic fibrosis, foreign body or tumor, defect in host defense, rheumatoid arthritis, Sjögren's syndrome, Young's syndrome, allergic bronchopulmonary aspergillosis, others ●*Procedure results:* No relevant procedures ●*Test findings:* Chest X-ray or high-resolution CT shows dilated airways, thickened bronchial walls

Bronchiolitis ●*Onset:* Insidious ●*Male:female ratio:* M>F ●*Ethnicity:* All ●*Character:* Dyspnea on exertion, cough ●*Location:* Chest ●*Pattern:* Inspiratory pops and squeaks ●*Precipitating factors:* Inhalational injury, infections, drugs, others ●*Relieving factors:* Bronchodilators, cough suppressants, supplemental oxygen, steroids and antibiotics in select cases ●*Clinical course:* Progressive over months-to-years ●*Co-morbidities:* Connective tissue disease, bone marrow transplantation ●*Procedure results:* Lung biopsy: shows small airway inflammation and fibrosis ●*Test findings:* Pulmonary function tests (PFTs) show irreversible obstructive ventilatory defect

Brucellosis ●*Onset:* Acute, subacute ●*Male:female ratio:* M=F ●*Ethnicity:* More common in developing nations ●*Character:* Progressive fever with night sweats, anorexia with weight loss, low back and large joint pain ●*Location:* Lumbar spine most common, other vertebrae, large joints (knee, hip, other), heart (endocardium, myocardium, pericardium), lung (pneumonia, lung nodule, associated adenopathy), liver (granulomatous hepatitis), female pelvis, male genitourinary tract, eye, skin ●*Pattern:* Osteomyelitis almost always vertebral, joint involvement is asymmetric ●*Precipitating factors:* Animal contact, unpasteurized dairy products, raw meat, workers in meat and dairy industry, rarely sexual and vertical transmission ●*Relieving factors:* Prolonged therapy is imperative, combination drug therapy preferred ●*Clinical course:* Incubation: 1 week-months, chronic progressive, untreated: low mortality but high morbidity (neurologic deficits, joint destruction), relapse rate is high and requires prolonged therapy ●*Co-morbidities:* None relevant ●*Procedure results:* Bone imaging: chronic osteomyelitis; joint fluid: 4000-40,000 WBC, granulocytes predominate, low-to-normal glucose, positive culture in 50%, Echo for endocarditis ●*Test findings:* Brucella isolation from blood, bone marrow, or tissue (requires prolonged incubation, special media, biohazard in the laboratory), elevated Brucella agglutinin, positive serology, elevated ESR

Bruxism ●*Onset:* Chronic ●*Male:female ratio:* M<F ●*Ethnicity:* All ●*Character:* Dull ache ●*Location:* Dentition and maxillary and mandibular regions ●*Pattern:* Chronic persistent pain; may be worse in the morning ●*Precipitating factors:* Stress ●*Relieving factors:* Warm compress; dental guard ●*Clinical course:* May persist or cycle with periods of waxing and waning ●*Co-morbidities:* Neurological disorders such as dystonia may be present ●*Procedure results:* No relevant procedures ●*Test findings:* Wear facets seen along the dentition; hypertrophy of the masseter muscle

Budd-Chiari syndrome ●*Onset:* Subacute, acute ●*Male:female ratio:* M=F ●*Ethnicity:* No predisposition ●*Character:* Right upper quadrant (RUQ) pain, hepatomegaly, ascites; may have jaundice, splenomegaly (less common) ●*Location:* Abdomen ●*Pattern:* Gradually increasing over days-to-weeks ●*Precipitating factors:* None relevant ●*Relieving factors:* Paracentesis ●*Clinical course:* Progresses to liver failure, with most patients dying within 3 years of diagnosis ●*Co-morbidities:* Myeloproliferative disorders, hypercoagulable states, malignancy, collagen-vascular diseases, contraceptive pill use, inflammatory bowel disease, cirrhosis ●*Procedure results:* Venography or Doppler ultrasound documenting obstruction of the hepatic veins ●*Test findings:* Ascites with an albumin gradient >1.1

Bulimia nervosa ●*Onset:* Late adolescence or early adulthood ●*Male:female ratio:* M(1):F(9) ●*Ethnicity:* All ●*Character:* Subtypes include purging and nonpurging types ●*Location:* Nonspecific ●*Pattern:* Typically bulimics are within a normal weight range, although some are slightly overweight or underweight ●*Precipitating factors:* Binge-eating typically begins during or after an episode of dieting ●*Relieving factors:* Psychotherapy and support ●*Clinical course:* May be chronic or intermittent, with periods of remission alternating with recurrence of binging ●*Co-morbidities:* Depression, anxiety disorders, substance abuse or dependence ●*Procedure results:* Serious dental abnormalities, enlarged salivary glands, menstrual abnormalities, esophageal tears, gastric rupture ●*Test findings:* Electrolyte abnormalities, elevated serum amylase

Bullous pemphigoid ●*Onset:* Subacute, insidious ●*Male:female ratio:* M<F ●*Ethnicity:* All ❶ *Character:* Itching ❷ *Location:* Trunk, proximal extremities ❸ *Pattern:* Tense blisters, urticarial plaques ●*Precipitating factors:* None relevant ●*Relieving factors:* Steroids, immunosuppressives ●*Clinical course:* Chronic ●*Co-morbidities:* None relevant ●*Procedure results:* Skin biopsy; hematoxylin-eosin: subepidermal blisters; immunofluorescence studies: immune complexes ●*Test findings:* No relevant tests

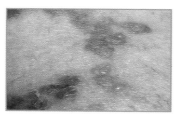

❶ *Character Multiple thick-walled blisters*

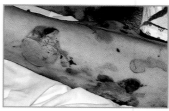

❷ *Location Erosions and crusts on the legs*

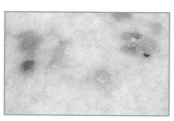

❸ *Pattern A tense, fluid-filled blister*

Burkitt's lymphoma ●*Onset:* Subacute ●*Male:female ratio:* M=F ●*Ethnicity:* Africa and New Guinea usually ●*Character:* Rapidly growing tumor mass (endemic/African type), abdominal pain or distention, bowel obstruction, CNS symptoms (nonendemic type), lymphadenopathy (immunodeficiency-related) ●*Location:* Mass in face or jaw (endemic type) ●*Pattern:* Nonspecific ●*Precipitating factors:* Epstein-Barr virus (EBV) infection ●*Relieving factors:* Aggressive combination chemotherapy ●*Clinical course:* Rapidly fatal (weeks to months) if untreated; 50% long-term survival with aggressive treatment ●*Co-morbidities:* HIV infection (immunodeficiency type) ●*Procedure results:* Biopsy of mass: 'starry sky' appearance of macrophages digesting tumor cells, monotonous sea of cells with oval/round nuclei and 4-5 nucleoli ●*Test findings:* Elevated lactate dehydrogenase (LDH), specific immunophenotype, genetic studies finding translocation of long arm of chromosome 8q24 t(8;14), t(2;8), t(8;22)

Burns ●*Onset:* Acute ●*Male:female ratio:* M=F ●*Ethnicity:* All ●*Character:* Erythema, pain, blisters, swelling; circumferential burns on extremities or digits may develop compartment syndrome ●*Location:* Nonspecific ●*Pattern:* Categorized as first degree (superficial), second degree (partial thickness), and third degree (full thickness) ●*Precipitating factors:* Flames, hot liquid or oil, steam, chemical or electrical exposure ●*Relieving factors:* ABCs first, oxygen, IV fluid hydration, narcotics for pain ●*Clinical course:* Dependent on extent and severity of burn ●*Co-morbidities:* Intoxication, major trauma ●*Procedure results:* No relevant procedures ●*Test findings:* Carboxyhemoglobin level: rule out carbon monoxide exposure; always estimate proportion of body surface area burned

Bursal swelling ●*Onset:* Variable ●*Male:female ratio:* M=F ●*Ethnicity:* All ●*Character:* Local tenderness, often exquisite ●*Location:* Subdeltoid, olecranon, trochanteric, prepatellar, anserine ●*Pattern:* Pain with rest or motion, with or without regional loss of active movement ●*Precipitating factors:* Obesity, local trauma, repetitive strain, direct pressure on specific joint ●*Relieving factors:* Rest, ice, elevation, anti-inflammatory medications, physical therapy ●*Clinical course:* Days to weeks, if remove precipitating agent ●*Co-morbidities:* Inflammatory joint disease; diabetes mellitus, alcohol use, immunosuppression (for olecranon) ●*Procedure results:* Bursal fluid aspiration revealing fluid itself, cell count, presence of crystals which can distinguish between different etiologies ●*Test findings:* X-ray is nondiagnostic; may show normal joint or arthritic changes

Cafe au lait spot ●*Onset:* Infancy ●*Male:female ratio:* M=F ●*Ethnicity:* Dark skin ●*Character:* Brown macule ●*Location:* Any site, mainly torso ●*Pattern:* Discrete well-circumscribed pale brown macule(s) ●*Precipitating factors:* None relevant ●*Relieving factors:* None relevant ●*Clinical course:* Variable ●*Co-morbidities:* Neurofibromatosis, Albright's syndrome ●*Procedure results:* No relevant procedures ●*Test findings:* Skin biopsy

Caffeine abuse ●*Onset:* Adolescence ●*Male:female ratio:* M=F ●*Ethnicity:* All ●*Character:* Need for caffeine as stimulant ●*Location:* Oral intake ●*Pattern:* Withdrawal symptoms without caffeine: headaches, irritation; caffeine effects: wakefulness, restlessness, decreased appetite; with severe ingestion: vomiting, seizures ●*Precipitating factors:* Prolonged caffeine intake ●*Relieving factors:* Cessation of caffeine intake ●*Clinical course:* Progressive unless stopped ●*Co-morbidities:* Other stimulant/drug usage ●*Procedure results:* No relevant procedures ●*Test findings:* No relevant tests

Callus ●*Onset:* Acquired, insidious ●*Male:female ratio:* M=F ●*Ethnicity:* All ●*Character:* Plaques of hyperkeratosis, broadbased, ill-defined, waxy/yellowish, dermatoglyphic markings become indistinct ●*Location:* Most commonly on plantar feet, overlying metatarsal heads, also on sides of arches, and heel; can occur anywhere repeated friction occurs ●*Pattern:* Can regress or progress depending on relief of friction/pressure ●*Precipitating factors:* Excessive local friction/pressure, faulty foot mechanics ●*Relieving factors:* Correction of abnormal weightbearing with the use of surgery or orthotics ●*Clinical course:* May become painful if hyperkeratosis prominent; reactive phenomenon of hyperproliferation secondary to friction ●*Co-morbidities:* Blistering seen at periphery of callus if autosomal dominant; callosity on dorsal hand may be associated with bulimia ●*Procedure results:* Biopsy reveals epidermal hyperplasia, thickened stratum corneum, prominent granular layer ●*Test findings:* No relevant tests

Campylobacter infection ●*Onset:* Acute ●*Male:female ratio:* M=F ●*Ethnicity:* All ●*Character:* >10 or more bowel movements: loose or bloody, abdominal cramping, fever (Campylobacter jejuni), relapsing fever (C. fetus), abscess formation (C. sputorum), dissemination, reactive arthritis, Guillain-Barré syndrome ●*Location:* GI tract (jejunum, ileum, colon), transient/sustained bacteremia, end-organ dissemination (gallbladder, pancreas, urinary bladder, meninges, heart, liver, other), immune complications (reactive arthritis, hemolytic-uremic syndrome, Guillain-Barré syndrome) ●*Pattern:* Panenteritis with fever and crampy abdominal pain ●*Precipitating factors:* Untreated water or dairy products, undercooked meat, farm animal contact, young pets, travel to endemic areas, clusters of infections common ●*Relieving factors:* Antibiotics early in course ●*Clinical course:* Gastroenteritis is self-limited but may persist for >1 week or relapse, prolonged course seen in AIDS and hypogammaglobulinemia, relapse and dissemination common with C. fetus, immunoreactive complications common ●*Co-morbidities:* Guillain-Barré syndrome, reactive arthritis, hemolytic-uremic syndrome, polyarthritis nodosa, Reiter's syndrome ●*Procedure results:* Fecal leukocytes and heme-positive stool, microscopic examination of stool for motile organism ●*Test findings:* Motile organism in stool examination by dark-field or phase microscopy, positive stool cultures, positive blood cultures are rare, occult blood and WBC in stool

Candida ●*Onset:* Subacute ●*Male:female ratio:* M(1):F(10) ●*Ethnicity:* All ●*Character:* Itching or burning ●*Location:* Vagina ●*Pattern:* Nonspecific ●*Precipitating factors:* Recent course of antibiotics; birth control pills; intercourse ●*Relieving factors:* Baths or creams may alleviate symptoms ●*Clinical course:* Usually will be self-limiting over days to weeks ●*Co-morbidities:* Diabetes ●*Procedure results:* Hyphae on wet preparation ●*Test findings:* Culture

Carbon monoxide poisoning ●*Onset:* Acute, subacute, chronic ●*Male:female ratio:* M=F ●*Ethnicity:* All ●*Character:* Most common: headache, dizziness, nausea, dyspnea, confusion, chest pain, palpitations; but symptoms may be very vague, and may affect any system ●*Location:* Nonspecific ●*Pattern:* Nonspecific ●*Precipitating factors:* Exposure to any carbon monoxide source: furnaces, heaters, stoves ●*Relieving factors:* 100% oxygen by mask, hyperbaric oxygen chambers ●*Clinical course:* Can cause coma and death; psychiatric and neurologic effects may be permanent ●*Co-morbidities:* Developing fetus in pregnant women and patients with pre-existing cardiac disease are most susceptible ●*Procedure results:* No relevant procedures ●*Test findings:* Carboxyhemoglobin level elevated

Carcinoid syndrome ●*Onset:* Subacute to insidious ●*Male:female ratio:* M=F ●*Ethnicity:* All ●*Character:* Facial flushing, diarrhea, abdominal cramps, bronchospasm ●*Location:* Nonspecific ●*Pattern:* Nonspecific ●*Precipitating factors:* Flushing precipitated by emotion, alcohol, eating, defecation, anesthesia ●*Relieving factors:* Somatostatin agonist (octreotide), surgical removal, chemotherapy (adjuvant) ●*Clinical course:* Depends on tumor type and stage of disease; often indolent ●*Co-morbidities:* None relevant ●*Procedure results:* No relevant procedures ●*Test findings:* Increased 24h urine 5-hydroxyindoleacetic acid (5-HIAA), positive octreotide scan

Carcinomatous meningitis ●*Onset:* Subacute/insidious ●*Male:female ratio:* M=F ●*Ethnicity:* All ●*Character:* Variable, headache, mental status changes, radiculopathy/polyradiculopathy, gait abnormality ●*Location:* Nonspecific ●*Pattern:* Nonspecific ●*Precipitating factors:* Metastatic cancer ●*Relieving factors:* Chemotherapy ●*Clinical course:* Poor ●*Co-morbidities:* None relevant ●*Procedure results:* No relevant procedures ●*Test findings:* CSF cytology study shows malignant cells

Cardiac tamponade ●*Onset:* Acute, subacute, insidious depending on etiology ●*Male:female ratio:* M=F ●*Ethnicity:* All ●*Character:* Shortness of breath, dyspnea on exertion, fatigue, light-headedness, hypotension, edema, hepatic engorgement, chest pain, elevated jugular venous pressures, distant heart sounds, pedal enema; Kussmaul sign is rare ●*Location:* Heart ●*Pattern:* The amount of pericardial fluid necessary to cause tamponade varies from 200cc if rapidly accumulated to 2000cc if slowly developing; symptoms may be present at rest and worsen with exertion ●*Precipitating factors:* Pericarditis, uremia, trauma, postcardiac surgical, infections such as tuberculosis ●*Relieving factors:* Removal of the pericardial fluid by pericardiocentesis ●*Clinical course:* If not acutely treated, can lead to pump failure, hypotension and possibly death ●*Co-morbidities:* Neoplastic diseases (i.e. lung, breast, lymphoma, leukemia, melanoma) ●*Procedure results:* Hypoxia, tachypnea; pulsus paradoxus of >10mm Hg suggestive of tamponade in the correct clinical setting ●*Test findings:* Echo: pericardial effusion with chamber compression; cardiac catheterization: equalization of pressures between the right atrial, right ventricular end-diastolic, pulmonary artery diastolic, pulmonary artery wedge pressures; ECG: electrical alternans may be present; chest X-ray: increased cardiopulmonary ratio

Cardiomyopathy ●*Onset:* Acute, subacute or insidious ●*Male:female ratio:* M=F ●*Ethnicity:* All ●*Character:* Shortness of breath, weakness, fatigue, exertional dyspnea, chest pain, orthopnea, paroxysmal nocturnal dyspnea, peripheral edema, weight gain, palpitations; symptoms depend on the classification of the cardiomyopathy (i.e. dilated, restrictive, constrictive or hypertrophic) ●*Location:* Nonspecific ●*Pattern:* Common findings in dilated cardiomyopathy: elevated neck veins, third heart sound, laterally displaced point of maximal impulse, pulmonary crackles/wheezes, pedal edema, hepatomegaly, cool extremities ●*Precipitating factors:* Fluid overload, excessive salt intake, alcohol and drug use, radiation or chemotherapy ●*Relieving factors:* For dilated cardiomyopathies, a decrease in fluid intake, salt restriction, cessation of alcohol and drug use, diuretics, vasodilator therapy; therapies for constrictive, restrictive, hypertrophic cardiomyopathies should be tailored to the underlying disease ●*Clinical course:* Generally progressive ●*Co-morbidities:* Dilated cardiomyopathy: ischemic heart disease, infections, valvular insufficiency, metabolic disorders, familial (i.e. glycogen storage diseases, hemochromatosis, Fabry's disease), nutritional deficiency, connective tissue disease (i.e. systemic lupus erythematosus, rheumatoid arthritis, dermatomyositis, systemic sclerosis), infiltrative (i.e. amyloid, sarcoid), toxic induced (i.e. alcohol, drugs, radiation) or neuromuscular (i.e. muscular dystrophy, myotonic dystrophy) in etiology; hypertrophic cardiomyopathy is familial; constrictive disease can be due to multiple etiologies affecting the pericardium; restrictive cardiomyopathy usually due to infiltrative disorders ●*Procedure results:* Decreased pulse pressure ●*Test findings:* ECG of dilated cardiomyopathy: low voltage with conduction abnormalities; chest X-ray: increased cardiopulmonary ratio and congestive heart failure; Echo: reduced ejection fraction; cardiac catheterization: elevated right and left heart cardiac filling pressures

Carotid-cavernous sinus fistula ●*Onset:* Subacute/insidious ●*Male:female ratio:* M=F ●*Ethnicity:* All ●*Character:* Headache, retro/periorbital pain, proptosis, conjunctival injection ●*Location:* Orbit/periorbital area ●*Pattern:* Variable ●*Precipitating factors:* Idiopathic; possibly head trauma ●*Relieving factors:* Endovascular surgery to embolize the connection ●*Clinical course:* Variable but usually progressive ●*Co-morbidities:* None relevant ●*Procedure results:* Cerebral angiogram shows fistula ●*Test findings:* No relevant tests

Carpal tunnel syndrome ●*Onset:* Insidious, subacute ●*Male:female ratio:* M(1):F(3-6) ●*Ethnicity:* All ●*Character:* Numbness, paresthesias, weakness, ill-defined pain in the wrist and hand ●*Location:* Thumb, index, middle, and lateral half of the ring fingers ●*Pattern:* Pain is usually worse at night; patient may massage hand for relief ●*Precipitating factors:* Occupational complication of repetitive percussion to the wrist or repetitive flexion and extension of the wrist, pregnancy, anemia, diabetes, rheumatological disorders, trauma ●*Relieving factors:* Remove etiology, wrist splints, corticosteroid injections, surgical decompression ●*Clinical course:* Good prognosis if the cause is removed or treated and the affected carpal tunnel is injected with corticosteroids or surgically decompressed ●*Co-morbidities:* Occupational complication of repetitive percussion to the wrist or repetitive flexion and extension of the wrist, pregnancy, anemia, diabetes, rheumatological disorders, trauma ●*Procedure results:* No relevant procedures ●*Test findings:* EMG reveals fibrillations in the muscles of the thenar eminence, distal latency of the median nerve is prolonged, and sensory nerve conduction velocities distal latency are prolonged

Cataract ●*Onset:* Insidious ●*Male:female ratio:* M=F ●*Ethnicity:* All ❶ *Character:* Blurred vision ●*Location:* Lens ❸ *Pattern:* Constant, painless visual loss, unilateral or bilateral ●*Precipitating factors:* None relevant ●*Relieving factors:* Glasses will improve vision when the cataract is immature ●*Clinical course:* Slowly progressive ●*Co-morbidities:* None relevant ●*Procedure results:* Lens opacity on slit lamp examination ●*Test findings:* No relevant tests

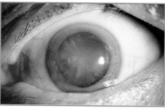

❶ *Character* White opacities in central superficial cortex and lens periphery

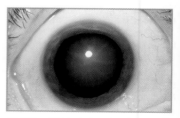

❸ *Pattern* The central, nuclear, lens opacity blends into the peripheral cortical lens

Cauda equina syndrome ●*Onset:* Acute, subacute ●*Male:female ratio:* M=F ●*Ethnicity:* All ●*Character:* Back pain, leg weakness, buttock, perineum paresthesias and numbness, urinary retention with overflow incontinence ●*Location:* Lumbosacral area ●*Pattern:* Nonspecific ●*Precipitating factors:* Penetrating spinal injury, spinal trauma, metastatic disease, infection ●*Relieving factors:* Variable, depending on etiology ●*Clinical course:* Once etiology is identified and removed, progression is arrested and return of function is poor ●*Co-morbidities:* None relevant ●*Procedure results:* No relevant procedures ●*Test findings:* MRI of the spinal cord

Cavernous hemangioma ●*Onset:* Birth ●*Male:female ratio:* M<F ●*Ethnicity:* All ●*Character:* Irregular bluish-red mass, lobulated, soft, subcutaneous ●*Location:* More often head/neck but other areas as well ●*Pattern:* Nonspecific ●*Precipitating factors:* Dilated blood vessels or sinusoidal blood spaces with endothelial cell lining ●*Relieving factors:* Usually spontaneous regression, intervention if complication (Kasabach-Merritt syndrome, ulceration) or near vital structure (eye, pharynx, auditory canal) with sclerosing agent, intralesional steroid, laser treatment; interferon treatment may help ●*Clinical course:* Present at

birth, grow rapidly in first year of life, then stationary phase followed by period of involution over 2-9 years ●*Co-morbidities:* Thrombocytopenia, Kasabach-Merritt syndrome, ulceration, infection if ulcerated ●*Procedure results:* Can be delineated by ultrasound or CT scan ●*Test findings:* No relevant tests

Cavernous sinus thrombosis ●*Onset:* Acute, subacute ●*Male:female ratio:* M=F ●*Ethnicity:* All ●*Character:* Pain, mydriasis, diplopia, noise in head, ptosis, proptosis ●*Location:* Orbit/retro-orbital ●*Pattern:* Nonspecific ●*Precipitating factors:* None relevant ●*Relieving factors:* Variable, depending on etiology ●*Clinical course:* Variable ●*Co-morbidities:* Aneurysm, infection, arteriovenous fistula ●*Procedure results:* No relevant procedures ●*Test findings:* MRI/magnetic resonance angiography of the brain, blood cultures, angiogram

Celiac disease ●*Onset:* Insidious ●*Male:female ratio:* M(2):F(3) ●*Ethnicity:* North European and Mediterranean. Rare in Asian and African-American ●*Character:* Watery diarrhea, weight loss, flatulence, fatigue, weakness ●*Location:* Intestinal ●*Pattern:* Fatigue and diarrhea are continuous; weight loss is progressive ●*Precipitating factors:* Gluten ingestion: wheat products primarily ●*Relieving factors:* Gluten-free diet ●*Clinical course:* Without dietary modification, childhood disease may remit in adolescence, then recur in adulthood; adult disease is progressive without treatment ●*Co-morbidities:* Dermatitis herpetiformis, diabetes mellitus, autoimmune thyroid disease, IgA deficiency ●*Procedure results:* Biopsy of small intestine showing blunted villi, deep crypts, intraepithelial lymphocytes ●*Test findings:* Positive antigliadin and antiendomysial antibodies. Often iron and calcium deficient

Cellulitis ●*Onset:* Acute ●*Male:female ratio:* M=F ●*Ethnicity:* All ❶ *Character:* Pain, swelling, fever ❷ *Location:* Most common: leg, face ❸ *Pattern:* Expanding red plaque ●*Precipitating factors:* Skin breakdown, venous disease ●*Relieving factors:* Antibiotics ●*Clinical course:* Resolves with treatment ●*Co-morbidities:* Stasis dermatitis; compromised venous drainage, e.g. after saphenous vein harvesting ●*Procedure results:* No relevant procedures ●*Test findings:* May have positive blood cultures

Images of ❶ *Character,* ❷ *Location,* ❸ *Pattern on page 444*

Cerebellar degeneration ●*Onset:* Subacute/insidious ●*Male:female ratio:* M=F ●*Ethnicity:* All ●*Character:* Hypotonia, asynergy, nystagmus, dysarthria, stance/gait abnormality, tremor ●*Location:* Nonspecific ●*Pattern:* Midline cerebellar abnormalities affect axial structures and lateral cerebellum control appendicular structures ●*Precipitating factors:* None relevant ●*Relieving factors:* Depends on the etiology ●*Clinical course:* Variable ●*Co-morbidities:* None relevant ●*Procedure results:* MRI/magnetic resonance angiography of the brain: paraneoplastic disorder ●*Test findings:* Genetic testing in young patients for Friedreich's ataxia/Huntington's chorea

Cerebellar hemorrhage ●*Onset:* Acute ●*Male:female ratio:* M=F ●*Ethnicity:* All ●*Character:* Headache, hypotonia, asynergy, nystagmus, dysarthria, stance/gait abnormality, tremor ●*Location:* Posterior headache and neck pain ●*Pattern:* Midline cerebellar abnormalities affect axial structures and lateraal cerebellum control appendicular structures ●*Precipitating factors:* Hypertension, vascular malformation ●*Relieving factors:* Supportive therapy; if hydrocephalus occurs, control pressure with a cerebral ventricular drain, and hyperosmotic agents, such as mannitol ●*Clinical course:* Variable ●*Co-morbidities:* None relevant ●*Procedure results:* MRI/magnetic resonance angiography of the brain ●*Test findings:* No relevant tests

Cerebral edema ●*Onset:* Acute ●*Male:female ratio:* M=F ●*Ethnicity:* All ●*Character:* Altered mental status ●*Location:* Brain ●*Pattern:* Nonspecific ●*Precipitating factors:* Trauma, hypoxia, cerebrovascular accident ●*Relieving factors:* None relevant ●*Clinical course:* Variable ●*Co-morbidities:* None relevant ●*Procedure results:* No relevant procedures ●*Test findings:* CT scan shows signs of edema

C

Cavernous sinus thrombosis • Celiac disease • Cellulitis • Cerebellar degeneration • Cerebellar hemorrhage • Cerebral edema

Cellulitis: Images *see text page 443*

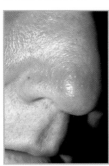

❶ *Character* Erythema and pustules on the nose

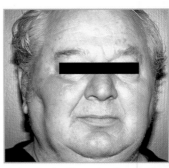

❷ *Location Swelling and erythema of the face*

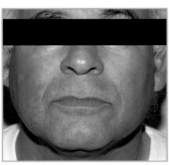

❷ *Location A red, warm, edematous plaque of acute onset on the right cheek*

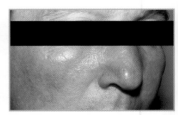

❸ *Pattern Unilateral, acute erythema is typical of cellulitis*

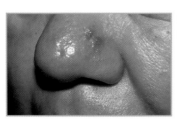

❸ *Pattern Red, warm, edematous plaque of acute onset, with crusted, oozing lesions*

Cerebral palsy ●*Onset:* Congenital/neonatal ●*Male:female ratio:* M(2):F(1) ●*Ethnicity:* All ●*Character:* Variable including: spastic hemiparesis, athetosis, dysarthria, however cognitive function frequently intact ●*Location:* Upper motor neurone lesion ●*Pattern:* Disability is usually stable, however functional achievement can be maximized by therapy ●*Precipitating factors:* Inutero insult is accepted as the most likely cause in the majority of cases ●*Relieving factors:* Intensive physical therapy, speech therapy, occupational therapy, and educational input from an early age improves functionality ●*Clinical course:* Disability is usually stable however functional achievement can be maximized by therapy ●*Co-morbidities:* Epilepsy; feeding difficulties with poor weight gain and failure to thrive; strabismus ●*Procedure results:* No relevant procedures ●*Test findings:* Abnormal reflexes in neonate with abnormal tone

Cerebrospinal fluid leak ●*Onset:* Acute ●*Male:female ratio:* M=F ●*Ethnicity:* All ●*Character:* Positional headache which is exacerbated by sitting up or standing; symptoms are improved when lying supine ●*Location:* Nonspecific ●*Pattern:* Positional headache ●*Precipitating factors:* Trauma, spontaneous ●*Relieving factors:* Blood patch, repair of dural tear, caffeine ●*Clinical course:* Overall good prognosis with treatment ●*Co-morbidities:* None relevant ●*Procedure results:* No relevant procedures ●*Test findings:* No relevant tests

Cervical disk syndrome ●*Onset:* Acute/subacute/insidious ●*Male:female ratio:* M=F ●*Ethnicity:* All ●*Character:* Aching pain in the neck and shoulder. Radicular pain in arm ●*Location:* Neck, shoulder ●*Pattern:* Nonspecific ●*Precipitating factors:* Degenerative disk disease, trauma, hyperextension injury ●*Relieving factors:* Rest, analgesics, tricyclic antidepressants ●*Clinical course:* Usually self-limited ●*Co-morbidities:* None relevant ●*Procedure results:* No relevant procedures ●*Test findings:* MRI of the cervical spine

Cervical dysplasia ●*Onset:* Insidious ●*Male:female ratio:* F ●*Ethnicity:* All ●*Character:* Asymptomatic; may be midmenstrual or postcoital bleeding ●*Location:* Nonspecific ●*Pattern:* Midmenstrual or postcoital bleeding ●*Precipitating factors:* Multiple sexual partners, unprotected intercourse leading to increased risk of human papillomavirus (HPV) infection ●*Relieving factors:* Treatment includes cryosurgery, office laser, large loop excision of transformation zone ●*Clinical course:* Very slowly progressive ●*Co-morbidities:* HPV infection, genital warts, risk of infertility increases after multiple treatments ●*Procedure results:* Colposcopy and endocervical curettage indicated for some abnormal PAPs ●*Test findings:* Abnormal PAP smear

Cervical ectropion ●*Onset:* Insidious ●*Male:female ratio:* F ●*Ethnicity:* All ●*Character:* Asymptomatic or increased nonirritating vaginal discharge (leukorrhea) ●*Location:* Nonspecific ●*Pattern:* Protusion of endocervical glandular cells onto surface of cervix ●*Precipitating factors:* Detected at birth during pregnancy and associated with oral contraceptive use ●*Relieving factors:* Resolution of hormonal changes: cessation of pregnancy, discontinuance of oral contraceptives ●*Clinical course:* Self-limited: squamous metaplasia covers columnar glandular cells ●*Co-morbidities:* None relevant ●*Procedure results:* Detected on speculum examination ●*Test findings:* PAP results: normal or benign cellular changes, e.g. squamous metaplasia

Cervical hyperextension injuries ●*Onset:* Acute ●*Male:female ratio:* M>F ●*Ethnicity:* All ●*Character:* Neck pain, dull occipital headache radiating to the bitemporal area ●*Location:* Neck ●*Pattern:* Nonspecific ●*Precipitating factors:* After sudden deceleration-acceleration usually in motor vehicle accident, cycling, fall ●*Relieving factors:* Rest, analgesics ●*Clinical course:* Depends on amount of damage to bony and ligamentous structures, nerve roots and if spinal cord is involved ●*Co-morbidities:* Cervical stenosis ●*Procedure results:* No relevant procedures ●*Test findings:* CT/MRI of the cervical spine

Cervical malignancy ●*Onset:* Insidious ●*Male:female ratio:* F ●*Ethnicity:* All ●*Character:* Vaginal bleeding; often postcoital ●*Location:* Vagina ●*Pattern:* Nonspecific ●*Precipitating factors:* Associated with human papilloma virus (HPV) infection ●*Relieving factors:* Early stage disease: surgery; later stage disease: radiotherapy ●*Clinical course:* Progresses to death if untreated ●*Co-morbidities:* Often anemia ●*Procedure results:* PAP smear and/or cervical biopsy revealing malignant cells ●*Test findings:* No relevant tests

Cervical polyp ●*Onset:* Insidious ●*Male:female ratio:* F ●*Ethnicity:* All ●*Character:* Intermenstrual bleeding, vaginal discharge ●*Location:* Nonspecific ●*Pattern:* Soft, red, friable, pedunculated lesion, usually 3-5mm ●*Precipitating factors:* None relevant ●*Relieving factors:* Removed by excision and curettage of base ●*Clinical course:* Progression to malignancy very rarely ●*Co-morbidities:* None relevant ●*Procedure results:* Detected on speculum examination ●*Test findings:* Pathology reveals benign cervical mucosa

Cervical spine injury ●*Onset:* Acute ●*Male:female ratio:* M>F ●*Ethnicity:* All ●*Character:* Neck pain, dull occipital headache radiating to the bitemporal area, weakness or paresthesias of the extremities ●*Location:* Neck ●*Pattern:* Nonspecific ●*Precipitating factors:* After sudden deceleration-acceleration usually in motor vehicle accident, cycling, fall ●*Relieving factors:* Steroids, analgesics, rest ●*Clinical course:* Depends on amount of damage to the spinal cord, bony and ligamentous structures, nerve roots, and vascular supply ●*Co-morbidities:* Carotid or vertebral dissection ●*Procedure results:* No relevant procedures ●*Test findings:* MRI of the cervical spine

Cervical spondylosis ●*Onset:* Subacute ●*Male:female ratio:* M=F ●*Ethnicity:* All ●*Character:* Spastic gait, arm weakness, muscle atrophy, hyperreflexia, increased tone, vibratory impairment, plantar extensor response in legs ●*Location:* Neurologic: extremities ●*Pattern:* Nonspecific ●*Precipitating factors:* Degenerative changes in intervertebral disk and anulus; bony osteophyte formation narrowing cervical canal ●*Relieving factors:* Soft collar, physical therapy, laminectomy ●*Clinical course:* Progressive, occasional spontaneous improvement ●*Co-morbidities:* None relevant ●*Procedure results:* Spine films show degenerative changes, osteophytes, disk space narrowed. Abnormal CT/myelography ●*Test findings:* No relevant tests

Cervicitis ●*Onset:* Subacute ●*Male:female ratio:* F ●*Ethnicity:* All ●*Character:* Asymptomatic or white/mucopurulent vaginal discharge ●*Location:* Lower abdominal discomfort or dyspareunia ●*Pattern:* Columnar eversion, nabothian cysts, friability, erythema ●*Precipitating factors:* Infection with Gardnerella, Trichomonas, Chlamydia, Candida ●*Relieving factors:* Appropriate antimicrobial treatment of patient and sexual partner ●*Clinical course:* Can progress to pelvic inflammatory disease ●*Co-morbidities:* Possible association with human papilloma virus infection ●*Procedure results:* Wet mount to detect clue cells or Trichomonas ●*Test findings:* Appropriate cultures, PAP smear to assess for dysplasia

Chagas' disease ●*Onset:* Acute infection, chronic late sequelae ●*Male:female ratio:* M=F ●*Ethnicity:* Africa ●*Character:* Early unilateral lid edema (Romana sign), indurated edematous skin at inoculation site (chagoma), late dilated cardiomyopathy, megaesophagus ●*Location:* Acute infection often asymptomatic, also: induration of inoculation site, unilateral lid edema, generalized edema, generalized lymphadenopathy and hepatosplenomegaly; meningoencephalitis, myocarditis are rare. Late (decades): dilated cardiomyopathy, cardiac arrhythmia, megaesophagus (mimicking achalasia), megacolon ●*Pattern:* Edema in early phase may be unilateral, lid edema is firm, late sequelae appear years-to-decades after primary infection ●*Precipitating factors:* Insect bite (usually reduviid or 'kissing' bug), blood transfusion, endemic in Central and South America ●*Relieving factors:* Nifurtimox or benznidazole for acute disease, symptomatic therapy for late sequelae ●*Clinical course:* Acute disease is often asymptomatic or self-limiting, chronic infection leads to symptoms in 10-30%, reactivation possible in the immunosuppressed individual ●*Co-morbidities:* None relevant ●*Procedure results:* Detection of parasite in wet- and Giemsa-stained blood and buffy coat smears (early), megacolon and megaesophagus on barium studies (late), dilated cardiomyopathy on Echo (late) ●*Test findings:* Detection of Trypanosoma cruzi in wet- and Giemsa-stained blood smears (early), T. cruzi IgG (late), new DNA and PCR-based assays

Chancroid ●*Onset:* Acute ●*Male:female ratio:* M(10):F(1) ●*Ethnicity:* More common in tropics ●*Character:* Tender nonindurated genital ulcer(s), tender inguinal adenopathy ●*Location:* Genital ulcer(s), inguinal lymph nodes, extragenital (mouth, fingers, breasts) rare ●*Pattern:* Single or multiple ulcers are tender, nonindurated, have a friable base, adenopathy is tender, usually unilateral ●*Precipitating factors:* Sexual contact, outbreaks, uncircumcised men ●*Relieving factors:* Azithromycin or ceftriaxone, aspiration of lymph nodes ●*Clinical course:* Clinical improvement within 7 days of therapy, healing complete in 2 weeks, adenitis may need aspiration ●*Co-morbidities:* HIV, syphilis, herpes simplex virus ●*Procedure results:* Large Gram-negative coccobacilli on Gram stain of ulcer base swab or lymph-node aspiration ('school of fish' pattern) ●*Test findings:* Demonstration (Gram stain) and isolation (culture) of Hemophilus ducreyi from ulcer or lymph node, PCR (polymerase chain reaction) assays

Charcot's joint ●*Onset:* Subacute ●*Male:female ratio:* M=F ●*Ethnicity:* All ●*Character:* Dull ache in affected joint area ●*Location:* Foot and ankle ●*Pattern:* Worse with use ●*Precipitating factors:* Weightbearing on affected joint ●*Relieving factors:* Casting ●*Clinical course:* Progressive loss of sensation, relaxation of supporting structure, chronic joint instability ●*Co-morbidities:* Diabetes, peripheral neuropathy, syphilis ●*Procedure results:* Plain radiographs show fractures, malalignment, and demineralization ●*Test findings:* No relevant tests

Charcot-Marie-Tooth disease ●*Onset:* Insidious ●*Male:female ratio:* M(3):F(1) ●*Ethnicity:* All ●*Character:* Peroneal muscle weakness and atrophy; patient presents with numbness or clumsiness ●*Location:* Small muscles of the hand and peroneal muscles of the calf ●*Pattern:* Chronic ●*Precipitating factors:* Autosomal dominant or autosomal recessive ●*Relieving factors:* Supportive ●*Clinical course:* Variable and depends on genetic predisposition ●*Co-morbidities:* None relevant ●*Procedure results:* Genetic testing is positive ●*Test findings:* Motor and sensory nerve conduction velocities are very slow in the peripheral nerve demyelinating type but are normal or only slightly delayed in other types

Chemical/ pesticide poisoning ●*Onset:* Acute ●*Male:female ratio:* M=F ●*Ethnicity:* All ●*Character:* Cholinergic symptoms most common: vomiting, diarrhea, urination, miosis, bradycardia, bronchospasm, salivation, muscle cramps or paralysis, diaphoresis, coma ●*Location:* Systemic ●*Pattern:* Nonspecific ●*Precipitating factors:* Exposure to organophosphate-type insecticides ●*Relieving factors:* General detoxification (remove clothing, wash skin), atropine IV, pralidoxime (2-PAM chloride) ●*Clinical course:* Varies according to exposure; heavy metals and pesticides may cause symptoms years after exposure ●*Co-morbidities:* None relevant ●*Procedure results:* No relevant procedures ●*Test findings:* Serum cholinesterase level is low in setting of poisoning

Chickenpox ●*Onset:* Acute ●*Male:female ratio:* M=F ●*Ethnicity:* All ●*Character:* Common: high fever, anorexia, malaise, vesicular skin rash, pruritus; less common (more in adults): cerebellar ataxia, encephalitis, transverse myelitis, pneumonitis, hepatitis ●*Location:* Nonspecific ●*Pattern:* Rash begins on trunk and face, spreads centripetally, crops of lesions in varying stages of evolution (macule, papule, vesicle, pustule, scab) are present ●*Precipitating factors:* Clusters of infections, more common in late winter and early spring ●*Relieving factors:* Bathing, topical antipruritic soaks, systemic therapy reserved for adolescents, adults, high-risk groups (infants, immunocompromised, bronchial dysplasia) ●*Clinical course:* Incubation 10-20 days, spontaneous recovery within 1-2 weeks in immunocompetent children; more severe in congenital disease, infants, adults, pregnant women ●*Co-morbidities:* Reye's syndrome (with aspirin ingestion) ●*Procedure results:* Interstitial pneumonitis on chest X-ray (rare) ●*Test findings:* Positive varicella IgM, positive direct fluorescent antigen of skin scraping, isolation of varicella in tissue culture (rarely needed), elevated hepatic transaminases (rare)

Child abuse ●*Onset:* Infant/toddler/adolescent ●*Male:female ratio:* M=F ●*Ethnicity:* Higher incidence in lower poverty groups ❶ *Character:* Emotional/physical ❷ *Location:* Whole body: bruises, trauma, burns, genital area ❸ *Pattern:* Injuries, trauma that are not consistent with child's developmental stage, possibly recurrent ●*Precipitating factors:* Poverty, spousal abuse, substance abuse, 'high risk' parent with 'high risk child' = prematurity, chronic medical condition, colic, child with behavior problem ●*Relieving factors:* Identification of abuse, removal of child from home, intervention by appropriate authorities: police, department of social services, appropriate counseling/therapy ●*Clinical course:* Worsening signs/symptoms without intervention/treatment ●*Co-morbidities:* Poverty, spousal abuse, substance abuse, 'high risk' parent with 'high risk child' = prematurity, chronic medical condition, colic, child with behavior problem ●*Procedure results:* Abnormal X-rays consistent with abuse: multiple healing fractures in otherwise healthy child, unlikely sites of fractures: rib, scapular, distal clavicle in prewalking child ●*Test findings:* Normal screening tests: prothrombin time, partial thromboplastin time, CBC to rule out bleeding disorder

Images of ❶ *Character,* ❷ *Location,* ❸ *Pattern on page 448*

C

Child abuse: Images *see text page 447*

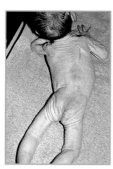

❶ *Character* Malnutrition from severe neglect

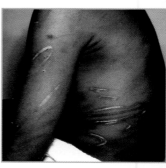

❷ *Location* Scars left from beating with a looped electrical cord

❸ *Pattern* Perineal burns from being set in scalding water

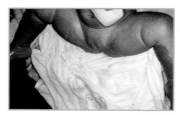

Childhood idiopathic immune thrombocytopenia ●*Onset:* Acute ●*Male:female ratio:* M=F ●*Ethnicity:* All ●*Character:* Sudden appearance of purpura and ecchymoses, mucocutaneous bleeding, no other systemic symptoms ●*Location:* Bleeding is usually mucocutaneous: epistaxis, gastrointestinal ●*Pattern:* Nonspecific ●*Precipitating factors:* Antiplatelet medications can worsen the symptoms, up to 80% of children have a preceding infection or vaccination ●*Relieving factors:* Usually spontaneously resolves, if severe bleeding: steroids, IVIG, IV anti-D immunoglobulin ●*Clinical course:* The majority of patients recover, a small percentage will have recurrent disease ●*Co-morbidities:* None relevant ●*Procedure results:* Bone marrow biopsy (unnecessary if typical presentation): normal appearance with increased erythroid and myeloid precursors and large megakaryocytes ●*Test findings:* Platelets usually <20,000, large platelets, otherwise normal laboratory tests

Chlamydia pneumoniae ●*Onset:* Acute, subacute ●*Male:female ratio:* M>F ●*Ethnicity:* All ●*Character:* Febrile illness with severe sore throat, hoarseness, cough, cervical adenopathy ●*Location:* Fever, pharynx, larynx, bronchi, lung, sinuses, other ●*Pattern:* Nonspecific ●*Precipitating factors:* None relevant ●*Relieving factors:* None relevant ●*Clinical course:* Incubation: 21 days, gradual onset, prolonged duration (weeks) even with antibiotic therapy ●*Co-morbidities:* None relevant ●*Procedure results:* Infiltrate on chest X-ray in some cases (diagnostic acute and convalescent specific IgG and IgM, pharyngeal swab for PCR or culture) ●*Test findings:* Normal-mildly elevated WBC

Chlamydia trachomatis infection ●*Onset:* Acute, subacute, chronic ●*Male:female ratio:* M=F ●*Ethnicity:* All ●*Character:* Asymptomatic most common; symptomatic: dysuria, clear/mucoid penile discharge (nongonococcal urethritis) in men, mucopurulent cervical discharge and cervical motion tenderness in women, mucoid rectal discharge; long-term sequelae: infertility, chronic pelvic pain; in neonates: conjunctivitis, pneumonitis ●*Location:* Women: cervix, fallopian tubes, uterus, adnexa, perihepatic, vagina, Bartholin cysts, other; men: urethra, rectum, epididymis, prostate, other; neonates: eye, lungs ●*Pattern:* Women: persistent mucopurulent cervical discharge and dyspareunia; men: persistent dysuria ●*Precipitating factors:* Sexual transmission, adolescents ●*Relieving factors:* None relevant ●*Clinical course:* Most commonly asymptomatic; can persist for months-years; can lead to infertility, chronic pain in women ●*Co-morbidities:* Reiter's syndrome, pelvic inflammatory disease, infertility, gonorrhea, syphilis, genital herpes, HIV, other STD ●*Procedure results:* WBC in urine sediment or cervical wet mount (Chlamydia trachomatis DNA in cervical/urethral swab/male urine, growth of C. trachomatis on specimen for other sites) ●*Test findings:* WBC observed in cervical discharge; cervical urethral, male urine, other site, swab for C. trachomatis DNA (probe, ligase chain reaction (LCR), PCR, other); rectum, other site, swab for tissue culture of C. trachomatis

Chlamydial conjunctivitis ●*Onset:* Subacute ●*Male:female ratio:* M=F ●*Ethnicity:* All ●*Character:* Scant mucoid discharge; ocular redness ●*Location:* Typically both eyes involved but can be unilateral ●*Pattern:* Variable degrees of disease severity can be seen that persist for months if untreated ●*Precipitating factors:* Hand to eye or ocular-genital contact with infected secretions ●*Relieving factors:* Antibiotics; artificial tears can relieve associated ocular discomfort ●*Clinical course:* Long protracted course with occasional corneal changes that almost never are visually significant; ultimately self-limited ●*Co-morbidities:* Sexually transmitted chlamydial diseases; in neonates, association with chlamydial pneumonitis ●*Procedure results:* No relevant procedures ●*Test findings:* Positive amplified gene probe test from conjunctival swab sample (detects chlamydial rRNA). Giemsa stain of conjunctiva reveals basophilic inclusion bodies in conjunctival epithelial cells

Chloasma ●*Onset:* Subacute ●*Male:female ratio:* M<F ●*Ethnicity:* Dark skin ●*Character:* Hyperpigmentation ●*Location:* Sunexposed, mainly face ●*Pattern:* Brown macules ●*Precipitating factors:* Pregnancy, sun exposure ●*Relieving factors:* Sun block, hydroquinones ●*Clinical course:* May persist postpartum ●*Co-morbidities:* None relevant ●*Procedure results:* No relevant procedures ●*Test findings:* No relevant tests

Choanal atresia ●*Onset:* Congenital ●*Male:female ratio:* M(1):F(2) ●*Ethnicity:* All ●*Character:* Nasal obstruction; purulent nasal discharge ●*Location:* Nasal cavity ●*Pattern:* Chronic ●*Precipitating factors:* None relevant ●*Relieving factors:* None relevant ●*Clinical course:* Symptoms persist until obstruction is corrected with surgery ●*Co-morbidities:* None relevant ●*Procedure results:* Inability to pass small nasogastric tube through either nasal cavity into the oropharynx ●*Test findings:* CT scan shows bony or membranous choanal obstruction with atresia plate

Cholecystitis ●*Onset:* Acute ●*Male:female ratio:* M(1):F(2) ●*Ethnicity:* All ●*Character:* Epigastric and right upper quadrant (RUQ) pain and tenderness, with fever and leukocytosis; Murphy's sign often present ●*Location:* Epigastrium and RUQ; pain may radiate to the back (under right scapula) ●*Pattern:* Nonspecific ●*Precipitating factors:* None relevant ●*Relieving factors:* Analgesics, antipyretics to relieve symptoms; cholecystectomy is curative ●*Clinical course:* Lasts hours-to-days, may be self-limited ●*Co-morbidities:* Gallstones or gallbladder sludge ●*Procedure results:* HIDA scan shows non-filling of gallbladder; U/S may show gallbladder wall thickening, pericholecystic fluid, gallstones ●*Test findings:* WBC usually elevated, liver function tests may be mildly elevated

Cholera ●*Onset:* Acute ●*Male:female ratio:* M=F ●*Ethnicity:* Common in developing countries ●*Character:* Painless, voluminous, watery diarrhea, followed by vomiting, muscle cramps (hypokalemia), postural dizziness ●*Location:* Small bowel, systemic (hypovolemia), kidney (secondary to hypovolemic shock) ●*Pattern:* 'Rice-water' stool (gray, cloudy, no blood), voluminous diarrhea, hypovolemic shock ●*Precipitating factors:* Residence in/travel to Latin America, Africa or Asia and ingestion of contaminated water/food; in the US, undercooked shellfish from the Gulf of Mexico ●*Relieving factors:* Rehydration (oral rehydration solution, IV fluids) and electrolyte replacement (most important) ●*Clinical course:* Variable ●*Co-morbidities:* None relevant ●*Procedure results:* Visualization of Vibrio by dark-field microscopy on a wet mount of fresh stool ●*Test findings:* Elevated hematocrit (hemoconcentration), mild neutrophilic leukocytosis, elevated blood urea nitrogen, elevated creatinine, low bicarbonate, high anion-gap acidosis, stool wet mount (dark-field microscope), stool culture

Cholesteatoma ●*Onset:* May be congenital, acute or chronic ●*Male:female ratio:* M=F ●*Ethnicity:* All ●*Character:* Ear drainage, ear fullness, hearing loss, dizziness, facial weakness ●*Location:* Extends from tympanic membrane into middle ear, possibly into bone, mastoid ●*Pattern:* Nonspecific ●*Precipitating factors:* Chronic infection, trauma, eustachian tube dysfunction ●*Relieving factors:* Antibiotics, ear cleaning, ear drops, surgery ●*Clinical course:* Intermittent drainage with signs/symptoms of infection and hearing loss; if untreated, bone destruction, deafness, facial nerve paralysis, dizziness, abscess, systemic infection, death ●*Co-morbidities:* Chronic middle ear infection, eustachian tube dysfunction ●*Procedure results:* Audiogram: conductive (and possible sensorineural) hearing loss; CT: extent of spread ●*Test findings:* No relevant tests

Cholesterol emboli ●*Onset:* Acute, subacute ●*Male:female ratio:* M>F ●*Ethnicity:* All ●*Character:* Pain, ulceration, gangrene ●*Location:* Distal digits, distal organs, kidneys ●*Pattern:* Livedo reticularis, ulceration, gangrene, cyanosis, preserved pulses ●*Precipitating factors:* Age, hypertension, hyperlipidemia, atherosclerosis, diabetes mellitus, peripheral vascular disease, instrumentation of the aorta, warfarin therapy ●*Relieving factors:* Stop anticoagulation ●*Clinical course:* Progressive with mortality approaching 40-80% ●*Co-morbidities:* Hypertension, diabetes mellitus, hyperlipidemia, atherosclerosis, peripheral vascular disease, carotid disease ●*Procedure results:* Biopsy shows needle-shaped clefts in arteriolar lumens in paraffin-fixed sections ●*Test findings:* Acute nonoliguric renal failure with increased creatinine, increased eosinophils, increased ESR, decreased complement levels

Chondromalacia patellae (patellofemoral pain syndrome) ●*Onset:* Insidious ●*Male:female ratio:* M=F ●*Ethnicity:* All ●*Character:* Dull ache ●*Location:* Anterior knee ●*Pattern:* Pain worst with first step ●*Precipitating factors:* Immobility or walking on a down slope ●*Relieving factors:* NSAIDs, strengthening of vastus medialis, physical therapy ●*Clinical course:* Gradual improvement ●*Co-morbidities:* Obesity ●*Procedure results:* Plain radiographs are normal ●*Test findings:* No relevant tests

Chorea ●*Onset:* Subacute/acute ●*Male:female ratio:* M=F ●*Ethnicity:* All ●*Character:* Abrupt, spasmodic, irregular movements of short duration ●*Location:* Fingers, hands, arms, face, tongue or head ●*Pattern:* Nonspecific ●*Precipitating factors:* Idiopathic, group A beta-hemolytic streptococci infection, pregnancy, benign hereditary chorea, Huntington's, Wilson's, familial calcification of the basal ganglia, stroke within the basal ganglia, medication (lithium, phenytoin, carbamazepine, amphetamines) ●*Relieving factors:* Treat underlying etiology; in some cases, haloperidol ●*Clinical course:* Variable depending on etiology ●*Co-morbidities:* None relevant ●*Procedure results:* The following tests may be useful to evaluate the underlying disorder: MRI of the brain, lumbar puncture, toxicology screen, genetic testing, liver function tests ●*Test findings:* Liver function tests

Chorioretinitis ●*Onset:* Acute/subacute/insidious ●*Male:female ratio:* M=F ●*Ethnicity:* All ●*Character:* Blurred vision; occasionally ocular pain ●*Location:* Uniocular; occasionally both eyes ●*Pattern:* Nonspecific ●*Precipitating factors:* Immunocompromised state contributes to some forms of chorioretinitis ●*Relieving factors:* Appropriate treatment directed at the cause ●*Clinical course:* Progresses slowly or rapidly without treatment ●*Co-morbidities:* Candidiasis and other fungal infections; sarcoidosis; toxoplasmosis ●*Procedure results:* Indirect ophthalmoscopic examination shows lesions in the retina and choroid ●*Test findings:* No relevant tests

Chronic allergic alveolitis ●*Onset:* Insidious ●*Male:female ratio:* M=F ●*Ethnicity:* All ●*Character:* Cough, dyspnea, fatigue, anorexia, weight loss ●*Location:* Respiratory: tachypnea, rales, digital clubbing in advanced cases ●*Pattern:* History of acute episodes lacking; cough and dyspnea without wheezing ●*Precipitating factors:* Exposure to inciting agents including agricultural dusts, bioaerosols, micro-organisms including fungal, bacterial or protozoal, certain reactive chemicals ●*Relieving factors:* Antigen avoidance; corticosteroids ●*Clinical course:* Reversible if detected and treated early; progressive irreversible pulmonary fibrosis in advanced cases ●*Co-morbidities:* Emphysema without history of smoking or other occupational exposure in 15% cases ●*Procedure results:* Bronchoalveolar lavage: lymphocytosis; biopsy results: granulomatous pneumonitis, interstitial pneumonitis, bronchiolitis obliterans, dense fibrosis ●*Test findings:* Pulmonary function tests: moderate-to-severe restrictive defect, reduced diffusing capacity; chest X-ray may be normal or show fibrosis with loss of lung volumes

Chronic bullous dermatosis ●*Onset:* Subacute ●*Male:female ratio:* M<F ●*Ethnicity:* All ●*Character:* Occurs after puberty, with most cases in fourth decade; combinations of grouped papules, vesicles and bullae, often crusted due to excoriations; can have mucosal changes as well ●*Location:* Symmetrically distributed on the extensor aspects of extremities (elbows, knees, buttocks) ●*Pattern:* Begin as erythematous papules and vesicles, and can present with tense bullae, often present as a 'string of pearls' around previously regressing lesion ●*Precipitating factors:* Vancomycin administration, lithium, diclofenac, lymphoid and nonlymphoid malignancies ●*Relieving factors:* Discontinue inciting drug; dapsone or sulfapyridine ●*Clinical course:* Self-limited disease, remission in 2 years; is milder if persistent into puberty ●*Co-morbidities:* Rare reports of gluten-sensitive enteropathy (like in dermatitis herpetiformis) ●*Procedure results:* Biopsy reveals subepidermal bulla with presence of a mixed inflammatory infiltrate; immunofluorescence reveals linear dermoepidermal junction staining with IgA ●*Test findings:* No relevant tests

Chronic fatigue syndrome ●*Onset:* Insidious ●*Male:female ratio:* M<F (slightly) ●*Ethnicity:* All ●*Character:* Fatigue ●*Location:* Polyarticular including elbows, shoulders, hips, knees ●*Pattern:* Nonspecific ●*Precipitating factors:* Exercise ●*Relieving factors:* NSAIDs, tricyclic antidepressants, SSRI antidepressants ●*Clinical course:* Self-limited ●*Co-morbidities:* Associated sleep disorders and headaches ●*Procedure results:* No relevant procedures ●*Test findings:* Normal laboratory examination

Chronic idiopathic neutropenia ●*Onset:* Insidious ●*Male:female ratio:* M=F ●*Ethnicity:* All ●*Character:* Generally asymptomatic ●*Location:* Nonspecific ●*Pattern:* Nonspecific ●*Precipitating factors:* Possibly drug- or immune-related ●*Relieving factors:* None relevant ●*Clinical course:* Usually persists for many years with a benign course ●*Co-morbidities:* None relevant ●*Procedure results:* Bone marrow biopsy: plentiful early myeloid precursors but reduced numbers of late metamyelocytes and mature granulocytes ●*Test findings:* Absolute neutrophil counts below 2000 per mcL

Chronic infection ●*Onset:* Chronic ●*Male:female ratio:* M=F ●*Ethnicity:* All ●*Character:* Prolonged fever, night sweats, weight loss, fatigue, wasting ●*Location:* Any organ or organ system ●*Pattern:* Drenching night sweats, involuntary weight loss, wasting, cachexia ●*Precipitating factors:* Travel, pets, abnormal heart valves, ill contacts, prosthetic devices; sometimes no factor identifiable ●*Relieving factors:* NSAIDs, acetaminophen provides temporary relief ●*Clinical course:* Slow progressive in most cases, self-limiting for some ●*Co-morbidities:* None relevant ●*Procedure results:* No relevant procedures ●*Test findings:* Elevated ESR, elevated platelet count

Chronic lead poisoning ●*Onset:* Chronic, encephalopathy acute ●*Male:female ratio:* M=F ●*Ethnicity:* All (urban poor) ●*Character:* Chronic abdominal pain, constipation ●*Location:* Nonspecific ●*Pattern:* Nonspecific ●*Precipitating factors:* Exposure to lead in old home (old paint) or other source ●*Relieving factors:* None relevant ●*Clinical course:* Progresses until treatment or removal from lead source ●*Co-morbidities:* Iron deficiency anemia, pica ●*Procedure results:* Lead lines on X-rays of distal femur, proximal tibia and fibula ●*Test findings:* High serum lead; microcytic anemia, basophilic stippling of RBCs

Chronic lymphadenitis ●*Onset:* Subacute or chronic ●*Male:female ratio:* M=F ●*Ethnicity:* All ●*Character:* Painful or painless swelling of a solitary lymph node, or group of nodes in one site (regional lymphadenitis), or several sites (generalized lymphadenitis) ●*Location:* A solitary lymph node, or group of nodes in one site (regional lymphadenitis), or several sites (generalized lymphadenitis) ●*Pattern:* Painful or painless swelling of lymph nodes of >several weeks duration ●*Precipitating factors:* Exposure to infection, travel, tick or animal bite ●*Relieving factors:* None relevant ●*Clinical course:* Depending on etiology may be self-limiting, persistent, or progressive; some may cause draining sinus tracts ●*Co-morbidities:* Chronic dermatitis, mycobacterial (e.g. TB), bacterial, fungal, or parasitic (e.g. toxoplasmosis) infections; HIV, lymphoproliferative disorder, STDs, autoimmune diseases (e.g. systemic lupus erythematosus) ●*Procedure results:* Lymph node biopsy showing chronic inflammatory changes (proliferation, hyperplasia, prominent germinal centres, mononuclear cells); may find caseating or non-caseating granulomata; may grow organism ●*Test findings:* Elevated ESR

Chronic lymphocytic leukemia ●*Onset:* Insidious ●*Male:female ratio:* M(2):F(1) ●*Ethnicity:* Rare in Chinese and related races ●*Character:* Fatigue, lymphadenopathy, can be asymptomatic ●*Location:* Nonspecific ●*Pattern:* Nonspecific ●*Precipitating factors:* None relevant ●*Relieving factors:* No treatment unless symptoms or progressive disease, then chemotherapy ●*Clinical course:* 25% >10-year survival, median survival 6 years, 5% develop Richter's syndrome (large cell lymphoma) with poor prognosis ●*Co-morbidities:* Autoimmune hemolytic anemia or thrombocytopenia ●*Procedure results:* Lymph node biopsy: positive for malignant cells ●*Test findings:* Elevated WBC, lymphocytosis (mature cells)

Chronic myelogenous leukemia ●*Onset:* Insidious, rarely acute ●*Male:female ratio:* M(1.3):F(1) ●*Ethnicity:* All ●*Character:* Fatigue, weight loss, fever, night sweats, abdominal fullness, bone pain, rarely blurry vision, pulmonary distress or priapism; if blast crisis, bleeding or infection ●*Location:* Nonspecific ●*Pattern:* Nonspecific ●*Precipitating factors:* None relevant ●*Relieving factors:* Hydroxyurea, alpha-interferon, bone marrow transplant and/or intensive chemotherapy for blast crisis ●*Clinical course:* Stable for years then transformation to acute leukemia, invariably fatal unless successful bone marrow transplant (60% cure) ●*Co-morbidities:* None relevant ●*Procedure results:* Bone marrow biopsy: hypercellular with marked left shift, blasts <5% ●*Test findings:* Increased WBC (usually >50,000), mature myeloid series with left shift, decreased leukosyte alkaline phosphotase, increased vitamin B12, increased uric acid, Philadelphia chromosome on cytogenetics

Chronic obstructive pulmonary disease ●*Onset:* Insidious ●*Male:female ratio:* M>F ●*Ethnicity:* All ●*Character:* Cough with phlegm (>1tbsp) daily for 2 or more months, 2 or more consecutive years, dyspnea ●*Location:* Chest ●*Pattern:* Morning worse than evening, dyspnea with exertion ●*Precipitating factors:* Tobacco, alpha-1 antitrypsin deficiency ●*Relieving factors:* Ipratropium, albuterol, salmeterol with or without theophylline, steroids, supplemental oxygen as needed; if severely decreased lung function: lung volume reduction surgery, transplant or bullectomy; pulmonary rehabilitation ●*Clinical course:* Progressive: can be slowed with smoking cessation and by preventing respiratory infections, hypoxemia and cor pulmonale ●*Co-morbidities:* Tobacco-related disorders, including coronary artery disease, atherosclerosis, malignancy plus sleep-disordered breathing ●*Procedure results:* No relevant procedures ●*Test findings:* Chest X-ray: hyperinflation, peribronchial cuffing; pulmonary function tests - obstructive ventilatory defect with decreased diffusion capacity of the lungs for carbon monoxide (DLCO)

Chronic otitis media ●*Onset:* Chronic ●*Male:female ratio:* M>F ●*Ethnicity:* All ●*Character:* Recurrent or persistent otorrhea with tympanic membrane perforation ●*Location:* Affected ear ●*Pattern:* Mucopurulent discharge, often foul-smelling ●*Precipitating factors:* None relevant ●*Relieving factors:* None relevant ●*Clinical course:* May be active for weeks-to-years with otorrhea as only symptom ●*Co-morbidities:* Cleft palate; eustachian tube dysfunction; tympanic membrane perforation; history of ear surgery ●*Procedure results:* Purulent discharge through tympanic membrane perforation on otoscopy ●*Test findings:* CT scan of ear may reveal mastoid opacification, cholesteatoma, bone erosion

Chronic pain disorder ●*Onset:* Subacute/insidious ●*Male:female ratio:* M=F ●*Ethnicity:* All ●*Character:* Pain persisting 1 month beyond usual course of an acute illness or injury, associated with chronic pathologic process or recurs at intervals of months or years ●*Location:* Variable ●*Pattern:* Variable: burning, shooting, lancinating ●*Precipitating factors:* Usually minor trauma ●*Relieving factors:* Variable: analgesics, sympathetic blockade, pain modulation with tricyclic antidepressants, psychological support ●*Clinical course:* Variable ●*Co-morbidities:* Depression, increased social stressors ●*Procedure results:* No relevant procedures ●*Test findings:* No relevant tests

Chronic renal failure ●*Onset:* Acute, subacute ●*Male:female ratio:* M=F ●*Ethnicity:* More common in African-Americans ●*Character:* Long-standing, irreversible impairment of renal function ●*Location:* Most causes of chronic renal failure are due to intrinsic renal disease including both glomerular and interstitial etiologies ●*Pattern:* Symptoms of uremia include anorexia, weight loss, dyspnea, fatigue, pruritus, sleep and taste disturbance, encephalopathy; physical findings: pericardial and pleural friction rub, muscle wasting, asterixis, excoriations/ecchymoses ●*Precipitating factors:* Diabetes, HIV, multiple myeloma, hypertension, glomerulonephritis, polycystic kidney disease, reflux nephropathy and other congenital disorders, interstitial nephritis especially due to analgesics ●*Relieving factors:* Aggressive treatment of hypertension can slowly progress to end-stage renal disease (ESRD); ACE inhibitors indicated in diabetic nephropathy; anemia treated with erythropoietin; dietary restriction of phosphate, potassium; dialysis for ESRD ●*Clinical course:* Gradual decline of renal function over months-to-years depending on underlying etiology ●*Co-morbidities:* Secondary hyperparathyroidism; amyloidosis; systemic lupus erythematosus ●*Procedure results:* Renal biopsy usually reveals glomerulosclerosis or interstitial fibrosis; renal U/S used to determine kidney size ●*Test findings:* Laboratory abnormalities include hyperkalemia, hyperphosphatemia, metabolic acidosis, hypocalcemia, hyperuricemia, anemia, hypoalbuminemia

Chronic sinusitis ●*Onset:* Insidious ●*Male:female ratio:* M=F ●*Ethnicity:* All ●*Character:* Dull pain and pressure over affected sinuses; purulent rhinorrhea; nasal congestion ●*Location:* Periorbital, facial ●*Pattern:* Symptoms persistent >3 months ●*Precipitating factors:* Allergy; nasal polyps ●*Relieving factors:* Topical or oral decongestants ●*Clinical course:* Chronic or chronic recurrent ●*Co-morbidities:* Allergy; nasal polyps ●*Procedure results:* Rhinoscopy may reveal pus, polyps, congestion; sinus CT: sinus outflow obstruction, mucosal thickening, air fluid levels ●*Test findings:* No relevant tests

Chronic tophaceous gout ●*Onset:* Insidious ●*Male:female ratio:* M(20):F(1) ●*Ethnicity:* All ●*Character:* Chronic dull joint pain; gouty tophi (subcutaneous nodules) ●*Location:* First metatarsophalangeal joint, wrist, metacarpophalangeal joints ●*Pattern:* Nonspecific ●*Precipitating factors:* Alcohol, diuretics, low-dose aspirin ●*Relieving factors:* Antihyperuricemic therapy (usually allopurinol) ●*Clinical course:* Recurrent acute attacks; if untreated, significant joint damage; good prognosis with antihyperuricemic therapy ●*Co-morbidities:* Hypertension, renal failure, obesity, hypothyroidism, hyperparathyroidism, hyperlipidemia, alcoholism, high cell turnover states (e.g. psoriasis, polycythemia) ●*Procedure results:* Periarticular joint erosions on plain film ●*Test findings:* High uric acid; negatively birefringent crystals (monosodium urate) on polarized microscopy of tophus aspiration

Chronic vibration exposure ●*Onset:* Insidious ●*Male:female ratio:* M(2):F(1) ●*Ethnicity:* All ●*Character:* Numbness and cold digits ●*Location:* Fingers and arms ●*Pattern:* Worse with vibratory stimulus ●*Precipitating factors:* Vibration, cold, wrist flexion ●*Relieving factors:* Removing vibratory stimulus and other vasoconstrictors (e.g. tobacco) ●*Clinical course:* Chronic, slowly progressive ●*Co-morbidities:* Tobacco use ●*Procedure results:* No relevant procedures ●*Test findings:* Electrodiagnostic tests with slowing of nerve conduction; cold water immersion test with vasospasm

Classic congenital adrenal hyperplasia ●*Onset:* Acute (adrenal crisis) or subacute (failure to thrive) ●*Male:female ratio:* M=F ●*Ethnicity:* All ●*Character:* Ambiguous genitalia in females, salt-wasting, dehydration in both sexes, accelerated growth and virilization in childhood; both nausea and vomiting, hyperpigmentation ●*Location:* Ambiguous genitalia in females ●*Pattern:* Nonspecific ●*Precipitating factors:* >90% of cases genetic: most common 21-hydroxylase deficiency ●*Relieving factors:* Hydration and glucocorticoids/mineralocorticoid; vaginal reconstructive surgery; if diagnosed inutero, dexamethasone prenatally to decrease virilization ●*Clinical course:* Progressive ●*Co-morbidities:* Hypertension with 11-b hydroxylase deficiency; infertility and short stature with inadequate treatment of all types ●*Procedure results:* Genotyping can be done; genetic counseling when considering pregnancy ●*Test findings:* Hyperkalemia, acidosis, hyponatremia, elevated urinary 17-ketosteroids for most common form, 21-hydroxylase, diagnosis is elevated 17-hydroxyprogesterone. For 11 beta-hydroxylase, diagnosis is elevated 11-deoxycortisol

Cluster headache ●*Onset:* Acute ●*Male:female ratio:* M(6):F(1) ●*Ethnicity:* All ●*Character:* Stabbing retro-orbital pain, lacrimation, nasal stuffiness, Horner's syndrome ●*Location:* Retro-orbital ●*Pattern:* Occurs in clusters; 3-5 times per day lasting a few minutes to hours ●*Precipitating factors:* None relevant ●*Relieving factors:* Oxygen therapy, calcium channel blockers, prednisone, lithium ●*Clinical course:* Variable ●*Co-morbidities:* None relevant ●*Procedure results:* No relevant procedures ●*Test findings:* Normal neurological examination

Coarctation of the aorta ●*Onset:* Birth; acute or asymptomatic ●*Male:female ratio:* M(1.7):F(1) ●*Ethnicity:* All ●*Character:* Weak/absent femoral pulses ●*Location:* Upper left sternal border heart murmur ●*Pattern:* Hypertension in otherwise well child ●*Precipitating factors:* Patent ductus arteriosus closes if duct-dependent ●*Relieving factors:* Prostaglandin if duct-dependent ●*Clinical course:* Progresses to hypertension if untreated and congestive heart failure ●*Co-morbidities:* Cardiac defects, Turner's syndrome ●*Procedure results:* Echo, ECG with left ventricular hypertrophy ●*Test findings:* Decreased or absent femoral pulses

Colic ●*Onset:* Age 3 weeks/acute ●*Male:female ratio:* M=F ●*Ethnicity:* All ●*Character:* Crying all evening in thriving infant ●*Location:* Nonspecific ●*Pattern:* Best in a.m., worse in p.m. ●*Precipitating factors:* Overstimulation worsens ●*Relieving factors:* Darkness, rhythmic activities, sounds, car rides, being held ●*Clinical course:* Lasts until 3 months of age; self-limiting ●*Co-morbidities:* None relevant ●*Procedure results:* All negative ●*Test findings:* Normal laboratory results

Collagen vascular disease ●*Onset:* Subacute; can be acute involving one organ system ●*Male:female ratio:* M<F ●*Ethnicity:* Typically Caucasian females ●*Character:* Cutaneous manifestations range from prominent telangiectasia (face, periungual), erythema with scaling (occasionally annular plaques), butterfly erythema, scarring alopecia, photosensitivity and sclerosis/Raynaud's phenomenon ●*Location:* Photodistributed; acral and periungual; upper trunk ●*Pattern:* Cutaneous lesions remit and recur with disease activity and sometimes parallel light exposure and rising antibody titers ●*Precipitating factors:* Sunlight, extreme cold ●*Relieving factors:* Photoprotection (including ultraviolet A); treatment with systemic steroids or steroid-sparing immunosuppressive agents ●*Clinical course:* Variable depending on specific disease entity; most collagen vascular disease responsive to immunesuppressive therapy, if treatment initiated prior to end-organ damage ●*Co-morbidities:* Paraneoplastic etiology in large number of dermatomyositic patients, swallowing disorder in progressive systemic sclerosis, bone marrow and renal failure in systemic lupus erythematosus (SLE) ●*Procedure results:* Biopsy reveals a lichenoid infiltrate with vacuolar interface dermatitis, and mucin present in the dermis ●*Test findings:* Wide range of serologic tests available that help narrow the diagnosis; antinuclear antigen (ANA) is positive at 1:40 titer in up to one-third of the US population

Collateral ligament sprain ●*Onset:* Acute ●*Male:female ratio:* M=F ●*Ethnicity:* All ●*Character:* Pain, swelling, or tenderness of ligament following injury to fingers or knee ●*Location:* Nonspecific ●*Pattern:* Nonspecific ●*Precipitating factors:* Acute stress of ligament ●*Relieving factors:* Splinting injured joint, anti-inflammatories for pain; complete ruptures usually require surgical repair ●*Clinical course:* Resolution in time is the norm although loss of function may result after severe sprain or rupture ●*Co-morbidities:* None relevant ●*Procedure results:* Radiographs to rule out associated fracture ●*Test findings:* Laxity on stress examination of the ligament indicates partial or complete rupture

Colles' fracture ●*Onset:* Acute ●*Male:female ratio:* M=F ●*Ethnicity:* All ●*Character:* Pain, swelling, or tenderness of distal forearm following injury ●*Location:* Distal forearm ●*Pattern:* Nonspecific ●*Precipitating factors:* Injury follows a fall on outstretched hand ●*Relieving factors:* Stabilization; in significantly displaced or angulated fractures, reduction followed by immobilization in splint or cast ●*Clinical course:* Some restriction in range of movement may persist after injury has healed, but overall good return of function ●*Co-morbidities:* None relevant ●*Procedure results:* Radiographs reveal distal radius fracture with dorsal displacement of distal fragment; ulnar styloid fracture present in 60% of cases ●*Test findings:* No relevant tests

Coloboma ●*Onset:* Congenital defect ●*Male:female ratio:* M=F ●*Ethnicity:* All ●*Character:* Blurred vision but sometimes asymptomatic ●*Location:* Almost always uniocular ●*Pattern:* Nonspecific ●*Precipitating factors:* None relevant ●*Relieving factors:* None relevant ●*Clinical course:* Not progressive; occasionally delayed onset retinal detachment ●*Co-morbidities:* Multiple chromosomal abnormalities; coloboma, heart disease, atresia choanae, retarded growth and retarded development (and/or CNS anomalies), genital hypoplasia, and ear anomalies and/or deafness (CHARGE) association; other multisystem disorders ●*Procedure results:* Comprehensive ophthalmic examination ●*Test findings:* Evidence of faulty development of ocular tissue along fetal fissure

Colon cancer ●*Onset:* Insidious ●*Male:female ratio:* M=F ●*Ethnicity:* All ●*Character:* Long asymptomatic period: may present as guaiac positive stools and/or iron deficiency anemia; lower GI bleeding may occur, obstructive symptoms include constipation, decreased stool caliber, colicky abdominal pain; postobstructive diarrhea may be seen; eventually anorexia and weight loss ●*Location:* Abdominal pain may be any location, but often hypogastric ●*Pattern:* Pain may worsen after meals if lesion is near-obstructing ●*Precipitating factors:* Meals in some cases ●*Relieving factors:* Tumor resection alleviates symptoms and may be curative in early lesions; chemotherapy may improve survival; radiotherapy in some cases ●*Clinical course:* Not self-limited; once symptomatic, usually progresses over months, with metastases and death ●*Co-morbidities:* Colonic polyps; hereditary polyposis syndromes (familial adenomatous polyposis [FAP], Gardner's); hereditary nonpolyposis colon cancer; inflammatory bowel disease (increased risk of colon cancer after 8-10 years) ●*Procedure results:* Colonoscopy reveals tumor; biopsy is diagnostic ●*Test findings:* Often iron-deficiency anemia

Colonic polyp ●*Onset:* Insidious growth of polyps over years, though symptoms can arise subacutely ●*Male:female ratio:* M=F ●*Ethnicity:* All ●*Character:* Usually asymptomatic; can have bleeding, constipation, change in stool caliber, bowel obstruction ●*Location:* Nonspecific ●*Pattern:* Nonspecific ●*Precipitating factors:* Family history of polyps or hereditary polyp syndrome; possibly a low-fiber, high-fat diet ●*Relieving factors:* Non-steroidal anti-inflammatory drugs (NSAIDs) may be preventative; small polyps: endoscopic removal; large polyps or invasive carcinoma: surgery ●*Clinical course:* Larger polyp: more likely to contain a focus of malignancy; adenomatous polyps: some become cancerous; hyperplastic and inflammatory polyps: benign ●*Co-morbidities:* If hereditary syndrome: other cancers (e.g. breast, genitourinary, small intestine, ovary); if inflammatory polyp: Crohn's or ulcerative colitis ●*Procedure results:* Colonoscopy or flexible sigmoidoscopy show polyps; barium enema or CT scan: polyp ●*Test findings:* Anemia, occult blood positive stools

Congenital abnormality of lymphatics ●*Onset:* Subacute ●*Male:female ratio:* M=F ●*Ethnicity:* All ●*Character:* Lymphangiectasia: dilation of lymphatics; pulmonary: respiratory distress; intestinal abdominal pain; lymphangioma; lymphatic dysplasia: lymphedema, chylous ascites, chylothorax, lymphangiomas of bone, lung ●*Location:* Lymph nodes, lungs, intestines, bones ●*Pattern:* Enlarging mass, worsening symptoms ●*Precipitating factors:* Genetic, postirradiation, infection, tumor compression ●*Relieving factors:* Surgical treatment ●*Clinical course:* Progresses until treated ●*Co-morbidities:* Lymphedema: Turner's/Noonan syndrome, Milroy disease; intestinal lymphangiectasia, cerebrovascular malformation, ptosis, dystrophic nails, distichiasis, cholestasis; postirradiation fibrosis, filiariasis ●*Procedure results:* CT scan of area, lymphangiogram ●*Test findings:* No relevant tests

Congenital dislocation of hip ●*Onset:* Acute ●*Male:female ratio:* M=F ●*Ethnicity:* All ●*Character:* Infants: decreased hip abduction, asymmetric thigh skin folds, shortening of leg, uneven knee levels (Galeazzi sign); older children: limping, increased lumbar lordosis, toe walking, uneven leg lengths ●*Location:* Hip ●*Pattern:* Nonspecific ●*Precipitating factors:* May have underlying neuromuscular condition: myelodysplasia, other syndromes; ligament laxity, prenatal posturing: breech position ●*Relieving factors:* Pavlik harness, Frejka splint, occasionally double/triple diapers; surgery includes: adductor tenotomy, closed/open reduction, spica cast, pelvic/femoral osteotomy ●*Clinical course:* Progressive unless treated ●*Co-morbidities:* Torticollis, metatarsus adductus, breech fetal position ●*Procedure results:* Abnormal hip U/S, X-rays, CT or MRI ●*Test findings:* Abnormal Ortolani-Barlot maneuver (hip clunk)

Congenital facial palsy ●*Onset:* Birth ●*Male:female ratio:* M=F ●*Ethnicity:* All ●*Character:* Facial assymetry ●*Location:* Face ●*Pattern:* More obvious with crying/smiling ●*Precipitating factors:* Congenital absence of depressor angularis oris muscle or in Mobius syndrome: bi/unilateral facial palsy from symmetrical calcified infarcts in the tegmentum of pons and medulla oblongata; possibly from trauma, drug exposure, illness during pregnancy ●*Relieving factors:* None ●*Clinical course:* Lifelong ●*Co-morbidities:* Mobius syndrome: ptosis, palatal/lingual palsy, hearing loss, pectoral/lingual muscle defects, esotropia, micrognathia, syndactyly ●*Procedure results:* No relevant procedures ●*Test findings:* No relevant tests

Congenital gonorrhea ●*Onset:* Acute ●*Male:female ratio:* M=F ●*Ethnicity:* All ●*Character:* Purulent conjunctivitis, chemoses, eyelid edema, rhinitis, anorectal infection, meningitis, sepsis, arthritis ●*Location:* Eye, CSF, joints, skin ●*Pattern:* 1 to 4 days after birth ●*Precipitating factors:* Infected pregnant mother ●*Relieving factors:* Antibiotic treatment ●*Clinical course:* Progressive if not treated ●*Co-morbidities:* Prior history of maternal venereal disease, unmarried state, premature rupture of membranes (PROM) in infected women ●*Procedure results:* Gram stain of conjunctival scraping showing intracellular Gram-negative diplococci, maternal cervical cultures; blood/CSF cultures showing organism if infected ●*Test findings:* No relevant tests

Congenital heart disease ●*Onset:* Acute/subacute depending on type ●*Male:female ratio:* M=F ●*Ethnicity:* All ●*Character:* Murmurs, cyanosis, hepatomegaly, failure to thrive, congestive heart failure (CHF) symptoms ●*Location:* Cardiac/respiratory systems ●*Pattern:* Progressive CHF symptoms, cyanosis, hypoxia ●*Precipitating factors:* Congenital defect ●*Relieving factors:* Surgical repair ●*Clinical course:* Progressive unless treated ●*Co-morbidities:* Multiple genetic disorders ●*Procedure results:* Abnormal chest X-ray/ECG/Echo/cardiac catheterization findings ●*Test findings:* No relevant tests

Congenital megacolon ●*Onset:* Acute/subacute ●*Male:female ratio:* M(4):F(1) ●*Ethnicity:* All ●*Character:* Delayed meconium passage, failure to thrive, constipation, abdominal distension ●*Location:* GI ●*Pattern:* Progressive constipation/GI obstructive symptoms ●*Precipitating factors:* Familial incidence ●*Relieving factors:* Surgery: excision of abnormal portion and reanastomosis, creation of neorectum or pull-through procedure ●*Clinical course:* Progressive unless treated ●*Co-morbidities:* Enterocolitis, Down syndrome, Waardenburg's or Lawrence-Moon-Bardet-Biedl syndromes ●*Procedure results:* Abnormal rectal manometry: high internal sphincter pressure with rectal distension; rectal biopsy: agangliosis, increased acetylcholinesterase staining; barium enema: transition zone, delayed evacuation ● *Test findings:* No relevant tests

Congenital middle ear defect ● *Onset:* Congenital ● *Male:female ratio:* M=F ● *Ethnicity:* All ● *Character:* Hearing loss in affected ear ● *Location:* Ear ● *Pattern:* Persistent hearing loss ● *Precipitating factors:* None ● *Relieving factors:* Compensation by listening with the 'good' ear ● *Clinical course:* Persistent, usually unchanging hearing loss ● *Co-morbidities:* May be associated with other syndromic head and neck congenital malformations ● *Procedure results:* Audiometry reveals a conductive hearing loss; CT scan may reveal the ossicular abnormality as well as abnormalities of the inner ear ● *Test findings:* No relevant tests

Congenital nasolacrimal duct stenosis ● *Onset:* Congenital ● *Male:female ratio:* M=F ● *Ethnicity:* All ● *Character:* Lifelong history of epiphora ● *Location:* Face/eyes ● *Pattern:* Chronic persistent epiphora ● *Precipitating factors:* None relevant ● *Relieving factors:* None relevant ● *Clinical course:* Symptoms persist until obstruction is corrected with surgery ● *Co-morbidities:* May suffer from chronic conjunctivitis ● *Procedure results:* Dye studies fail to reveal rapid passage of material from conjunctiva into nasal cavity indicating stenosis ● *Test findings:* No relevant tests

Congenital nystagmus ● *Onset:* Congenital defect ● *Male:female ratio:* M=F ● *Ethnicity:* All ● *Character:* Typical congenital nystagmus is purely horizontal ● *Location:* Both eyes ● *Pattern:* Some have a 'null zone' in eccentric gaze ● *Precipitating factors:* None relevant ● *Relieving factors:* Head turn to keep eyes in 'null zone' ● *Clinical course:* Not progressive ● *Co-morbidities:* Hyperopic astigmatism ● *Procedure results:* Comprehensive ophthalmic examination to rule out secondary cause ● *Test findings:* Horizontal nystagmus in all fields of gaze

Congenital rubella syndrome ● *Onset:* Congenital ● *Male:female ratio:* M=F ● *Ethnicity:* All ● *Character:* Congenital cataract, deafness, heart diseases ● *Location:* Common: CNS, cranial nerves, ears, lenses, liver, spleen, platelets, bone, heart ● *Pattern:* Manifestations are inborn or delayed (2-4 years), isolated deafness possible, pulmonic valve stenosis, patent ductus arteriosus ● *Precipitating factors:* Maternal infection early in pregnancy (before the 20th week) ● *Relieving factors:* None relevant ● *Clinical course:* Syndrome is inborn or presents within 2-4 years of birth ● *Co-morbidities:* Subacute sclerosing panencephalitis (SSPE) ● *Procedure results:* Isolation of virus from tissue, specific serology ● *Test findings:* Thrombocytopenia

Congenital syphilis ● *Onset:* Pregnancy/newborn ● *Male:female ratio:* M=F ● *Ethnicity:* All ● *Character:* Stillbirth, hydrops fetalis, prematurity; early: hepatosplenomegaly, jaundice, lymphadenopathy, periostitis, osteochondritis, mucocutaneous rash (red/maculopapular/bullous lesions with desquamation of palms/soles), rhinitis, condylomatous lesions, chorioretinitis, nephritis; late: frontal bossing, Olympian brow, thickened clavicle, Higoumenakis sign, Hutchinson teeth, saddle nose, keratitis, corneal opacification, blindness, eighth nerve deafness ● *Location:* Multiple organ systems: skin, liver, eye, kidney; bones, teeth ● *Pattern:* Irritability/refusal to move extremity due to pain: pseudoparalysis of Parrot; failure to thrive ● *Precipitating factors:* Maternal infection ● *Relieving factors:* Maternal treatment during pregnancy: at least one month prior to delivery with penicillin; treatment of newborn with penicillin ● *Clinical course:* If live birth, late manifestations develop if not treated ● *Co-morbidities:* Other STDs ● *Procedure results:* X-ray: osteochondritis - wrists/elbows/ankles/knees; periostitis - long bones ● *Test findings:* Elevated liver function tests, abnormal liver biopsy, Coombs' negative hemolytic anemia, thrombocytopenia, maternal testing; during pregnancy: venereal disease research laboratory (VDRL) or rapid plasma reagin; in high-risk patient: also fluorescent treponemal antibody-absorbed test (FTA-ABS) or microhemagglutination assay for Treponema pallidum (MHA-TP); in newborn: serum VDRL or RPR and FHA-ABS or MHA-TP, CSF VDRL/cell analysis/protein; spirochetes on darkfield microscopy or direct fluorescent antibody (DFA) of tissue sample

Congestive heart failure ●*Onset:* Acute, subacute, insidious ●*Male:female ratio:* M>F (M=F after age 75) ●*Ethnicity:* All ●*Character:* Shortness of breath, weakness, fatigue, exertional dyspnea, chest pain, orthopnea, paroxysmal nocturnal dyspnea, peripheral edema, weight gain, palpitations ●*Location:* Elevated neck veins, third heart sound, laterally displaced point of maximal impulse, with or without pulmonary crackles/wheezes with or without pedal edema, with or without hepatomegaly, with or without cool extremities, decreased pulse pressure ●*Pattern:* Progressive worsening if untreated ●*Precipitating factors:* Fluid overload, excessive salt intake, alcohol and drug use, radiation or chemotherapy, malnutrition and occasionally pregnancy (i.e. postpartum cardiomyopathy) ●*Relieving factors:* Decrease in fluid intake, salt restriction, cessation of alcohol and drug use, diuretics, vasodilator medication ●*Clinical course:* Untreated, patients develop worsening symptoms ●*Co-morbidities:* Constrictive or restrictive cardiomyopathy; hypertrophic cardiomyopathy ●*Procedure results:* No relevant procedures ●*Test findings:* ECG may reveal ischemic ST/T: wave changes; chest X-ray: increased cardiopulmonary ratio and congestive heart failure

Connective tissue disease ●*Onset:* Insidious ●*Male:female ratio:* M(3):F(1) ●*Ethnicity:* All ●*Character:* Dull ache ●*Location:* Joints ●*Pattern:* Worse in morning ●*Precipitating factors:* Inactivity ●*Relieving factors:* Anti-inflammatory medicines ●*Clinical course:* Chronic, slowly progressive ●*Co-morbidities:* None relevant ●*Procedure results:* Inflammatory synovial fluid analysis ●*Test findings:* Elevated acute phase reactants

Constipation ●*Onset:* Subacute ●*Male:female ratio:* M<F ●*Ethnicity:* All ●*Character:* Abdominal pain, soiling in underwear, passage of large and/or hard stools ●*Location:* Abdomen, rectum ●*Pattern:* Recurrent crampy abdominal/rectal pain ●*Precipitating factors:* Behavioral: control issues, prior passage of hard/painful stool ●*Relieving factors:* Bowel movement, laxative/stool softeners, high fiber diet, behavioral modification/toilet training in children ●*Clinical course:* Usually resolves with appropriate intervention ●*Co-morbidities:* None relevant ●*Procedure results:* Plain abdominal films with retained stool in rectum/large intestine ●*Test findings:* No relevant tests

Contact dermatitis ●*Onset:* Acute ●*Male:female ratio:* M=F ●*Ethnicity:* All ❶ *Character:* Itching ❷ *Location:* Any area of contact ❸ *Pattern:* Papules, vesicles in demarcated pattern ●*Precipitating factors:* Contact with skin ●*Relieving factors:* Topical and/or systemic steroids, antihistamines ●*Clinical course:* Resolves in weeks ●*Co-morbidities:* None relevant ●*Procedure results:* No relevant procedures ●*Test findings:* No relevant tests

Images of ❶ *Character,* ❷ *Location,* ❸ *Pattern on page 459*

Conversion disorder ●*Onset:* Usually acute or subacute ●*Male:female ratio:* M<F ●*Ethnicity:* Usually rural, uneducated Caucasian ●*Character:* Unusual and dramatic loss of physical function (paralysis, blindness) not consistent with known medical disease ●*Location:* Limbs, voice, sight ●*Pattern:* Usually sudden loss of some physical function following a stressful event ●*Precipitating factors:* Stressful experience ●*Relieving factors:* Patient can do little but others can be reassuring and patient can be encouraged to resume normal activities ●*Clinical course:* Acute condition usually resolves but same or new symptoms tend to recur ●*Co-morbidities:* Depression, personality disorders ●*Procedure results:* Normal medical and neurologic workup ●*Test findings:* No relevant tests

Cor pulmonale ●*Onset:* Insidious ●*Male:female ratio:* M>F ●*Ethnicity:* All ●*Character:* Dyspnea on exertion, fatigue, lethargy, chest pain, syncope with exertion ●*Location:* Nonspecific ●*Pattern:* Increased P2 on heart examination, jugular venous distension, tricuspid regurgitation murmur, right-sided S3, hepatojugular reflux, edema, ascites (rare) ●*Precipitating factors:* Hypoxemia, flare of underlying pulmonary disease, exertion, dietary indiscretion ●*Relieving factors:* Oxygen, treatment of underlying lung

Contact dermatitis: Images *see text page 458*

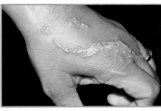

❶ *Character* Acute onset of small vesicles arranged linearly. Pruritus is intense

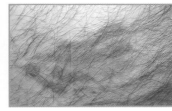

❶ *Character* Linear erythema and vesicles are typical

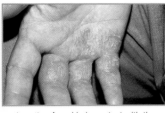

❷ *Location* Any skin in contact with the environment may be affected

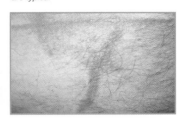

❸ *Pattern* Linear lesions are very typical in allergic contact dermatitis

disease, diuretics only if volume overloaded; vasodilators ●*Clinical course:* Poor prognosis: majority of patients die within 3-5 years ●*Co-morbidities:* Chronic obstructive pulmonary disease, pulmonary hypertension, sleep apnea ●*Procedure results:* Pulmonary hypertension on right heart catheterization ●*Test findings:* Right ventricle enlargement and right pulmonary artery >2cm in diameter on chest X-ray. ECG may show right ventricular strain, right-axis deviation, tall R in V1 and P pulmonale. Echo: right atrial and ventricle dilation, tricuspid regurgitation and elevated PA pressure

Corneal abrasion ●*Onset:* Acute ●*Male:female ratio:* M=F ●*Ethnicity:* All ●*Character:* Sharp eye pain ❷ *Location:* Cornea ●*Pattern:* Usually unilateral ●*Precipitating factors:* Preceding ocular trauma; exposure to breaking glass or windy conditions ●*Relieving factors:* Topical anesthetic relieves pain ●*Clinical course:* Will heal in 24-48 hours with treatment ●*Co-morbidities:* Other facial/ocular trauma ●*Procedure results:* After topically applied fluorescein, corneal epithelial staining with cobalt blue light or Wood's lamp ●*Test findings:* No relevant tests

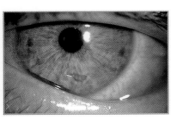

❷ *Location* Oval-shaped area of corneal distortion inferiorly. Definite ciliary injection present

Corns ●*Onset:* Chronic ●*Male:female ratio:* M=F ●*Ethnicity:* All ●*Character:* Hyperkeratotic plaque, smaller than callus, well-defined, usually ring-shaped with a central prominent translucent core, devoid of the thrombosed capillaries seen in a wart ●*Location:* Over bony prominences; under metatarsal heads on plantar surfaces, underneath the nail (onychoclavus); interdigital (between the toes) ●*Pattern:* Once corns occur, they tend to persist as the provoking stimulus also persists, i.e. friction ●*Precipitating factors:* Friction, repetitive trauma, problem with weight distribution on plantar foot ●*Relieving factors:* Orthotics help redistribute weight and reduce friction ●*Clinical course:* Do well if treated appropriately ●*Co-morbidities:* None relevant ●*Procedure results:* Biopsy reveals prominent hyperkeratosis ●*Test findings:* No relevant tests

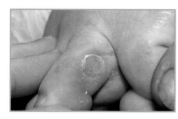

❶ *Character A painful, hyperkeratotic papulonodule between the toes. Classic for a corn*

Corrosive acid ingestion ●*Onset:* Acute ●*Male:female ratio:* M=F ●*Ethnicity:* All ●*Character:* Facial or oropharyngeal burns, dysphagia, odynophagia, drooling and dyspnea; may develop hematemesis, gastric perforation ●*Location:* Symptoms mainly involve mouth, esophagus, stomach ●*Pattern:* Nonspecific ●*Precipitating factors:* Ingestion of acids (commomly in household products): toilet bowl cleaners; drain openers ●*Relieving factors:* Dilution with water or milk may be helpful, but can lead to vomiting and is controversial; Ipecac contraindicated; steroids may prevent scarring and stricture formation ●*Clinical course:* May lead to gastric perforation and peritonitis; later, can develop fibrosis and gastric outlet obstruction ●*Co-morbidities:* None relevant ●*Procedure results:* Endoscopy: esophageal and gastric burns or perforation; chest X-ray: rule out esophageal, gastric perforation or aspiration pneumonitis ●*Test findings:* No relevant tests

Costochondritis ●*Onset:* Acute ●*Male:female ratio:* M<F ●*Ethnicity:* All ●*Character:* Sharp pain ●*Location:* Chest wall ●*Pattern:* Pain worse with deep inspiration and palpation ●*Precipitating factors:* None relevant ●*Relieving factors:* NSAIDs ●*Clinical course:* Self-limited ●*Co-morbidities:* Rheumatoid arthritis, ankylosing spondylitis, psoriatic arthritis ●*Procedure results:* Negative aspirate from costochondral junction ●*Test findings:* Erosions on plain films if chronic

Cough ●*Onset:* Acute, subacute, insidious ●*Male:female ratio:* M=F ●*Ethnicity:* All ●*Character:* May be productive of sputum ●*Location:* Chest or upper airway ●*Pattern:* Intermittent ●*Precipitating factors:* Infection, asthma, allergies, gastroesophageal reflux disease, industrial/chemical exposures, lung cancer, other lung masses ●*Relieving factors:* Treatment of underlying etiology, bronchodilator and inhaled steriods for asthma; antibiotics for infection, cough suppressants ●*Clinical course:* Self-limited or chronic ●*Co-morbidities:* May cause cough syncope, urinary incontinence, rib fractures, muscle strain ●*Procedure results:* Pulmonary function tests and chest X-ray often helpful, results dependent on underlying etiology ●*Test findings:* Dependent on underlying etiology

Coxa valga ●*Onset:* Congenital, possibly subacute if related to injury ●*Male:female ratio:* M=F ●*Ethnicity:* All ●*Character:* Deformity of neck/shaft relationship of femur, with progressive increase in the angle between the femoral neck and shaft ●*Location:* Hips, usually bilateral ●*Pattern:* Femoral angling away from the midline distally ●*Precipitating factors:* Congenital, trauma ●*Relieving factors:* None relevant ●*Clinical course:* May lead to superior dislocation in the immature hip (if congenital); unilateral results in leg length discrepancy and limp ●*Co-morbidities:* Congenital spinal muscular atrophy, dwarfism ●*Procedure results:* X-ray demonstrates deformity ●*Test findings:* No relevant tests

Coxa vara ●*Onset:* Congenital, developmental (early childhood), or due to injury; in adults, postpelvic radiation therapy pathologic fracture ●*Male:female ratio:* M=F ●*Ethnicity:* All ●*Character:* Deformity of neck/shaft relationship of femur, with progressive decrease in angle between femoral neck and shaft; progressive shortening of the limb resulting in limping and pain ●*Location:* Hips, usually bilateral ●*Pattern:* Femoral angling toward the midline distally ●*Precipitating factors:* Congenital, trauma/fracture, radiation therapy ●*Relieving factors:* Corrective surgery (age 4-5) ●*Clinical course:* Deformity develops after walking is begun; unilateral results in leg length discrepancy and limp ●*Co-morbidities:* None relevant ●*Procedure results:* X-ray demonstrates deformity ●*Test findings:* No relevant test

Creutzfeldt-Jakob disease ●*Onset:* Subacute ●*Male:female ratio:* M=F ●*Ethnicity:* All ●*Character:* Rapidly progressive dementia, myoclonus (startle myoclonus), mental disorientation, behavioral disturbances, visual deficits, loss of coordination ●*Location:* Cortex, cerebellum, striata, thalamus, cranial nerves ●*Pattern:* Dementia, behavioral changes progress rapidly; gradual loss of coordination; myoclonus is common and is aggravated by startle ●*Precipitating factors:* Sporadic (most), familial (some), iatrogenic transmission is rare (transplantation, dural grafts, contaminated surgical equipment, contact with infected tissue), possible bovine to human transmission (new variant CJD) ●*Relieving factors:* None relevant ●*Clinical course:* Rapidly progressive; average duration from onset to death 7-9 months ●*Co-morbidities:* Psychiatric disorders ●*Procedure results:* Abnormal EEG, acellular CSF, elevated CSF 14-3-3 protein, increased T2 signals on brain MRI, spongiform changes and positive immunohistochemistry for prion protein on brain biopsy ●*Test findings:* Normal CBC and ESR

Crohn's disease ●*Onset:* Insidious ●*Male:female ratio:* M<F (slightly) ●*Ethnicity:* Increased incidence in Caucasians and Jewish populations ●*Character:* Recurrent episodes of right lower quadrant pain and diarrhea: pain is colicky and may be relieved after bowel movements; diarrhea is usually watery, but may be bloody if colon is involved; low-grade fever may be present; weight loss; perianal disease (fissures, fistulas, abscesses) in up to one third of patients; ileal disease may lead to intestinal obstruction; extraintestinal signs include episcleritis, uveitis, aphthous ulcers, erythema nodosum, arthritis ●*Location:* Right lower quadrant of the abdomen ●*Pattern:* Nonspecific ●*Precipitating factors:* None relevant ●*Relieving factors:* Mesalamine and steroids are effective; antibiotics or immunosuppressives may be helpful; infliximab is used in difficult or refractory cases; surgery is not curative, but limited resection can be helpful ●*Clinical course:* Intermittent symptoms over years ●*Co-morbidities:* Primary sclerosing cholangitis; colon cancer; thromboembolic disease ●*Procedure results:* Barium studies reveal diseased ileum; colonoscopy with ileal intubation reveals inflammation; biopsies show acute and chronic inflammation; granulomas are diagnostic ●*Test findings:* ESR and WBC elevated; anemia is common

Croup ●*Onset:* Acute ●*Male:female ratio:* M=F ●*Ethnicity:* All ●*Character:* Stridor; shortness of breath; cough ●*Location:* Breathing/respiration ●*Pattern:* Progressive shortness of breath, may progress to severe respiratory distress ●*Precipitating factors:* Antecedent upper respiratory infection ●*Relieving factors:* Upright position, slow breathing, reluctant to swallow ●*Clinical course:* Symptoms may plateau or progress to respiratory distress; overall, self-limited ●*Co-morbidities:* Dangerous in the setting of subglottic stenosis ●*Procedure results:* No relevant procedures ●*Test findings:* Steeple sign in subglottis on plain films of the neck

Cryoglobulinemia ●*Onset:* Insidious to subacute ●*Male:female ratio:* M=F ●*Ethnicity:* All ●*Character:* Purpuric rash, arthralgias, abdominal pain, lymphadenopathy, hepatosplenomegaly, peripheral neuropathy; signs of underlying disease including chronic liver disease, lymphoproliferative disorder, HIV, or chronic inflammatory or autoimmune disorder ●*Location:* Rash is often on the lower extremities ●*Pattern:* Nonspecific ●*Precipitating factors:* Underlying infection (hepatitis C virus [HCV]), malignancy (lymphoproliferative), autoimmune disease (systemic lupus erythematosus) ●*Relieving factors:* Fair results with steroids and immunosuppressive medications ●*Clinical course:* Generally good prognosis but depends on treatment of the underlying disorder ●*Co-morbidities:* Chronic liver disease (especially HCV), lymphoproliferative disorder, HIV, or chronic inflammatory or autoimmune disorder ●*Procedure results:* Skin or renal biopsy: IgM deposition, precipitated cryoglobulins ●*Test findings:* Low complement levels, circulating cryoglobulins, spuriously high WBC and platelets

Cubital tunnel syndrome ●*Onset:* Gradual ●*Male:female ratio:* M=F ●*Ethnicity:* All ●*Character:* Paresthesias along lateral forearm, wrist, fourth and fifth fingers; pain at elbow ●*Location:* Compression of ulnar nerve in fibro-osseous canal formed by medial condyle, ulnar collateral ligament and flexor carpi ulnaris muscle ●*Pattern:* Atrophy of intrinsic hand muscles weak pinch and grasp; sensory loss at fifth finger laterally ●*Precipitating factors:* Occupational stress, repetitive movements, e.g. hammering, unusual positioning e.g. using elbows to arise from chair ●*Relieving factors:* Avoidance of prolonged elbow flexion; corticosteroid injection at ulnar groove; surgery for decompression ●*Clinical course:* Slow progression to weakness and disability if untreated; may be irreversible if symptoms present >1 year ●*Co-morbidities:* Rheumatoid arthritis; disabilities leadng to overuse of elbows e.g. stroke and spinal cord injuries ●*Procedure results:* Nerve conduction studies localize site of ulnar nerve compression ●*Test findings:* Hoffman-Tinel test: tapping on nerve at ulnar groove reproduces pain/paresthesia

Cushing's syndrome ●*Onset:* Gradual ●*Male:female ratio:* M<F ●*Ethnicity:* All ●*Character:* Central obesity, weight gain, striae, moon facies, supraclavicular fat pad, easy bruising, proximal muscle weakness, hyperpigmentation ●*Location:* Central fat, moon face, supraclavicular fat pad ●*Pattern:* Nonspecific ●*Precipitating factors:* Exogenous steroids, endogenous steroid overproduction ●*Relieving factors:* Removal of source of steroid excess (or stimulating); in rare cases (e.g. cancer) may use ketoconazole, metyrapone, mitotane ●*Clinical course:* Progressive ●*Co-morbidities:* Infection, osteoporosis, impaired wound healing, diabetes mellitus ●*Procedure results:* If central Cushing's, MRI or CT may show pituitary tumor; if ectopic, X-ray, chest CT or MRI may show lung mass ●*Test findings:* Elevated 24-hour free cortisol, failure to suppress cortisol production in response to 1mg overnight dexamethasone suppression test

Cutaneous T cell lymphoma ●*Onset:* Insidious ●*Male:female ratio:* M>F ●*Ethnicity:* African-American ●*Character:* Scaling, erythematous macular rash, then barely palpable, erythematous and eczematous plaques, then definitive plaques; painful erythroderma ●*Location:* Nonspecific ●*Pattern:* Early phase rash in a 'bathing suit' distribution/nonsunexposed areas ●*Precipitating factors:* None relevant ●*Relieving factors:* Depending on stage: topical chemotherapy, psoralens and ultraviolet application/A-range (PUVA) therapy, localized radiation, total skin electron beam therapy, interferon, systemic chemotherapy ●*Clinical course:* Depends on stage and % total skin involvement; early stages, 80-90% 5-yr survival, more advanced stages 20-50% ●*Co-morbidities:* None relevant ●*Procedure results:* Imaging: lymphadenopathy; skin biopsy: neoplastic T cells with invasion, clonal T cell population, Pautrier's microabscesses (epidermal collections of lymphocytes) ●*Test findings:* Circulating neoplastic T cells; flow cytometry positive for CD4, CD8, CD3, CD45RO, CD20 antigens; elevated CD4/CD8 ratio

Cyclic neutropenia ●*Onset:* Subacute ●*Male:female ratio:* M=F ●*Ethnicity:* All ●*Character:* Fatigue, malaise, mouth sores, stomatitis, vaginitis, proctitis, skin infections ●*Location:* Nonspecific ●*Pattern:* Cyclic every 10-35 days, lasting 3-4 days ●*Precipitating*

factors: Autosomal dominant with variable expression ●*Relieving factors:* Antibiotics ●*Clinical course:* Cyclical, usually begins in early childhood and lasts decades ●*Co-morbidities:* None relevant ●*Procedure results:* Bone marrow biopsy during granulocytopenia usually shows hypoplasia or an arrest in maturation at the myelocyte stage ●*Test findings:* Neutropenia, compensatory monocytosis, also cyclic variation in reticulocytes and platelets

Cystic fibrosis ●*Onset:* Acute at birth to subacute ●*Male:female ratio:* M=F ●*Ethnicity:* Caucasian ●*Character:* Persistent productive cough, meconium ileus in the newborn or episodic small bowel obstruction in older children and adults, malabsortion of fat, diarrhea, infertility ●*Location:* Bronchiectasis, sinusitis, pancreatic insufficiency, primary biliary cirrhosis ●*Pattern:* Clubbing, bilateral expiratory rhonchi and inspiratory crackles, sinus tenderness to percussion ●*Precipitating factors:* Recurrent infections, dehydration ●*Relieving factors:* Antibiotics, hydration, bronchodilators, mucolytics, chest physical therapy, postural drainage, exercise ●*Clinical course:* Lifelong ●*Co-morbidities:* None relevant ●*Procedure results:* Genetic mutation in cystic fibrosis transmembrane regulator ●*Test findings:* Elevated sweat chloride (>60mEq/L); genetic mutation in cystic fibrosis transmembrane regulator; chest X-ray: hyperinflation and bronchiectasis; pulmonary function tests: obstructive ventilatory defects

Cystitis ●*Onset:* Acute ●*Male:female ratio:* M<F ●*Ethnicity:* All ●*Character:* Painful urination ●*Location:* Suprapubic pain, urethral spasm, flank pain ●*Pattern:* Frequency, urgency voiding in small amounts, fever, chills ●*Precipitating factors:* Failure to void following intercourse ●*Relieving factors:* Appropriate antibiotic medication usually 1-3 days in uncomplicated cases without comorbidities, increased fluid intake ●*Clinical course:* Can progress to pyelonephritis and systemic sepsis especially in elderly or diabetics ●*Co-morbidities:* Vaginitis or urethritis due to STDs ●*Procedure results:* No relevant procedures ●*Test findings:* Bacteriuria and pyuria on urinalysis, urine culture varyingly positive with colony counts 100-100,000 range

Cytomegalovirus ●*Onset:* Acute, subacute, chronic ●*Male:female ratio:* M>F ●*Ethnicity:* All ●*Character:* Mononucleosis-like illness (fever, sore throat, lymphadenopathy), increasing dyspnea in bone marrow transplant patients; in AIDS patients: 'floaters' and decreased vision, unremitting explosive watery diarrhea with or without blood, progressive ascending flaccid paralysis ●*Location:* CMV-mononucleosis: lymph nodes, spleen, liver, throat; complications: lungs (interstitial pneumonitis), brain, spinal cord, meninges, retina, GI tract: oral mucosa, esophagus, stomach, small intestines, large intestines; heart, bone marrow, skin ●*Pattern:* Asymptomatic in young children, progressive blindness and ascending lower extremity weakness in AIDS patients, progressive dyspnea in transplant patients ●*Precipitating factors:* Contact with infants and children (daycare), kissing, sexual contact, blood transfusion, breast-feeding, immunosuppression ●*Relieving factors:* None relevant ●*Clinical course:* Self-limited in immunocompetent, may cause congenital syndrome if acquired in pregnancy, reactivation with immunosuppression may lead to blindness, malnutrition, death ●*Co-morbidities:* AIDS, transplantation ●*Procedure results:* Antigen detection in white blood cells, CMV-DNA detection in blood or CSF, growth of CMV from culture, cells with nuclear inclusions from clinical specimen, interstitial infiltrates on chest X-ray (in pneumonitis), shallow ulcers on esophagogastroduodenoscopy (EGD) or colonoscopy, acellular bone marrow ●*Test findings:* Relative lymphocytosis (CMV mononucleosis), atypical lymphocytes, elevated hepatic transaminases (immunocompetent), anemia thrombocytopenia, neutropenia (in immunosuppressed)

Daily headache ●*Onset:* Insidious ●*Male:female ratio:* M=F ●*Ethnicity:* All ●*Character:* Non-throbbing tightness, vice-like ●*Location:* Bitemporal, occipital, on top of the head ●*Pattern:* Waxes and wanes thourought the day; never goes away completely ●*Precipitating factors:* Stress, fatigue, anxiety, caffeine withdrawal ●*Relieving factors:* Stress management, use of tricyclic antidepressants ●*Clinical course:* Overall prognosis is good when the stressor is identified and relieved ●*Co-morbidities:* Anxiety, stress ●*Procedure results:* No relevant procedures ●*Test findings:* Normal neurological examination

de Quervain's contracture ●*Onset:* Subacute/recurrent ●*Male:female ratio:* M(1):F(10) ●*Ethnicity:* All ●*Character:* Pain and tenderness, weakness of grip, possible palpable thickening of underlying fibrous sheath ●*Location:* Radial styloid of wrist ●*Pattern:* Nonspecific ●*Precipitating factors:* Overuse of thumb in grasping while twisting hand radially, rheumatoid arthritis, pregnancy ●*Relieving factors:* Rest, temporary splint immobilization, corticosteroid injections, surgery, NSAIDs ●*Clinical course:* Usually resolves with rest, frequently recurs, may last months ●*Co-morbidities:* Rheumatoid arthritis ●*Procedure results:* No relevant procedures ●*Test findings:* Finkelstein's sign: with thumb folded into the palm and held with the fingers, forced flexion of the wrist in the ulnar direction elicits sharp pain at the radial styloid

Decreased cortical inhibition ●*Onset:* Usually acquired ●*Male:female ratio:* M=F ●*Ethnicity:* All ●*Character:* Also called pyramidal, corticospinal or upper motor neuron lesions; cerebral lesions that involve corticospinal tracts can result in contralateral paralysis of volitional movements, and fixed posturing with arm flexed and leg extended; also characterized by 'clasp-knife' spasticity, absence of involuntary movements, increased tendon reflexes and paralysis of voluntary movement; the Babinski reflex is present ●*Location:* The lesion usually occurs at any level, with descending corticospinal tracts affected; fibers decussate in the medulla most of the time, hence ipsilateral paralysis occurs if fibers are affected above the medulla; if fibers affected above the pons, hand and arm muscles are more severely affected than the foot and the leg; on the face, lower face and tongue muscles more affected ●*Pattern:* Paralysis is never permanent; muscles with bilateral innervation such as larynx, pharynx, eyes, neck, thorax and jaw are rarely affected ●*Precipitating factors:* Ischemic or toxic injury or space-occupying lesion ●*Relieving factors:* Decompression if space-occupying lesion ●*Clinical course:* Usually sudden onset; can improve with time ●*Co-morbidities:* Spasticity; irradiation of reflexes ●*Procedure results:* Removal of space-occupying lesion may result in improvement ●*Test findings:* Nerve conduction normal; no denervation potentials in electromyogram

Deep vein thrombosis ●*Onset:* Acute, subacute ●*Male:female ratio:* M(1):F(1.2) ●*Ethnicity:* All ●*Character:* Ache or pain in the calf or thigh with or without swelling; can be asymptomatic; distension of superficial veins, slight elevation in temperature, tenderness to palpation, and Homan's sign may be present ●*Location:* Calf or thigh most common; can occur in upper extremities, especially after IV catheter placement ●*Pattern:* Pain in the calf or thigh may be associated with swelling; sometimes worse with walking; if untreated, increased risk for pulmonary embolism ●*Precipitating factors:* Postoperative state, cancer (e.g. adenocarcinomas), hypercoagulable states, oral contraceptive use in smokers; obesity; immobility ●*Relieving factors:* Anticoagulation, leg elevation ●*Clinical course:* Increased risk of pulmonary emboli and chronic venous insufficiency if untreated ●*Co-morbidities:* Cancer (e.g. adenocarcinomas), hypercoagulable states, obesity ●*Procedure results:* No relevant procedures ●*Test findings:* Contrast venography or Doppler U/S can demonstrate thrombosis

Degenerative arthritis of hip ●*Onset:* Insidious ●*Male:female ratio:* M=F ●*Ethnicity:* African-American ●*Character:* Dull ache ●*Location:* Lateral hip into the groin ●*Pattern:* Worse with walking and weightbearing ●*Precipitating factors:* Weightbearing ●*Relieving factors:* Weight loss, acetaminophen, NSAIDs, total hip replacement ●*Clinical course:* Chronic and slowly progressive ●*Co-morbidities:* Obesity, slipped capital femoral epiphysis, congenital hip dysplasia ●*Procedure results:* Joint space narrowing on plan radiograph ●*Test findings:* No relevant tests

Dehydration ●*Onset:* Acute/subacute/chronic ●*Male:female ratio:* M=F ●*Ethnicity:* All ●*Character:* Graded as mild, moderate, or severe; may see lethargy, dry membranes, sunken eyes or fontanelle, hypotension, tachycardia, decreased skin turgor ●*Location:* Nonspecific ●*Pattern:* Nonspecific ●*Precipitating factors:* Intravascular volume depletion, usually from vomiting/diarrhea; may follow prolonged high fevers or urinary losses (diuretics) ●*Relieving factors:* Oral (for selected mild cases) or intravenous hydration; replace potassium losses ●*Clinical course:* Rapid progression to death in infants may occur without intervention ●*Co-morbidities:* Very young and old, diabetics, use of diuretics ●*Procedure results:* No relevant procedures ●*Test findings:* Elevated blood urea nitrogen and/or creatinine, low potassium or serum bicarbonate, hypo/hypernatremia

Delirium ●*Onset:* Acute/subacute/chronic ●*Male:female ratio:* M=F ●*Ethnicity:* All ●*Character:* Impaired cognitive function with associated altered level of consciousness; rapid fluctuations in consciousness and activity, visual hallucinations common ●*Location:* Nonspecific ●*Pattern:* Symptoms fluctuate rapidly ●*Precipitating factors:* Neurologic (CNS trauma, mass, infections) and systemic (infections, sepsis, metabolic, endocrine, drugs, medications, alcohol) ●*Relieving factors:* Treat underlying cause, tranquilizers if necessary, supportive care ●*Clinical course:* Varies depending on cause ●*Co-morbidities:* Elderly, diabetics, renal or liver failure, drug use ●*Procedure results:* No relevant procedures ●*Test findings:* Depends on cause but thorough evaluation with blood tests, cultures, and X-rays usually indicated

Dementia ●*Onset:* Onset varies with dementia subtype ●*Male:female ratio:* M=F ●*Ethnicity:* All ●*Character:* Multiple cognitive deficits, including memory disturbance and aphasia, apraxia, agnosia, or disturbance in executive funtioning ●*Location:* Nonspecific ●*Pattern:* Nonspecific ●*Precipitating factors:* Deterioration may follow medical illness and psychosocial stress ●*Relieving factors:* Treatment of reversible dementias ●*Clinical course:* Progressive, static, or remitting ●*Co-morbidities:* Motor disturbances, inhibited behavior, mood disorders, anxiety disorders, sleep disturbances, psychoses, especially persecutory delusions and visual hallucinations ●*Procedure results:* No relevant procedures ●*Test findings:* Abnormal thyroid function, megaloblastic anemia and intoxication should be excluded

Dental infection ●*Onset:* Subacute ●*Male:female ratio:* M=F ●*Ethnicity:* All ●*Character:* Dull aching pain in tooth socket ●*Location:* Usually affected tooth, but may radiate to cheek or neck ●*Pattern:* Persistent pain, worse with eating ●*Precipitating factors:* Poor dental hygiene ●*Relieving factors:* Cold pack, aspirin or NSAIDs ●*Clinical course:* Persistence of symptoms until treated ●*Co-morbidities:* Radiation therapy, alcohol use, cigarette smoking ●*Procedure results:* X-ray may reveal apical abscess ●*Test findings:* Pain on palpation of infected tooth; gingival swelling around tooth

Dental occlusion defects ●*Onset:* Infant/child/adolescent ●*Male:female ratio:* M=F ●*Ethnicity:* All ●*Character:* Cross bite: mandibular teeth positioned outside of maxillary teeth, incisors or molars; open bite: anterior teeth apart when posterior mandibular/maxillary teeth make contact; closed bite: mandibular anterior teeth occlude inside of maxillary anterior teeth; dental crowding: incisor overlap; digit sucking: open bite with incisor flaring ●*Location:* Jaw and teeth ●*Pattern:* Cross bite: mandibular teeth positioned outside of maxillary teeth, incisors or molars; open bite: anterior teeth apart when posterior mandibular/maxillary teeth make contact; closed bite: mandibular anterior teeth occlude inside of maxillary anterior teeth; dental crowding: incisor overlap; digit sucking: open bite with incisor flaring ●*Precipitating factors:* Thumb sucking, jaw growth pattern ●*Relieving factors:* Spacing, braces, cessation of digit sucking, orthodontic correction ●*Clinical course:* Persists unless treated ●*Co-morbidities:* Micrognathia ●*Procedure results:* Abnormal oral examination, dental X-rays ●*Test findings:* No relevant tests

Depression ●*Onset:* Typically develops over days-to-weeks ●*Male:female ratio:* M(1):F(2) ●*Ethnicity:* In different cultures, depression may be expressed in mostly somatic terms (e.g. 'bad heart') ●*Character:* Significant sadness and/or irritability and/or loss of interest or pleasure in almost all activites plus somatic symptoms ●*Location:* Nonspecific ●*Pattern:* Often mood and affect vary during course of day; symptoms may intensify in women around time of menses ●*Precipitating factors:* Often follows psychosocial stressor(s), especially loss; postpartum depression common and serious ●*Relieving factors:* Antidepressant therapy, relief of stress, support from family and friends ●*Clinical course:* In majority, there is complete remission; in remainder, there are either repeated episodes, or chronic impairment ●*Co-morbidities:* Substance abuse disorders, eating disorders, anxiety disorders, other mood disorders, coexisting medical conditions may be worsened ●*Procedure results:* No relevant procedures ●*Test findings:* Sleep EEG abnormalities common

Dermatitis herpetiformis ●*Onset:* Acute/subacute ●*Male:female ratio:* M(1.5):F(1) ●*Ethnicity:* All ●*Character:* Intense itching ●*Location:* Knees, elbows, buttocks, scalp ●*Pattern:* Symmetrical grouped vesicles ●*Precipitating factors:* HLAB8, ingestion of gluten ●*Relieving factors:* Dapsone ●*Clinical course:* Chronic ●*Co-morbidities:* Gluten enteropathy ●*Procedure results:* Skin biopsy: IgA in basement membrane ●*Test findings:* No relevant tests

Dermoid cyst ●*Onset:* Infancy/toddler ●*Male:female ratio:* M=F ●*Ethnicity:* All ●*Character:* Firm, round, smooth lesion, yellowish-white to fleshy pink color ●*Location:* Superficially on body, various locations including sacral area and conjunctiva ●*Pattern:* Appearance with some growth ●*Precipitating factors:* Aberrant development of dermal components ●*Relieving factors:* Surgery ●*Clinical course:* Stable unless removed ●*Co-morbidities:* None relevant ●*Procedure results:* Biopsy consistent with various dermal tissue: glands, hair follicles, hair shafts ●*Test findings:* No relevant tests

Developmental delay ●*Onset:* Insidious ●*Male:female ratio:* M=F ●*Ethnicity:* All ●*Character:* Delay in obtaining developmental milestones, language skills and social skills, gross motor function or fine motor function ●*Location:* Nonspecific ●*Pattern:* Nonspecific ●*Precipitating factors:* Premature birth, perinatal infection, cerebral palsy ●*Relieving factors:* Supportive care ●*Clinical course:* Depends on severity and therapy given ●*Co-morbidities:* None relevant ●*Procedure results:* No relevant procedures ●*Test findings:* Normal MRI of the brain

Deviated nasal septum ●*Onset:* Insidious ●*Male:female ratio:* M=F ●*Ethnicity:* All ●*Character:* Persistent nasal obstruction ●*Location:* Airflow usually worse on side of deviation ●*Pattern:* Constant obstruction, perhaps worse at night or during allergy season ●*Precipitating factors:* Nasal fracture ●*Relieving factors:* Use (abuse) of over-the-counter topical nasal decongestants or oral decongestants ●*Clinical course:* May progress slowly throughout life ●*Co-morbidities:* Allergic rhinitis; chronic sinusitis ●*Procedure results:* Nasal endoscopy/rhinoscopy discloses obstruction due to deviation ●*Test findings:* No relevant tests

Diabetes insipidus ●*Onset:* Gradual or acute ●*Male:female ratio:* M=F ●*Ethnicity:* All ●*Character:* Polyuria, polydipsia, change in mental status ●*Location:* Hypothalamus ●*Pattern:* Nonspecific ●*Precipitating factors:* Pituitary surgery, head trauma, pituitary tumor, granulomatous disease, rarely pregnancy ●*Relieving factors:* Hydration, desmopressin ●*Clinical course:* Progressive though may resolve completely if postoperative or pregnancy-related ●*Co-morbidities:* Pituitary tumor ●*Procedure results:* MRI may show tumor; water deprivation test shows high serum osmolality with low urine osmolality ●*Test findings:* Hypernatremia, hyperosmolality in the setting of polyuria with dilute urine, vasopressin low in central diabetes insipidus, administer vasopressin to rule out nephrogenic diabetes insipidus

Diabetes mellitus in children ●*Onset:* Acute/subacute/may be insidious ●*Male:female ratio:* M=F ●*Ethnicity:* All ●*Character:* Polyuria, polydipsia, polyphagia, failure to thrive, weight loss ●*Location:* Nonspecific ●*Pattern:* Nonspecific ●*Precipitating factors:* Autoimmune, possibly viral, infection may precipitate diabetic ketoacidosis (DKA); may have family history but less common than with Type 2 ●*Relieving factors:* Insulin, hydration ●*Clinical course:* Polyuria, polydipsia, polyphagia, failure to thrive, weight loss ●*Co-morbidities:* Polyglandular failure syndrome ●*Procedure results:* No relevant procedures ●*Test findings:* Hyperglycemia, ketonuria, acidosis, elevated Hb A1c

Diabetes mellitus type 1 ●*Onset:* Acute or subacute, may be insidious ●*Male:female ratio:* M=F ●*Ethnicity:* All ●*Character:* Polyuria, polydipsia, polyphagia, failure to thrive, weight loss ●*Location:* Nonspecific ●*Pattern:* Nonspecific ●*Precipitating factors:* Autoimmune, possibly viral, infection may precipitate ketoacidosis (DKA), may have family history but less common than with Type 2 ●*Relieving factors:* Insulin, hydration ●*Clinical course:* Progressive but may have 'honeymoon' period after initial presentation ●*Co-morbidities:* Polyglandular failure syndrome ●*Procedure results:* No relevant procedures ● *Test findings:* Hyperglycemia, ketonuria, acidosis, elevated Hb A1c

Diabetes mellitus type 2 ●*Onset:* Insidious ●*Male:female ratio:* M<F ●*Ethnicity:* Increased in non-Caucasians ●*Character:* Polyuria, polydipsia, polyphagia, visual changes and blindness (cataracts and retinopathy), numbness, tingling and pain particularly in stocking glove distribution (nephropathy), renal failure ●*Location:* Nonspecific ●*Pattern:* Nonspecific ●*Precipitating factors:* Steroids, obesity, physical inactivity, family history of diabetes mellitus ●*Relieving factors:* Weight loss, exercise, insulin sensitizers or hypoglycemic agents ●*Clinical course:* Progressive ●*Co-morbidities:* Obesity, Cushing's disease or syndrome, syndrome X (dyslipidemia, hypertension) ●*Procedure results:* Two or more elevated values on 75g oral glucose tolerance test ●*Test findings:* Elevated blood glucose and hemoglobin A1c

Diabetic enteropathy ●*Onset:* Acute or subacute ●*Male:female ratio:* M=F ●*Ethnicity:* All ●*Character:* Nausea, vomiting, constipation, abdominal pain, dysphagia, fecal incontinence, gastric splash hours past meal ●*Location:* Abdomen ●*Pattern:* May be intermittent ●*Precipitating factors:* Poor glucose control ●*Relieving factors:* Improvement in glucose control, metoclopramide, antireflux therapy, occasionally course of antibiotic for bacterial overgrowth ●*Clinical course:* Fluctuating and intermittent ●*Co-morbidities:* Esophagitis, erratic glucose control; other diabetic neuropathics and diabetic complications ●*Procedure results:* Abnormal esophageal motility ●*Test findings:* Radiolabeled scintigraphy: delayed gastric emptying; radiolabeled marker study: slow colonic transit (in constipation)

Diabetic hypoglycemia ●*Onset:* Acute ●*Male:female ratio:* M=F ●*Ethnicity:* All ●*Character:* Sweating, palpitations, lightheadedness, hunger, syncope, mental status change, seizure, tremulousness ●*Location:* Nonspecific ●*Pattern:* Nonspecific ●*Precipitating factors:* Insulin use with inadequate food intake, alcohol intake without food, early pregnancy, adrenal insufficiency, autonomic dysfunction, gastroparesis ●*Relieving factors:* Glucose, glucagon can be administered by family member in emergency out of hospital ●*Clinical course:* Rapid resolution of symptoms with glucose administration (unless previous prolonged hypoglycemia and permanent brain damage) ●*Co-morbidities:* Diabetic autonomic dysfunction and/or gastroparesis, adrenal insufficiency, renal insufficiency, liver failure ●*Procedure results:* No relevant procedures ●*Test findings:* Low blood sugar

Diabetic ketoacidosis ●*Onset:* Subacute ●*Male:female ratio:* M=F ●*Ethnicity:* All ●*Character:* Lethargy, hyperpnea, dehydration, changes in sensorium, nausea and vomiting, weight loss ●*Location:* Abdominal pain: diffuse ●*Pattern:* Progressive to coma ●*Precipitating factors:* Infection or other physiologic stress ●*Relieving factors:* Hydration, insulin ●*Clinical course:* Progresses to coma/death ●*Co-morbidities:* Existing history of diabetes in majority of cases; can be presenting sign of diabetes in some cases ●*Procedure results:* No relevant procedures ●*Test findings:* Hyperglycemia, ketonuria, acidosis, hyponatremia

Diabetic mononeuritis ●*Onset:* Acute ●*Male:female ratio:* M=F ●*Ethnicity:* All ●*Character:* Cranial nerve: unilateral opthalmoplegia sparing eye movement and pupillary function, headache, paresthesias, thigh motor weakness with pain ●*Location:* Cranial nerve palsy especially (III, IV, VI, VII), sites of nerve compression, intercostal neuropathy, femoral neuropathy ●*Pattern:* Pain may be worse at night ●*Precipitating factors:* Hyperglycemia ●*Relieving factors:* Often spontaneously remits (week-to-months), improve glucose control, analgesics ●*Clinical course:* Usually resolves in weeks-to-months ●*Co-morbidities:* Entrapment injuries ●*Procedure results:* Slowing of nerve conduction ●*Test findings:* No relevant tests

Diabetic neuropathy ●*Onset:* Subacute but may present acutely ●*Male:female ratio:* M=F ●*Ethnicity:* All ●*Character:* Starts at toes and moves centrally ●*Location:* Stocking-glove neuropathy, sensory greater than motor initially ●*Pattern:* Some sensory symptoms worse at night ●*Precipitating factors:* Poor glucose control ●*Relieving factors:* Improvement in glucose control, tricyclic antidepressants, some anticonvulsants ●*Clinical course:* Progressive with fluctuations, can have spontaneous improvement ●*Co-morbidities:* Ulcerations, skin infections, other diabetic complications ●*Procedure results:* Nerve condition studies show diffuse damage but sensory > motor and proximal > distal ●*Test findings:* Decreased pinprick, vibratory, position sense and light touch

Diabetic retinopathy ●*Onset:* Insidious ●*Male:female ratio:* M=F (type 1); M<F (type 2) ●*Ethnicity:* All ●*Character:* Unilateral or bilateral blurred vision ●*Location:* Retina ●*Pattern:* Typically affects both eyes; neovascularization in retina, dot and blot hemorrhage, retinal exudate ●*Precipitating factors:* Duration of hyperglycemia ●*Relieving factors:* None relevant ●*Clinical course:* Progressive ●*Co-morbidities:* Cataract, glaucoma, cranial neuropathy, peripheral neuropathy, renal disease ●*Procedure results:* No relevant procedures ●*Test findings:* No relevant tests

Diaper dermatitis ●*Onset:* Acute, subacute ●*Male:female ratio:* M=F ●*Ethnicity:* All ●*Character:* Erythema ●*Location:* Diaper area ●*Pattern:* Erythema, occasional scale and pustules ●*Precipitating factors:* Moisture, irritants ●*Relieving factors:* Topical steroids, nystatin ●*Clinical course:* Self-limited ●*Co-morbidities:* None relevant ●*Procedure results:* No relevant procedures ●*Test findings:* No relevant tests

Diaphragmatic paralysis ●*Onset:* Acute, subacute ●*Male:female ratio:* M=F ●*Ethnicity:* All ●*Character:* Recumbent and exertional dyspnea ●*Location:* Chest and abdomen ●*Pattern:* Paradoxical movement of the chest and abdomen, bibasilar inspiratory rales ●*Precipitating factors:* Neurologic injury or disease at C3-C5 or to the phrenic nerve(s), cold cardioplegia during coronary artery bypass graft surgery can injure phrenic nerve ●*Relieving factors:* Noninvasive ventilation if bilateral paralysis, otherwise chest physical therapy and deep respirations to clear basilar secretions ●*Clinical course:* Months: chronic ●*Co-morbidities:* Cervical spine disease, systemic lupus erythematosis, amyotrophic lateral sclerosis, many other neurologic and systemic diseases ●*Procedure results:* No relevant procedures ●*Test findings:* Fluoroscopy or U/S of the diaphragms while breathing (sniff test)

Diarrhea ●*Onset:* Acute to chronic ●*Male:female ratio:* M=F ●*Ethnicity:* All ●*Character:* Stools are loose, often watery, large volume, frequent, usually nonbloody; persist despite fasting; weight loss possible ●*Location:* GI tract ●*Pattern:* Not related to meals ●*Precipitating factors:* Three common categories: infection/enterotoxin e.g. cholera, noninvasive E.coli; humoral agent e.g. vasoactive intestinal peptide, calcitonin; detergents e.g. bile salts, laxatives, fatty acids ●*Relieving factors:* Antibiotics if infectious (cholera); antisecretory or antimotility agents ●*Clinical course:* Depends on etiology, most infectious diarrhea is self-limited ●*Co-morbidities:* Depends on etiology; paraneoplastic syndrome is a common cause of humoral agent-induced diarrhea; terminal ileal resection: bile salt diarrhea ●*Procedure results:* Colonoscopy: normal mucosa ●*Test findings:* No fecal leukocytes, stool pH >7, osmolality 260-300mosm/L, osmotic gap <20-40

Dietary weight gain ●*Onset:* Usually insidious ●*Male:female ratio:* M=F ●*Ethnicity:* All ●*Character:* Hypertension, insulin resistance or diabetes mellitus, hyperlipidemia; obstructive sleep apnea, osteoarthritis also possible ●*Location:* Central obesity confers increased risk of cardiovascular sequelae ●*Pattern:* Nonspecific ●*Precipitating factors:* Family history; depression may predispose; hypothyroidism can cause weight gain; other rare hereditary metabolic disorders of lipid or glycogen metabolism ●*Relieving factors:* Exercise, dietary weight loss; medical therapies can help with up to 5% total body weight loss; surgical therapies including gastroplasty available for morbidly obese ●*Clinical course:* Obesity beginning earlier than age 18 carries greatest risk of morbidity; degree and rate of associated medical sequelae depend on genetic predispositions, severity of dietary indiscretions ●*Co-morbidities:* Hypertension, insulin resistance, diabetes mellitus, hyperlipidemia, obstructive sleep apnea, osteoarthritis ●*Procedure results:* Check BMI (height in meters squared/weight in kg squared) ●*Test findings:* BMI >25: overweight; BMI >30: obese; BMI >35 morbidly obese

Diphtheria ●*Onset:* Acute, subacute ●*Male:female ratio:* M=F ●*Ethnicity:* All ●*Character:* Progressive sore throat with dysphagia, hoarseness, neck swelling, later ascending paralysis, syncope, dyspnea on exertion and chest pain ●*Location:* Local: anterior nose, pharynx, tonsils, larynx, trachea, bronchi, skin (cutaneous diptheria), ear, vagina; systemic (toxin-mediated): fever, heart, nerves (ascending paralysis) ●*Pattern:* Gray-white exudates coalescing to a pseudomembrane, exudate removal causes bleeding, skin disease involves, in decreasing order of frequency, the lower extremities, upper extremities, head, trunk; nerve damage involves multiple motor nerves (polyneuritis), causing ascending paralysis ●*Precipitating factors:* Crowded conditions, partial or no immunization, residence in the former Soviet Union (Russia, Ukraine) and central Asia (epidemic since 1990), homelessness and residence in tropical areas (cutaneous diphtheria) ●*Relieving factors:* None relevant ●*Clinical course:* Incubation: 2-5 days, untreated would last 2-4 weeks or longer ●*Co-morbidities:* Homelessness, eczema (for cutaneous), no immunization, alcoholism ●*Procedure results:* Gram stain (club-shaped Gram-variable: positive rod) and culture of nasal/pharyngeal/skin material (isolation of Corynebacterium diphtheria requires special culture media), testing of C. diphtheria isolates for toxin production ●*Test findings:* Gram stain (irregularly staining, club-shaped, Gram-positive rod), growth of C. diphtheria in culture (requires special media), production of toxin by C. diphtheria isolate

Direct hyperbilirubinemia ●*Onset:* Acute/subacute/insidious ●*Male:female ratio:* M=F ●*Ethnicity:* All ●*Character:* Greenish yellow ●*Location:* Skin, eyes ●*Pattern:* Nonspecific ●*Precipitating factors:* Hepatic cellular damage or damaged biliary tract by sepsis, metabolic disorders, endocrine abnormalities ●*Relieving factors:* Treatment of underlying disease and transplantation ●*Clinical course:* Variable and chronic ●*Co-morbidities:* Portal hypertension, xanthomas, pruritus, ascites, encephalopathy, endocrine abnormalities, renal failure and bleeding ●*Procedure results:* Liver biopsy by percutaneous needle to determine etiology; U/S and CT scan to evaluate liver size, consistency and for masses; radionuclide studies and cholangiography to visualize the intrahepatic and extrahepatic biliary tree ●*Test findings:* Elevated direct or conjugated bilirubin >2-3mg/dL, elevated alanine transaminase, aspartate transaminase and gamma glutamyl transferase and alkaline phosphatase, prothrombin, bile acids, cholesterol and low albumin; viral studies for hepatitis A, B, and C

Discoid lupus erythematosus ●*Onset:* Subacute ●*Male:female ratio:* M(1):F(3-9) ●*Ethnicity:* African-American population more commonly affected than Caucasian ●*Character:* Lesions, patchy alopecia ●*Location:* Scalp, ears, face ●*Pattern:* Annular red plaques with central scale ●*Precipitating factors:* Sun exposure ●*Relieving factors:* Topical and intralesional steroids, antimalarials ●*Clinical course:* Progressive ●*Co-morbidities:* Rarely systemic lupus erythematosus ●*Procedure results:* No relevant procedures ●*Test findings:* Positive skin biopsy

Disseminated intravascular coagulation ●*Onset:* Usually acute, rarely indolent ●*Male:female ratio:* M=F ●*Ethnicity:* All ●*Character:* Multiple bleeding sites, vasospasm with acrocyanosis, hypotension ●*Location:* Bleeding: skin, mucous membranes, sites of minor trauma ●*Pattern:* Follows the course of the underlying disorder ●*Precipitating factors:* Trauma, infection (bacterial), obstetrical catastrophes, metastatic malignancies ●*Relieving factors:* Treatment of the underlying disorder, red cell transfusions, depending on scenario: anticoagulants vs fresh frozen plasma ●*Clinical course:* Follows course of underlying disorder ●*Co-morbidities:* Trauma, infection (bacterial), obstetrical catastrophes, metastatic malignancy ●*Procedure results:* No relevant procedures ●*Test findings:* Schistocytes (fragmented red blood cells), thrombocytopenia, prolonged prothrombin (PT) and partial thromboplastin time (PTT) and thrombin time, reduced fibrinogen level, increased fibrinogen degradation products

Distended urinary bladder ●*Onset:* Acute/subacute ●*Male:female ratio:* M<F to age 65; M>F at 65+ ●*Ethnicity:* All ●*Character:* Difficulty in voiding, pain and discomfort ●*Location:* Bladder/suprapubic area ●*Pattern:* Nonspecific ●*Precipitating factors:* UTI, prostatitis, acute spinal cord injury, trauma ●*Relieving factors:* Bladder drainage: catheter or surgical ●*Clinical course:* Progressive to azotemia when not treated ●*Co-morbidities:* UTI, prostatitis, spinal cord injury, trauma, diabetes, neurogenic bladder, benign prostatic hypertrophy, urethral strictures, meatal stenosis, congenital abnormalities in newborns ●*Procedure results:* Ultrasound, CT: distended bladder, possible bilateral hydroureteronephrosis ●*Test findings:* Urine analysis: possible hematuria and pyuria; urine culture and sensitivities: possible bacterial growth

Diuretic abuse ●*Onset:* Chronic ●*Male:female ratio:* M<F ●*Ethnicity:* All ●*Character:* Frequent use of diuretics, usually in attempt to lose water weight ●*Location:* One weight loss technique used by a minority of patients with bulimia ●*Pattern:* Bulimic individual uses diuretics as one way to lose fluid and, therefore, weight ●*Precipitating factors:* Desire to experience a relatively quick weight loss ●*Relieving factors:* Weight loss ●*Clinical course:* Chronic problem resembling other addictive behaviors ●*Co-morbidities:* Bulimia, depressed mood, chemical dependency ●*Procedure results:* ECG may show arrhythmia even with normal electrolytes ●*Test findings:* Depressed levels of CSF-5-hydroxyindoleacetic acid suggest bulimia; electrolyte abnormalities suggest diuretic abuse and/or purging

Diverticular disease ●*Onset:* Insidious ●*Male:female ratio:* M=F ●*Ethnicity:* All ●*Character:* Diverticular bleeding: painless rectal bleeding, often profuse; diverticulitis: left lower quadrant pain and tenderness, fever, WBC usually elevated; IBS-like symptoms which may or may not be related to the diverticula ●*Location:* Left lower quadrant typically ●*Pattern:* Nonspecific ●*Precipitating factors:* There is a theory that seedy foods and nuts may predispose to diverticulitis by becoming lodged in diverticula ●*Relieving factors:* A high fiber diet may be helpful in preventing diverticula formation and in preventing fecal impaction in diverticula; diverticular bleeding usually stops on its own, but may require endoscopic therapy, angiography, or surgical resection if bleeding is prolonged; diverticulitis requires antibiotic therapy, bowel rest ●*Clinical course:* Usually self-limited, but may recur (both bleeding and diverticulitis have 20-30% recurrence rates) ●*Co-morbidities:* None relevant ●*Procedure results:* Diverticular bleeding can be diagnosed via angiography or in some cases by endoscopy; diverticulitis can be diagnosed via CT scan, showing thickening of a segment of colon or a pericolonic abscess ●*Test findings:* WBC usually elevated in diverticulitis

Down syndrome ●*Onset:* Acute - at birth ●*Male:female ratio:* M=F ●*Ethnicity:* All ❶ *Character:* Hypotonia, flat facies, slanted palpebral fissure, small ears, mental deficiency, iris speckling (Brushfield spots), Simian crease, ventricular septal defect (VSD), atrial septal defect (ASD), atrioventricular canal) ●*Location:* Face, CNS, cardiac ●*Pattern:* Nonspecific ●*Precipitating factors:* Trisomy 21 ●*Relieving factors:* None relevant ●*Clinical course:* Lifelong ●*Co-morbidities:* Congenital heart defects, atlantioaxial dislocation, leukemia, lymphocytic thyroiditis ●*Procedure results:* Abnormal amniocentesis, prenatal ultrasound ●*Test findings:* Chromosomal analysis: trisomy 21, low maternal alpha fetoprotein

Image of ❶ *Character on page 471*

Down syndrome: Image *see text page 470*

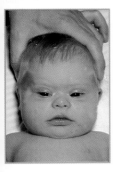

❶ *Character Characteristic facial features of an infant with Down syndrome*

Drug fever ●*Onset:* Acute, subacute, or chronic ●*Male:female ratio:* M=F ●*Ethnicity:* All ●*Character:* Fever, malaise, rash, pruritis, arthralgias. Fever may occur without other symptoms ●*Location:* Nonspecific ●*Pattern:* Nonspecific ●*Precipitating factors:* Many medications implicated: multiple antibiotics, salicylates, cocaine, amphetamines, neuroleptics the most common. Mechanism may be allergic reaction, increased metabolism, altered thermoregulation ●*Relieving factors:* Discontinuing the medication. Treating physiologic effect also helpful (e.g. using benzodiazepines for cocaine induced fever) ●*Clinical course:* Fever may be acute (cocaine, amphetamines), but usually seen after 1-2 weeks of starting drug. May take several weeks to resolve after discontinuing drug ●*Co-morbidities:* None relevant ●*Procedure results:* No relevant procedures ●*Test findings:* Must rule out infectious cause of fever (check blood count, cultures) before making definitive diagnosis

Drug reaction ●*Onset:* Acute ●*Male:female ratio:* M=F ●*Ethnicity:* All ❶ *Character:* Rash, pruritus, swelling of tongue or lips ●*Location:* Nonspecific ●*Pattern:* Nonspecific ●*Precipitating factors:* Medication administration ●*Relieving factors:* Discontinuation of medication ●*Clinical course:* Variable ●*Co-morbidities:* None relevant ●*Procedure results:* No relevant procedures ●*Test findings:* No relevant tests

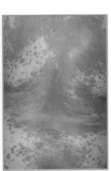

❶ *Character The typical drug reaction is symmetric and diffuse*

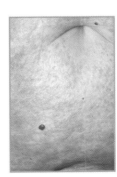

❶ *Character Urticarial papules and plaques are typical*

Drug reaction, ACE inhibitors ●*Onset:* Acute ●*Male:female ratio:* M=F ●*Ethnicity:* All ●*Character:* Non-productive cough ●*Location:* Chest ●*Pattern:* Nonspecific ●*Precipitating factors:* Any ACE inhibitor, but not angiotensin II receptor blocker ●*Relieving factors:* Stop ACE inhibitor ●*Clinical course:* Onset over days to months, resolution within a week after discontinuation of ACE inhibitor ●*Co-morbidities:* Cough hypersensitivity, angioedema ●*Procedure results:* No relevant procedures ●*Test findings:* No relevant tests

Drug reaction, allergic ●*Onset:* Immediate: within 60 min; accelerated: within 1-72 h; late: >72 h ●*Male:female ratio:* M=F ●*Ethnicity:* All ●*Character:* Immediate anaphylactoid reaction or late systemic illness ●*Location:* Cutaneous: urticaria, maculopapular eruptions, exfoliative dermatitis, Stevens-Johnson syndrome. Respiratory: rhinitis, bronchospasm, laryngedema. Systemic: fever ●*Pattern:* Immediate: anaphylactoid urticaria, wheezing, rhinitis, anaphylaxis. Accelerated: urticaria. Late: maculopapular eruptions, fever, hemolytic anemia, nephritis, serum sickness, Stevens-Johnson syndrome ●*Precipitating factors:* Previous exposure to allergens necessary. Most common drugs: beta-lactam antibiotics, ASA, IV contrast, local anesthesia. Elicited by minute dose. Reappears with challenge with shortening of latency period ●*Relieving factors:* Discontinue drug. Antihistamines, systemic corticosteroids. Drug desensitization ●*Clinical course:* Anaphylactoid reactions life-threatening. Late systemic reactions usually resolve within days after stopping drug. Urticaria may persist weeks ●*Co-morbidities:* HIV patients have high incidence of cutaneous reaction to sulfa drugs ●*Procedure results:* Skin testing: reagents to PCN minor determinant not widely available but highly predictive of anaphylaxis ●*Test findings:* Presence of IgE antibodies

Drug reaction, delirium and confusional states ●*Onset:* Acute, subacute, or chronic ●*Male:female ratio:* M=F ●*Ethnicity:* All ●*Character:* Impaired cognitive function with associated altered level of consciousness. Rapid fluctuations in consciousness and activity, visual hallucinations common ●*Location:* Nonspecific ●*Pattern:* Nonspecific ●*Precipitating factors:* Many medications implicated: narcotics (therapeutic or social use), benzodiazepines, barbiturates, cimetidine, glucocorticoids, anticholinergics, phenothiazines ●*Relieving factors:* Discontinuing the medication. Always rule out other treatable causes of altered mental status ●*Clinical course:* Varies on etiology ●*Co-morbidities:* Elderly and patients with impaired liver or renal function most susceptible ●*Procedure results:* No relevant procedures ●*Test findings:* No relevant tests

Drug reaction, lithium ●*Onset:* Acute, subacute, or chronic ●*Male:female ratio:* M=F ●*Ethnicity:* All ●*Character:* Common side effects: thirst, anorexia, diarrhea, polyuria, polydipsia. Toxicity indicated by muscle hyperirritablity, sedation, ataxia, confusion, ventricular arrhythmias, seizures, coma, or death ●*Location:* Nonspecific ●*Pattern:* Nonspecific ●*Precipitating factors:* Overdose, concurrent use of diuretics or nonsteroidal anti-inflammatory drugs, low sodium diet all increase risk of toxicity ●*Relieving factors:* Intravenous normal saline, alkalinization of urine and osmotic diuresis. Hemodialysis in severe toxicity ●*Clinical course:* Up to 10-20% mortality in severe poisonings ●*Co-morbidities:* Elderly patients, hypertension, diabetes mellitus, renal failure increase risk of toxicity ●*Procedure results:* No relevant procedures ●*Test findings:* Toxic lithium level above 2.0mEq/L. ST-T wave and QT interval changes on electrocardiogram. May have abnormal electrolytes and renal function

Drug reaction, peptic ulcer ●*Onset:* Subacute to acute ●*Male:female ratio:* M=F ●*Ethnicity:* All ●*Character:* Abdominal pain, black stools, hematemesis, lightheadedness, fatigue ●*Location:* Nonspecific ●*Pattern:* Nonspecific ●*Precipitating factors:* Nonsteroidal anti-inflammatory medications especially with old age, use of corticosteroids, history of peptic ulcers, anticoagulant usage ●*Relieving factors:* Endoscopic therapy for severe bleeding, withdrawal of medication, proton pump inhibitors or misoprostol ●*Clinical course:* Self-limited with treatment ●*Co-morbidities:* None relevant ●*Procedure results:* Upper endoscopy: ulcer crater or craters, erythema, bleeding ●*Test findings:* Barium study: ulcer crater; anemia, increased RDW and mean corpuscular volume, increased BUN

Drug reaction, skin ●*Onset:* Acute ●*Male:female ratio:* M=F ●*Ethnicity:* All ●*Character:* Itching, erythema ❷ *Location:* Generalized ●*Pattern:* Erythematous macules, papules ●*Precipitating factors:* Medications ●*Relieving factors:* Antihistamines ●*Clinical course:* Self-limited ●*Co-morbidities:* None relevant ●*Procedure results:* No relevant procedures ●*Test findings:* No relevant tests

Image of ❷ *Location on page 473*

Drug reaction, skin: Image *see text page 472*

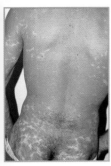

❷ *Location Near total body erythema of acute onset*

Drug reaction, tinnitus ●*Onset:* Subacute ●*Male:female ratio:* M=F ●*Ethnicity:* All ●*Character:* Fullness, tightness, ringing in the ear ●*Location:* Ear ●*Pattern:* Nonspecific ●*Precipitating factors:* Drug induced; many drugs can cause this symptom ●*Relieving factors:* Remove offending drug ●*Clinical course:* Variable ●*Co-morbidities:* None relevant ●*Procedure results:* MRI/CT of brain, biochemical tests for toxins, vitamin deficiencies, endocrine disturbances, vasculopathies affecting the brain, and CNS infections ●*Test findings:* No relevant tests

Drug reaction, uremia ●*Onset:* Acute or chronic ●*Male:female ratio:* M=F ●*Ethnicity:* All ●*Character:* Drug-induced renal failure may occur in many forms including glomerular injury (membranous glomerulonephritis), tubular disease/interstitial nephritis, papillary necrosis, prerenal azotemia ●*Location:* Nonspecific ●*Pattern:* Drug-induced uremia suggests rise in creatinine and BUN, reflecting decreased creatinine clearance. May see associated drug rash, fever, and eosinophilia or eosinophiluria ●*Precipitating factors:* Inadequate hydration, exposure to offending medications including: heroine, analgesics, NSAIDs, aminoglycosides, Penicillins, trimethoprim/sulfamethoxazole, rifampin, pentamidine, amphotericin, allopurinol, ranitidine, ACE inhibitors ●*Relieving factors:* Hydration. Some drug-induced injury can be limited with specific therapy (i.e. N-acetylcysteine for acetaminophen toxicity) ●*Clinical course:* Varies. Acute fulminant renal failure with some drug-induced injury to insidious, slowly progressive renal disease with chronic exposure to other medications. Spontaneous resolution with withdrawal of drug in some cases, residual renal impairment in others ●*Co-morbidities:* Depends on drug; i.e. hepatotoxicity with acetaminophen overdose ●*Procedure results:* Serology ●*Test findings:* Increased creatinine and BUN

Drug withdrawal ●*Onset:* Acute or subacute ●*Male:female ratio:* M=F ●*Ethnicity:* All ●*Character:* Syndromes specific to particular drugs. Most common are alcohol (autonomic hyperactivity, hallucinations, seizures, confusion) and opiates (vomiting, diarrhea, abdominal cramps, chills, diaphoresis) ●*Location:* Nonspecific ●*Pattern:* Nonspecific ●*Precipitating factors:* Clinical syndromes induced by cessation or reduction in use of substance of abuse ●*Relieving factors:* Alcohol withdrawal: intravenous hydration, thiamine, dextrose, sedation with benzodiazepines, close monitoring. Opiate withdrawal: clonidine, symptomatic treatment ●*Clinical course:* Alcohol withdrawal life-threatening whereas opiate withdrawal is not ●*Co-morbidities:* None relevant ●*Procedure results:* No relevant procedures ●*Test findings:* No relevant tests

Dry eye ●*Onset:* Insidious ●*Male:female ratio:* M<F ●*Ethnicity:* All ●*Character:* Foreign body sensation ●*Location:* Ocular adnexa (lids, lacrimal gland, conjunctiva) ●*Pattern:* Typically affects both eyes ●*Precipitating factors:* Worse in heat, wind, low humidity; exacerbated by smoke and other environmental irritants; worsened by antihistamines, antidepressants ●*Relieving factors:* Artificial tears; self-induced yawns also relieve symptoms ●*Clinical course:* Can remit or recur ●*Co-morbidities:* Sjögren's syndrome; rarely Riley-Day syndrome or hypovitaminosis A ●*Procedure results:* Anesthetized Shirmer test result: <5mm wetting in 5 min ●*Test findings:* No relevant tests

Dubin-Johnson syndrome ● *Onset:* Subacute ● *Male:female ratio:* M=F ● *Ethnicity:* All ● *Character:* Mild jaundice ● *Location:* Liver ● *Pattern:* Nonspecific ● *Precipitating factors:* Autosomal recessive - defect in hepatocyte secretion of bilirubin glucuronide, absent function of multiple drug-resistant protein and adenosine triphosphate-dependent canicular transporter ● *Relieving factors:* None relevant ● *Clinical course:* Lifelong ● *Co-morbidities:* None relevant ● *Procedure results:* Gallbladder X-ray abnormal; IV cholangiography shows no biliary tract ● *Test findings:* Normal serum bile acids and urinary coproporphyrin but coproporphyrin I is 80% of the total (coproporphyrin III is normally 75% of total) normal LFTs

Duodenal atresia ● *Onset:* Subacute ● *Male:female ratio:* M=F ● *Ethnicity:* All ● *Character:* Premature birth, feeding intolerance, nausea/vomiting, upper abdominal distention, aspiration, failure to thrive ● *Location:* Nonspecific ● *Pattern:* Symptoms worse postprandially ● *Precipitating factors:* Oral intake ● *Relieving factors:* Vomiting, nasogastric tube placement, surgical correction ● *Clinical course:* Usually recognized shortly after birth and good prognosis if surgically treated ● *Co-morbidities:* 50% have associated congenital defects - trisomy 21, annular pancreas, malrotation, congenital bands, imperforate anus, esophageal atresia, congenital cardiac and renal disease ● *Procedure results:* No relevant procedures ● *Test findings:* Neonatal ultrasound - polyhydramnios; noncontrast radiography - 'double-bubble' sign with air in stomach and first portion of duodenum; contrast radiography demonstrating atresia of second portion of duodenum

Dupuytren's contracture ● *Onset:* Insidious ● *Male:female ratio:* M(10):F(1) ● *Ethnicity:* All ❶ *Character:* Chronic stiffness ● *Location:* Palm ● *Pattern:* Tender fibrous nodule in palm ● *Precipitating factors:* None relevant ● *Relieving factors:* Heat, stretching, ultrasound, cortisone injection ● *Clinical course:* Slowly progressive ● *Co-morbidities:* Alcohol use, diabetes mellitus, epilepsy ● *Procedure results:* No relevant procedures ● *Test findings:* No relevant tests

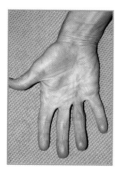

❶ *Character Thickened, fibrous band involving the flexor tendon and contracting the finger*

Dysbarism and barotrauma ● *Onset:* Acute ● *Male:female ratio:* M=F ● *Ethnicity:* All ● *Character:* Barotrauma of descent ('squeeze') effects sinuses or ears with pain, tympanic membrane rupture, bleeding, tinnitus, deafness, vertigo. Ascent can affect ears, teeth, bowel, lungs, joints (the bends), skin, neurologic system ● *Location:* Systemic ● *Pattern:* Symptoms occur during dive or immediately following dive ● *Precipitating factors:* Ascending from dive too quickly ● *Relieving factors:* 100% oxygen, hyperbaric oxygen chamber ● *Clinical course:* Treat as soon as possible to prevent long-term effects ● *Co-morbidities:* None relevant ● *Procedure results:* No relevant procedures ● *Test findings:* No relevant tests

Dysfunctional uterine bleeding ● *Onset:* Subacute ● *Male:female ratio:* F ● *Ethnicity:* Nonspecific ● *Character:* Heavier than usual vaginal bleeding ● *Location:* Nonspecific ● *Pattern:* Usually subacute; progressive over several days ● *Precipitating factors:* Anovulation; polycystic ovary syndrome ● *Relieving factors:* Oral contraceptive, cyclic progestins ● *Clinical course:* Usually self-limiting ● *Co-morbidities:* Anemia; polycystic ovary syndrome ● *Procedure results:* Proliferative endometrium on biopsy ● *Test findings:* Anemia

Dyslexia ●*Onset:* Subacute ●*Male:female ratio:* M(3):F(1) ●*Ethnicity:* All ●*Character:* Difficulty with reading in person with normal intelligence/motivation/opportunities without other learning disabilities. Difficulty with decoding, word recognition with mispronunciations, hesitations, limited comprehension ●*Location:* Nonspecific ●*Pattern:* Nonspecific ●*Precipitating factors:* Familial: 23-65% have parent with dyslexia. Thought to be associated with chromosome 6 ●*Relieving factors:* Combined teaching methods specifically tailored for dyslexia including phonologic methods, educational aids (laptop computers with spell checkers), tutorial services, alternative tests ●*Clinical course:* Lifelong ●*Co-morbidities:* Attention deficit hyperactivity disorder ●*Procedure results:* No relevant procedures ●*Test findings:* Educational testing: specific for dyslexia

Dysmenorrhea ●*Onset:* Subacute, insidious ●*Male:female ratio:* F ●*Ethnicity:* All ●*Character:* Crampy, waxes and wanes ●*Location:* Pelvic pain, may be associated with nausea, vomiting, diarrhea, dizziness ●*Pattern:* Cyclic pelvic pain occurring just before or at onset of menses, lasting 48-72 hours ●*Precipitating factors:* Primary dysmenorrhea has no underlying pathologic process ●*Relieving factors:* NSAIDs, oral contraceptives, gonadotrophin-releasing hormone agonist analogues, e.g. Leuprolide depot ●*Clinical course:* Variable, depending on underlying cause and age at onset ●*Co-morbidities:* Endometriosis, adenomyosis, cervical stenosis, pelvic inflammatory disease cause secondary amenorrhea ●*Procedure results:* Laparoscopy for direct visualization of endometriosis ●*Test findings:* Pelvic ultrasound, MRI, hysterosalpingogram to diagnose adenomyosis

Dyspareunia ●*Onset:* Acute, subacute ●*Male:female ratio:* M<F ●*Ethnicity:* All ●*Character:* Sharp pain associated with vaginal penetration ●*Location:* Introital, pelvic ●*Pattern:* Vulvovaginal with insertion or pelvic pain with deep penetration ●*Precipitating factors:* Inadequate lubrication, incomplete hymen rupture, inadequate episiotomy, vaginismus, Bartholin cyst ●*Relieving factors:* Adequate lubrication, treatment of infectious or atrophic vaginitis ●*Clinical course:* Unremitting unless appropriately treated ●*Co-morbidities:* Pelvic inflammatory disease (PID), endometriosis, ovarian cyst, leiomyomas, history of sexual abuse ●*Procedure results:* Laparoscopy to assess endometriosis, adnexal mass, lysis of adhesions ●*Test findings:* Pelvic U/S to assess structural abnormalities

Dystonia ●*Onset:* Subacute/acute ●*Male:female ratio:* M=F ●*Ethnicity:* All ●*Character:* Abnormal sustained movement or posture due to a disturbance of muscle tone in agonists and antagonists ●*Location:* Involves fingers, hands, arms, legs, toes, and face ●*Pattern:* Nonspecific ●*Precipitating factors:* Idiopathic, Huntington's disease, Wilson's disease, familial calcification of the basal ganglia, stroke within the basal ganglia, medications: lithium, phenytoin, carbamazepine, amphetamines ●*Relieving factors:* Treat the underlying etiology. In some cases, haloperidol is used ●*Clinical course:* Variable depending on etiology ●*Co-morbidities:* None relevant ●*Procedure results:* No relevant procedures ●*Test findings:* No relevant tests

Eaton-Lambert (myasthenic) syndrome ●*Onset:* Insidious ●*Male:female ratio:* M=F ●*Ethnicity:* All ●*Character:* Weakness, ptosis, diplopia, myalgias, stiffness ●*Location:* Weakness is usually in the hip-girdle, less commonly in shoulders ●*Pattern:* Worse in the morning and improves throughout the day ●*Precipitating factors:* None relevant ●*Relieving factors:* Plasmapheresis, immunosuppression, variable response to anticholenergics ●*Clinical course:* Poor prognosis when associated with small-cell lung cancer ●*Co-morbidities:* Small-cell lung cancer, less commonly associated with autoimmune disease ●*Procedure results:* No relevant procedures ●*Test findings:* EMG-repetitive stimulation produces incremental response, antibody against P/Q type presynaptic channels

Echinococcosis ●*Onset:* Chronic ●*Male:female ratio:* M=F ●*Ethnicity:* All ●*Character:* Pain or discomfort in the upper abdominal region, weight loss, hives, anaphylaxis ●*Location:* Liver, lungs, brain, kidney, spleen, other (any organ) ●*Pattern:* Incidental radiographic finding of large cysts, RUQ pain with or without a palpable mass ●*Precipitating factors:* Areas where livestock and dogs, worldwide distribution but more in the Middle East, South America, Africa, Eastern Europe, Mediterranean ●*Relieving factors:* None relevant ●*Clinical course:* Slowly progressive over years-decades, asymptomatic early, rupture or leakage may cause anaphylaxis or death ●*Co-morbidities:* None relevant ●*Procedure results:* Irregular cysts, sometimes with mural calcifications, on abdominal ultra-sound, chest X-ray, or CT of the head, chest, or abdomen (specific serology) ●*Test findings:* Rare eosinophilia, rare elevation in alkaline phosphatase, usually normal

Eclampsia ●*Onset:* Subacute, acute ●*Male:female ratio:* F ●*Ethnicity:* Nonspecific ●*Character:* Seizure in the third trimester of pregnancy ●*Location:* Vascular/placental ●*Pattern:* Usually progressive from pre-eclampsia though not always; associated hypertension, edema, proteinuria ●*Precipitating factors:* None relevant ●*Relieving factors:* Delivery of fetus ●*Clinical course:* Usually self-limiting though potentially lethal; resolves with delivery ●*Co-morbidities:* Lupus, hypertension, renal disease, diabetes ●*Procedure results:* Reduction in amniotic fluid, fetal growth, umbilical blood flow on fetus ●*Test findings:* Proteinuria, thrombocytopenia, elevated transaminases, elevated uric acid

Ectodermal dysplasia ●*Onset:* Congenital ●*Male:female ratio:* X-linked recessive anhydrotic variant M>F; hydrotic variant M=F ●*Ethnicity:* Hydrotic variant seen in French Canadians (Clouston's syndrome) ●*Character:* Alopecia, hypohidrosis and anodontia in the anhydrotic variant; alopecia, nail dystrophy, palmoplantar hyperkeratosis, cataracts characterize the hydrotic variant ●*Location:* Various clinical features by location, including scalp, mouth and dry/warm/anhydrotic or hypohydrotic skin ●*Pattern:* As this is a genodermatosis, there is no progression or regression of disease; anhydrosis can cause overheating problems ●*Precipitating factors:* Heat exposure ●*Relieving factors:* None relevant ●*Clinical course:* Alopecia is permanent and can be treated with hair pieces; anodontia can be treated with prostheses; anhydrosis can pose an emergency due to heat exhaustion and heat stroke ●*Co-morbidities:* Mental retardation, absent mammary glands occasionally ●*Procedure results:* No relevant procedures ●*Test findings:* No relevant tests

Ectopic pregnancy ●*Onset:* Subacute, acute ●*Male:female ratio:* F ●*Ethnicity:* Nonspecific ●*Character:* Stabbing pain or intermittent pain associated with bleeding per vagina ●*Location:* Lower abdominal pain ●*Pattern:* Nonspecific ●*Precipitating factors:* None relevant ●*Relieving factors:* Surgery; methotrexate ●*Clinical course:* Significant cause of maternal death; if untreated rupture and significant blood loss may occur. Loss of tube following surgery may afffect fertility ●*Co-morbidities:* Previous PID; pelvic adhesions ●*Procedure results:* Ectopic pregnancy or ultrasound; absence of intrauterine pregnancy on vaginal probe ultrasound with HCG>1500 ●*Test findings:* HCG positive

Ectopic ureter ●*Onset:* Acute/subacute/or insidious ●*Male:female ratio:* M=F ●*Ethnicity:* Any ●*Character:* Can be asymptomatic, or result in symptoms and signs of urinary tract obstruction (pain, azotemia, hypertension) ●*Location:* Ectopic ureter most commonly in retrocaval position. If results in renal obstruction, pain typically in flank region; may radiate down to groin ●*Pattern:* Colicky/visceral pain if obstruction occurs ●*Precipitating factors:* Congenital ●*Relieving factors:* Surgical correction ●*Clinical course:* If ectopic ureter results in obstruction, can have long-term sequelae including chronic hydronephrosis and renal failure ●*Co-morbidities:* Obstruction due to congenital anomalies can result in urinary reflux, chronic infection, hydronephrosis, and renal failure ●*Procedure results:* Intravenous pyelogram (IVP) ●*Test findings:* May be evident on CT scan or other imaging

Ehlers-Danlos syndrome ●*Onset:* Subacute ●*Male:female ratio:* M=F ●*Ethnicity:* All ●*Character:* Skin hyperelastic, skin fragile, joint hypermobility ●*Location:* Skin able to be stretched, easy bruising and keloid formation, joints dislocatable ●*Pattern:* Minor lacerations result in severe wounds ●*Precipitating factors:* Minor lacerations. Valsalva maneuver can lead to rupture of great vessels ●*Relieving factors:* None relevant ●*Clinical course:* Chronic ●*Co-morbidities:* Aortic anuerysm ●*Procedure results:* Collagen abnormality ●*Test findings:* Decreased enzyme activity in fibroblasts

Ehrlichiosis ●*Onset:* Acute ●*Male:female ratio:* M=F ●*Ethnicity:* All ●*Character:* Abrupt onset of fever, headache, myalgia, malaise, and less often anorexia, nausea, and vomiting, followed by confusion ●*Location:* Systemic infection of granulocytes or monocytes, involving bloodstream, CNS, liver, conjunctivae, and less often skin, lungs, kidneys, coagulation cascade (DIC), other organ systems ●*Pattern:* Illness is nonspecific and flu-like; headache is pronounced; rash is uncommon (10%); symptoms are more severe in the elderly ●*Precipitating factors:* Tick bite, northeastern and midwestern USA between April and November for human granulocytic ehrlichiosis; south-central, mid-Atlantic, and southeastern USA, Europe and Africa for human monocytic ehrlichiosis; northwestern USA for E. Ewingii, rural areas ●*Relieving factors:* Acetaminophen ●*Clinical course:* Abrupt onset, lasts 3-30 days, self-limiting in most cases but severe illness may be fatal, rapid response to antimicrobial therapy ●*Co-morbidities:* Lyme disease, babesiosis (for HGE) ●*Procedure results:* Intragranulocytic or intramonocytic inclusions (morulae) on peripheral blood smear, detection of Ehrlichia DNA in blood by PCR (polymerase chain reaction), positive serologic tests ●*Test findings:* Normal or low WBC, thrombocytopenia, elevated hepatic transaminases

Elbow dislocation ●*Onset:* Acute ●*Male:female ratio:* M=F ●*Ethnicity:* All ●*Character:* May be posterior (most common) or anterior. Marked swelling and pain at elbow joint. Elbow may be held in flexion (posterior type) or full extension (anterior type) ●*Location:* Elbow joint ●*Pattern:* Nonspecific ●*Precipitating factors:* Fall on extended arm (posterior) or direct blow to olecranon with elbow in flexion (anterior) ●*Relieving factors:* Pain medication, reduction of dislocation, splinting ●*Clinical course:* Some restriction in range of movement may persist after injury has healed ●*Co-morbidities:* Brachial artery, ulnar and median nerve injuries common ●*Procedure results:* No relevant procedures ●*Test findings:* Radiographs will reveal dislocation and any fractures around joint

Elbow injury ●*Onset:* Acute ●*Male:female ratio:* M=F ●*Ethnicity:* All ●*Character:* Pain and limited range of motion following injury. May see swelling or deformity around joint. May cause neurovascular compromise distal to injury ●*Location:* Nonspecific ●*Pattern:* Nonspecific ●*Precipitating factors:* Most common: falls on joint, direct blows and falls on outstretched. Abrupt traction on arm causes subluxation in children (nursemaids' elbow) ●*Relieving factors:* Immobilization with splint and/or sling. Ice, analgesics. Reduction of dislocations. Fractures may require open reduction and fixation ●*Clinical course:* Some restriction in range of movement may persist after injury has healed ●*Co-morbidities:* None relevant ●*Procedure results:* X-ray diagnoses fractures/dislocations ●*Test findings:* Posterior fat pad or displaced anterior fat pad indicate probable fracture

Empyema ● *Onset:* Acute, subacute ● *Male:female ratio:* M=F ● *Ethnicity:* All ● *Character:* Fever, dyspnea, chest discomfort ● *Location:* Chest ● *Pattern:* Dullness to percussion and decreased breath sounds ● *Precipitating factors:* Pneumonia, chest surgery or procedure (fine needle aspirate or biopsy), Borhaave's syndrome ● *Relieving factors:* Thoracostomy, antibiotics ● *Clinical course:* Weeks-months ● *Co-morbidities:* Pneumonia, upper abdominal infectious disorder, chest trauma or procedure ● *Procedure results:* Bacteria present on pleural fluid Gram stain or culture ● *Test findings:* Exudative pleural effusion. Commonly, pleural fluid leukocytosis (neutrophilia) and low glucose

Encephalitis ● *Onset:* Acute, subacute ● *Male:female ratio:* M=F ● *Ethnicity:* All ● *Character:* Confusion, focal neurologic exam, fever ● *Location:* Nonspecific ● *Pattern:* Nonspecific ● *Precipitating factors:* Exposure to infectious agent ● *Relieving factors:* Supportive and treatment of herpes encephalitis with acyclovir ● *Clinical course:* Variable ● *Co-morbidities:* None relevant ● *Procedure results:* Lumbar puncture. CSF pleocytosis predominate with lymphs ● *Test findings:* Variable CT/MRI findings, abnormal CSF pleocytosis with a predominance of lymph

Encephalitis lethargica ● *Onset:* Subacute ● *Male:female ratio:* M=F ● *Ethnicity:* All ● *Character:* Somnolence and ophthalmoplegia ● *Location:* Inflammation of thalamus and midbrain thought to be due to viral infection ● *Pattern:* Occurred during and 10 years following World War 1 ● *Precipitating factors:* Causative viral agent never identified ● *Relieving factors:* Supportive care ● *Clinical course:* Progression to Parkinsonism months-to-years following illness in high proportion of survivors ● *Co-morbidities:* None relevant ● *Procedure results:* Lumbar puncture usually positive for leukocytosis and elevated protein; MRI shows changes of localized infection prior to CT ● *Test findings:* Examination consistent with viral infection of the thalamus and midbrain

Encephalopathy ● *Onset:* Acute ● *Male:female ratio:* M=F ● *Ethnicity:* All ● *Character:* Altered brain function due to metabolic abnormalities ● *Location:* Disruption of cerebral metabolism ● *Pattern:* Cognitive impairment, alteration of level of arousal, sleep disturbance, asterixis, hyperactive deep tendon reflexes, papilledema (hypercapnea) ● *Precipitating factors:* Hepatic insufficiency, malignant hypertension, uremia, hypoglycemia, drug intoxication, hypoxemia, hypercapnea ● *Relieving factors:* Identification and reversal of underying cause. Dialysis, reversal of electrolyte abnormalities ● *Clinical course:* Potentially reversible depending on duration of symptoms and severity ● *Co-morbidities:* Emphysema, diabetes, hepatic failure, renal failure, thyroid disorders, Cushing's disease ● *Procedure results:* CT indicated to rule out other causes; may show generalized cerebral edema ● *Test findings:* Electrolyte disturbance, hypoglycemia, uremia, elevated ammonia levels, elevated drug levels, abnormal liver function tests

Enchondroma ● *Onset:* Subacute ● *Male:female ratio:* M=F ● *Ethnicity:* All ● *Character:* Pain and swelling ● *Location:* Proximal fingers ● *Pattern:* Nonspecific ● *Precipitating factors:* None relevant ● *Relieving factors:* Surgical curettage ● *Clinical course:* Chronic with occasional transformation to malignant chondrosarcoma ● *Co-morbidities:* None relevant ● *Procedure results:* Biopsy of involved bone shows mature cartilage within bone ● *Test findings:* Radiographs show thinning of the cortex with calcifications

Encopresis ● *Onset:* Subacute ● *Male:female ratio:* M>F ● *Ethnicity:* All ● *Character:* Loose watery stools leaking around hard retained stools, abdominal pain ● *Location:* Rectum ● *Pattern:* History of constipation/withholding stools leading to distension of rectum/colon with decreased sensitivity of defecation reflex and ineffective peristalsis ● *Precipitating factors:* Constipation/withholding of stools - behavioral or underlying organic problem ● *Relieving factors:* Behavioral modification, treatment of underlying cause, enemas/suppositories/stool softeners/dietary changes ● *Clinical course:* Persists until underlying cause treated ● *Co-morbidities:* Hypothyroidism, cystic fibrosis, Hirschsprung's disease, neuronal dysgenesis, anal stricture ● *Procedure results:* Rectal exam showing large amount stool in rectal vault ● *Test findings:* Kidneys, ureter and bladder X-ray showing large amount of retained stool

Endemic typhus ●*Onset:* Abrupt ●*Male:female ratio:* M=F ●*Ethnicity:* Common in Asia ●*Character:* Fever, chills, and vomiting lasting about 12 days; occasionally accompanied by rash, pneumonia, or other organ system involvement ●*Location:* Systemic (bloodstream), generalized skin, including face, palms, soles, lungs; less commonly CNS, liver, kidneys, other ●*Pattern:* Fever higher at night; rash macular (rarely petechial) and generalized, involving palms, soles, face; lung involvement interstitial; encephalopathy nondistinctive and rare ●*Precipitating factors:* Flea bite or exposure to fleas, occupational or other exposure to animals carrying fleas such as cats, rats, raccoons, skunks, possums ●*Relieving factors:* Symptoms respond rapidly to antimicrobial therapy. Ten percent require hospitalization ●*Clinical course:* Incubation period: 8-16 days; prodrome of headache and myalgia 1-3 days, followed by abrupt and prolonged high fever with chills which last 9-18 days with rash, when present, appearing on second day ●*Co-morbidities:* None relevant ●*Procedure results:* Pulmonary infiltrates on chest X-ray in 25% ●*Test findings:* Early leukopenia followed by leukocytosis, anemia, thrombocytopenia, hyponatremia, hypoalbuminemia, elevated hepatic transaminases. Four-fold rise in antibody titer or single titer >=1:128, detection of R. typhi or R. felis DNA in blood by PCR

Endometrial cancer ●*Onset:* Insidious ●*Male:female ratio:* F ●*Ethnicity:* All ●*Character:* Vaginal bleeding ●*Location:* Uterine ●*Pattern:* Irregular bleeding, abnormal Pap test ●*Precipitating factors:* Unopposed estrogen therapy ●*Relieving factors:* None relevant ●*Clinical course:* Progression to invasion and malignancy ●*Co-morbidities:* Obesity ●*Procedure results:* Endometrial biopsy shows atypical, dysplastic cells on pathology ●*Test findings:* No relevant tests

Endometrial scarring ●*Onset:* Insidious ●*Male:female ratio:* F ●*Ethnicity:* All ●*Character:* Amenorrhea ●*Location:* Intrauterine ●*Pattern:* Absence of menses after surgical procedure ●*Precipitating factors:* Usually associated with postpartum sharp curettage ●*Relieving factors:* Hysteroscopic resection of scar tissue ●*Clinical course:* Relieved only surgically ●*Co-morbidities:* Associated with miscarriages ●*Procedure results:* Hysteroscopic visualization of scarring. Hysterosalpingram revealing scarring ●*Test findings:* No relevant tests

Endometriosis ●*Onset:* Subacute onset over months/years ●*Male:female ratio:* F ●*Ethnicity:* Nonspecific ●*Character:* Cramping, aching ●*Location:* Pain below umbilicus, tenderness, nodularity of uterosacral ligaments on exam ●*Pattern:* Pelvic pain just before and during menses ●*Precipitating factors:* Peak incidence age 25, more frequent in nulliparous women ●*Relieving factors:* NSAIDs, oral contraceptives, GnRH agonist analogues, e.g. Leuprolide depot ●*Clinical course:* Persistent, progressive ●*Co-morbidities:* Infertility, pelvic mass due to endometrioma ●*Procedure results:* Laparoscopy definitive diagnosis. Pelvic ultrasound normal ●*Test findings:* No relevant tests

Enterobiasis ●*Onset:* Acute, persistent until treated ●*Male:female ratio:* M=F ●*Ethnicity:* All ●*Character:* Perianal itching, rarely vaginal itching, may be asymptomatic ●*Location:* Duodenum, intestines, perianal area, vagina (rare) ●*Pattern:* Nocturnal symptoms, pruritic perianal area, rarely pruritic vulvar area ●*Precipitating factors:* Contact, day care, family clusters, no hand washing ●*Relieving factors:* None relevant ●*Clinical course:* Persistent until treated, can be asymptomatic, relapse and reinfection common ●*Co-morbidities:* None relevant ●*Procedure results:* Pinworms on Sellotape pressed against perianal area at night or early morning, visualization of worms in perianal area at night ●*Test findings:* Pinworms eggs on Sellotape pressed against perianal area at night or early morning, visualization of pinworms in perianal area, worms and eggs in stool

Enuresis ● *Onset:* Subacute ● *Male:female ratio:* M(3):F(1) ● *Ethnicity:* All ● *Character:* Voluntary/involuntary repeated urination into clothes/bed after age when bladder control should be established (usually by age 5) ● *Location:* Bladder ● *Pattern:* Primary (persistent): never dry at night. Secondary (regressive): dry for at least 1 year and then wet again ● *Precipitating factors:* Secondary: stress, strong genetic predisposition for nocturnal enuresis, sleep apnea/disorder, obstructive uropathy, delayed maturation of bladder function, reduced bladder capacity, abnormal antidiuretic hormone secretion ● *Relieving factors:* Treat underlying problem if present, behavior modification, including conditioning device (bell-pad alarm), imipramine, desmopressin, biofeedback ● *Clinical course:* Spontaneous resolution or usually self-limited once underlying issue treated or behavior modification used ● *Co-morbidities:* UTI, micturition deferral, chemical urethritis, constipation, diabetes (mellitus/insipidus), giggle incontinence, uninhibited bladder, infrequent voiding, Hinman syndrome, posterior urethral valves, neurologic disorder ● *Procedure results:* Renal ultrasound, voiding cystourethrogram ● *Test findings:* Urinalysis normal/abnormal

Eosinophilic pneumonias ● *Onset:* Acute, insidious ● *Male:female ratio:* M=F ● *Ethnicity:* All ● *Character:* Dyspnea, cough ● *Location:* Chest ● *Pattern:* Bilateral inspiratory rales ● *Precipitating factors:* Parasitic infection, drug reaction, idiopathic ● *Relieving factors:* Specific antibiotics if infection identified, withdrawal of suspect drug, steroids ● *Clinical course:* Weeks-months ● *Co-morbidities:* Vasculitis (rarely) ● *Procedure results:* Chest X-ray: fleeting pulmonary infiltrates or, in chronic eosinophilic pneumonia, peripheral dense infiltrates ('photographic negative' of pulmonary edema) with peripheral blood or bronchoalveolar lavage eosinophilia ● *Test findings:* Peripheral blood and/or bronchoalveolar lavage eosinophilia, PFT: restrictive ventilatory defect (in acute or chronic eosinophilic pneumonia or tropical eosinophilic pneumonia) or obstructive ventilatory defect (in allergic bronchopulmonary aspergillosis, Churg-Strauss vasculitis, asthma), stool or sputum for ova and parasites positive for ascaris or strongyloides, p-ANCA positive with vasculitis

Epicondylitis ● *Onset:* Subacute ● *Male:female ratio:* M=F ● *Ethnicity:* All ● *Character:* Sharp pain ● *Location:* Medial or lateral aspect of elbow ● *Pattern:* Focal pain ● *Precipitating factors:* Stress of the associated tendons ● *Relieving factors:* NSAIDs, rest, ice, corticosteroid injection, splint ● *Clinical course:* Pain continues if tendon is chronically stressed ● *Co-morbidities:* None relevant ● *Procedure results:* No relevant procedures ● *Test findings:* No relevant tests

Epidermolysis bullosa ● *Onset:* Acute ● *Male:female ratio:* M=F ● *Ethnicity:* All ● *Character:* Mechanobullous disorder with skin fragility, tense bullae; noninflammatory, present mainly on acral skin, heal with scarring and milia formation ● *Location:* Acral; another variant characterized by a widespread eruption involving the trunk, central body and skin folds ● *Pattern:* Begins with vesicles and bullae on acral skin areas; hard to treat, but does well with attention to skin care; heals with scarring and milia ● *Precipitating factors:* Frictional trauma to skin can result in lesions ● *Relieving factors:* Alleviation of trauma with the use of protective dressings over bony prominences ● *Clinical course:* Resistant to treatment; with proper education on skin care, and newer therapies including intravenous immunoglobulin, patients remain disease-free for extended periods of time ● *Co-morbidities:* Inflammatory bowel disease, lupus erythematosus, thyroiditis, pulmonary fibrosis, chronic lymphocytic leukemia, thymoma, diabetes ● *Procedure results:* Skin biopsy reveals subepidermal bulla; direct immunofluorescence staining with antibody to collagen VII reveals a linear pattern at the base of the bulla ● *Test findings:* Indirect immunofluorecence on salt-split skin shows staining of the base of the bulla; titers not helpful in following disease progression

Epididymitis ● *Onset:* Subacute ● *Male:female ratio:* M ● *Ethnicity:* All ● *Character:* Pain, swelling, induration ● *Location:* Scrotum, inguinal canal ● *Pattern:* Usually unilateral ● *Precipitating factors:* STD, UTI, indwelling Foley catheter, urethral stricture, urethral and transurethral surgery ● *Relieving factors:* Antibiotics, anti-inflammatory medications, scrotal elevation, surgical intervention (rarely used) ● *Clinical course:* Progressive if untreated

Possibly leading to abscess formation, testicular necrosis or infertility ● *Co-morbidities:* STD, UTI, urethral strictures, BPH, TB, prostatitis, hydrocele ● *Procedure results:* Doppler scrotal ultrasound or nuclear scan ruling out acute testicular torsion ● *Test findings:* Gram stain and culture of midstream urine or urethral swab: any or all possibly positive

Epidural abscess ● *Onset:* Subacute/acute ● *Male:female ratio:* M=F ● *Ethnicity:* All ● *Character:* Severe back pain ● *Location:* Pain is located above the area of abscess ● *Pattern:* Nonspecific ● *Precipitating factors:* Immunocompromised, trauma, systemic infection, spinal anesthesia ● *Relieving factors:* Surgical debridement and antibiotics ● *Clinical course:* Good prognosis with treatment ● *Co-morbidities:* None relevant ● *Procedure results:* MRI/CT of spinal canal will reveal abscess location ● *Test findings:* Complete blood count, blood cultures

Epiglottitis ● *Onset:* Acute ● *Male:female ratio:* M>F (slightly) ● *Ethnicity:* All ● *Character:* Severe sore throat, fever, odynophagia ● *Location:* Pharynx, hypopharynx, larynx ● *Pattern:* Steady, perhaps rapid, progressive throat pain and shortness of breath, reluctant to swallow secretions ● *Precipitating factors:* None relevant ● *Relieving factors:* Upright position, leaning forward ● *Clinical course:* Variable: may be rapid progression in children ● *Co-morbidities:* None relevant ● *Procedure results:* Swollen epiglottis on fiberoptic endoscopy ● *Test findings:* Swollen epiglottis on lateral view of the neck; fever

Epilepsy ● *Onset:* Acute ● *Male:female ratio:* M=F ● *Ethnicity:* All ● *Character:* Generalized tonic-tonic, complex partial, simple partial, focal motor ● *Location:* Nonspecific ● *Pattern:* Nonspecific ● *Precipitating factors:* Idiopathic, infection, tumor, genetic, trauma ● *Relieving factors:* Depends on etiology ● *Clinical course:* Variable ● *Co-morbidities:* None relevant ● *Procedure results:* No relevant procedures ● *Test findings:* Variable CT/MRI findings. CSF profile depending on etiology

Episcleritis ● *Onset:* Acute ● *Male:female ratio:* M=F ● *Ethnicity:* All ❶ *Character:* Mild to moderate achy pain, tearing foreign body sensation ● *Location:* Episclera ● *Pattern:* Usually unilateral ● *Precipitating factors:* None relevant ● *Relieving factors:* NSAIDs may relieve pain ● *Clinical course:* Self-limited without treatment in 1 to 2 weeks ● *Co-morbidities:* Work-up usually negative; connective tissue disease for recurrent or atypical attacks ● *Procedure results:* Slit lamp exam; sectoral conjunctival, episcleral injection ● *Test findings:* Residual episcleral injection after application of 2.5% phenylephrine

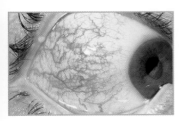

❶ *Character Conjunctival injection blanches with pressure and with phenylephrine hydrochloride eye drops*

Epistaxis ● *Onset:* Acute ● *Male:female ratio:* M=F ● *Ethnicity:* All ❶ *Character:* Bleeding from nose ● *Location:* Usually unilateral nares ● *Pattern:* Epistaxis occurs more often in the evening ● *Precipitating factors:* Strenuous activity; nose picking; trauma ● *Relieving factors:* Icepack; pinching the nose; packing the nose ● *Clinical course:* May start and stop spontaneously or may persist, requiring therapy on an urgent basis ● *Co-morbidities:* Blood thinners (coumadin, aspirin); septal deviation ● *Procedure results:* Anterior rhinoscopy will often disclose bleeding from the anterior septum ● *Test findings:* No relevant tests

Epithelial cell ovarian cancer ●*Onset:* Insidious ●*Male:female ratio:* F ●*Ethnicity:* BRCA1 and BRCA2 carriers may have up to a 50% lifetime risk ●*Character:* Vague abdominal discomfort; bloating; constipation ●*Location:* Abdomen ●*Pattern:* About 75% present with advanced stage disease ●*Precipitating factors:* BRCA1 and BRCA2 carriers may have up to a 50% lifetime risk ●*Relieving factors:* None relevant ●*Clinical course:* Progression to invasion and distant metastases ●*Co-morbidities:* None relevant ●*Procedure results:* Adnexal mass with or without ascites on ultrasound or CT scan ●*Test findings:* Elevated CA-125

Epitrochlear lymphadenitis ●*Onset:* Acute ●*Male:female ratio:* M=F ●*Ethnicity:* All ●*Character:* Unilateral tender swelling, erythema and induration along medial aspect of elbow, pain on moving the elbow ●*Location:* Peritrochlear area (medial aspect of elbow area), may spread to medial arm and forearm ●*Pattern:* Unilateral tender swelling medial to elbow, erythema and induration along medial aspect of elbow, pain on moving the elbow ●*Precipitating factors:* Infection of little, ring or middle finger, skin infection of medial hand, rarely joint or bone infection of medial hand/elbow ●*Relieving factors:* Drainage is suppurative, antibiotics, treating underlying infection ●*Clinical course:* Acute ●*Co-morbidities:* Pyoderma, skin infection, arthritis, osteomyelitis ●*Procedure results:* Pus upon incision and drainage ●*Test findings:* Leukocytosis, positive drainage culture (usually Staphylococcus aureus or group A Streptococcus)

Erysipelas ●*Onset:* Acute ●*Male:female ratio:* M=F ●*Ethnicity:* All ●*Character:* Abrupt onset; sharply demarcated; painful, bright red, warm, swelling; induration on face or extremities ●*Location:* Lower extremities, malar areas of the face, nasal bridge, other ●*Pattern:* Rash has well-defined, raised, indurated borders, bright red, warm, associated intense pain, superficial bullae may form and later desquamate ●*Precipitating factors:* Venous staxis, lymphedema, skin ulcer, umbilical stump in neonate as portal of entry, prior erysipelas ●*Relieving factors:* None relevant ●*Clinical course:* Abrupt onset over a few hours, bullae appear after 2-3 days, desquamation may occur after 5-7 days ●*Co-morbidities:* Lymphedema, venous insufficiency, nephrotic syndrome, CABG surgery, mastectomy, eczema, nonintact skin ●*Procedure results:* No relevant procedures ●*Test findings:* Leukocytosis with a left shift, rarely positive blood cultures for Streptococcus pyogenes

Erythema infectiosum ●*Onset:* Acute ●*Male:female ratio:* M=F ●*Ethnicity:* All ●*Character:* Rash, fever ●*Location:* Cheeks, proximal extremities ●*Pattern:* Red 'slapped' cheeks, reticulate exanthem proximal extremities ●*Precipitating factors:* Infection with parvovirus b19 ●*Relieving factors:* Symptomatic relief ●*Clinical course:* Resolves in weeks: may wax and wane ●*Co-morbidities:* Rare anemia/leukopenia, pregnancy: increased fetal risk ●*Procedure results:* No relevant procedures ●*Test findings:* Test for parvovirus b19

Erythema multiforme ●*Onset:* Acute ●*Male:female ratio:* M(3):F(2) ●*Ethnicity:* All ❶ *Character:* Skin lesions ●*Location:* Acral/extremities, rare mucous membranes ❸ *Pattern:* Red purpuric macules, target lesions, bullae ●*Precipitating factors:* Infection, medication ●*Relieving factors:* Antihistamines, rarely systemic steroids ●*Clinical course:* Self-limited episodes ●*Co-morbidities:* None relevant ●*Procedure results:* No relevant procedures ●*Test findings:* Positive skin biopsy

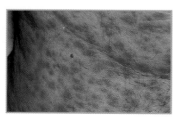

❶ *Character* These lesions are atypical targets

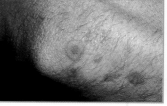

❸ *Pattern* A very typical target lesion

Erythema nodosum ●*Onset:* Acute ●*Male:female ratio:* M(1):F(3) ●*Ethnicity:* All **❶** *Character:* Pain **❷** *Location:* Pretibial **❸** *Pattern:* Tender, warm, red, bruise-like nodules ●*Precipitating factors:* Infection, medication ●*Relieving factors:* Heat, rest, NSAIDs, saturated potassium iodine ●*Clinical course:* Self-limited, 3-6 weeks ●*Co-morbidities:* Arthritis, inflammatory bowel disease ●*Procedure results:* Positive skin biopsy ●*Test findings:* No relevant tests

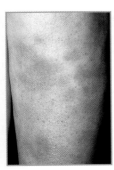

❶ *Character* A nodule (above) and a plaque (below)

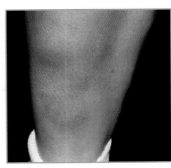

❷ *Location* Multiple erythematous nodules on the shin

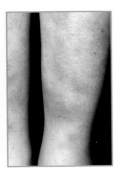

❸ *Pattern* Multiple painful erythematous nodules are typical

Erythema toxicum ●*Onset:* Acute ●*Male:female ratio:* M=F ●*Ethnicity:* All ●*Character:* Evanescent firm yellow-white papulo-pustular lesions with surrounding erythema, splotchy redness, few to many lesions ●*Location:* Over body usually sparing palms/soles ●*Pattern:* Evanescent, peak incidence on second day of life ●*Precipitating factors:* Unknown - found in 50% of full-term infants, less in pre-term infants ●*Relieving factors:* Resolves spontaneously ●*Clinical course:* Waxes/wanes from days to weeks, resolves without treatment ●*Co-morbidities:* None relevant ●*Procedure results:* Eosinophils around pilosebaceous follicle eosinophils found in Wright-stained smears of lesions; cultures areas sterile ●*Test findings:* No relevant tests

Erythroderma ●*Onset:* Acute, subacute ●*Male:female ratio:* M=F ●*Ethnicity:* All ●*Character:* Itching, burning ●*Location:* Generalized ●*Pattern:* Diffuse redness, some scale ●*Precipitating factors:* Infection, medication, atopic dermatitis, lymphoma ●*Relieving factors:* Topical soaks and steroids ●*Clinical course:* Self-limited, chronic ●*Co-morbidities:* None relevant ●*Procedure results:* No relevant procedures ●*Test findings:* Skin biopsy

Escherichia coli infection ●*Onset:* Acute; rarely subacute ●*Male:female ratio:* M=F ●*Ethnicity:* All ●*Character:* Diarrhea in a traveler, any form of acute diarrhea (maybe with cramps, or bloody), dysuria and increasing frequency, fevers, chills, localizing symptoms to involved area ●*Location:* Intestines (colon>small), urinary tract (urethra, bladder, kidneys), prostate, epididymis, abdominal cavity, biliary tract, liver, blood stream, abscess, any other organ ●*Pattern:* Abdominal cramps and watery diarrhea in a traveler, bloody diarrhea, uncomplicated or complicated urinary tract infection, other ●*Precipitating factors:* Travel, fecal oral transmission, eating undercooked beef, anal sex, urinary obstruction, bowel perforation ●*Relieving factors:* Hydration for diarrheal illness, specific antibiotic therapy ●*Clinical course:* Usually acute illness that resolves with specific antimicrobial therapy, Ecoli-0157 may result in hemolytic uremic syndrome in young children and the elderly ●*Co-morbidities:* Perforated viscus, hemolytic uremic syndrome ●*Procedure results:* Finding of gram negative rods on Giemsa stain or culture, blood in stool ●*Test findings:* Isolation of gram negative rods from culture, isolation of E.coli 0157 from stool, pyuria, WBC in stool, leukocytosis

Esophageal cancer ●*Onset:* Insidious ●*Male:female ratio:* M(3):F(1) ●*Ethnicity:* High incidence in southern Africa and northern Asia ●*Character:* Progressive dysphagia to solids, then liquids, with anorexia and significant weight loss. Chest pain may be present ●*Location:* Mid-chest and epigastric pain in some cases ●*Pattern:* Progressive over weeks or months ●*Precipitating factors:* None relevant ●*Relieving factors:* Eating smaller and smaller pieces of solid food, eventually changing over to a puree or liquid diet. Medical therapy can include surgical resection, chemotherapy, and/or radiotherapy ●*Clinical course:* Progressive over weeks to months ●*Co-morbidities:* Smoking, alcohol use. Achalasia is associated with squamous cell cancer, while GERD and Barrett's esophagus are associated with adenocarcinoma ●*Procedure results:* EGD reveals mass lesion in the esophagus - biopsy is diagnostic ●*Test findings:* Barium swallow often shows obstructing lesion in the esophagus

Esophageal candidiasis ●*Onset:* Variable ●*Male:female ratio:* M=F ●*Ethnicity:* All ●*Character:* Dull to severe burning retrosternal/chest pain; difficulty swallowing ●*Location:* Chest, mediastinum, neck ●*Pattern:* May be worse with supine position ●*Precipitating factors:* Immunocompromised state ●*Relieving factors:* Decreased oral intake ●*Clinical course:* May progress to be severe or fatal ●*Co-morbidities:* Immunocompromised state; HIV infection; radiation therapy ●*Procedure results:* Mucosal damage/inflammation/ulceration on esophagoscopy ●*Test findings:* Mucosal abnormalities on barium esophagram; thickening of esophagus on CT scan

Esophageal spasm ●*Onset:* Acute ●*Male:female ratio:* M=F ●*Ethnicity:* All ●*Character:* Dysphagia (intermittent, shortlived), substernal chest pain (mimics angina, usually lasts 5min-1h, induced by food and emotional tension), no weight loss ●*Location:* Pain is substernal ●*Pattern:* Nonspecific ●*Precipitating factors:* Emotional tension, food ●*Relieving factors:* Reassurance, sublingual nitroglycerin or long-acting nitrates, anxiolytics, calcium channel blockers (minimally effective), esophageal dilation ●*Clinical course:* Often selfresolving, overall a benign course ●*Co-morbidities:* Anxiety, gastroesophageal reflux disease ●*Procedure results:* Esophageal manometry: frequent, simultaneous contractions ●*Test findings:* Barium swallow: tertiary contractions

Esophageal varices ●*Onset:* Development of varices is insidious, but hemorrhage is acute ●*Male:female ratio:* M>F ●*Ethnicity:* All ●*Character:* Asymptomatic until hemorrhage occurs - painless hematemesis and/or melena ●*Location:* Esophagus ●*Pattern:* No specific pattern ●*Precipitating factors:* None relevant ●*Relieving factors:* Emergency evaluation with EGD and band ligation or sclerotherapy of varices; intravenous infusion of octreotide also indicated ●*Clinical course:* Varices enlarge over months-years, and bleeding risk increases with increasing size ●*Co-morbidities:* Cirrhosis of any etiology; Budd-Chiari syndrome; portal vein thrombosis; congenital hepatic fibrosis; schistosomiasis ●*Procedure results:* EGD shows varices in the esophagus ●*Test findings:* No specific findings, though low platelets (<100,000/mm^3) is often an indication of portal hypertension and possible varices

Esophagitis ●*Onset:* Often subacute ●*Male:female ratio:* M=F ●*Ethnicity:* All ●*Character:* Esophageal or chest pain, pain with swallowing, fever, dehydration, weight loss, nausea, melena or hematemesis ●*Location:* Nonspecific ●*Pattern:* Nonspecific ●*Precipitating factors:* Most commonly due to severe gastroesophageal (GERD) or infection with candida or herpes; other causes: medications (fosamex, KCL, tetracycline), CMV, graft-vs-host disease, chemotherapy, radiation to the mediastinum ●*Relieving factors:* Depends on etiology: if GERD, high-dose proton pump inhibitors; treatment of inciting infection; removal of pills, chemotherapy. Also for symptoms can use viscous lidocaine, and other topical medications ●*Clinical course:* Depends on etiology - GERD is easily treated; infections can also be treated. However, often the underlying disease (e.g. HIV) determines overall prognosis ●*Co-morbidities:* HIV, cancer, GERD ●*Procedure results:* Esophagogastroduodenoscopy: inflamed, often ulcerated mucosa, exact appearance depends on etiology; pathology and/or culture is often diagnostic ●*Test findings:* Barium swallow: ragged mucosa

Essential hypertension ●*Onset:* Subacute, insidious ●*Male:female ratio:* M>F ●*Ethnicity:* African-Americans at higher risk ●*Character:* Often asymptomatic. Symptoms can include headache, tinnitus, dizziness ●*Location:* Signs/symptoms of longstanding hypertension include left ventricular hypertrophy, stroke, vascular changes in the fundus, renal failure ●*Pattern:* Symptoms become more prominent with higher BPs ●*Precipitating factors:* Essential hypertension is idiopathic. Alcohol, drugs, smoking, increased salt intake may further elevate BP ●*Relieving factors:* Antihypertensive medications. Cessation of smoking, alcohol, drug use. Exercise and weight loss in inactive or obese patients ●*Clinical course:* Untreated longstanding hypertension may lead to end-organ damage: stroke, heart disease/failure, renal failure, visual loss, dissections ●*Co-morbidities:* Obesity, sleep apnea, physical inactivity ●*Procedure results:* No relevant procedures ●*Test findings:* Defined as BP >140/90mm Hg for most patients. If elevated, BP should be rechecked to rule out 'white coat hypertension'

Estrogen deficient vulvovaginitis ●*Onset:* Gradual onset following menopause ●*Male:female ratio:* F ●*Ethnicity:* All ●*Character:* Drying, thinning, shrinking of vagina leading to painful splitting, tearing, bleeding, itching, burning ●*Location:* Vagina, bladder ●*Pattern:* Vaginal epithelium becomes dry and secretion is alkaline ●*Precipitating factors:* Estrogen deficiency either endogenous or surgically induced ●*Relieving factors:* Nonpharmacologic: vaginal lubricants; HRT or estrogen vaginal creams or new estrogen vaginal 'ring' ●*Clinical course:* Unrelenting unless treated ●*Co-morbidities:* Estrogen deficiency associated with osteoporosis, atherosclerosis ●*Procedure results:* Diagnosed on pelvic speculum exam ●*Test findings:* Pap shows atrophic changes

Eustachian tube dysfunction ●*Onset:* Chronic ●*Male:female ratio:* M=F ●*Ethnicity:* All ●*Character:* Intermittent ear blockage ●*Location:* Affected ear; may be bilateral ●*Pattern:* Blockage or pressure worse with supine position, airplane flight, scuba diving ●*Precipitating factors:* None relevant ●*Relieving factors:* Oral decongestants; Valsalva maneuver; ear popping ●*Clinical course:* Usually chronic, but may be self-limited ●*Co-morbidities:* Allergic rhinitis; chronic sinusitis ●*Procedure results:* Normal ear examination ●*Test findings:* May have abnormal tympanometry

Excessive anticoagulation ●*Onset:* Insidious, subacute ●*Male:female ratio:* M=F ●*Ethnicity:* All ●*Character:* Bleeding (bloody stools, hematemesis, hemoptysis, hematuria, epistaxis), easy bruising ●*Location:* Nonspecific ●*Pattern:* Nonspecific ●*Precipitating factors:* Drug interaction; dosage error; intercurrent disease; alcohol consumption ●*Relieving factors:* Temporary decrease in therapy ●*Clinical course:* Identification of the cause, correction of anticoagulation dosage, treatment of complications will usually result in resolution ●*Co-morbidities:* Diabetes, old age, ischemic heart disease, polypharmacy ●*Procedure results:* No relevant procedures ●*Test findings:* INR, clotting studies outside target range

Esophagitis • Essential hypertension • Estrogen deficient vulvovaginitis • Eustachian tube dysfunction • Excessive anticoagulation

Exfoliative dermatitis ● *Onset:* Subacute, acute ● *Male:female ratio:* M=F ● *Ethnicity:* All ● *Character:* Red/scaly, thickened/crusted skin, may or may not be itchy, lymphadenopathy, occasional temperature elevation ● *Location:* Entire skin surface ● *Pattern:* Nonspecific ● *Precipitating factors:* May have underlying dermatitis: atopic/psoriatic/contact or from drugs: penicillin, sulfa, isoniazid, phenytoin or from lymphoma, mycosis fungoides ● *Relieving factors:* Stop offending medication, topical/oral steroids, antihistamines ● *Clinical course:* Progressive if not treated ● *Co-morbidities:* Dermatitis: atopic/psoriatic/contact; drugs: penicillin, sulfa, isoniazid, phenytoin or lymphoma, mycosis fungoides ● *Procedure results:* Biopsy may help rule out other causes ● *Test findings:* No relevant tests

Exostosis (osteochondroma) ● *Onset:* Insidious ● *Male:female ratio:* M=F ● *Ethnicity:* All ● *Character:* Usually painless ● *Location:* Humerus, tibia, and femur ● *Pattern:* Nonspecific ● *Precipitating factors:* Pressure over osteochondroma ● *Relieving factors:* Surgical excision ● *Clinical course:* Rarely transform to malignant osteosarcoma; occasionally recur after surgical excision ● *Co-morbidities:* None relevant ● *Procedure results:* Surgical biopsy shows characteristic pathology ● *Test findings:* No relevant tests

Extrapyramidal lesion ● *Onset:* Congenital or acquired ● *Male:female ratio:* M=F ● *Ethnicity:* All ● *Character:* Generally divided into basal ganglia involvement (unilateral plastic rigidity with static tremor, unilateral hemiballismus, hemichorea, athetosis and dystonia, decerebrate rigidity, palatal and facial myoclonus and eventually diffuse myoclonus) and cerebellar (incoordination and imbalance) ● *Location:* Striatopallidonigral system (basal ganglia) and cerebellum ● *Pattern:* Generalized involvement, predominates in flexors of limbs and trunk; slight hyper-reflexia, absent Babinski sign, plasticity (equal resistance throughout movement) ● *Precipitating factors:* Depletion of dopamine in the substantia nigra and striatum, e.g. by drugs such as reserpine and phenothiazines ● *Relieving factors:* Discontinuation of medications, administration of dopamine precursors ● *Clinical course:* Generally progressive, with some response to therapy with dopamine precursors ● *Co-morbidities:* Chemical and metabolic imbalance (decreased production of dopamine in the substantia nigra and striatum) ● *Procedure results:* No standardized surgical solution (experimentally implanted dopamine-producing cells may be of some benefit) ● *Test findings:* No relevant tests

Extrinsic airway compression ● *Onset:* Acute, subacute ● *Male:female ratio:* M=F ● *Ethnicity:* All ● *Character:* Chest tightness, dyspnea ● *Location:* Chest or throat ● *Pattern:* Inspiratory stridor or expiratory rhonchi or wheeze ● *Precipitating factors:* (A) neck, laryngeal or vocal cord injury, infection or tumor; (B) mediastinal mass or enlargement of lymph nodes or vascular structures, or (C) intrathoracic mass ● *Relieving factors:* Consider heliox, tracheostomy and treatment of underlying disease for upper airway obstruction. For thoracic airways, treatment of underlying disease. Consider mechanical airway stenting as needed ● *Clinical course:* Variable ● *Co-morbidities:* Tumor, granulomatous disease, lymphoma, others ● *Procedure results:* Extrinsic narrowing of the airway evident upon direct inspection (e.g. during bronchoscopy) ● *Test findings:* Plateau on the inspiratory or expiratory limb of the pressure-volume loop during routine spirometry, lateral neck film, or chest CT may be abnormal

Eyelid edema ● *Onset:* Acute, subacute, or chronic depending on the cause ● *Male:female ratio:* M=F ● *Ethnicity:* All ● *Character:* Depends on the cause of eyelid edema ● *Location:* Can involve any combination of all four lids depending on the cause(s) ● *Pattern:* Generally worse after lying prone ● *Precipitating factors:* Allergy, infection, insect bite, chemical reaction ● *Relieving factors:* NSAIDs, antihistamines depending on cause ● *Clinical course:* Depends on the cause; eyelid edema due to allergy tends to be self-limited ● *Co-morbidities:* Allergy and blepharitis ● *Procedure results:* Depends on the cause; often nothing more than a comprehensive eye examination is necessary ● *Test findings:* Loss of eyelid creases; ptosis

Factor II deficiency ●*Onset:* Acute ●*Male:female ratio:* M=F ●*Ethnicity:* Consanguinity ●*Character:* Often does not present until hemostatic challenge (often a minor procedure such as venopuncture or circumcision) then presents with unexplained bleeding or hematomas. Rarely presents in infancy ●*Location:* Nonspecific ●*Pattern:* Nonspecific ●*Precipitating factors:* Trauma (often minor) ●*Relieving factors:* Oten no treatment necessary. If persistent bleeding, replacement of factor IIC, if not available fresh frozen plasma ●*Clinical course:* Rare disorder. Usually does not cause significant or life-threatening bleeding ●*Co-morbidities:* None relevant ●*Procedure results:* No relevant procedures ●*Test findings:* Low plasma levels of factor II; abnormal partial thromboplastin time (PTT) and PT (prothrombin time)

Factor V deficiency ●*Onset:* Acute to insidious depending on severity of coagulation defect ●*Male:female ratio:* M=F ●*Ethnicity:* Autosomal recessive ●*Character:* Mild bleeding disorder often presents with poor hemostasis during minor surgery or with menarche, sometimes mucocutaneous bleeding, rare hemarthroses ●*Location:* Nonspecific ●*Pattern:* Nonspecific ●*Precipitating factors:* Surgery, trauma ●*Relieving factors:* Fresh frozen plasma ●*Clinical course:* Mild course ●*Co-morbidities:* None relevant ●*Procedure results:* No relevant procedures ●*Test findings:* Prolonged prothrombin time (PT) and thromboplastin time (PTT), lack of factor V activity on functional assay

Factor VII deficiency ●*Onset:* Acute ●*Male:female ratio:* M=F ●*Ethnicity:* Autosomal recessive ●*Character:* Bleeding tendencies which are highly variable; severe disease often results in intracranial hemorrhage at birth ●*Location:* Nonspecific ●*Pattern:* Nonspecific ●*Precipitating factors:* Surgery, trauma (often mild) ●*Relieving factors:* Prothrombin complex concentrates, factor VII concentrates if available for severe bleeding ●*Clinical course:* Depends on severity of bleeding tendency ●*Co-morbidities:* None relevant ●*Procedure results:* No relevant procedures ●*Test findings:* Prolonged prothrombin time (PT), normal thromboplastin (PTT), normal thrombin time, reduced plasma factor VII:C activity

Factor X deficiency ●*Onset:* Subacute ●*Male:female ratio:* M=F ●*Ethnicity:* Rare, autosomal recessive ●*Character:* Post-traumatic musculoskeletal bleeding and/or menorrhagia ●*Location:* Nonspecific ●*Pattern:* Nonspecific ●*Precipitating factors:* Trauma ●*Relieving factors:* Fresh frozen plasma ●*Clinical course:* Lifelong, but rarely severe ●*Co-morbidities:* None relevant ●*Procedure results:* No relevant procedures ●*Test findings:* No relevant tests

Familial dysautonomia ●*Onset:* Congenital (autosomal recessive) ●*Male:female ratio:* M=F ●*Ethnicity:* Ashkenazi Jews, IKAP mutation ●*Character:* Autonomic neuropathy characterized by postural hypotension, lability of blood pressure, faulty temperature regulation, diminished hearing, hyperhidrosis, skin blotchiness, insensitivity to pain, emotional lability and vomiting ●*Location:* Deficiency of neurons in superior cervical ganglia and lateral horns of the spinal cord ●*Pattern:* Infant presents with poor suckling, failure to thrive, unexplained fever and episodes of pneumonia; subsequently loss of pain and temperature and preservation of pressure and tactile sense ●*Precipitating factors:* Temperature regulation and attention to prevention of burns needed ●*Relieving factors:* Protected environment; no specific treatment ●*Clinical course:* Keratitis needs prevention with artificial tears; aspiration problems can lead to death; nephropathy develops with time ●*Co-morbidities:* Breech presentation; aseptic necrosis ●*Procedure results:* Nerve biopsy with diminution of small myelinated and unmyelinated fibers ●*Test findings:* Decrease in serum dopamine beta hydroxylase, increased urinary excretion of homovanillic acid and decreased amounts of vanillylmandelic acid and methoxyhydroxyphenylglycol

Familial Mediterranean fever ●*Onset:* Episodic acute attacks ●*Male:female ratio:* M(3):F(2) ●*Ethnicity:* Predominantly in Sephardic Jews, Turks, Armenians, and Arabs, but occurs in others ●*Character:* Recessively inherited disorder characterized by episodes of fever and abdominal pain, possibly with pleurisy, arthritis, and skin erythema/swelling, with rare pericarditis and aseptic meningitis ●*Location:* Abdominal pain initially focal then spreads to entire abdomen. Skin signs commonly in lower legs and foot. Arthritis in large joints ●*Pattern:* Nonspecific ●*Precipitating factors:* Genetic link ●*Relieving factors:* Long-term prophylactic colchicine decreases frequency and severity of episodes, and may prevent amyloidosis ●*Clinical course:* Episodes last 1-2 days, up to 1 week. Frequency of episodes commonly every 2-4 weeks, ranging from twice a week to yearly. Remissions for years are possible. Between attacks, asymptomatic ●*Co-morbidities:* Some patients develop concurrent amyloidosis. Depression ●*Procedure results:* Laparotomy, if performed for acute abdomen, demonstrates inflamed peritoneum and a neutrophilic exudate ●*Test findings:* Genotypic test for the MEFV gene can identify three mutations known to be responsible for large proportion of cases

Familial short stature ●*Onset:* Insidious ●*Male:female ratio:* M=F ●*Ethnicity:* All ●*Character:* Short stature ●*Location:* Height ●*Pattern:* Nonspecific ●*Precipitating factors:* Genetic ●*Relieving factors:* None relevant ●*Clinical course:* Permanent ●*Co-morbidities:* None relevant ●*Procedure results:* Normal growth hormone (GH) response to insulin-induced hypoglycemia or arginine infusion ●*Test findings:* Stable growth curve; normal growth rate; normal IgF

Fanconi's anemia ●*Onset:* Insidious ●*Male:female ratio:* M=F ●*Ethnicity:* All ●*Character:* Aplastic anemia resulting in hemorrhage (bleeding gums, nose, skin, vagina, GI tract, due to thrombocytopenia), neutropenia (and increased susceptibility to bacterial infection), weakness/fatigue due to anemia ●*Location:* Systemic condition. Chromosomal abnormality resulting in bone marrow failure ●*Pattern:* Anemia, leukopenia, and thrombocytopenia (all three cell lines typically depressed) ●*Precipitating factors:* Congenital (autosomal recessive) ●*Relieving factors:* Supportive care including transfusion, infection prevention. Bone marrow transplant may help ●*Clinical course:* Lifelong problem. Slow progression to marrow failure. Increased risk of developing leukemia or other malignancy in setting of marrow failure ●*Co-morbidities:* Multiple congenital somatic anomalies: renal and cardiac malformations, skin hyperpigmentation, bony abnormalities (especially hypoplastic or absent thumbs or radii). Leukemia can be a long-term complication ●*Procedure results:* Bone marrow biopsy; chromosomal analysis ●*Test findings:* Anemia, leukopenia, thrombocytopenia

Fanconi's syndrome ●*Onset:* Insidious ●*Male:female ratio:* M=F ●*Ethnicity:* All ●*Character:* Hypophosphatemia, diabetes mellitus, gonadal atrophy, osteomalacia, short stature ●*Location:* Bone ●*Pattern:* Nonspecific ●*Precipitating factors:* Autosomal recessive inherited, secondary to heavy metal poisoning, hematological malignancies and connective tissue diseases ●*Relieving factors:* Treatment of underlying disorder ●*Clinical course:* Progressive ●*Co-morbidities:* Genetic diseases such as cystinosis, galactosemia, tyrosemia, Wilson's disease, underlying hematological malignancy or connective tissue disease ●*Procedure results:* X-ray of bones, compared with osteomalacia/rickets pseudofractures ●*Test findings:* Low serum phosphorus

Fatty liver ●*Onset:* Insidious ●*Male:female ratio:* M=F ●*Ethnicity:* All ●*Character:* Usually asymptomatic - patients have abnormal AST/ALT; may have vague right upper quadrant pain and hepatomagaly ●*Location:* Right upper quadrant ●*Pattern:* No pattern ●*Precipitating factors:* None relevant ●*Relieving factors:* Weight loss - 10% or more of body weight may decrease symptoms ●*Clinical course:* Usually not progressive, but in 15% of patietns, may cause progressive liver damage and cirrhosis ●*Co-morbidities:* Obesity; diabetes; high cholesterol ●*Procedure results:* Liver biopsy with fat deposition, with or without associated inflammation and fibrosis ●*Test findings:* AST and ALT elevated; U/S and CT may show fatty infiltration (not sensitive)

Febrile seizure ●*Onset:* Acute ●*Male:female ratio:* M=F ●*Ethnicity:* All ●*Character:* Generalized seizure, brief (less than 20 min), fever ●*Location:* Generalized ●*Pattern:* Occurs with quickly rising temperature ●*Precipitating factors:* Fever ●*Relieving factors:* Antipyretics, time ●*Clinical course:* Single episode less than 20 min. Self-limiting. One third of patients will have another in lifetime ●*Co-morbidities:* Seizure disorder ●*Procedure results:* LP if done normal ●*Test findings:* Nl, EEG

Fecal impaction ●*Onset:* Subacute ●*Male:female ratio:* M=F ●*Ethnicity:* All ●*Character:* Abdominal pain and distension in the pattern of intestinal obstruction - cramping pain for several minutes, followed by a pain-free interval of several minutes. There may be small volume diarrhea due to leakage of liquid stool around the impaction ●*Location:* Diffuse abdominal pain ●*Pattern:* Episodes of crampy pain lasting minutes, with 5-10 min periods of respite between paroxysms ●*Precipitating factors:* Constipation ●*Relieving factors:* If the impaction is distal, manual disimpaction may be helpful. Enemas may also resolve the obstruction ●*Clinical course:* May be self-limited, but usually requires treatment for relief of symptoms ●*Co-morbidities:* Constipation ●*Procedure results:* No relevant procedures ●*Test findings:* KUB may show stool in colonic segments, with proximal dilation of bowel loops

Fecal mass ●*Onset:* Subacute ●*Male:female ratio:* M=F ●*Ethnicity:* All ●*Character:* Patients often but not always complain of constipation. No associated weight loss or bloody stools ●*Location:* Mass anywhere in the abdomen ●*Pattern:* Nonspecific ●*Precipitating factors:* Constipation ●*Relieving factors:* Laxatives to induce bowel movements lead to resolution of the mass: disappearance of the mass after BM is diagnostic ●*Clinical course:* Self-limited: resolves with BM ●*Co-morbidities:* Constipation, more easily detected in thin or wasted patients ●*Procedure results:* No relevant procedures ●*Test findings:* Examination: mass in colon detectable

Felon ●*Onset:* Acute ●*Male:female ratio:* M=F ●*Ethnicity:* All ●*Character:* Also called staphylococcal whitlow; purulent infection/abscess of bulbous distal end of finger (finger pulp); common causes are Herpes simplex and Staphylococcus aureus; finger is hot, tender and edematous with a pus collection visible ●*Location:* Finger tip ●*Pattern:* Requires analgesics and therapy with systemic antibiotics, incision and drainage of abscess ●*Precipitating factors:* Trauma ●*Relieving factors:* Systemic antibiotics, incision and drainage ●*Clinical course:* Can be complicated by osteomyelitis; does well with therapy early, with antibiotics ●*Co-morbidities:* Can be associated with a pyogenic granuloma ●*Procedure results:* Incision and drainage with pus from finger tip ●*Test findings:* Culture of pus commonly yields S. aureus; if recurrent problem, culture for H. simplex

Female stress incontinence ●*Onset:* Subacute ●*Male:female ratio:* F ●*Ethnicity:* All ●*Character:* Inability to control urination when pressure is exerted on the bladder ●*Location:* Perineum, genitalia ●*Pattern:* Worse with increased activity ●*Precipitating factors:* Any activity that increases abdominal pressure: laughing, sneezing, coughing, lifting, jogging, etc; hysterectomy; menopause; vaginal deliveries ●*Relieving factors:* Resting positions (sitting, supine, sleeping); surgical correction; alpha-adrenergic agonists, estrogens; pelvic floor exercises and biofeedback ●*Clinical course:* Progressive if untreated ●*Co-morbidities:* Atrophic vaginitis, cystocele, obesity, COPD and other respiratory disease ●*Procedure results:* Cystourethroscopy with urodynamics: urethral hypermobility and/or intrinsic sphincter deficiency ●*Test findings:* No relevant tests

Femoral artery aneurysm ●*Onset:* Chronic ●*Male:female ratio:* M=F ●*Ethnicity:* All ●*Character:* Pathologic dilatation of a segment of the femoral artery ●*Location:* Most commonly occurs at bifurcation ●*Pattern:* May be asymptomatic or painful due to occlusion or rupture ●*Precipitating factors:* Atherosclerosis, trauma, vasculitis ●*Relieving factors:* Operative excision with replacement with a graft ●*Clinical course:* Gradual progression requiring surgical repair ●*Co-morbidities:* Hyperlipidemia, hypertension, age, smoking, IV drug use ●*Procedure results:* Doppler blood flow analysis, angiography ●*Test findings:* Clinical examination may reveal pulsatile lesion, femoral bruit and decreased pedal pulses

Femoral hernia ●*Onset:* Subacute, acute ●*Male:female ratio:* M(1):F(3) ●*Ethnicity:* All ●*Character:* May be asymptomatic, may present with painfull or painless lump. Presentation with abdominal pain and obstruction may occur ●*Location:* Femoral ring, below and lateral to the pubic ramus ●*Pattern:* Risk of strangulation is significant ●*Precipitating factors:* Cough, heavy lifting ●*Relieving factors:* Manual reduction may be possible but recurrance inevitable. Surgical correction is the treatment of choice ●*Clinical course:* Risk of strangulation is significant. Prophylactic repair should be considered ●*Co-morbidities:* None relevant ●*Procedure results:* No relevant procedures ●*Test findings:* Cough impulse and bowel sounds may be present. Hernia may be reducable manually

Fever ●*Onset:* Abrupt, insidious, or chronic ●*Male:female ratio:* M=F ●*Ethnicity:* All ●*Character:* Elevated temperature ●*Location:* Any body organ may be involved ●*Pattern:* Usually not predictive of cause but includes remittent, intermittent, saddleback, quartan, persistent or sustained, with a diurnal pattern, with reversal of the diurnal pattern, with pulse temperature dissociation ●*Precipitating factors:* Infection, malignancy, drug, toxin or medication, hospitalization (nosocomial fever), immunodeficiency, HIV, connective tissue disease, chronic illness ●*Relieving factors:* Antipyretic therapy (such as aspirin, nonsteroidal anti-inflammatory drugs, or acetaminophen); sponging with tepid water or cooling blankets only in combination with an antipyretic, disease-specific therapy ●*Clinical course:* Most fevers are brief and self-limited; some fevers represent a serious illness - most can be diagnosed and effectively treated with disease-specific therapy; a small proportion of fevers are persistent and difficult to diagnose (fever of unknown origin) or represent an uncurable illness ●*Co-morbidities:* Infection, malignancy, hospitalization (nosocomial fever), immunodeficiency, HIV, connective tissue disease, chronic illness ●*Procedure results:* Depend on cause ●*Test findings:* Depend on cause

Fibroadenosis ●*Onset:* Insidious/cyclic ●*Male:female ratio:* F (with rare exceptions) ●*Ethnicity:* All ●*Character:* Diffuse lumpiness of breast tissue accompanied by tenderness in the days prior to menses ●*Location:* Most commonly bilateral upper lateral breasts ●*Pattern:* Pain and tenderness in the days prior to menses; improves with the onset of menses ●*Precipitating factors:* Menses ●*Relieving factors:* Breast support with firm brassiere. Analgesics ●*Clinical course:* Tenderness and pain cycle with menstrual periods. May spontaneously improve over time ●*Co-morbidities:* None relevant ●*Procedure results:* Fine needle aspiration (FNA) and/or open biopsy (if done for suspicion of malignancy) shows normal tissue ●*Test findings:* No relevant tests

Fibrocystic breast disease ●*Onset:* Subacute ●*Male:female ratio:* M<F ●*Ethnicity:* All ●*Character:* Asymptomatic or dull ache, heaviness in breast ●*Location:* Diffuse or localized most commonly to upper outer breast, unilateral or bilateral ●*Pattern:* Palpable thickening or discrete mass, can be cyclic related to menses; nipple discharge may be present ●*Precipitating factors:* Cyclic pain relieved with onset of menses, can be worsened with HRT or oral contraceptives ●*Relieving factors:* NSAIDs, d/c of HRT, relief with danazol, bromocriptine, tamoxifen ●*Clinical course:* Symptoms resolve/improve after menses ●*Co-morbidities:* Breast pain rarely associated with malignancy; proliferative lesions increase risk of malignancy ●*Procedure results:* Biopsy specimen reveals nonproliferative lesion ●*Test findings:* Ultrasound distinguishes solid mass or cyctic lesion, mammogram positive for non-specific abnormality

Fibromyalgia ●*Onset:* Subacute ●*Male:female ratio:* M(1):F(9) ●*Ethnicity:* All ●*Character:* Dull ache ●*Location:* Polyarticular including elbows, shoulders, hips and knees; pain sometimes localized to 'tender points' ●*Pattern:* Pain is constant ●*Precipitating factors:* Psychological or physical stress, lack of sleep ●*Relieving factors:* Tricyclic antidepressants, aerobic exercise, psychological support ●*Clinical course:* Waxing and waning ●*Co-morbidities:* Depression, substance abuse, physical or sexual abuse, obstructive sleep apnea ●*Procedure results:* No relevant procedures ●*Test findings:* Normal laboratory examination

Fibrosing alveolitis ●*Onset:* Insidious or subacute ●*Male:female ratio:* M=F ●*Ethnicity:* All ●*Character:* Dyspnea on exertion ●*Location:* Lungs ●*Pattern:* Nonspecific ●*Precipitating factors:* Smoking, chemical exposures, drugs (e.g. nitrafurantoin) ●*Relieving factors:* Oxygen ●*Clinical course:* Progressive ●*Co-morbidities:* Right heart failure ●*Procedure results:* Lung biopsy: variegated alveolitis and inflammatory cells, fibrosis ●*Test findings:* Chest X-ray: bilateral interstitial/alveolar infiltrates; pulmonary function tests: diminished diffusion, restriction; CT: same as chest X-ray with honeycomb changes

Fifth disease ●*Onset:* Subacute ●*Male:female ratio:* M=F ●*Ethnicity:* All ●*Character:* Headache, malaise, low-grade fever ●*Location:* Face: 'slapped cheek' appearance ●*Pattern:* Low-grade fever followed by 'slapped cheek' appearance followed by truncal rash ●*Precipitating factors:* Infection with parvovirus B19 ●*Relieving factors:* Supportive care, e.g. acetaminophen ●*Clinical course:* 1-3 weeks ●*Co-morbidities:* Aplastic crisis in sickle cell or hemolytic anemia ●*Procedure results:* No relevant procedures ●*Test findings:* Parvovirus B19 antibodies, anemia and reticulocytopenia in aplastic crisis

Filariasis ●*Onset:* Subacute, chronic ●*Male:female ratio:* M>F ●*Ethnicity:* Tropical areas ●*Character:* Progressive localized edema (of scrotum or limb) followed by skin thickening, fissuring. Rarely paroxysmal cough, wheezing with fever and weight loss (tropical pulmonary eosinophilia) ●*Location:* Subcutaneous tissue and lymphatics of scrotum, lower extremity, other. Lung (tropical pulmonary eosinophilia) - rare, other ●*Pattern:* Hydrocele or retrogradely evolving (descending) localized pitting edema with thickening and fissuring of the skin (elephantiasis); paroxysmal nocturnal cough and wheezing are rare ●*Precipitating factors:* Residence or prolonged stay in endemic areas (tropics and subtropics) and repeated mosquito bites ●*Relieving factors:* Elevation of affected limb, elastic stockings ●*Clinical course:* Slowly progressive ●*Co-morbidities:* None relevant ●*Procedure results:* Early - visualization of microfilaria in blood or hydrocele fluid, lymphatic obstruction by worm on lymphoscintigraphy, nodules and lymphatic dilation on scrotal ultrasound, worm movement in lymphatics on Doppler, restrictive lung disease on PFTs in tropical pulmonary eosinophilia, assays for circulating antigens, specific serology ●*Test findings:* Eosinophilia, elevated serum IgE (early)

Fitz-Hugh-Curtis syndrome (ascending PID) ●*Onset:* Subacute ●*Male:female ratio:* F ●*Ethnicity:* Nonspecific ●*Character:* Right upper quadrant/pleurisy with or without pelvic pain associated with fever, sweats, chills ●*Location:* Right upper quadrant/pleuritic ●*Pattern:* Progressive over several days, usually starting within 2 weeks of menses ●*Precipitating factors:* Infection with gonorrhea or chlamydia ●*Relieving factors:* Antibiotics ●*Clinical course:* Fevers resolves within 72 hours of antibiotics though pain can persist for weeks ●*Co-morbidities:* None relevant ●*Procedure results:* 'Violin string' adhesions over the liver seen at laparoscopy ●*Test findings:* Elevated WBC; elevated transaminases

Flat foot ●*Onset:* Subacute, insidious, can be congenital ●*Male:female ratio:* M=F ●*Ethnicity:* More common in African-Americans ●*Character:* Occasionally painful ●*Location:* Midfoot ●*Pattern:* Nonspecific ●*Precipitating factors:* Congenital, high heel use, stroke, trauma, neuromuscular disease, peripheral neuropathy, spastic Achilles tendon, posterior tibial tendon rupture ●*Relieving factors:* Orthotics, shoe modifications, plantar inserts, arch supports ●*Clinical course:* Progressive ●*Co-morbidities:* Hallux valgus with hammer toe formation, anterior shin splints, chondromalacia patellae, chronic low back pain ●*Procedure results:* No relevant procedures ●*Test findings:* X-ray shows loss of normal medial longitudinal arch

Flow murmur ●*Onset:* Typically insidious ●*Male:female ratio:* M=F (but increased in pregnancy) ●*Ethnicity:* All ●*Character:* Usually asymptomatic and detected incidentally on physical examination ●*Location:* Aortic region or right sternal border ●*Pattern:* Soft (grade I or II/VI) midsystolic ejection murmur (crescendo/decrescendo) heard best at the aortic region or right sternal border/pulmonic region. Usually does not radiate and usually not associated with extra heart sounds, clicks, opening snaps, knocks, or rubs ●*Precipitating factors:* Can be a benign condition of childhood or pregnancy. Typically heard in a young adult or child with a thin chest and high velocity of blood flow. Anemia, hemorrhage, pregnancy, or hypermetabolic state can precipitate a flow murmur ●*Relieving factors:* None relevant; correct underlying cause if secondary to anemia or other condition ●*Clinical course:* Flow murmur of childhood or pregnancy often resolves spontaneously; otherwise usually self-limiting. If secondary to underlying cause (anemia, hemorrhage) which worsens, can rarely result in high output heart failure ●*Co-morbidities:* None relevant ●*Procedure results:* Echo can confirm absence of pathologic valvular disease and demonstrate increased flow through aortic valve ● *Test findings:* Low murmur should diminish with valsalva. Aortic stenosis murmur typically harsher sounding, (sometimes 'musical'), and can be associated with (carotid) pulsus parvus et tardus. Typically affects older patients (65+ unless bicuspid aortic valve: 55+).

Fluid overload ●*Onset:* Acute ●*Male:female ratio:* M=F ●*Ethnicity:* All ●*Character:* Shortness of breath, edema, weight gain ●*Location:* Pedal edema, periorbital can be seen with nephrotic syndrome or pre-ecclampsia. Increased abdominal girth in congestive heart failure (CHF) or cirrhosis ●*Pattern:* Orthopnea, paroxysmal nocturnal dypsnea with CHF ●*Precipitating factors:* Dietary indiscretion (high salt load), alcoholism or other causes of cirrhosis, nephrotic syndrome, pre-eclampsia, congenital heart disease or valvular disease ●*Relieving factors:* Diuresis, correction of underlying disorder, paracentesis may be necessary in cirrhotic patient ●*Clinical course:* Continues as long as underlying cause persists. Depending on severity of underlying condition, can cause acute or subacute decompensation (shortness of breath) ●*Co-morbidities:* CHF ●*Procedure results:* No relevant procedures ●*Test findings:* Increased jugular venous pressure, hepatomegaly possible in CHF. Crackles at lung bases. Peripheral edema

Folate deficiency ●*Onset:* Subacute (days-to-months) ●*Male:female ratio:* M<F ●*Ethnicity:* All ●*Character:* Pallor, shortness of breath (manifestations of anemia); neural tube defects if deficient in first trimester. Hypercoaguable state may result from elevated homocysteine, seen with folate deficiency ●*Location:* Anemia: bone marrow, peripheral blood. Neural tube defects: prenatal CNS ●*Pattern:* Megaloblastic anemia. Smear may also show hypersegmented polymorphs ●*Precipitating factors:* Alcoholism, exfoliative skin disease, hemolytic anemia predispose to folate deficiency. States of increased folate requirements: pregnancy, lactation. Dietary: lack of animal products or leafy green vegetables. Some drugs interfere with folate metabolism (phenytoin, trimethoprim, methotrexate). Small bowel surgery or disease may result in malabsorption of folate ●*Relieving factors:* Replenish stores; dietary modification. Supplement during pregnancy (0.8-1mg folate per day) ●*Clinical course:* Body stores (5-10mg) can be depleted in days/months (e.g. 2-4 days in alcoholics). Megaloblastic anemia develops in 4-5 months; responds well to folate repletion ●*Co-morbidities:* May coexist with B12 deficiency; important to rule out, as deficiency can have neurologic sequelae. Hypercoagulable state due to hyperhomocysteinemia ●*Procedure results:* No relevant procedures ●*Test findings:* Blood smear with macro-ovalocytes, hypersegmented polymorphs. CBC with low hematocrit, elevated mean corpuscular volume. Serum homocysteine level may be elevated

Follicular adenoma ●*Onset:* Insidious ●*Male:female ratio:* M<F ●*Ethnicity:* All ●*Character:* Benign thyroid tumor noticeable as lump or nodule ●*Location:* Thyroid ●*Pattern:* Nonspecific ●*Precipitating factors:* Iodine exposure, e.g. from contrast media, may accelerate progression to hyperthyroidism ●*Relieving factors:* Surgical excision, radioactive iodine ablation, suppressive thyroid hormone treatment ●*Clinical course:* Slowly growing, typically autonomous nodule, may lead to eventual suppression of thyroid-stimulat-

ing hormone (TSH) and atrophy of the rest of the thyroid, then later to hyperthyroidism ●*Co-morbidities:* None relevant ●*Procedure results:* Fine needle aspiration (FNA) demonstrates benign cytology ●*Test findings:* Initially TSH and thyroid hormone levels normal, later TSH may be suppressed, then T4 and T3 may be elevated. Radionuclide scan initially may show cold, warm or hot nodule, later likely hot, with suppression in the rest of thyroid

Folliculitis ●*Onset:* Acute ●*Male:female ratio:* M>F ●*Ethnicity:* All ❶ *Character:* Pustules ❷ *Location:* Hairy regions: beard, axilla, groin, legs ❸ *Pattern:* Scattered red pustules ●*Precipitating factors:* Shaving ●*Relieving factors:* Antibiotics ●*Clinical course:* Self-limited, can recur ●*Co-morbidities:* None relevant ●*Procedure results:* No relevant procedures ●*Test findings:* Positive skin culture

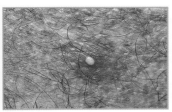

❶ *Character A pustule pierced by a hair*

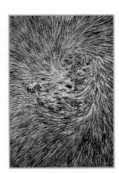

❷ *Location Bacterial folliculitis of the scalp*

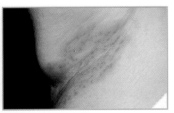

❷ *Location Multiple grouped pustules in the armpit are typical*

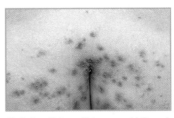

❸ *Pattern Note multiple grouped inflamed papules and erosions*

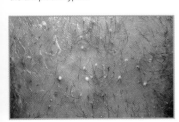

❸ *Pattern Multiple follicular pustules are typical*

Foreign body ●*Onset:* Acute ●*Male:female ratio:* M=F ●*Ethnicity:* All ●*Character:* Pain or foreign body sensation in involved area. In respiratory tract, wheezing, stridor, difficulty breathing. In esophagus, vomiting, drooling ●*Location:* Nonspecific ●*Pattern:* Nonspecific ●*Precipitating factors:* Swallowing or placing foreign body in any orifice ●*Relieving factors:* Most swallowed objects will pass uneventfully. Sharp or pointy objects may need to be removed with direct visualization (endoscopy). All respiratory tract, ear, nose, and rectal objects require removal ●*Clinical course:* Dependent on object and location ●*Co-morbidities:* None relevant ●*Procedure results:* No relevant procedures ●*Test findings:* X-rays often reveal foreign object

Foreign body in foot ●*Onset:* Acute ●*Male:female ratio:* M=F ●*Ethnicity:* All ●*Character:* Sharp or dull pain, skin laceration or entry point, signs of local infection ●*Location:* Superficial or deep soft tissue, bone ●*Pattern:* Persistent pain after trauma, infection without identified source ●*Precipitating factors:* None ●*Relieving factors:* Surgical aseptic exploration and removal ●*Clinical course:* May be a nucleus for cellulitis ●*Co-morbidities:* None ●*Procedure results:* None relevant ●*Test findings:* X-ray showing foreign body

Fracture ●*Onset:* Acute ●*Male:female ratio:* M=F ●*Ethnicity:* All ●*Character:* Pain, swelling, tenderness or ecchymosis at fracture site. May palpate bone deformity ●*Location:* Any bone may be broken. Extremities and digits most common ●*Pattern:* Nonspecific ●*Precipitating factors:* Falls or direct blow to bone most common mechanisms ●*Relieving factors:* Immobilization with splint or cast. Ice, analgesics, elevation of involved extremity. Reduction, either open or closed, of displaced fractures. Spinal precautions and immobilization with spinal fractures ●*Clinical course:* Some restriction in range of movement may persist after injury has healed ●*Co-morbidities:* Elderly more prone to fractures with minor injuries. Always check neurovascular function distal to fractures of the extremities or digits ●*Procedure results:* No relevant procedures ●*Test findings:* Radiographs required to diagnose fractures

Fragile X syndrome ●*Onset:* Congenital: usually detected after age 3 ●*Male:female ratio:* More F carriers, M often worse affected ●*Ethnicity:* All ●*Character:* Hyperactivity and mental retardation ●*Location:* Gross motor delays and speech delays ●*Pattern:* Hypotonia in infancy ●*Precipitating factors:* None relevant ●*Relieving factors:* Special education and treatment of attention deficit hyperactivity disorder (ADHD) ●*Clinical course:* Chronic ●*Co-morbidities:* ADHD, mitral valve prolapse, scoliosis, pes planus, macroorchidism ●*Procedure results:* No relevant procedures ●*Test findings:* Mutation of X chromosome

Friedreich's ataxia ●*Onset:* Insidious ●*Male:female ratio:* M=F ●*Ethnicity:* All ●*Character:* Ataxia of all extremities and with neuropathy ●*Location:* Spinal cord and peripheral nerves ●*Pattern:* Nonspecific ●*Precipitating factors:* Autosomal recessive ●*Relieving factors:* None relevant ●*Clinical course:* Progressive ●*Co-morbidities:* Cardiac and pulmonary complications ●*Procedure results:* No relevant procedures ●*Test findings:* Normal MRI and lumbar puncture. Abnormal electromyogram (EMG)/nerve conduction study (NCS), positive genetic testing

Frontotemporal lobe degeneration (Pick's disease) ●*Onset:* Insidious ●*Male:female ratio:* M=F ●*Ethnicity:* All ●*Character:* Progressive dementia with behavioral abnormalities ●*Location:* Nonspecific ●*Pattern:* Nonspecific ●*Precipitating factors:* None relevant ●*Relieving factors:* Supportive ●*Clinical course:* Progressive ●*Co-morbidities:* None relevant ●*Procedure results:* No relevant procedures ●*Test findings:* Frontotemporal lobe atrophy, normal lumbar puncture

Frostbite environmental hypothermia ●*Onset:* Acute ●*Male:female ratio:* M=F ●*Ethnicity:* All ●*Character:* Characterized as superficial or deep tissue injury. Superficial: erythema, clear blisters, edema, black, hard eschars eventually form. Deep: hemorrhagic blisters, blue-gray skin color, nonviable structures turn black (mummified) and slough off (in weeks to months) ●*Location:* Any skin surface, but most common on nose, ears, face, hands and feet ●*Pattern:* Nonspecific ●*Precipitating factors:* Prolonged cold exposure to skin surface ●*Relieving factors:* Rapid rewarming in circulating heated water (40-42°C). Tetanus prophylaxis, analgesia. Debride or aspirate clear blisters (not hemorrhagic ones), dress open wounds, antibiotics ●*Clinical course:* 3 to 4 weeks for full demarcation of injury to occur. May require tissue grafting or amputation. Prognosis is good with superficial injuries, poor with deep injuries ●*Co-morbidities:* Alcohol intoxication ●*Procedure results:* No relevant procedures ●*Test findings:* No relevant tests

Frozen shoulder ●*Onset:* Subacute ●*Male:female ratio:* M<F ●*Ethnicity:* All ●*Character:* Dull ache ●*Location:* Unilateral shoulder involvement ●*Pattern:* Constant. Loss of shoulder

range of motion ●*Precipitating factors:* None relevant ●*Relieving factors:* NSAIDs, ultrasound, corticosteroid injection, physical therapy ●*Clinical course:* Slowly progressive ●*Co-morbidities:* Diabetes, hypothyroidism ●*Procedure results:* No relevant procedures ●*Test findings:* No relevant tests

Functional benign ovarian tumor ●*Onset:* Subacute; onset of acute pain indicates rupture ●*Male:female ratio:* F ●*Ethnicity:* All ●*Character:* Usually asymptomatic. May result in delayed or abnormal menses ●*Location:* Pain localized to pelvis usually unilateral ●*Pattern:* Cyst leakage/rupture causes pelvic pain with peritoneal signs ●*Precipitating factors:* Ovulation induction medications can lead to functional theca-lutein cysts ●*Relieving factors:* NSAIDs, oral contraceptives to prevent recurrence ●*Clinical course:* Most commonly spontaneously regress during the next subsequent menstrual period ●*Co-morbidities:* Infertility, polycystic ovary syndrome ●*Procedure results:* U/S findings: <6cm, unilocular 'simple' cyst with low-level internal echoes, no ascites. Pathology shows follicular and luteal cyst ●*Test findings:* Frequently found on routine pelvic examination

Fungal infection ●*Onset:* Chronic; occasionally subacute ●*Male:female ratio:* M<F ●*Ethnicity:* All ●*Character:* Erythematous, annular plaques with central regression and overlying scale ●*Location:* Scalp, trunk; commonly on intertriginous skinfold areas ●*Pattern:* Begin as erythematous papules, and progress to become annular lesions; can involve deeper appendages such as the hair follicle (Majocchi's granuloma) ●*Precipitating factors:* Presence of excessive moist macerated skin (intertriginous); immunesuppression (diabetes mellitus, HIV/AIDS, organ transplant, carcinoma) ●*Relieving factors:* Intertriginous areas kept dry and clean ●*Clinical course:* Can be self-limiting in immunocompetent hosts; usually progress to become larger ●*Co-morbidities:* None relevant ●*Procedure results:* No relevant procedures ●*Test findings:* No relevant tests

Furunculosis ●*Onset:* Acute ●*Male:female ratio:* M=F ●*Ethnicity:* All ●*Character:* Tender nodules ●*Location:* Hairy regions: beard, axilla, groin, legs ❸ *Pattern:* Tender, warm, red, fluctuant nodules ●*Precipitating factors:* Shaving ●*Relieving factors:* Antibiotics, incision, drainage ●*Clinical course:* Self-limited, can recur ●*Co-morbidities:* None relevant ●*Procedure results:* Gram stain positive ●*Test findings:* Culture of drainage pos

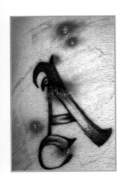

❸ *Pattern* Pustules with surrounding inflammation. Tattoo possibly opened skin, allowing bacteria to enter

Galactorrhea ●*Onset:* Subacute, insidious ●*Male:female ratio:* M<F ●*Ethnicity:* All ●*Character:* Bilateral milky nipple discharge ●*Location:* Pituitary macroadenomas can produce headache and visual field cut ●*Pattern:* Nonspecific ●*Precipitating factors:* Use of oral contraceptives, prior pregnancy, local breast stimulation, other drugs include phenothiazines, metoclopramide, reserpine, methyldopa, haloperidol, isoniazid, imipramine ●*Relieving factors:* Discontinue causative medications, discontinue local breast stimulation, bromocriptine for pituitary microadenomas, radiotherapy considered for macroadenomas unresponsive to bromocriptine ●*Clinical course:* Normoprolactinemic galactorrhea can be self-limited ●*Co-morbidities:* Oligomenorrhea, amenorrhea, infertility, hypothyroidism, osteoporosis ●*Procedure results:* Surgical resection of rapidly growing pituitary lesions ●*Test findings:* Elevated serum prolactin; MRI demonstrating pituitary micro- or macroadenoma

Ganglion ●*Onset:* Subacute/recurrent ●*Male:female ratio:* M<F ●*Ethnicity:* All ●*Character:* Firm, smooth, pea-sized mass. May be fluctuant. Rarely with clicking or weakness ●*Location:* Wrist, hand, fingers (especially dorsum of wrist, volar-radial side of wrist, flexor crease at metacarpal proximal joint) ●*Pattern:* Nonspecific ●*Precipitating factors:* Acute or recurrent injury ●*Relieving factors:* May be ruptured by pressure or hitting with a book, aspiration, corticosteroid injections (but not definitive treatment) ●*Clinical course:* Rarely self resolving ●*Co-morbidities:* None relevant ●*Procedure results:* No relevant procedures ●*Test findings:* Aspiration (not necessary) yields benign synovial fluid

Gangrene ●*Onset:* Acute ●*Male:female ratio:* M=F ●*Ethnicity:* All ●*Character:* Acute pain in site of wound or acute abdominal pain, followed by edema, erythema, induration, bullae formation, discoloration of the skin (red to purple to black). Crepitus may be present in gas gangrene ●*Location:* Skin, fascia, muscles of lower extremities, upper extremities, perineum, surgical sites, site of trauma, other skin, GI or genitourinary mucosa, systemic complications ●*Pattern:* Extreme pain at site of skin inflammation, bullae formation, discoloration of skin/bullae fluid from red to purple to black. Pronounced tachycardia, diaphoresis. Crepitus may be present (in gas gangrene/myonecrosis) ●*Precipitating factors:* Breach to skin/mucosal integrity, penetrating injury, trauma, surgery, injection drug use, diabetes, peripheral vascular disease, neutropenia, GI malignancy ●*Relieving factors:* None relevant ●*Clinical course:* Rapidly progressive over hours-to-several days, mutilating, potentially fatal if not immediately treated ●*Co-morbidities:* Trauma, skin disease, surgery, peripheral vascular disease, diabetes, neutropenia, GI malignancy, injection drug use ●*Procedure results:* Gas in soft tissue on X-ray, necrosis of fascia or muscle with infiltration of polymorphic neutrophils and positive Gram stain on frozen section/biopsy material ●*Test findings:* Leukocytosis, left shift, elevated creatine phosphokinase (CPK) (if muscle involved), elevated creatinine, hemolytic anemia (Clostridia), positive Gram stain and culture of bullae fluid/biopsy material/blood

Gastric cancer ●*Onset:* Insidious ●*Male:female ratio:* M(1.7):F(1) ●*Ethnicity:* Increased incidence among Japanese ●*Character:* Dull midepigastric pain, with anorexia, early satiety and weight loss; may have nausea and vomiting ●*Location:* Epigastrium ●*Pattern:* Slowly progressive over months ●*Precipitating factors:* Eating ●*Relieving factors:* Small meals may ameliorate symptoms; medical treatment is with chemotherapy and/or surgery ●*Clinical course:* Progresses over 3-12 months, typically ●*Co-morbidities:* Helicobacter pylori infection; history of gastric resection; pernicious anemia ●*Procedure results:* EGD (esophagogastroduodenoscopy) reveals gastric mass in most cases; a variant form has diffuse infiltration of stomach with tumor, best seen with endoscopic U/S. Biopsy is diagnostic ●*Test findings:* Barium upper gastrointestinal series may reveal mass or show poor distensibility of stomach suggesting tumor infiltration

Gastric dilation ●*Onset:* Subacute to insidious ●*Male:female ratio:* M=F ●*Ethnicity:* All ●*Character:* Early satiety, indigestion, anorexia, nausea, vomiting, epigastric pain, weight loss ●*Location:* Nonspecific ●*Pattern:* Worse after meals ●*Precipitating factors:* Duodenal or prepyloric ulcer, congenital abnormalities of the duodenum, delayed gastric emptying, postabdominal surgery ●*Relieving factors:* Nasogastric decompression for acute severity, small meals, treatment of underlying ulcer if exists, endoscopic dilation of web/stricture, surgery, promotility agents if delayed emptying (not if obstruction) ●*Clinical course:* Depends on the etiology: ulcers are generally curable, motility problems tend to be chronic ●*Co-morbidities:* Diabetes, cancer ●*Procedure results:* Radionuclide study: poor gastric emptying; esophago-gastroduodenoscopy (EGD): pyloric obstruction ●*Test findings:* Barium study: dilated stomach with slow transit or obstruction

Gastritis ●*Onset:* Acute, subacute ●*Male:female ratio:* M=F ●*Ethnicity:* All ●*Character:* Gastritis is a pathologic diagnosis, but patients may have a number of upper GI symptoms including epigastric pain or discomfort, and nausea (with or without vomiting). Patients do not typically lose weight. Many are asymptomatic, with gastritis diagnosed on upper endoscopy for other indications ●*Location:* Epigastric burning pain is often seen, or vague upper abdominal discomfort ●*Pattern:* Nonspecific ●*Precipitating factors:* Eating certain foods (spicy or fatty foods most commonly) may worsen symptoms. Use of NSAIDs can also exacerbate symptoms ●*Relieving factors:* Antacids, H2-blockers, or proton pump inhibitors may be helpful. Treatment of Helicobacter pylori infection (if present) may also relieve symptoms, but this is not universal. Discontinuing NSAIDs is often helpful ●*Clinical course:* Chronic illness with waxing and waning symptoms ●*Co-morbidities:* Any disorder requiring NSAID use; H. pylori infection ●*Procedure results:* Esophagogastroduodenoscopy (EGD) shows erythematous mucosa in the stomach, perhaps with erosions. Biopsy is diagnostic, showing inflammatory cells in the mucosa and lamina propria ●*Test findings:* H. pylori serology may be positive

Gastroenteritis ●*Onset:* Acute ●*Male:female ratio:* M=F ●*Ethnicity:* All ●*Character:* Varies depending on the infectious agent: may be primarily nausea/vomiting and abdominal pain, or diarrhea and abdominal pain. Stools may be watery, with blood or mucus. Fever is variable. Malaise is almost universal, as is anorexia ●*Location:* Abdomen ●*Pattern:* Nonspecific ●*Precipitating factors:* Exposure to ill persons or contaminated foods ●*Relieving factors:* Antiemetics (e.g. perchlorperazine) and antidiarrheals (e.g. loperamide) are often useful; antidiarrheals should not be used if there is fever or bloody diarrhea. Bacterial colitis may respond to antibiotic therapy ●*Clinical course:* Self-limited over days ●*Co-morbidities:* Immunosuppressed patients are at greater risk ●*Procedure results:* Stool cultures may be diagnostic, although most cases are viral and have negative cultures. In colitis, a sigmoi-doscopy may be diagnostic ●*Test findings:* Patients often have an elevated WBC

Gastroesophageal reflux disease ●*Onset:* Often subacute ●*Male:female ratio:* M=F ●*Ethnicity:* All ●*Character:* Epigastric or retrosternal burning discomfort, radiating to the neck. May have regurgitation of bitter liquid into the throat. Usually occurs after meals, or in the supine position ●*Location:* Epigastrium, mediastinum, neck ●*Pattern:* Worse when supine or after meals ●*Precipitating factors:* Food intake - especially spicy or fatty food, citrus, mint, chocolate, caffeine. Lying supine - especially after meals. Bending forward or lifting objects ●*Relieving factors:* Antacids give temporary relief; H2 blockers and PPIs give lasting relief. Patients should avoid foods that induce symptoms, lying down for 2 hours after eating, and being overweight; the head of their bed should be elevated at 30 degrees ●*Clinical course:* Not self-limited - varies from chronic to progressive ●*Co-morbidities:* Esophageal cancer; asthma; hoarseness; chest pain; hiatus hernia; peptic ulcer disease ●*Procedure results:* Esophagogastroduodenoscopy (EGD) shows inflammation of the esophagus in only 15% of patients; barium swallow may show mucosal abnormalities; a 24-hour pH study is the best diagnostic test ●*Test findings:* No relevant tests

Gaucher's disease ●*Onset:* Subacute ●*Male:female ratio:* M=F ●*Ethnicity:* Type 1: Ashkenazi Jews; type 3: Swedish ●*Character:* Type 1: easy bruising, fatigue, hepatosplenomegaly, bone pain, growth retardation; type 2: increased tone in infancy, strabismus, organomegaly, failure to thrive, neurodegenerative; type 3; symptoms of 1 and 2 with neurologic involvement ●*Location:* Liver, spleen, bone marrow, bones ●*Pattern:* Nonspecific ●*Precipitating factors:* Autosomal recessive, deficient lysosomal hydrolase, acid B-glucosidase on chromosome 1(q21-q31) ●*Relieving factors:* Symptomatic, blood transfusions, splenectomy, analgesics for bone pain, bone marrow transplant, enzyme replacement ●*Clinical course:* Progressive; type 2: death within 2 years; type 3: death by 10-15 years ●*Co-morbidities:* None relevant ●*Procedure results:* Radiological changes: Erlenmeyer flask deformity of distal femur, lytic lesions of femur, ribs, pelvis ●*Test findings:* Thrombocytopenia, anemia, elevated liver function tests, Gaucher cell in bone marrow

Genital herpes ●*Onset:* Acute ●*Male:female ratio:* M<F ●*Ethnicity:* All ●*Character:* First episode: painful vesicular or ulcerative eruption in genital organs/perineum, tender lymphadenopathy, dysuria, clear vaginal discharge, fever, and rarely urinary retention. Reactivation: single or few vesicles associated with tingling ●*Location:* Women: vulva, vagina, cervix. Men: penile shaft, glans, scrotum. Both: perianal area, thighs, buttocks, rectum, urethra. Rare: dissemination to other skin or internal organs (lungs, liver, esophagus, CSF, brain, other) ●*Pattern:* Vesicular, ulcerative rash. Primary rash is more extensive and extremely painful. Recurrent outbreaks are milder, single or few vesicles associated with tingling ●*Precipitating factors:* Sexual exposure (genital, anal, and oral for primary infection), HIV, immunosuppression (more frequent outbreaks) ●*Relieving factors:* None relevant ●*Clinical course:* Primary eruption is self-limiting within days-to-several weeks. Pain syndrome may last months. Recurrences are common (especially with HSV-2) ●*Co-morbidities:* Erythema multiforme, HIV ●*Procedure results:* Intranuclear inclusions in epithelial cell from base of a vesicle. Positive direct fluorescent antigen for HSV on smeared material from vesicles. Growth of HSV in culture ●*Test findings:* With severe primary infection: lymphocytosis, atypical lymphocytes

Genital warts ●*Onset:* Chronic ●*Male:female ratio:* M=F ●*Ethnicity:* All ●*Character:* Skin-colored papules, some with cauliflower-like appearance, usually painless, rarely itching or bleeding ●*Location:* Women: vulva (most common in posterior introitus/labia), vagina, cervix. Men: penis (most common near meatus, frenum). Both: perianal. Other ●*Pattern:* Papules are flesh or skin-colored, cauliflower-like, usually painless, but may itch or bleed ●*Precipitating factors:* Multiple sex partners, unprotected sexual intercourse, men who have sex with men, HIV, other STD (syphilis, genital herpes, gonorrhea, chlamydia) ●*Relieving factors:* None relevant ●*Clinical course:* Prolonged infection (months), some self-limiting, some progressive, more progressive in immunocompromised hosts (HIV, transplantation), some types are associated with anogenital/cervical dysplasia and anal/cervical carcinoma ●*Co-morbidities:* HIV, AIDS, transplantation, other STDs ●*Procedure results:* Application of 3-5% acetic acid causes lesions to turn white, visualization of vaginal and cervical lesions on colposcopy ●*Test findings:* No relevant tests

Genitofemoral neuralgia ●*Onset:* Subacute ●*Male:female ratio:* M=F ●*Ethnicity:* All ●*Character:* Pain/dysesthesia in groin ●*Location:* Can include iliolingual, iliohypogastric and genital branch of genitofemoral nerve ●*Pattern:* Injury or entrapment of nerves innervating groin ●*Precipitating factors:* Postoperative following hernia repair, traumatic injury such as due to motor vehicle accident/seatbelt ●*Relieving factors:* Injection of local anesthetic into groin; re-exploration and neurolysis ●*Clinical course:* Complete resolution of pain in most cases adequately treated locally or with repeat surgery ●*Co-morbidities:* Hernia ●*Procedure results:* Injection of local anesthetic is diagnostic as well as therapeutic ●*Test findings:* No relevant tests

Geographic tongue ●*Onset:* Chronic ●*Male:female ratio:* M=F ●*Ethnicity:* All ●*Character:* Migratory areas of depapillation on the dorsal tongue surrounded by sharply demarcated whitish hyperkeratotic areas ●*Location:* Dorsal tongue; also on buccal mucosa (geographic mucositis)

●*Pattern:* Persistent migratory areas ●*Precipitating factors:* No relevant procedures ●*Relieving factors:* None relevant ●*Clinical course:* Rarely remits spontaneously; occasionally waxes and wanes with cutaneous psoriasis lesions ●*Co-morbidities:* Psoriasis, 40% associated with fissured tongue ●*Procedure results:* Biopsy reveals hyperkeratosis at the edge of the whitish areas with spongiosis and transmigration of neutrophils and occasionally microabscesses in the epidermis ●*Test findings:* Superimposed oral candidiasis must be ruled out with a potassium hydroxide preparation of a curetted tongue specimen

Germ cell ovarian cancer ●*Onset:* Insidious ●*Male:female ratio:* F ●*Ethnicity:* Nonspecific ●*Character:* Abdominal pain with palpable mass ●*Location:* Pelvis ●*Pattern:* Nonspecific ●*Precipitating factors:* None relevant ●*Relieving factors:* None relevant ●*Clinical course:* Progression to invasion and distant metastases ●*Co-morbidities:* None relevant ●*Procedure results:* No relevant procedures ●*Test findings:* Elevated alfa-fetoprotein (AFP) - endodermal sinus tumors; elevated human chorionic gonadotropin (hCG) - choriocarcinoma; elevated lactate dehydrogenase (LDH) - dysgerminoma

Gestational trophoblastic neoplasm ●*Onset:* Usually insidious but can be acute ●*Male:female ratio:* F ●*Ethnicity:* Higher incidence in Asians ●*Character:* Nausea/vomiting, uterus larger than dates, uterine bleeding, vaginal passage of vesicles ●*Location:* Nonspecific ●*Pattern:* Bleeding begins at 6-8 weeks gestation ●*Precipitating factors:* History of molar pregnancy ●*Relieving factors:* Evacuation of the uterus, chemotherapy (for more advanced cases), birth control for 1 year afterwards ●*Clinical course:* Normal lifespan for hydatiform mole, 85% 5-year survival for choriocarcinoma ●*Co-morbidities:* Pre-eclampsia ●*Procedure results:* No relevant procedures ●*Test findings:* Very elevated human chorionic gonadotrophin (hCG) beta subunit (>40.000). Ultrasound - multiple echoes, large uterus, no fetus or placenta

Giant cell arteritis ●*Onset:* Acute, subacute ●*Male:female ratio:* M(1):F(2) ●*Ethnicity:* Caucasian almost exclusively ●*Character:* Pain over temporal arteries, jaw claudication, visual disturbances, polymyalgia rheumatica ●*Location:* Large vessels, mainly extracranial arteries ●*Pattern:* Nonspecific ●*Precipitating factors:* None relevant ●*Relieving factors:* Corticosteroids ●*Clinical course:* Progressive with occasional spontaneous remissions ●*Co-morbidities:* Polymyalgia rheumatica ●*Procedure results:* Temporal artery biopsy with disruption of internal elastic lamina, granulomas, and panarteritis ●*Test findings:* ESR over 100

Giardiasis ●*Onset:* Sudden or gradual ●*Male:female ratio:* M=F ●*Ethnicity:* All ●*Character:* Diarrhea with abdominal pain and bloating, occasional flatus, nausea, and vomiting ●*Location:* Duodenum, small intestines > large intestines ●*Pattern:* Diarrhea is nonbloody and voluminous, associated with bloating and flatulence, may last longer than one week ●*Precipitating factors:* Waterborne transmission (mountain streams, reservoirs), person-to-person transmission in institutions and day-care centers, anal sex, hypogammaglobulinemia, travel ●*Relieving factors:* Hydration, specific antibiotics, reduced lactose in diet during recovery ●*Clinical course:* Acute or gradual onset, usually lasts 1-3 weeks but may persist longer, and result in malabsorption, more severe in hypogammaglobulinemia ●*Co-morbidities:* AIDS, hypogammaglobulinemia, cystic fibrosis, anterior uveitis, arthritis, urticaria, malabsorption ●*Procedure results:* No relevant procedures ●*Test findings:* Finding of cysts or trophozoites (pear-shaped with two nuclei) in stool (for ova and parasites), trophozoites in duodenal/small intestinal fluid sample or biopsy, finding of antigen-antigen in stool

Gilbert's disease ●*Onset:* Subacute ●*Male:female ratio:* M(3):F(1) ●*Ethnicity:* All ●*Character:* Intermittent jaundice, abdominal pain, malaise ●*Location:* Skin/liver ●*Pattern:* Nonspecific ●*Precipitating factors:* Low enzyme levels of hepatic glucuronyl transferase activity: missense mutation in transferase gene (UGTI); fatigue/stress may precipitate symptoms ●*Relieving factors:* None relevant ●*Clinical course:* Lifelong/intermittent ●*Co-morbidities:* None relevant ●*Procedure results:* No relevant procedures ●*Test findings:* Unconjugated hyperbilirubinemia more than 1.5 mg/dL but less than 6 mg/dL, normal liver function tests, absence of urinary bile, signs of hemolysis, no anemia

Gingivitis ●*Onset:* Insidious ●*Male:female ratio:* M=F ●*Ethnicity:* All ●*Character:* Bleeding painful gums ●*Location:* Oral cavity, periodontal ●*Pattern:* Worse after eating or brushing teeth ●*Precipitating factors:* Poor dental hygiene ●*Relieving factors:* Topical oral anesthetics ●*Clinical course:* Chronic ●*Co-morbidities:* Dental caries ●*Procedure results:* No relevant procedures ●*Test findings:* No relevant tests

Glaucoma ●*Onset:* Insidious, subacute, acute ●*Male:female ratio:* M<F (primary angle-closure glaucoma) ●*Ethnicity:* All ❶ *Character:* Some forms of glaucoma produce browache and halos but most forms are asymptomatic ❷ *Location:* Blurred vision ❸ *Pattern:* Unilateral, bilateral, asymmetric ●*Precipitating factors:* Precipitating factor depends on subtype of glaucoma ●*Relieving factors:* Therapy to lower intraocular pressure ●*Clinical course:* Rate of progression depends on the level of intraocular pressure ●*Co-morbidities:* None relevant ●*Procedure results:* No relevant procedures ●*Test findings:* Characteristic optic nerve changes (pathalogic cupping of optic nerve), visual field loss

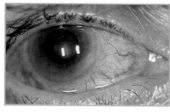

❶ *Character Mildly edematous cornea, with dilated and fixed pupil. Ciliary injection prominent*

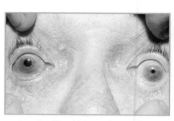

❷ *Location The right eye shows ciliary injection and a dilated, fixed pupil*

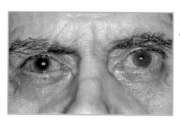

❸ *Pattern Right eye is red, showing a dilated and fixed pupil*

Glenohumeral joint instability ●*Onset:* Subacute ●*Male:female ratio:* M=F ●*Ethnicity:* All ●*Character:* Pain ●*Location:* Shoulder ●*Pattern:* Worse with weightbearing in affected shoulder ●*Precipitating factors:* Labral tear ●*Relieving factors:* Physical therapy or surgical repair of labrum ●*Clinical course:* Progressive ●*Co-morbidities:* None relevant ●*Procedure results:* Demonstrated by plain radiograph ●*Test findings:* No relevant tests

Glomus tumor (paraganglioma) ●*Onset:* Insidious ●*Male:female ratio:* M=F ●*Ethnicity:* All ●*Character:* Frequently asymptomatic; symptoms come from either local mass effect with or without invasion of local structures, or else from catecholamine secretion (1-3% of tumors are 'functional') ●*Location:* Symptoms depend on location of tumor (mainly in head and neck); can include ear 'fullness', hearing loss, tinnitus, facial nerve weakness, vertigo, vocal cord paralysis, dysphagia; rarely systemic catecholamine effects, asymptomatic neck mass ●*Pattern:* Gradual progression of symptoms from slowgrowing tumor ●*Precipitating factors:* Symptoms are spontaneous, insidiously progressive, and unrelated to patient's activities ●*Relieving factors:* Symptoms of local invasion/compression are only relieved by reduction or excision of tumor mass by surgery or radiation therapy; beta-blockers may attenuate symptoms related to the rare functional tumor ●*Clinical course:* Most paragangliomas are nonfunctional, benign, with very slow inexorable growth; rarely malignant with invasion and/or metastasis (also associated with very slow progression); can see multiple tumors, whether familial or not ●*Co-morbidities:* May be familial disorder (autosomal dominant); associated pheochromocytoma; associated with multiple endocrine neoplasia complex, parathyroid, thyroid, other neural crest tumors ●*Procedure results:* Arteriography may show splaying of internal and external carotid arteries in case of carotid body paraganglioma; increased vascularity of tumor may be seen; fine needle aspiration may reveal typical cytology of paraganglioma ●*Test findings:* CT or MRI scan will show tumor and define its extent, local effects, invasion, and possibly metastasis

Glossitis ●*Onset:* Insidious ●*Male:female ratio:* M>F ●*Ethnicity:* All ●*Character:* Burning tongue pain ●*Location:* Oral cavity ●*Pattern:* Ulcerated or inflamed appearance of tongue ●*Precipitating factors:* Acid foods, spicy foods ●*Relieving factors:* Topical oral anesthetics, cough drops ●*Clinical course:* Usually chronic persistent ●*Co-morbidities:* Numerous: autoimmune disease, steroid asthma inhaler, lichen planus ●*Procedure results:* Mucosal inflammation on tongue biopsy ●*Test findings:* Mucosal inflammation on tongue biopsy

Gonorrhea ●*Onset:* Acute ●*Male:female ratio:* M=F ●*Ethnicity:* In the US higher in minorities ●*Character:* Men: purulent urethral discharge, dysuria, meatal erythema. Women: asymptomatic, pelvic and lower abdominal pain (acute or chronic), dysuria, vaginal discharge ●*Location:* Men: urethra, epididymis, prostate. Women: endocervix, urethra, fallopian tubes, endometrium, Bartholin's glands (unilateral), perihepatitis. Both: anal canal and rectum, pharynx. Dissemination (disseminated gonococcal infection [DGI]): one or more joints/tendons (tenosynovitis, most common are wrists, fingers, ankles, knees), skin (pustular lesions) ●*Pattern:* In men, dysuria and meatal erythema in addition to discharge, In women, cervical motion tenderness and dyspareunia, In DGI, rash in pustular on red (petechial) base. Joint diseases with multiple polyarthralgia and mono- or oligoarthritis ●*Precipitating factors:* Multiple sex partners, unprotected sexual intercourse, crack cocaine use, genitourinary chlamydia, syphilis, HIV, men who have sex with men, deficiency in complement C5-8 predisposes to DGI ●*Relieving factors:* None relevant ●*Clinical course:* Acute disease in men. May be asymptomatic, acute or subacute in women. Resolves with therapy. Untreated may lead to chronic pelvic pain, infertility in women ●*Co-morbidities:* Chlamydia, syphilis, crack cocaine use, HIV, terminal complement deficiency (for DGI), infertility, chronic pelvic pain ●*Procedure results:* Gram stain of ureteral endocervical swab: Gram-negative diplococci in leukocytes, joint aspiration: >10,000 polymorphonuclear neutrophils (PMN), organisms rarely recovered, U/S in pelvic inflammatory disease (PID) may reveal a tubo-ovarian abscess, positive DNA probe/ligase chain reaction (LCR) for gonorrhea with or without chlamydia, positive culture for gonorrhea ●*Test findings:* Leukocytosis (in disseminated diseases), intracellular Gram-negative diplococci in clinical specimen, joint aspiration: >10,000 PMN

Goodpasture's syndrome ●*Onset:* Acute, subacute ●*Male:female ratio:* M(6):F(1) with early onset disease. Later onset has equal sex distribution ●*Ethnicity:* All ●*Character:* Cough, fever, dyspnea, oliguria (hemoptysis is absent in >50% of patients) ●*Location:* Lungs, kidney ●*Pattern:* Bilateral inspiratory rales ●*Precipitating factors:* Idiopathic (common), infection or hydrocarbon exposure (rare). Note: pulmonary hemorrhage is usually associated with cigarette smoking or other concomitant lung injury ●*Relieving factors:* Plasmapheresis, steroid therapy, cyclophosphamide ●*Clinical course:* If creatinine >5mg/dL prior to treatment, then endstage renal disease requiring maintenance dialysis is likely ●*Co-morbidities:* Anemia, acute renal failure ●*Procedure results:* Renal biopsy positive for crescentic glomerulonephritis, linear immunofluorescence along glomerular capillaries ●*Test findings:* Serum antiglomerular basement membrane antibodies; urinalysis: proteinuria, RBC, WBC, granular casts; hemosiderin-laden macrophages in sputum; anemia

Gram negative septicemia ●*Onset:* Most are of acute or abrupt onset although rarely may be insidious, persistent, or chronic ●*Male:female ratio:* M=F ●*Ethnicity:* All ●*Character:* Evidence of systemic response to infection with fever or hypothermia, chills, rapid heart rate, hyperventilation, sometimes with low blood pressure and acral cyanosis (hypoperfusion), may be associated with altered mental status, oliguria, jaundice, congestive high output heart failure, may be associated with skin lesions (ecthyma, petechia, bullous lesions) ●*Location:* Systemic (by definition), bloodstream, multiorgan systems including: lungs, CNS, liver, kidneys, skin, any other organ ●*Pattern:* The patient appears critically ill with: fever with chills or hypothermia, hyperventilation and vasodilation (early), then hypoperfusion, low blood pressure, change in mental status, tachycardia, acrocyanosis, oliguric renal failure, discolored skin lesions (ecthyma, petechia, bollous lesions), disseminated intravascular coagulation (DIC) ●*Precipitating factors:* Neutropenia, hypogammaglobulinemia, immunosuppression, transplantation, chemotherapy, hospitalization, indwelling catheters, localized infection (urinary tract infection [UTI], cholecystitis, peritonitis, pneumonia or aspiration, meningitis, other), bowel perforation, aspiration, surgery, trauma, burn ●*Relieving factors:* Supportive care, fluid replacement to maintain adequate tissue perfusion, removal of infection source, specific antimicrobial therapy, pressors (such as norepinephrine and epinephrine) ●*Clinical course:* Some patients have transient hypotension and respond quickly to fluid replacement and antimicrobial therapy. However many progress rapidly to warm then cold shock (20-35%) which is associated with a high mortality rate (40-55%) ●*Co-morbidities:* Immunodeficiency, cancer, neutropenia, chemotherapy, transplantation, chronic indwelling catheters, injection drug use, burn, trauma, surgery, bowel perforation, aspiration, localized infection (urinary infection, cholecystitis, pneumonia, meningitis, endocarditis, other) ●*Procedure results:* Isolation of Gram-negative organisms from blood cultures; Swan Ganz: early normal or elevated cardiac index and decreased vascular resistance with a relatively preserved or low pulmonary wedge pressure on Swan Ganz catheterization (not always true given myocardial suppression) ●*Test findings:* Leukocytosis or leukopenia, left shift (band forms), thrombocytopenia, early respiratory alkalosis (high pH, low CO_2), later metabolic acidosis (low pH), lactatemia, later increased creatinine

Granuloma annulare ●*Onset:* Subacute ●*Male:female ratio:* M(1):F(2) ●*Ethnicity:* All ●*Character:* Skin lesions ●*Location:* Dorsal hands, feet, knees, elbows. Rarely generalized ●*Pattern:* Rings of skin-colored indurated papules ●*Precipitating factors:* None relevant ●*Relieving factors:* Intralesional steroids ●*Clinical course:* Frequently resolves in months-to-years ●*Co-morbidities:* Possibly diabetes ●*Procedure results:* No relevant procedures ●*Test findings:* Positive skin biopsy

Granuloma inguinale (donovanosis) ●*Onset:* Subacute, chronic ●*Male:female ratio:* M=F ●*Ethnicity:* More common in developing nations ●*Character:* Painless genital papules that ulcerate then turn into areas of irregularly raised, beefy-red, friable granulation tissue ●*Location:* Women: vulva progressing anteriorly from the fourchette. Men: glans penis, penile shaft. Both: perianal, inguinal skin, subcutaneous tissue (pseudobubo), mouth, face, neck, other ●*Pattern:* Lesions evolve from papules to ulcers to areas of friable, beefy-red, painless, granulation tissue, then spread by autoinoculation. Inguinal lymph nodes are not involved. Lymphedema and sinus tracts form late ●*Precipitating factors:* Sex partners with donovanosis, repeated unprotected sexual intercourse, other STD (particularly syphilis), men who have sex with men, HIV, endemic in the tropics (Papua New Guinea, southern India, southern Africa, Australia, Brazil, Caribbean) ●*Relieving factors:* None relevant ●*Clinical course:* Incubation of days-to-weeks, slow indolent progression by autoinoculation causing local tissue destruction ●*Co-morbidities:* Syphilis, AIDS, other STD, secondary bacterial infection, sinus tract formation, lymphedema ●*Procedure results:* Donovan bodies (intracellular rod-shaped bacteria) on Giemsa/Wright-stained crush preparation from lesion ●*Test findings:* No relevant tests

Graves' disease ●*Onset:* Insidious, acute ●*Male:female ratio:* M(1):F(10) ●*Ethnicity:* All ●*Character:* Palpitations, sweating, tremor, weight loss ●*Location:* Enlarged thyroid, exophthalmous, brisk reflexes, tremor on outstretched hands, pretibial myxedema ●*Pattern:* Nonspecific ●*Precipitating factors:* First trimester of pregnancy and postpartum state

●*Relieving factors:* Antithyroid medication and beta blockade, permanent treatment: radioactive iodine or surgery ●*Clinical course:* Usually worsens but may spontaneously remit, 20% of patients on antithyroid treatment remit within 1 year ●*Co-morbidities:* Eye disease (including exophthalmus), systolic hypertension, atrial tachyarrhythmias, bone loss, may be associated with polyglandular autoimmune syndrome ●*Procedure results:* Elevated I-123 uptake ●*Test findings:* Suppressed thyroid-stimulating hormone (TSH), high T4 (and T3), thyroid stimulating immunoglobulin (TSI) usually high but not clinically indicated

Group A beta hemolytic streptococcus
●*Onset:* Acute ●*Male:female ratio:* M=F ●*Ethnicity:* All ●*Character:* Pyogenic infections sometimes associated with toxin-mediated disease including: pharyngitis; scarlet fever; impetigo; erysipelas; cellulitis; necrotizing fasciitis; pneumonia and empyema; puerperal sepsis; toxic shock syndrome ●*Location:* Most common: pharynx, skin, fascial planes, muscle, vagina, endometrium, bloodstream, joint, lung, pleural space, other; toxin-mediated disease is systemic. Late complications involve the heart, joints, central nervous system, and kidneys ●*Pattern:* Pharyngitis is associated with sore throat, fever, erythema and swelling of pharyngeal mucosa, and white exudates; impetigo: skin lesions are pustular with a honeycomb-like crust; erysipelas: erythema is sharply demarcated, bright red, and tender; cellulitis progresses rapidly. In necrotizing fasciitis erythema is rapidly progressive, painful, associated with systemic symptoms and toxic appearance, and the late formation of bullae; toxic shock syndrome requires a localized infection with group A streptococci as well as toxic appearance, hypotension, evidence of endorgan demmage, and generalized erythroderm that may desquamate ●*Precipitating factors:* Skin injury, trauma, dermatosis, sick contact, surgery, trauma, lymphedema, mastectomy, childbirth, possibly NSAID use (in toxic shock syndrome) ●*Relieving factors:* Specific antimicrobial therapy, fluid replacement, supportive care, and intravenous immunoglobulin in toxic shock ●*Clinical course:* Most are mild-to-moderate and respond rapidly to specific therapy. Some, especially necrotizing fasciitis, toxic shock syndrome, empyema, and sepsis, may be rapidly progressive and fatal. Some lead to late complications such as rheumatic fever and glomerulonephritis ●*Co-morbidities:* Surgery, lymphedema, broken or nonintact skin, mastectomy, diabetes, alcoholism, varicella, rheumatic fever, glomerulonephritis ●*Procedure results:* Isolation of group A Streptococci from infected site, positive rapid diagnostic test from a pharyngeal swab, Gram-positive cocci in chains on Gram stain from infected site ●*Test findings:* Isolation of group A Streptococci from infected site, positive rapid diagnostic test from a pharyngeal swab, Gram-positive cocci in chains on Gram stain from infected site, leukocytosis with a left shift, in toxic shock syndrome and necrotizing fasciitis: elevated creatinine, low calcium, low albumin, high creatine kinase, thrombocytopenia, elevated hepatic transaminases

Group B beta hemolytic streptococcus
●*Onset:* Newborn/infancy ●*Male:female ratio:* M=F ●*Ethnicity:* More common in African-Americans ●*Character:* Colonizes maternal genitourinary (GU)/gastrointestinal (GI) tract, 4-40% of pregnant women and 40-70% of infants born to colonized mothers ●*Location:* Neonatal disease: early onset (inutero): fetal asphyxia, coma, shock, pneumonia, bacteremia (asymptomatic to sepsis), pulmonary hypertension, meningitis; late onset: bacteremia, meningitis, osteoarthirits, cellulitis ●*Pattern:* Pregnant women usually asymptomatic; urinary tract infection (UTI) ●*Precipitating factors:* Maternal colonization, low birth weight infant (abnormal host defense mechanisms.), premature rupture of fetal membranes, prolonged labor, chorioamnionitis, maternal UTI, prior delivery with group B streptococcus disease, from other contaminated people (adults/infants), opsonophagocytic defects due to deficient maternally derived type-specific antibodies ●*Relieving factors:* Intrapartum prophylaxis if risk factors present: prior infant with group B streptococcal disease, group B streptococcal disease bacteruria during pregnancy, premature delivery, maternal fever during delivery >38°C; treatment of infant with appropriate antibiotics ●*Clinical course:* Severe illness unless treated ●*Co-morbidities:* None relevant ●*Procedure results:* Chest X-ray: pneumonia; bone film: osteomyelitis ●*Test findings:* Culture positive CSF, blood, skin; Gram-positive cocci in gastric/tracheal aspirates; group B streptococcal latex particle agglutination; increased bands/WBCs on CBC. I/T ratio >0.2, decreased platelets

Growth hormone deficiency ●*Onset:* Insidious ●*Male:female ratio:* M=F ●*Ethnicity:* All ●*Character:* Low energy, decreased ability to concentrate ●*Location:* Increased body fat, decreased muscle strength ●*Pattern:* Nonspecific ●*Precipitating factors:* Pituitary surgery/tumor/irradiation ●*Relieving factors:* Growth hormone (GH) replacement may be indicated in some ●*Clinical course:* Permanent ●*Co-morbidities:* Hyperlipidemia; decreased bone density ●*Procedure results:* No or decreased GH response to intravenous insulin-induced hypoglycemia or infused arginine ●*Test findings:* Low insulin-like growth factor (IGF), elevated lipids

Growth hormone deficiency in children ●*Onset:* Insidious, but pituitary apoplexy acute ●*Male:female ratio:* M=F ●*Ethnicity:* All ●*Character:* Fall-off growth curve ●*Location:* Pituitary ●*Pattern:* Nonspecific ●*Precipitating factors:* Pituitary tumor, pituitary surgery, pituitary irradiation ●*Relieving factors:* Growth hormone (GH) replacement, glucose for hypoglycemia ●*Clinical course:* Progressive ●*Co-morbidities:* None relevant ●*Procedure results:* No relevant procedures ●*Test findings:* Low somatomedin C level. Failure of GH to rise in response to insulin-induced hypoglycemia

Growth hormone excess ●*Onset:* Toddler/adolescence (rarely infancy) ●*Male:female ratio:* M=F ●*Ethnicity:* All ●*Character:* Rapid linear and head growth, coarse facies, enlarged hands/feet; behavioral/visual problems ●*Location:* Pituitary, hypothalamus; face, head, hands, feet ●*Pattern:* Worsening symptoms without treatment ●*Precipitating factors:* Pituitary adenoma, hypothalamic (rarely, pancreatic) tumor secreting growth hormone-releasing hormone (GHRH), mutation of G protein gene in McCune-Albright syndrome ●*Relieving factors:* Surgery, radiation, suppression with octreotide ●*Clinical course:* Worsening symptoms without treatment ●*Co-morbidities:* McCune-Albright syndrome ●*Procedure results:* Abnormal CT/MRI e.g. pituitary, normal osseous maturation ●*Test findings:* Elevated growth hormone (GH) and prolactin level, no GH suppression by glucose tolerance test, elevated insulin-like growth factor (IGF)-1, IGF binding protein (IGFBP)-3 (acromegaly)

Guillain-Barré syndrome (acute infective polyneuritis) ●*Onset:* Acute, subacute ●*Male:female ratio:* M(1.5):F(1) ●*Ethnicity:* All ●*Character:* Weakness and paresthesias of the extremities ●*Location:* Nonspecific ●*Pattern:* Nonspecific ●*Precipitating factors:* Postviral syndrome, postdiarrheal illness ●*Relieving factors:* IgG or plasmaphoresis ●*Clinical course:* Variable, usually self-limited ●*Co-morbidities:* Campylobacter jejuni infection ●*Procedure results:* Lumbar puncture with protein cytologic dissociation (normal WBC and elevated protein) ●*Test findings:* Delayed nerve conduction velocities

Hallux valgus (bunion) ●*Onset:* Insidious ●*Male:female ratio:* M=F ●*Ethnicity:* All ●*Character:* Pain ●*Location:* Pain over bunion ●*Pattern:* Nonspecific ●*Precipitating factors:* Worse with shoes and weightbearing ●*Relieving factors:* Wide toe box shoes, correctional surgery ●*Clinical course:* Progressive ●*Co-morbidities:* Arthritides, upper motor neuron lesions ●*Procedure results:* Plain radiograph demonstrates angulation ●*Test findings:* No relevant procedures

Hand injury ●*Onset:* Acute ●*Male:female ratio:* M=F ●*Ethnicity:* All ●*Character:* Pain, swelling at site of injury. Weakness or pain with flexion or extension of digits. Diminished sensation distal to injury ●*Location:* Nonspecific ●*Pattern:* Weak or absent flexion/extension or pain with passive flexion/extension of digits indicate tendon injury ●*Precipitating factors:* Fractures, lacerations, puncture or bite wounds, burns ●*Relieving factors:* Irrigating all wounds well. Repair lacerations. Nerve and tendon lacerations may also require repair. Splinting, analgesics, antibiotics for some wounds ●*Clinical course:* Close followup usually required ●*Co-morbidities:* None relevant ●*Procedure results:* Explore all wounds in bloodless field to remove foreign bodies and identify tendon or bone injuries ●*Test findings:* Radiographs required to identify fractures, foreign bodies

Hand-foot-and-mouth disease ●*Onset:* Acute ●*Male:female ratio:* M=F ●*Ethnicity:* All ●*Character:* Fever, malaise, sore throat, followed by a painful vesicular rash in oropharynx and tongue, then hands, then (not always) feet ●*Location:* Buccal mucosa, dorsum of hands, less frequently palms, feet (including soles), buttocks, palate, uvula, tonsils. Systemic involvement (viremia, fever, malaise) ●*Pattern:* Painful vesicular rash begins in the mouth, then on the hands, and less commonly on the feet; vesicles rapidly ulcerate ●*Precipitating factors:* Outbreaks ●*Relieving factors:* Acetaminophen ●*Clinical course:* Acute onset of fever and sore throat, followed by rash. Self-limiting within 1 week ●*Co-morbidities:* IgA deficiency ●*Procedure results:* Detection of coxsackievirus A16 in stool or blood (not needed) ●*Test findings:* Normal-to-low WBC

Head and neck carcinoma ●*Onset:* Insidious ●*Male:female ratio:* M>F ●*Ethnicity:* All ●*Character:* Growth or mass in the head/neck, pain, bleeding; dysarthria, dysphagia, hoarseness, stridor, aspiration, otalgia, ocular symptoms, nasal obstruction are all possible depending on the location of the tumor ●*Location:* Head and neck ●*Pattern:* Nonspecific ●*Precipitating factors:* None relevant ●*Relieving factors:* Many potential carcinogens including alcohol, poor dentition, cigarettes, viral infections (Epstein-Barr virus [EBV]), nutritional deficiencies, genetic predisposition ●*Clinical course:* Surgery, radiation therapy, chemotherapy: often in combination ●*Co-morbidities:* Depends on type/location of cancer and stage at diagnosis ●*Procedure results:* No relevant procedures ●*Test findings:* Direct laryngoscopy, rigid esophagoscopy, or bronchoscopy revealing a mass; biopsy revealing squamous cell cancer of the upper aerodigestive tract

Head injury ●*Onset:* Acute ●*Male:female ratio:* M>F ●*Ethnicity:* All ●*Character:* From asymptomatic, through mild headache, to coma at presentation ●*Location:* Head ●*Pattern:* Nonspecific ●*Precipitating factors:* Trauma ●*Relieving factors:* Neurosurgical intervention, control incranial pressure, supportive care ●*Clinical course:* Variable ●*Co-morbidities:* Cervical spine fracture, chest/abdomen/pelvis trauma, cardiac contusion ●*Procedure results:* MRI/CT of the brain ranges from normal to massive hemorrhage ●*Test findings:* No relevant tests

Head lice ●*Onset:* Acute, insidious ●*Male:female ratio:* M<F ●*Ethnicity:* All ●*Character:* Head itch and discomfort with presence of eggs, nymphs, adult lice in head ●*Location:* Scalp, hair, rarely generalized rash, fever (allergic reaction) ●*Pattern:* Tingling sensation of something moving in the hair, itching; eggs (to be viable) within 6mm of scalp ●*Precipitating factors:* Contact with an infested person, usually during play at school and at home (slumber parties, camp, playground), wearing infested clothing (such as hats), sharing hair brushes ●*Relieving factors:* Shampooing with over-the-counter pediculicide, combing eggs and lice out of the hair, hot-cycle (130°F) machine washing of all clothing, bedlinens ●*Clinical course:* Chronic persistent and transmissible if untreated ●*Co-morbidities:* Secondary bacterial infections ●*Procedure results:* Finding eggs within 6mm of the scalp, a live nymph or adult louse on the scalp or in the hair of a person ●*Test findings:* No relevant tests

Healthy athlete ●*Onset:* Subacute ●*Male:female ratio:* M=F ●*Ethnicity:* All ●*Character:* Clinical picture varies from asymptomatic to symptomatic to sudden death ●*Location:* Nonspecific ●*Pattern:* Nonspecific ●*Precipitating factors:* High level of athletic training can result in cardiac hypertrophy. This should be differentiated from hypertrophic cardiomyopathy ●*Relieving factors:* In athlete's heart, there is a decrease in the cardiac hypertrophy with deconditioning. Rest is advised. Therapy may include beta-blockers or calcium channel blockers, rarely pacemaker insertion ●*Clinical course:* Can be asymptomatic. First manifestation may be syncope or sudden death; other manifestations may include dyspnea, angina, fatigue, palpitations, congestive heart failure (CCF) ●*Co-morbidities:* Heavy athletic activities can be associated with athlete's heart ●*Procedure results:* Possible findings: ECG, evidence for hypertrophy; Echo, hypertrophic changes and aortic outflow tract gradient; chest X-ray, cardiomegaly with or without congestive heart failure (CHF); cardiac catheterization, elevated right and left heart filling pressures and suggest outflow tract gradient ●*Test findings:* Examination variable; may reveal left ventricular lift, displaced point of maximal impulse (PMI), third or fourth heart sounds, CHF, elevated jugular venous pressure, systolic ejection murmur which may worsen with maneuvers that decrease left ventricular cavity size or alter the preload/afterload/contractility

Hearing loss ●*Onset:* Usually subacute ●*Male:female ratio:* M=F ●*Ethnicity:* All ●*Character:* Decreased hearing ●*Location:* Affected ear (often bilateral) ●*Pattern:* Nonspecific ●*Precipitating factors:* Extensive noise exposure ●*Relieving factors:* None relevant ●*Clinical course:* Generally progresses gradually over years ●*Co-morbidities:* Family history of hearing loss ●*Procedure results:* No relevant procedures ●*Test findings:* Abnormal audiogram showing sensorineural hearing loss or conducted hearing loss, depending on type

Heat stroke and heat exhaustion ●*Onset:* Acute ●*Male:female ratio:* M=F ●*Ethnicity:* All ●*Character:* Heat exhaustion: fatigue, headache, nausea, sweating, normal or slightly elevated temperature. Heat stroke: triad of fever (>40.5°C), CNS dysfunction and absence of sweat ●*Location:* Nonspecific ●*Pattern:* May see sweating early in course of heat stroke ●*Precipitating factors:* Exercising in hot, humid climate. May occur without exertion ●*Relieving factors:* Exhaustion: rest, cool environment, IV fluid/electrolyte replacement. Stroke: rapid cooling with ice packs or apply water and cool with fan ●*Clinical course:* Heat stroke potentially fatal ●*Co-morbidities:* Elderly more susceptible. Also pre-existing cardiovascular disease, use of anticholinergic medications ●*Procedure results:* No relevant procedures ●*Test findings:* Laboratory tests may reveal renal or liver dysfunction. Rule out other causes of fever and altered mental status

Heavy metal poisoning ●*Onset:* Acute, subacute, chronic ●*Male:female ratio:* M=F ●*Ethnicity:* All ●*Character:* Encephalopathy, cognitive or behavioral changes, paresthesias, anemias, abdominal pain, vomiting, renal effects, arrhythmias ●*Location:* Systemic ●*Pattern:* Nonspecific ●*Precipitating factors:* Ingestion of lead, arsenic, or mercury-containing products ●*Relieving factors:* Supportive management in acute toxicity. Chelating agents: BAL (dimercaprol), EDTA, D-penicillamine, DMSA ●*Clinical course:* Many effects may be permanent, especially CNS effects ●*Co-morbidities:* None relevant ●*Procedure results:* No relevant procedures ● *Test findings:* Anemia on complete blood count, 'lead bands' on bone radiographs, radiopaque material in intestines on abdominal radiographs. Elevated blood lead levels and 24-hour urine levels of arsenic or mercury

Helicobacter pylori ● *Onset:* Gradual, occasionally acute ● *Male:female ratio:* M=F ● *Ethnicity:* Less common in more affluent socioeconomic groups ● *Character:* Most infections are asymptomatic, chronic dyspepsia, recurrent epigastric pain (if gastritis or peptic ulcer), weight loss and anemia (for malignancy) ● *Location:* Gastric mucosa (antrum > other), duodenal bulb ● *Pattern:* Episodic epigastric pain, usually sharp or burning, may be relieved or accentuated by food ● *Precipitating factors:* Older age, low income, developing countries, clusters in families ● *Relieving factors:* Antacids, H2 blockers, food (temporary relief) ● *Clinical course:* Most are asymptomatic, few develop chronic gastritis or peptic ulcer disease (duodenal or gastric ulcer). May lead to adenocarcinoma of the stomach, gastric lymphoma, or mucosa-associated lymphoid tissue, and may result in vitamin B12 deficiency ● *Co-morbidities:* Gastritis, peptic ulcer, gastric carcinoma, gastric non-Hodgkin's lymphoma (NHL), mucosa-associated lymphoid tissue, vitamine B12 deficiency, iron deficiency ● *Procedure results:* Gastric or duodenal ulcer on barium swallow or endoscopy, a positive biopsy urease test, finding of bacteria in gastric or duodenal biopsy, positive serologic test, positive urea breath test ● *Test findings:* Positive biopsy urease test, finding of bacteria in gastric or duodenal biopsy, positive serologic test, positive urea breath test

Hemangioma of the liver ● *Onset:* Insidious ● *Male:female ratio:* M(1):F(5) ● *Ethnicity:* All ● *Character:* Usually asymptomatic, incidental finding on imaging study; if tumor large, may cause abdominal pain, nausea, early satiety; rupture usually heralded by severe abdominal pain, hypotension ● *Location:* Upper abdomen ● *Pattern:* Usually asymptomatic ● *Precipitating factors:* None relevant ● *Relieving factors:* If symptomatic, resection is recommended; hemorrhage requires urgent surgery or angiography with plans to embolize feeding vessels ● *Clinical course:* May grow slowly over time, but often remains unchanged ● *Co-morbidities:* None relevant ● *Procedure results:* MRI of liver shows characteristic signal characteristics. U/S and CT less useful ● *Test findings:* No relevant tests

Hemarthrosis ● *Onset:* Acute to subacute ● *Male:female ratio:* M>F ● *Ethnicity:* All ● *Character:* Prodromal joint stiffness and warmth, then joint swelling and pain. Affected joint held in flexion. Small children may only show irritability and decreased use of the affected limb ● *Location:* Most often affects large joints (ankles in children, knees, elbows, ankles, shoulders and hips in adults) ● *Pattern:* Nonspecific ● *Precipitating factors:* Spontaneous hemarthroses are virtually diagnostic of hemophilia. Trauma is required in mild hemophilia or in the absence of a clotting disorder ● *Relieving factors:* Infusion of clotting factors in hemophilia. Rest, analgesics. For chronic arthritis surgery may be indicated ● *Clinical course:* Gradual resolution of acute episode in approximately 2 weeks. With hemophilia, recurrent episodes lead to a chronic arthritis with joint deformities and limited motion ● *Co-morbidities:* Hemophilia ● *Procedure results:* No relevant procedures ● *Test findings:* No relevant tests

Hemifacial spasm ● *Onset:* Fifth and sixth decades ● *Male:female ratio:* M<F ● *Ethnicity:* All ● *Character:* Painless, irregular clonic contractions of varying degrees of one side of the face ● *Location:* Facial nerve involvement ● *Pattern:* Muscular spasm usually begins in the orbicularis oculi and gradually spreads to other muscles, ipsilaterally, including the platysma ● *Precipitating factors:* Nerve root compression, compression of facial nerve by aberrant artery, or vein, or acoustic neuroma; could also be sequelae of Bell's palsy ● *Relieving factors:* Surgical decompression of a vascular loop which involves posterior fossa exploration; carbamazepine or baclofen may be tried first; botulinum toxin injections every six months may be beneficial ● *Clinical course:* Persistent problem, does not resolve spontaneously ● *Co-morbidities:* Acoustic neuroma, aberrant vasculature around facial nerve ● *Procedure results:* Surgical decompression of vascular loop with exploration of posterior fossa; complicated by deafness, and recurrence of the spasms in 2 years ● *Test findings:* No relevant tests

Hemochromatosis ●*Onset:* Insidious ●*Male:female ratio:* M=F ●*Ethnicity:* Western European or Mediterranean descent ●*Character:* Autosomal recessive mutation of HFE gene on HLA locus of chromosome 6. Leads to increased intestinal iron absorption, iron overload, and deposition in tissues ●*Location:* Liver: hepatomegaly, elevated liver enzymes, cirrhosis, hepatocellular cancer; pancreas: diabetes mellitus; joints: arthropathy; heart: dilated cardiomyopathy, conduction disturbances; pituitary: hypogonadism, loss of libido; thyroid: hypothyroidism; GI: esophageal varices ●*Pattern:* Iron deposition in parenchymal cells of affected organs. Late in disease into reticuloendothelial cells. Clinical manifestations uncommon in heterozygotes ●*Precipitating factors:* Family member, clinical manifestations occur earlier in men ●*Relieving factors:* Phlebotomy results in improvement or reversal of esophageal varices, left ventricular dysfunction, hypogonadism. Chelation therapy with desferoxamine ●*Clinical course:* Increased mortality in patients with cirrhosis and diabetes mellitus ●*Co-morbidities:* Potentiation of alcoholic liver disease. Increased risk of infection with Listeria and Yersinia enterocolitica ●*Procedure results:* Endoscopy to detect esophageal varices. Liver biopsy to detect cirrhosis ●*Test findings:* Fasting transferrin % saturation (serum iron/total iron binding capacity[TIBC]) >60% in men, >50% in women, 95% accurate. Elevated ferritin, abnormal liver function tests. Family screening with genetic testing for C282Ymutation. X-ray findings of hook-like osteophytes of second and third metocarpophalangeal joint

Hemoglobin C disease ●*Onset:* Insidious ●*Male:female ratio:* M=F ●*Ethnicity:* African ●*Character:* Fatigue ●*Location:* Nonspecific ●*Pattern:* Nonspecific ●*Precipitating factors:* None relevant ●*Relieving factors:* None relevant ●*Clinical course:* Mild, lifelong ●*Co-morbidities:* Hemoglobin S (sickle cell trait) ●*Procedure results:* No relevant procedures ●*Test findings:* Mild anemia, hemoglobin electropheresis abnormality

Hemolysis ●*Onset:* Insidious to subacute ●*Male:female ratio:* M=F ●*Ethnicity:* All ●*Character:* Symptoms of anemia (fatigue, dyspnea, pallor), jaundice, red-brown urine ●*Location:* Nonspecific ●*Pattern:* Nonspecific ●*Precipitating factors:* Certain drugs, infections, toxins and malignancies; immune-related (drugs, antibodies), hereditary defects in RBC, prosthetic vascular graphs or heart valves, blood transfusion reactions, splenomegaly ●*Relieving factors:* Removal of precipitant, folic acid, blood transfusions in severe cases, other treatment based on etiology (splenectomy, immunosuppression) ●*Clinical course:* Depends on etiology; if toxin-, infection- or drug-related usually resolves with removal of precipitant; hereditary cell defects and immune disorders are more refractory ●*Co-morbidities:* Autoimmune diseases, cancer ●*Procedure results:* Bone marrow biopsy: erythroid hyperplasia ●*Test findings:* Blood smear: abnormal red cells (schistocytes, sickled cells, target cells); anemia, elevated aspartate transaminase (AST) and bilirubin (unconjugated), elevated lactate dehydrogenase (LDH), + Coombs test, low haptoglobin, elevated reticulocyte count, elevated urine hemosiderin if intravascular hemolysis

Hemolytic disease of the newborn (erythroblastosis fetalis) ●*Onset:* Acute ●*Male:female ratio:* M=F ●*Ethnicity:* If disease due to D antigen more common in Caucasian vs African-American ●*Character:* Jaundice, icterus, kernicterus, hepatosplenomegaly; if extreme, may have pallor, cardiac decompensation = hydrops fetalis ●*Location:* Skin/liver ●*Pattern:* Worsening jaundice ●*Precipitating factors:* Transplacental passage of maternal antibody active against RBC antigens of infant - commonly D antigen of the Rh group and with ABO incompatibility; usually caused by prior delivery of Rh+ infant leading to disease of subsequent pregnancies ●*Relieving factors:* Prevention due to Rh+ infant: Rhogam immunization after delivery; intrauterine transfusion, phototherapy, exchange transfusion ●*Clinical course:* Progressive unless treated ●*Co-morbidities:* Hydrops fetalis ●*Procedure results:* Antenatal: test parental blood types, check maternal IgG antibodies to D, fetal Rh status by amnio or U/S percutaneous umbilical blood sampling ●*Test findings:* Positive direct Coombs' test, anemia, blood smear shows hemolysis, elevated unconjugated bilirubinemia

Hemolytic transfusion reaction ●*Onset:* Acute ●*Male:female ratio:* M<F ●*Ethnicity:* All ●*Character:* Fever, chills, back pain, difficulty breathing, renal failure. Delayed reactions may occur ●*Location:* Nonspecific ●*Pattern:* Nonspecific ●*Precipitating factors:* Result from

transfusion of RBCs that are incompatible in the ABO blood group system ●*Relieving factors:* Discontinue transfusion, IV hydration, supportive care ●*Clinical course:* Hypotension and shock may lead rapidly to death ●*Co-morbidities:* Most severe reactions occur in anesthetized or comatose patients ●*Procedure results:* No relevant procedures ●*Test findings:* Hemoglobinuria, elevated bilirubin

Hemolytic uremic syndrome ●*Onset:* Subacute ●*Male:female ratio:* M=F ●*Ethnicity:* All ●*Character:* Bloody diarrhea ●*Location:* Abdominal pain ●*Pattern:* Diarrhea to colitis ●*Precipitating factors:* Infection with Escherichia coli 0157:H7 ●*Relieving factors:* Blood transfusions, hemodialysis ●*Clinical course:* Potentially fatal, may lead to chronic renal insufficiency ●*Co-morbidities:* None relevant ●*Procedure results:* Stool culture E. coli 0157:H7 ●*Test findings:* Microangiopathic hemolytic anemia, thrombocytopenia, elevated blood urea nitrogen and creatinine

Hemophilia A ●*Onset:* Acute, often diagnosed in infancy, if mild disease diagnosed later in childhood ●*Male:female ratio:* M ●*Ethnicity:* Caucasian ●*Character:* Bleeding after mild injury, symptoms often precede evidence of bleeding ●*Location:* Any site of injury, hemarthrosis (tends to recur in same joint), hematuria, bleeding in oropharynx and CNS ●*Pattern:* Nonspecific ●*Precipitating factors:* Minor trauma, use of antiplatelet medications; bleeding can be spontaneous in severe disease ●*Relieving factors:* Factor VIII concentrates, cryoprecipitate ●*Clinical course:* Lifelong, often chronic complications related to bleeding and risks of treatment (e.g. HIV, hepatitis C) ●*Co-morbidities:* HIV and hepatitis C (contaminated blood products), osteoarthritis (chronic hemarthroses) ●*Procedure results:* No relevant procedures ●*Test findings:* Prolonged partial thromboplastin time (PTT), decreased factor VIII on assay, defective allele on genetic testing

Hemophilia B ●*Onset:* Acute ●*Male:female ratio:* M ●*Ethnicity:* X-linked recessive ●*Character:* Bleeding, commonly into large joints (spontaneous hemarthroses), muscles and gastrointestinal tract; bleeding in response to minor trauma or surgery ●*Location:* Bleeding commonly into large joints, muscles and GI tract ●*Pattern:* Nonspecific ●*Precipitating factors:* Minor trauma or surgery ●*Relieving factors:* Transfusion of factor IX concentrates, aminocaproic acid for persistent bleeding ●*Clinical course:* Prognosis is good in the absence of HIV, hepatitis B, C which were commonly acquired in tainted blood products ●*Co-morbidities:* HIV, hepatitis B, C acquired through blood product transfusions ●*Procedure results:* No relevant procedures ●*Test findings:* Prolonged partial prothrombin time (PTT), low levels of factor IX or dysfunctional factor IX

Hemorrhage into tissue ●*Onset:* Acute ●*Male:female ratio:* M=F ●*Ethnicity:* All ●*Character:* Swelling, ecchymosis, pain ●*Location:* Soft tissue ●*Pattern:* Nonspecific ●*Precipitating factors:* Trauma, subcutaneous or intramuscular injection, surgery ●*Relieving factors:* None relevant ●*Clinical course:* Resolution over days ●*Co-morbidities:* Anticoagulation, thrombocytopenia ●*Procedure results:* No relevant procedures ●*Test findings:* No relevant tests

Hemorrhagic disease of newborn ●*Onset:* Acute ●*Male:female ratio:* M=F ●*Ethnicity:* All ●*Character:* Severe bleeding ●*Location:* Bleeding: nasal, gastrointestinal, intracranial, procedure site: circumcision ●*Pattern:* 2nd to 7th day of life ●*Precipitating factors:* Normal decrease in vitamin K-dependent clotting factors II, VII, IX, X 48-72 hours after birth, decreased bacterial intestinal flora that normally synthesize vitamin K in infant, decreased availability of vitamin K in breast milk; maternal use of phenobarbital/phenytoin/warfarin/rifampin/isoniazid ●*Relieving factors:* 1mg vitamin K injection after birth prevents; if symptoms occur - infusion of vitamin K; possible fresh frozen plasma infusion ●*Clinical course:* Progressive if not treated ●*Co-morbidities:* Late onset disease 1-6 months associated with biliary atresia, cystic fibrosis, hepatitis abetalipoprotein deficiency, warfarin ingestion ●*Procedure results:* No relevant procedures ●*Test findings:* Prolonged prothrombin time (PT) and partial thromboplastin time (PTT), decreased factors II (prothrombin), VII, IX, X with normal bleeding time, fibrinogen, factors V and VIII

Hemorrhoids ●*Onset:* Subacute ●*Male:female ratio:* M=F ●*Ethnicity:* All ●*Character:* Bleeding: bright red blood separate from stool, either as streaks on the outside of stool, drops of blood from the anus after a bowel movement, or blood on the toilet paper. Prolapsing hemorrhoids are felt as an anal mass after defecation; usually, this can be reduced manually. Anal pain occurs if the hemorrhoids are thrombosed, and anal itching may occur ●*Location:* Anus ●*Pattern:* Usually worse with defecation, but no set pattern ●*Precipitating factors:* Defecation ●*Relieving factors:* Over-the-counter preparations (Anusol, preparation H) and Sitz baths may relieve symptoms. Bulk agents and stool softeners may prevent prolapse. In difficult cases, surgical hemorrhoidectomy, band ligation, or sclerotherapy may be used ●*Clinical course:* Waxing and waning symptoms - may be self-limited ●*Co-morbidities:* Constipation ●*Procedure results:* Anoscopy or flexible sigmoidoscopy reveals hemorrhoids ●*Test findings:* No relevant tests

Hemothorax ●*Onset:* Acute, subacute ●*Male:female ratio:* M=F ●*Ethnicity:* All ●*Character:* Dyspnea, chest discomfort ●*Location:* Chest ●*Pattern:* Dullness to percussion and decreased breath sounds ●*Precipitating factors:* Trauma (including postoperative bleeding), pulmonary embolism, tumor, endometriosis ●*Relieving factors:* Thoracostomy and consider evacuation of hematoma if traumatic or large, medical treatment of tumor or pulmonary emboli if relevant ●*Clinical course:* Weeks-to-months, danger is the risk for a trapped lung ●*Co-morbidities:* None relevant ●*Procedure results:* Bloody pleural effusion ●*Test findings:* Pleural fluid hematocrit >50% peripheral blood hematocrit

Henoch-Schönlein purpura ●*Onset:* Subacute ●*Male:female ratio:* M(2):F(1) ●*Ethnicity:* All ●*Character:* Palpable purpura, nonmigratory arthralgias, GI complaints (bleeding, pain, diarrhea, constipation) ●*Location:* Nonspecific ●*Pattern:* Purpura commonly on extensor surfaces of extremities and on the buttocks ●*Precipitating factors:* Possibly upper respiratory infection, certain medications, insect bites, immunizations ●*Relieving factors:* Glucocorticoid therapy, though many resolve without therapy ●*Clinical course:* Usually self-limited, but can recur for years, in adults involvement can be lifethreatening ●*Co-morbidities:* Strong history of atopy in one-third ●*Procedure results:* Skin biopsy: small vessel vasculitis with IgA deposition; renal biopsy: deposition of IgA in mesangial region ●*Test findings:* Mild leukocytosis, normal platelet count, occasionally eosinophilia, elevated IgA levels with normal complement, hematuria, proteinuria

Hepatic encephalopathy ●*Onset:* Subacute, insidious ●*Male:female ratio:* M=F ●*Ethnicity:* All ●*Character:* Disturbances of mood and personality, asterixis, hyperreflexia, increased muscle tone ●*Location:* Nonspecific ●*Pattern:* Nonspecific ●*Precipitating factors:* Alcohol abuse, viral hepatitis, toxic liver damage, GI bleeding ●*Relieving factors:* Treating etiology, lactulose, decrease dietary protein ●*Clinical course:* Variable ●*Co-morbidities:* Liver disease, alcohol abuse, hepatitis ●*Procedure results:* No relevant procedures ●*Test findings:* Normal MRI/magnetic resonance angiography (MRA) of the brain

Hepatocellular jaundice ●*Onset:* Subacute to insidious ●*Male:female ratio:* M=F ●*Ethnicity:* All ●*Character:* Jaundice (usually painless), anorexia, malaise, if more advanced: ascites, asterixis, confusion ●*Location:* If pain if present, is in the right upper quadrant (RUQ) ●*Pattern:* Depends on etiology ●*Precipitating factors:* Exposure to hepatotoxin, infectious exposure (viral), family history of cholestatic liver disease ●*Relieving factors:* Treatment of underlying etiology: elimination of toxin, viral treatment, supportive measures ●*Clinical course:* Depends on etiology ●*Co-morbidities:* Alcohol abuse, intravenous drug abuse ●*Procedure results:* Liver biopsy: cholestasis, other findings specific to etiology ●*Test findings:* Elevated transaminases as well as alkaline phosphatase and bilirubin, prolonged prothrombin time (PT) that does not correct with vitamin K, normal intra- and extraheptic ducts on imaging

Hepatoma ●*Onset:* Insidious ●*Male:female ratio:* M>F ●*Ethnicity:* Most common in endemic areas for hepatitis B: southeast Asia, Africa ●*Character:* Right upper quadrant (RUQ) or epigastric pain, usually a dull aching, accompanied by weight loss, anorexia, and progressive weakness. Patients may have early satiety or abdominal distension. The liver is usually enlarged, tender, and firm. An hepatic bruit may be heard in the RUQ. Patients may have intermittent fevers ●*Location:* Epigastrium and RUQ ●*Pattern:* Progressive symptoms without pattern ●*Precipitating factors:* None relevant ●*Relieving factors:* Ablation of tumor with cryotherapy, alcohol injection, or radiotherapy may palliate pain, but does not prolong survival. Chemotherapy is rarely helpful. Surgery may be curative if the tumor is less than 2cm in size (usually asymptomatic and picked up on screening) ●*Clinical course:* Progressive over months, nearly always fatal when symptomatic ●*Co-morbidities:* Cirrhosis of any cause - especially from hepatitis B and C, and hemochromatosis. Hepatitis B may lead to hepatoma even without cirrhosis ●*Procedure results:* Biopsy of the hepatic mass is definitive ●*Test findings:* Alpha-fetoprotein is often elevated (but not always); CT and MR show a hypervascular hepatic mass

Hepatomegaly ●*Onset:* Depends on etiology. Subacute if due to acute vascular congestion or infection. Insidious if due to infiltrative disease or chronic congestion ●*Male:female ratio:* M=F ●*Ethnicity:* All ●*Character:* Right upper quadrant (RUQ) pain and fullness. Other signs of liver failure such as easy bleeding, confusion, fatigue, jaundice ●*Location:* Pain is RUQ in location ●*Pattern:* Nonspecific ●*Precipitating factors:* Viral infection (hepatitis A, herpes simpex virus [HSV]), toxic ingestion or overdose (acetaminophen), ethanol abuse, hepatic vein thrombosis, right-sided heart failure ●*Relieving factors:* Resolution of infection, withdrawal of toxic agent, relief of vascular congestion ●*Clinical course:* Depends on etiology. Some infections are self-limited and some toxic injuries resolve. Tumor infiltration and vascular occlusion have a less optimistic prognosis ●*Co-morbidities:* None relevant ●*Procedure results:* Liver biopsy: varied, depends on etiology ●*Test findings:* Elevated transaminases, coagulopathy, hyperbilirubinemia, low albumin; abdominal ultrasound or CT: enlarged, congested liver

Hereditary hemorrhagic telangectasia ●*Onset:* Insidious with manifestations increasing with age ●*Male:female ratio:* M=F ●*Ethnicity:* All ●*Character:* Telangectasias and arteriovenous malformations leading to epistaxis, hemoptysis, dyspnea, fatigue, stroke, brain abscess, GI bleeding, seizures, subarachnoid and intracerebral bleeding ●*Location:* Telangectasias in lips, tongue, face, trunk, arms, nail beds. Nasal, pulmonary, cerebral, spinal, hepatic arteriovenous malformations ●*Pattern:* Recurrent episodes of bleeding ●*Precipitating factors:* Autosomal dominant inheritance ●*Relieving factors:* Percutaneous catheter embolization of arteriovenous malformations, laser therapy of telangectasias, estrogen plus progesterone therapy for arteriovenous malformations ●*Clinical course:* Epistaxis manifests in first two decades of life, followed by telangectasias in the fourth, and GI bleeding in the sixth. Pulmonary and cerebral arteriovenous malformations can occur at any time. Significant pulmonary arteriovenous malformations can lead to cyanosis, polycythemia, stroke secondary to right to left shunting ●*Co-morbidities:* Anemia, polycythemia, stroke ●*Procedure results:* High resolution CT, angiogram, magnetic resonance angiography (MRA): evidence of arteriovenous malformations. Skin biopsy: telangectasia ●*Test findings:* Orthodeoxia and low oxygen saturation on pulse oximetry and arterial blood gas

Hereditary neuropathy of liability to pressure palsies ●*Onset:* Acute, subacute ●*Male:female ratio:* M(2):F(1) ●*Ethnicity:* All ●*Character:* Peripheral neuropathy secondary to nerve damage or compression; gradual worsening over many years of nerve function ●*Location:* Common peroneal nerve most commonly affected, sensory and motor loss. ●*Pattern:* Sudden loss of function and sensation after compression injury leads to gradual and partial recovery over 8 to 12 weeks ●*Precipitating factors:* Pressure or injury to nerve ●*Relieving factors:* Avoidance of persistent pressure ●*Clinical course:* While recovery after each episode of compression injury is common and partial, accumulative damage occurs over time ●*Co-morbidities:* None relevant ●*Procedure results:* Genetic: autosomal dominant, changes occuring on chromosome 17 ●*Test findings:* No relevant tests

Hereditary spherocytosis ●*Onset:* Insidious ●*Male:female ratio:* M=F ●*Ethnicity:* Caucasians ●*Character:* Icterus, fatigue, possibly abdominal fullness due to splenomegaly ●*Location:* Nonspecific ●*Pattern:* Nonspecific ●*Precipitating factors:* Folate deficiency, infection ●*Relieving factors:* Folic acid, splenectomy ●*Clinical course:* Good prognosis after splenectomy; without treatment chronic hemolytic anemia ●*Co-morbidities:* Pigment gallstones ●*Procedure results:* No relevant procedures ●*Test findings:* Variable degrees of anemia, increased reticulocytes, mean corpuscular hemoglobin concentration (MCHC) and bilirubin, negative Coomb's test, spherocytes on blood smear, positive osmotic fragility test

Herpangina ●*Onset:* Acute ●*Male:female ratio:* M=F ●*Ethnicity:* All ●*Character:* Sudden onset of fever, sore throat, painful swallowing, tender oropharyngeal papules, vesicles with erythematous base ●*Location:* Oropharynx: soft palate, uvula, tonsils, posterior buccal mucosa, not gingiva (unlike herpes), lymph nodes, systemic (fever) ●*Pattern:* Lesions are papular, vesicular and involve the posterior oropharyngeal mucosa but not the gingiva ●*Precipitating factors:* Outbreaks ●*Relieving factors:* None relevant ●*Clinical course:* Acute onset, self-limiting, may last days-to-weeks ●*Co-morbidities:* None relevant ●*Procedure results:* No relevant procedures ●*Test findings:* No relevant tests

Herpes simplex ●*Onset:* Acute ●*Male:female ratio:* M=F ●*Ethnicity:* All ❶ *Character:* Pain, burning ❷ *Location:* Genitalia, labia, gingiva ❸ *Pattern:* Grouped vesicles on a red base ●*Precipitating factors:* Sun, stress, menstruation ●*Relieving factors:* Acyclovir ●*Clinical course:* Resolves over weeks, recurrent ●*Co-morbidities:* Erythema multiforme ●*Procedure results:* Giant cells on Tzanck preparation ●*Test findings:* Culture positive

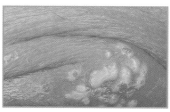

❶ *Character Multiple vesicular lesions of upper lid, characteristic of herpes simplex*

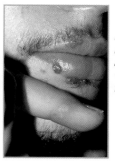

❷ *Location Vesicles on upper and lower lips, along with vesicle on finger*

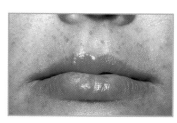

❸ *Pattern Grouped yellow vesicles on both upper and lower lips*

Herpes zoster, shingles ●*Onset:* Acute ●*Male:female ratio:* M=F ●*Ethnicity:* All ❶ *Character:* Pain: frequently severe ●*Location:* Any dermatome. Most common: thoracic, cervical, trigeminal, lumbosacral ❸ *Pattern:* Grouped vesicles red base, crusting, dermatomal distribution ●*Precipitating factors:* Immunosuppression, local nerve pressure ●*Relieving factors:* Acyclovir, prednisone, capsaicin ●*Clinical course:* Self-limited, weeks-to-months ●*Co-morbidities:* Malignancies ●*Procedure results:* Giant cells on Tzanck preparation ●*Test findings:* Culture positive

Images of ❶ *Character,* ❸ *Pattern* on page 513

Hiatal hernia ●*Onset:* Insidious ●*Male:female ratio:* M(1):F(2) ●*Ethnicity:* Western countries; uncommon in Africa and Asia ●*Character:* Usually asymptomatic. Heartburn (esophageal burning, substernal pain, sore taste, halitosis, cough). Can present with symptoms of chronic blood loss ●*Location:* Nonspecific ●*Pattern:* Symptoms tend to be worse at night or after a large meal ●*Precipitating factors:* Same as for heartburn: straining, bending or reclining; smoking; eating, especially prior to reclining; weight gain/obesity; certain foods such as mint, chocolate, citrus and fat ●*Relieving factors:* Antacids, acid-reducing medications, behavior modification, uncommonly surgery ●*Clinical course:*

Herpes zoster, shingles: Images *see text page 512*

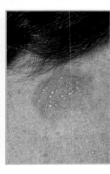

❶ *Character* Early lesion that shows an edematous plaque with vesicles

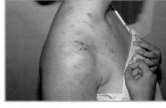

❸ *Pattern* Inflammatory papules and vesicles, covering several dermatomes across the shoulders

Chronic, benign condition ●*Co-morbidities:* Obesity, pregnancy ●*Procedure results:* Upper endoscopy: squamocolumnar junction and diaphragmatic indentation at disparate levels. Barium study: esophageal buldge above the diaphram. Evidence of heartburn such as esophagitis or Barrett's mucosa is occasionally seen ●*Test findings:* No relevant tests

Hidradenitis suppurativa ●*Onset:* Subacute ●*Male:female ratio:* M<F ●*Ethnicity:* All ●*Character:* Pain, skin drainage ❷ *Location:* Axilla, perineum, breasts, neck, scalp ●*Pattern:* Tender draining nodules sinus tracts, comedones ●*Precipitating factors:* None relevant ●*Relieving factors:* Antibiotics, intralesional steroids, surgical excision ●*Clinical course:* Persistent with exacerbations ●*Co-morbidities:* Acne; rarely, squamous cell cancer ●*Procedure results:* No relevant procedures ●*Test findings:* No relevant tests

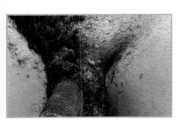

❷ *Location* This irregular scar is a typical remnant of an active lesion

Hip fracture ●*Onset:* Acute ●*Male:female ratio:* M=F ●*Ethnicity:* All ●*Character:* Following injury, pain in hip with any movement or weightbearing. Leg most commonly is shortened and externally rotated ●*Location:* Most common are femoral neck or intertrochanteric fractures ●*Pattern:* Nonspecific ●*Precipitating factors:* Mechanism of injury: fall onto hip or direct trauma ●*Relieving factors:* Analgesics, surgical repair ●*Clinical course:* Requires repair ●*Co-morbidities:* Most common in elderly ●*Procedure results:* No relevant procedures ●*Test findings:* Radiographs of hip are diagnostic. May be seen on MRI or bone scan if initial radiographs are normal

Hip injury ●*Onset:* Acute ●*Male:female ratio:* M=F ●*Ethnicity:* All ●*Character:* Pain on movement at hip joint or with weightbearing. In fractures, leg may be shortened, externally rotated. In posterior dislocations, leg is internally rotated ●*Location:* Nonspecific ●*Pattern:* Nonspecific ●*Precipitating factors:* Falls onto affected side. Motor vehicle accidents most common cause of dislocations ●*Relieving factors:* Fractures require operative repair. Dislocations require early reduction. Analgesics ●*Clinical course:* Some restriction in range of movement may persist after injury has healed ●*Co-morbidities:* Elderly most prone to hip fractures ●*Procedure results:* Radiographs required to diagnose fractures or dislocations. MRI or bone scan may be required to diagnose some nondisplaced fractures ●*Test findings:* No relevant tests

Hip synovitis ● *Onset:* Acute ● *Male:female ratio:* M=F ● *Ethnicity:* All ● *Character:* Sudden onset of limp and pain in the hip in a child ● *Location:* Hip ● *Pattern:* Often brief and intermittent episodes ● *Precipitating factors:* Possible viral etiology ● *Relieving factors:* Rest ● *Clinical course:* Spontaneous resolution within days is the norm ● *Co-morbidities:* None relevant ● *Procedure results:* Hip X-ray normal ● *Test findings:* CBC, ESR normal

Hirschsprung's disease ● *Onset:* Acute enterocolitis or chronic constipation ● *Male:female ratio:* M=F ● *Ethnicity:* All ● *Character:* Chronic constipation and failure to thrive. Enterocolitis: bilious emesis, diarrhea, fever, toxic ● *Location:* Anal sphincter with increased tone with empty rectal vault. Failure to pass meconium in first 24h of life ● *Pattern:* Chronic constipation ● *Precipitating factors:* None relevant ● *Relieving factors:* Laxatives may help temporarily ● *Clinical course:* Chronic unless treated ● *Co-morbidities:* Down syndrome ● *Procedure results:* Biopsy of anal mucosa reveals absence of ganglion cells ● *Test findings:* Anorectal manometry reveals decreased pressure

Histoplasmosis ● *Onset:* Acute, subacute, chronic ● *Male:female ratio:* M(4):F(1) ● *Ethnicity:* All ● *Character:* Acute pulmonary histoplasmosis: flu-like illness; chronic pulmonary histoplasmosis: fever, dry cough, hemoptysis, weight loss; disseminated histoplasmosis: fever, night sweats, weight loss, diffuse lymphadenopathy, other ● *Location:* Lungs, skin, oropharyngeal mucosa, liver, spleen, lymph nodes, bone marrow, pericardium, brain and CSF, GI tract, adrenal glands, heart valves, eye, other ● *Pattern:* Acute disease: acute flu-like illness with a dry cough; chronic pulmonary disease: gradual onset of fever with night sweats, weight loss, productive cough with occasional hemoptysis; disseminated disease: progressive fever, papular skin rash, oral ulcers, weight loss, generalized lymphadenopathy, enlarged liver and spleen ● *Precipitating factors:* Spelunking (cave exposure), exposure to bat and bird droppings in soil, residence in or travel to the midwestern, eastern, or central USA ● *Relieving factors:* None relevant ● *Clinical course:* Acute histoplasmosis is usually asymptomatic or mild, self-limiting within 1-2 weeks; rarely mediastinal fibrosis leads to restrictive lung disease. Chronic pulmonary histoplasmosis is progressive over months-to-years, and may be fatal if untreated; spontaneous recovery is less common. Disseminated histoplasmosis is progressive over weeks-to-months, may be fatal ● *Co-morbidities:* Erythema nodosum, erythema multiforme, AIDS ● *Procedure results:* Hilar adenopathy with or without infiltrates on chest X-ray in acute disease. Nodular infiltrates in the upper lobes, less commonly cavities on chest X-ray in chronic pulmonary disease. Hepatosplenomegaly on abdominal sonar or CT in disseminated disease ● *Test findings:* Only in disseminated disease: pancytopenia (leukopenia, anemia, thrombocytopenia), elevated alkaline phosphatase, hyperbilirubinemia, elevated ESR

Hodgkin's disease ● *Onset:* Usually insidious, can be subacute ● *Male:female ratio:* M(1.4):F(1) ● *Ethnicity:* More common in Caucasians and developed nations ● *Character:* Painless mass, fever, weight loss, drenching night sweats, pruritus ● *Location:* Mass is usually in the neck, pruritus is generalized ● *Pattern:* Nonspecific ● *Precipitating factors:* Pain in lymph nodes after drinking alcohol ● *Relieving factors:* Depends on stage: radiation, chemotherapy, autologous bone marrow transplant ● *Clinical course:* Stages IA-IIA: 10-year survival >80%; Stages IIIB, IV: 5-year survival 50-60% ● *Co-morbidities:* None relevant ● *Procedure results:* Lymph node biopsy finding typical cells ● *Test findings:* No relevant tests

Hordeolum, chalazion, blepharitis ● *Onset:* Acute, subacute ● *Male:female ratio:* M=F ● *Ethnicity:* All ❶ *Character:* Hordeolum and chalazion present as lid lump ❷ *Location:* Lids ● *Pattern:* Typically bilateral; worse in morning ● *Precipitating factors:* None relevant ● *Relieving factors:* Warms, compresses ● *Clinical course:* Usually not progressive ● *Co-morbidities:* None relevant ● *Procedure results:* Slit lamp examination of eyelid margins shows plugged meibomian glands ● *Test findings:* No relevant tests

Images of ❶ *Character,* ❷ *Location on page 515*

Hordeolum, chalazion, blepharitis: Images *see text page 514*

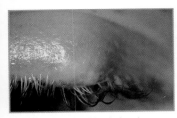

❶ *Character Internal hordeolum (common stye). Localized swelling is red and tender*

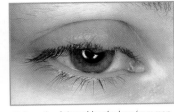

❷ *Location Internal hordeolum (common stye). Diffuse swelling involves most of the eyelid*

Horner's syndrome ● *Onset:* Acute, subacute ● *Male:female ratio:* M=F ● *Ethnicity:* All ● *Character:* Miosis, ptosis, anhydrosis ● *Location:* Eye ● *Pattern:* Nonspecific ● *Precipitating factors:* Cervical trauma, lung mass, brainstem stroke ● *Relieving factors:* Supportive care ● *Clinical course:* Variable ● *Co-morbidities:* Stroke, lung tumor, cervical trauma ● *Procedure results:* No relevant procedures ● *Test findings:* No relevant tests

Huntington's disease ● *Onset:* Insidious ● *Male:female ratio:* M=F ● *Ethnicity:* All ● *Character:* Involuntary choreoathetotic movements and dementia ● *Location:* Nonspecific ● *Pattern:* Nonspecific ● *Precipitating factors:* Autosomal dominant ● *Relieving factors:* Supportive care ● *Clinical course:* Progressive ● *Co-morbidities:* None relevant ● *Procedure results:* No relevant procedures ● *Test findings:* Genetic testing positive, MRI of the brain shows ventricular flattening of the caudate nuclei in established cases

Hurler's syndrome ● *Onset:* Insidious ● *Male:female ratio:* M=F ● *Ethnicity:* All ● *Character:* Facial dysmorphism ● *Location:* Face, bones, eyes ● *Pattern:* Nonspecific ● *Precipitating factors:* None relevant ● *Relieving factors:* Physical therapy ● *Clinical course:* Progressive ● *Co-morbidities:* Autosomal recessive ● *Procedure results:* No relevant procedures ● *Test findings:* Increased urinary excretion of dermatan and heparan sulfate

Hydrocele ● *Onset:* Subacute, acute ● *Male:female ratio:* M ● *Ethnicity:* All ● *Character:* Painless swelling ● *Location:* Scrotum, inguinal canal ● *Pattern:* Fluctuation in size with communicating hydrocele ● *Precipitating factors:* Infection, tumors, trauma, ipsilateral renal transplantation, peritoneal dialysis ● *Relieving factors:* Surgical correction, percutaneous aspiration ● *Clinical course:* Frequent resolution by age 1 with the infantile type; mostly progressive in all other age categories ● *Co-morbidities:* Ventriculoperitoneal shunt, extrophy of the bladder, Ehlers-Danlos syndrome ● *Procedure results:* High rate of recurrence with aspiration, high rate of success with surgical correction ● *Test findings:* Abdominal X-ray, scrotal U/S ruling out associated pathologies

Hydrocephalus ● *Onset:* Acute, insidious ● *Male:female ratio:* M=F ● *Ethnicity:* All ● *Character:* Enlargement of the head ● *Location:* CNS ● *Pattern:* Fontanelle bulging, setting sun eyes with downward displacement, spasticity, clonus, and increased DTRs, papilledema, headaches ● *Precipitating factors:* Obstruction within the ventricle system, or obliteration of subarachnoid cisterns, or abnormal villi secondary to tumor, infection, bleeding, or congenital development ● *Relieving factors:* Medical treatment with acetazolamide and furosemide initially, then permanent extracranial ventriculoperitoneal shunt ● *Clinical course:* Increased risk for infection. Children have variety of developmental disabilities with lower IQ, abnormal vision, social difficulties, and premature pubertal development ● *Co-morbidities:* Chiari and Dandy-Walker malformation, X-linked hydrocephalus, prematurity with hemorrhage or CNS infection, neurofibromatosis, and spina bifida ● *Procedure results:* Skin examination, abnormal increase in head size with positive 'cracked pot' or 'Macewen's sign', audible cranial bruit, abnormal optic exam with papilledema, CT, U/S, or MRI scan indicates hydrocephalus ● *Test findings:* No relevant tests

Hyperaldosteronism ●*Onset:* Gradual but hypertension may accelerate acutely ●*Male:female ratio:* M(1):F(2) ●*Ethnicity:* All ●*Character:* Headache, easy fatiguability, muscle weakness ●*Location:* Adrenal gland ●*Pattern:* Nonspecific ●*Precipitating factors:* Diuretics may exacerbate hypokalemia ●*Relieving factors:* Removal of adrenal adenoma, spironolactone, amiloride, triamterene; if glucocorticoid-remediable hyperaldosteronism, then glucocorticoid may treat ●*Clinical course:* Progressive ●*Co-morbidities:* Hypertension ●*Procedure results:* CT or MRI of adrenal may show solitary or multiple nodules; failure to suppress aldosterone with saline load; failure of renin to rise with prolonged upright posture ●*Test findings:* Suppressed renin, elevated aldosterone, hypokalemia

Hypercalcemia ●*Onset:* Insidious ●*Male:female ratio:* M=F ●*Ethnicity:* All ●*Character:* Fatigue, lethargy, confusion, nausea, constipation, renal stones leading to renal colic, polyuria ●*Location:* Nonspecific ●*Pattern:* Nonspecific ●*Precipitating factors:* Milk/alkali syndrome, hyperparathyroidism, vitamin D intoxication, malignancy, symptoms often precipitated by dehydration ●*Relieving factors:* Hydration, treatment of underlying cause, steroids, bisphosphonates ●*Clinical course:* Progressive ●*Co-morbidities:* For hyperparathyroidism as cause of MEN-1, malignancy ●*Procedure results:* No relevant procedures ●*Test findings:* High serum and urine calcium, elevated/nonsuppressed parathyroid hormone level for hyperparathyroidism, high 25-hydroxyvitamin D3 level for vitamin D intoxication, high 1,25-dihydroxyvitamin D3 for granulomatous disease

Hypercapnia ●*Onset:* Acute ●*Male:female ratio:* M=F ●*Ethnicity:* All ●*Character:* Elevated CO2 level ●*Location:* Nonspecific ●*Pattern:* Nonspecific ●*Precipitating factors:* Decrease in respiratory rate, decrease in tidal volume, administration of oxygen ●*Relieving factors:* None relevant ●*Clinical course:* Variable ●*Co-morbidities:* COPD, asthma ●*Procedure results:* No relevant procedures ●*Test findings:* Blood gas shows elevated PCO2

Hyperkalemia ●*Onset:* Insidious, acute ●*Male:female ratio:* M=F ●*Ethnicity:* All ●*Character:* Weakness ●*Location:* Nonspecific ●*Pattern:* Nonspecific ●*Precipitating factors:* Adrenal insufficiency, hypoaldosteronism, renal failure, potassium oversupplementation, converting enzyme inhibitors, spironolactone, hemolysis, acidosis, hyporenin-hyperaldosteronism, cyclosporin, heparin, nonsteriodal anti-inflammatory drugs ●*Relieving factors:* Relieving factors: calcium gluconate, potassium-binding resin, glucose and insulin temporarily move potassium into cells, loop diuretics, dialysis, treatment of underlying cause ●*Clinical course:* Progressive or self-limited, depending on cause ●*Co-morbidities:* Adrenal insufficiency, renal failure, hyporenin-hypoaldosteronism, acidosis ●*Procedure results:* Depends on etiology ●*Test findings:* Elevated plasma potassium, peaked T waves on EKG

Hypermetropia ●*Onset:* Insidious ●*Male:female ratio:* M=F ●*Ethnicity:* All ●*Character:* Inability for the eyes to focus on close objects, also known as far- or long-sightedness ●*Location:* Eyes ●*Pattern:* May be symmetric or asymmetric ●*Precipitating factors:* None relevant ●*Relieving factors:* Convex corrective lenses ●*Clinical course:* Typically worsens with age as progressive presbyopia with age decreases ability to accommodate ●*Co-morbidities:* None relevant ●*Procedure results:* No relevant procedures ●*Test findings:* Visual acuity exam demonstrates

Hypernatremia ●*Onset:* Insidious, acute ●*Male:female ratio:* M=F ●*Ethnicity:* All ●*Character:* Mental status change, somnolence, coma ●*Location:* CNS symptoms ●*Pattern:* Nonspecific ●*Precipitating factors:* Dehydration, baseline dementia or other factors limiting free water intake, diabetes insipidus, diabetes mellitus, lithium (nephrogenic diabetes insipidus) ●*Relieving factors:* Free water repletion with hypotonic or isotonic saline; treatment of diabetes insipidus if that is cause ●*Clinical course:* Progressive or maybe self-limited ●*Co-morbidities:* Dementia or being bed-ridden ●*Procedure results:* No relevant procedures ●*Test findings:* High serum sodium and osmolality

Hyperparathyroidism ●*Onset:* Insidious ●*Male:female ratio:* M=F ●*Ethnicity:* All ●*Character:* Fatigue, lethargy, confusion, nausea, constipation, renal stones leading to renal colic, polyuria, osteoporosis, and fractures ●*Location:* Nonspecific ●*Pattern:* Nonspecific ●*Precipitating factors:* Thiazides may worsen hypercalcemia ●*Relieving factors:* Hydration, parathyroidectomy ●*Clinical course:* Progressive ●*Co-morbidities:* Multiple endocrine neoplasia (MEN) 1, MEN 2A ●*Procedure results:* No relevant procedures ●*Test findings:* High serum and urine calcium, elevated/nonsuppressed parathyroid hormone level, high 1, 25 vitamin D

Hyperprolactinemia ●*Onset:* Subacute or insidious ●*Male:female ratio:* M<F ●*Ethnicity:* All ●*Character:* Galactorrhea; oligomenorrhea; infertility in a female; impotency in a male; headaches or visual changes if large pituitary adenoma ●*Location:* Milky breast discharge or headache or visual change ●*Pattern:* Nonspecific ●*Precipitating factors:* Pregnancy, Dopamine antagonist drugs such as phenothiazines, tricyclic antidepressants and metoclopromide, Pituitary tumor producing prolactin or other pituitary tumor compressing pituitary stalk, Renal failure, Breast stimulation ●*Relieving factors:* If drug induced ñ stop drug; other options dopamine agonists bromocriptine and carbegoline for prolactinoma or if other pituitary tumor causing stalk compression may need surgery. ●*Clinical course:* Stable or progressive or may remit depending on cause ●*Co-morbidities:* Pregnancy, lactation, renal failure, MEN-1, pituitary tumors ●*Procedure results:* MRI may show tumor ●*Test findings:* Elevated prolactin (rule out pregnancy)

Hypersomnia ●*Onset:* Usually gradual progression, from weeks to months ●*Male:female ratio:* M=F ●*Ethnicity:* All ●*Character:* Excessive sleepiness for at least a month, as evidenced by prolonged nighttime sleep episodes or daytime sleep episodes daily ●*Location:* Nonspecific ●*Pattern:* Nonspecific ●*Precipitating factors:* Depression, drug abuse ●*Relieving factors:* Stimulants (use may lead to addiction) ●*Clinical course:* Usually chronic ●*Co-morbidities:* Major depression, substance abuse disorders, psychosocial consequences of excessive sleepiness ●*Procedure results:* Supporting polysomnography ●*Test findings:* No relevant tests

Hypertensive retinopathy ●*Onset:* Acute, subacute or insidious ●*Male:female ratio:* M>F ●*Ethnicity:* More common in African Americans ●*Character:* Varies from no symptoms to blurred vision and headache ●*Location:* When blurred vision develops it is usually in both eyes ●*Pattern:* Hypertensive retinopathy manifests itself in the optic nerve, macula, the retinal vascular arcades, and choroid ●*Precipitating factors:* Generally no; occasionally symptomatic patients have accelerated hypertension secondary to acute renal failure, renal vascular disease, or other conditions ●*Relieving factors:* Lowering blood pressure gradually can reverse some retinal changes ●*Clinical course:* The condition progresses until the blood pressure is controlled ●*Co-morbidities:* There are many causes of arterial hypertension but essential hypertension is the most common ●*Procedure results:* Fundus exam and measurement of blood pressure ●*Test findings:* Retinal arteriolar narrowing; AV nicking; copper wiring; silver wiring; cotton wool spots; in acute cases there is retinal exudate and optic disc edema

Hyperthyroidism ●*Onset:* Insidious, acute ●*Male:female ratio:* M(1):F(10) ●*Ethnicity:* All ●*Character:* Palpitations, sweating, tremor, weight loss ●*Location:* Enlarged thyroid if not exogenous cause, exophthalmos in Graves' disease, brisk reflexes, tremor of outstretched hands ●*Pattern:* Nonspecific ●*Precipitating factors:* First trimester pregnancy (Graves' disease) and postpartum state (Graves' disease and hyperthyroid phase of postpartum thyroiditis) iodine load for hyperthyroidism associated with multinodular goiter ●*Relieving factors:* Antithyroid medication and beta blockade, permanent treatment radioactive iodine (RAI) or more rarely surgery ●*Clinical course:* Usually worsens but may spontaneously remit occasionally for Graves' disease; routinely for thyroiditis ●*Co-morbidities:* Eye diseases in Graves' disease, systolic hypertension, atrial tachyarrhthymias, bone loss, Graves' disease may be associated with polyglandular autoimmune syndrome ●*Procedure results:* Elevates 1-123 uptake for Graves' disease and sometimes with multinodular goiter; low for thyroiditis ●*Test findings:* Suppressed TSH, high T4 (and T3), TSI usually high in Graves' disease but not clinically indicated

Hyperventilation ●*Onset:* Acute or chronic ●*Male:female ratio:* M=F ●*Ethnicity:* All ●*Character:* Defined as condition when carbon dioxide ($PaCO_2$) level decreases below normal range. Usually see tachypnea and dyspnea, but not always; also dizziness, circumoral numbness, carpopedal spasm, and weakness ●*Location:* Nonspecific ●*Pattern:* Nonspecific ●*Precipitating factors:* Many causes: anxiety, hypoxia, pneumonia, pneumothorax, pulmonary embolus, pregnancy, salicylates, fever, pain, acidosis ●*Relieving factors:* Treat underlying cause: inhaling low concentration of carbon dioxide (breathing in paper bag or face mask) may relieve symptoms.; treat anxiety ●*Clinical course:* Resolves with treatment of underlying cause ●*Co-morbidities:* Lung disease, anxiety disorders ●*Procedure results:* No relevant procedures ●*Test findings:* Arterial blood gas will show respiratory alkalosis (high pH) and low $PaCO_2$; may also see metabolic acidosis as primary disorder (low pH)

Hyperviscosity syndrome ●*Onset:* Subacute ●*Male:female ratio:* M=F ●*Ethnicity:* All ●*Character:* Hemorrhage (bruising, mucosal bleeding), blurred vision, weakness, fatigue, headache, nystagmus, vertigo, confusion, shortness of breath, distended neck veins ●*Location:* Nonspecific ●*Pattern:* Nonspecific ●*Precipitating factors:* Plasma cell dyscrasias: macroglobulinemia, less commonly multiple myeloma ●*Relieving factors:* Plasmapheresis, systemic chemotherapy for the underlying disorder ●*Clinical course:* Poor prognosis without treatment, though plasmapheresis is only temporizing and the underlying disorders are difficult to cure ●*Co-morbidities:* None relevant ●*Procedure results:* Bone marrow biopsy consistent with macroglobulinemia or multiple myeloma; ocular exam: retinal hemorrhages, papilledema ●*Test findings:* Serum hyperviscosity (>4.0cP); elevated levels of IgM, plasmacytosis

Hypoalbuminemia ●*Onset:* Insidious ●*Male:female ratio:* M=F ●*Ethnicity:* All ●*Character:* Ascites (abdominal distension), peripheral edema ●*Location:* Nonspecific ●*Pattern:* Edema is in dependent areas ●*Precipitating factors:* Malnourishment, liver disease, protein-losing gastropathy, nephrotic syndrome, hypercatabolic state ●*Relieving factors:* Weight gain (sufficient protein in diet), improved hepatic function, resolution of nephropathy ●*Clinical course:* Poor prognosis when due to serious underlying or irreversible disease; otherwise, good prognosis with reversal of precipitant ●*Co-morbidities:* Congestive heart failure, systemic infections, advanced malignancy ●*Procedure results:* No relevant procedures ●*Test findings:* Low serum albumin (usually less than 3g/L), most commonly associated abnormalities are abnormal liver function or renal function

Hypocalcemia ●*Onset:* Insidious, acute ●*Male:female ratio:* M=F ●*Ethnicity:* All ●*Character:* Numbness, tingling, irritability, carpopedal spasm, tetany ●*Location:* Carpopedal spasm ●*Pattern:* Nonspecific ●*Precipitating factors:* Parathyroid surgery and hypoparathyroidism, vitamin D deficiency, magnesium deficiency (may be in setting of alcohol abuse), acute pancreatitis ●*Relieving factors:* Calcium repletion and/or vitamin D, magnesium repletion ●*Clinical course:* Progressive ●*Co-morbidities:* Hypoparathyroidism ●*Procedure results:* No relevant procedures ●*Test findings:* Low serum calcium, prolonged QTc on EKG

Hypochondriasis ●*Onset:* Can begin at any age, but typically early adulthood ●*Male:female ratio:* M(1):F(2) ●*Ethnicity:* All ●*Character:* Preoccupation with idea that one has a serious disease, based on misinterpretation of bodily symptoms ●*Location:* Nonspecific ●*Pattern:* Nonspecific ●*Precipitating factors:* Past experience with disease in family; medical disease in childhood; stressors, especially death of loved one ●*Relieving factors:* Reassurance and negative findings only briefly relieve ●*Clinical course:* Usually chronic; acute onset associated with better prognosis ●*Co-morbidities:* Iatrogenic complications from repeated diagnostic tests. Often real medical conditions are missed, because complaints are dismissed; depression; anxiety disorders ●*Procedure results:* No relevant procedures ●*Test findings:* Findings do not support individual's preoccupation

Hypokalemia ●*Onset:* Usually insidious ●*Male:female ratio:* M=F ●*Ethnicity:* All ●*Character:* Weakness, fatigue, myalgias, eventual paralysis ●*Location:* Nonspecific ●*Pattern:* Nonspecific ●*Precipitating factors:* Diuretics, diarrhea, renal potassium wasting (i.e. from amphotericin), primary hyperaldosteronism, Cushing's disease or syndrome, exogenous glucocorticoids ●*Relieving factors:* Potassium repletion ●*Clinical course:* Progressive ●*Co-morbidities:* Primary hyperaldosteronism, Liddle's syndrome, Bartter's syndrome, renal tubular acidosis, Cushing's disease or syndrome ●*Procedure results:* No relevant procedures ●*Test findings:* Low serum potassium

Hyponatremia ●*Onset:* Insidious, acute ●*Male:female ratio:* M=F ●*Ethnicity:* All ●*Character:* Mental status change, somnolence, seizure, coma ●*Location:* CNS symptoms ●*Pattern:* Nonspecific ●*Precipitating factors:* Free water overload, inappropriate antidiuretic secretion (malignancy, thiazides, chlorpropamide, CNS lesions, pulmonary disease), dehydration with free water replacement, hypoadrenalism, hypothyroidism, pain, hyperglycemia, and hypertriglyceridemia may also cause apparent hyponatremia ●*Relieving factors:* Free water restriction, hydration if dehydrated; occasionally medication (e.g. demeclocycline) ●*Clinical course:* Progressive, may be self-limited ●*Co-morbidities:* Hypothyroidism, hypoadrenalism, CNS, or pulmonary disease ●*Procedure results:* No relevant procedures ●*Test findings:* Low serum sodium and osmolality

Hypoparathyroidism ●*Onset:* Insidious but can be acute following parathyroid surgery ●*Male:female ratio:* M=F ●*Ethnicity:* All ●*Character:* Weakness, fatigue, numbness, carpopedal spasm ●*Location:* Nonspecific ●*Pattern:* Nonspecific ●*Precipitating factors:* Following parathyroid surgery ●*Relieving factors:* Calcium and vitamin D supplementation ●*Clinical course:* Progressive ●*Co-morbidities:* Polyglandular autoimmune syndrome ●*Procedure results:* No relevant procedures ●*Test findings:* Low serum calcium and low parathyroid hormone level

Hypopituitarism ●*Onset:* Insidious, acute ●*Male:female ratio:* M=F ●*Ethnicity:* All ●*Character:* Depends on which deficiencies predominate in a given patient; symptoms of cortisol insufficiency include fatigue, weight loss, loss of appetite, thyroid deficiency (fatigue, weight gain, delayed reflexes, cold intolerance); symptoms of gonadotropin insufficiency include secondary amenorrhea in women and impotence in men; no hyperpigmentation ●*Location:* Pituitary ●*Pattern:* Nonspecific ●*Precipitating factors:* Pituitary tumor, pituitary surgery, brain/pituitary irradiation, autoimmune, Sheehan's syndrome ●*Relieving factors:* Replacement of insufficient hormones ●*Clinical course:* Progressive ●*Co-morbidities:* Autoimmune, associated with polyglandular failure syndrome ●*Procedure results:* CT/MRI may show empty sella, enlarged pituitary, or tumor, or be normal ●*Test findings:* Low morning cortisol and adrenal corticotropic hormone, low thyroid profile and thyroid-stimulating hormone, low gonadotropins and estradiol/testosterone

Hypothermia ●*Onset:* Acute ●*Male:female ratio:* M=F ●*Ethnicity:* All ●*Character:* Temperature <35C (95F); hypotension, cardiac dysrhythmias, confusion, coma ●*Location:* Nonspecific ●*Pattern:* Nonspecific ●*Precipitating factors:* Environmental exposures most common; also hypoglycemia, hypothyroidism, ethanol use, sepsis ●*Relieving factors:* Resuscitate if required; passive rewarming in mild cases; active rewarming in more severe cases: warming blankets, warm water immersion, warmed humidified oxygen or IV fluids; peritoneal lavage or cardiopulmonary bypass for most severe cases ●*Clinical course:* Full recovery with appropriate treatment ●*Co-morbidities:* Ethanol or drug use, very young or elderly, debilitated patients most susceptible ●*Procedure results:* No relevant procedures ●*Test findings:* Osborn or J waves on EKG

Hypothyroidism ●*Onset:* Insidious ●*Male:female ratio:* M(1):F(5-10) ●*Ethnicity:* All ●*Character:* Fatigue, sluggishness, weight gain, dry skin, constipation ●*Location:* Enlarged symmetric thyroid, though may be normal size ●*Pattern:* Nonspecific ●*Precipitating factors:* Radioactive iodine, thyroid surgery, postpartum state, viral infection ●*Relieving factors:* Thyroid hormone replacement ●*Clinical course:* Progressive, though subacute thyroiditis and postpartum thyroiditis may spontaneously resolve ●*Co-morbidities:* Diastolic hypertension, hypercholesterolemia ●*Procedure results:* None indicated ●*Test findings:* Elevated TSH, low T4 (T3 not indicated), thyroid peroxidase antibodies elevated in Hashimoto's disease

Hypoxia ●*Onset:* Acute, insidious ●*Male:female ratio:* M=F ●*Ethnicity:* All ●*Character:* Dyspnea ●*Location:* Systemic ●*Pattern:* Cyanosis if > 5g/dL deoxyhemoglobin ●*Precipitating factors:* Cardiopulmonary disease ●*Relieving factors:* Supplemental oxygen ●*Clinical course:* Variable ●*Co-morbidities:* None relevant ●*Procedure results:* No relevant procedures ●*Test findings:* PaO_2 is decreased, alveolar-arterial O_2 difference is increased, and oxygen saturation is usually decreased

Idiopathic hypertrophic subaortic stenosis ●*Onset:* Acute, insidious ●*Male:female ratio:* M=F ●*Ethnicity:* All ●*Character:* Shortness of breath, chest pain, presyncope/syncope ●*Location:* Chest ●*Pattern:* Symptoms usually experienced with exertion ●*Precipitating factors:* Autosomal dominant inheritance, hypertension, exercise, volume depletion/dehydration, atherosclerosis ●*Relieving factors:* Beta-blockers, calcium channel blockers, disopyramide in patients with diastolic dysfunction; myomectomy or ethanol injection of septum in those with symptoms and inadequate response to medical therapy; amiodarone in those with atrial fibrillation; implantable cardioverter defibrillator in those at high risk for sudden death; antibiotic prophylaxis for dental and surgical procedures ●*Clinical course:* Can be asymptomatic to more symptomatic; symptoms tend to increase with age; sudden death not related to gradient.; sudden death increased with young age, history of syncope, family history of sudden death, certain genetic mutations, ventricular tachycardia (VT) on ambulatory monitoring, ischemia, marked left ventricular hypertrophy (LVH) ●*Co-morbidities:* Hypertension, Wolff-Parkinson-White syndrome, atrial fibrillation, VT ●*Procedure results:* Myocardial biopsy with hypertrophy, myocardial fiber disarray, fibrosis; echo with or without asymmetric hypertrophy, with or without increased intraventricular gradient, abnormal systolic anterior motion of the anterior mitral leaflet, diastolic dysfunction, with or without systolic dysfunction ●*Test findings:* In patients with gradient, examination with harsh, crescendo-decrescendo midsystolic murmur, loudest between the left sternal border and apex, which is increased by Valsalva and standing and decreased by squatting, passive leg raising, etc; + S4; triple-apical impulse, brisk carotid upstroke with bifid pulse; narrow vs paradoxically split S2; ECG with LVH, Q waves in inferior and precordial leads, giant negative T waves in mid-precordial leads; chest X-ray with cardiomegaly

Idiopathic myelofibrosis ●*Onset:* Insidious ●*Male:female ratio:* M=F ●*Ethnicity:* All ●*Character:* Severe fatigue, fever, night sweats, weight loss, left upper quadrant fullness (due to splenomegaly), ascites (due to hepatomegaly) ●*Location:* Pain is generally in the left upper quadrant and sometimes in the left shoulder ●*Pattern:* Nonspecific ●*Precipitating factors:* None relevant ●*Relieving factors:* Allogeneic bone marrow transplantation is potentially curative, splenectomy in some cases if severe complications; radiation therapy, androgens, chemotherapy or anagrelide as palliative options ●*Clinical course:* If poor prognostic factors (e.g. severe anemia, constitutional symptoms, advanced age) median survival is <5 yrs, without these risk factors it can be 15 yrs ●*Co-morbidities:* Essential polycythemia transforms into myelofibrosis in 5%, polycythemia vera in 10-20% ●*Procedure results:* Bone marrow biopsy: extensive fibrosis and osteosclerosis; bone marrow aspirate: 'dry tap' ●*Test findings:* Anemia; high or low platelet and WBC counts; peripheral blood smear with teardrop and nucleated RBCs and early WBC forms; increases in LDH, alkaline phosphatase, uric acid, and vitamin B12

Idiopathic pulmonary interstitial fibrosis ●*Onset:* Insidious ●*Male:female ratio:* M=F ●*Ethnicity:* All ●*Character:* Dyspnea, especially with exertion ●*Location:* Chest ●*Pattern:* Bilateral inspiratory rales, clubbing; signs of cor pulmonale late in course of disease ●*Precipitating factors:* None relevant ●*Relieving factors:* Corticosteroids (with or without azathioprine if incomplete response to steroids), supplemental oxygen, pulmonary rehabilitation; consider lung transplantation ●*Clinical course:* Usually progressive ●*Co-morbidities:* Pneumoconiosis, sarcoidosis, chronic hypersensitivity, drug reaction, radiation therapy, connective tissue disease, eosinophillic granuloma ●*Procedure results:* Lung biopsy reveals usual, desquamative, or nonspecific interstitial pneumonitis ●*Test findings:* Pulmonary function tests: restrictive ventilatory defect with decreased diffusion capacity for carbon monoxide (DLCO); hypoxemia; chest X-ray and high resolution computed tomography: increased interstitial markings progresses to fibrotic changes with honeycombing

Idiopathic thrombocythemia ●*Onset:* Acute ●*Male:female ratio:* M=F ●*Ethnicity:* All ●*Character:* Easy bruising, petechial rash, mucosal bleeding ●*Location:* Nonspecific ●*Pattern:* Follows recovery from a viral illness ●*Precipitating factors:* Viral illness, including EBV and CMV, toxoplasmosis ●*Relieving factors:* Self-limited ●*Clinical course:* Majority resolve spontaneously in weeks to months ●*Co-morbidities:* None relevant ●*Procedure results:* Bone marrow biopsy: evidence of increased platelet production ●*Test findings:* Thrombocytopenia, large thrombocytes, and if recent bleeding: mild normocytic anemia

Idiopathic thrombocytopenic purpura ●*Onset:* Usually insidious though can be acute ●*Male:female ratio:* M=F (acute); 1(M):3(F) (chronic) ●*Ethnicity:* All ●*Character:* Easy bruising, menometrorrhagia, epistaxis, hematuria, petechial rash ●*Location:* Systemic ●*Pattern:* Nonspecific ●*Precipitating factors:* No recognizable precipitant (in contrast to other causes of thrombocytopenia) ●*Relieving factors:* No specific therapy unless bleeding or very low platelet count, glucocorticoids, IVIG in severe cases, splenectomy ●*Clinical course:* Weeks-years ●*Co-morbidities:* Typically none ●*Procedure results:* Bone marrow biopsy - evidence of increased platelet production ●*Test findings:* Thrombocytopenia, large thrombocytes, and if recent bleeding - mild normocytic anemia

Iliac apophysitis ●*Onset:* Acute ●*Male:female ratio:* M=F ●*Ethnicity:* All ●*Character:* Localized pain and swelling, can be dull, decreased range of movement, muscle weakness ●*Location:* Near hip, over iliac crest ●*Pattern:* None ●*Precipitating factors:* Repetitive activity, such as long distance running, dancing; sudden forceful muscle traction ●*Relieving factors:* Rest, ice, compression, elevation, NSAIDs, relaxation of involved tendons by local heat or ultrasound ●*Clinical course:* Variable ●*Co-morbidities:* None ●*Procedure results:* None relevant ●*Test findings:* X-ray to rule out other diagnoses such as fracture

Immunodeficiency diseases ●*Onset:* Subacute ●*Male:female ratio:* M>F ●*Ethnicity:* All ●*Character:* Cough, purulent sputum, dyspnea ●*Location:* Chest, sinus, infertility in select disorders ●*Pattern:* Recurrent sinopulmonary infections with sinus tenderness and congestion; inspiratory rales, expiratory rhonchi ●*Precipitating factors:* None relevant ●*Relieving factors:* If recurrent infections and deficient humoral immunity (i.e. decreased IgA, IgG2, IgG4) supplemental gammaglobulin; otherwise, antibiotics as indicated, chest physiotherapy, postural drainage, exercise to improve pulmonary toilet; sinus drainage (decongestants, surgery in severe disease), lavage with saline ●*Clinical course:* Slowly progressive over months to years, exacerbations last days to weeks ●*Co-morbidities:* Male or female infertility secondary to immotile cilia ●*Procedure results:* Cilia biopsy may reveal structural abnormality by electron microscopy ●*Test findings:* Deficient immunoglobulin levels (IgA, IgG2, IgG4)

Impacted cerumen ●*Onset:* Insidious ●*Male:female ratio:* M=F ●*Ethnicity:* All ●*Character:* Decreased hearing; ear blockage ●*Location:* Affected ear; may be bilateral ●*Pattern:* Persistent blockage ●*Precipitating factors:* Manipulation with Q-tip ●*Relieving factors:* None relevant ●*Clinical course:* Usually recurrent accumulation of wax requiring cleaning ●*Co-morbidities:* None relevant ●*Procedure results:* Wax seen to include canal on otoscopy ●*Test findings:* No relevant tests

Imperforate anus ●*Onset:* Acute/at birth ●*Male:female ratio:* M=F ●*Ethnicity:* All ●*Character:* Blind rectum found approximately 2cm above perineal skin; meconium in vagina/rugal folds of scrotum ●*Location:* Perineal/rectal area ●*Pattern:* Nonspecific ●*Precipitating factors:* Abnormal prenatal development ●*Relieving factors:* Colostomy, surgical repair ●*Clinical course:* Corrected after surgical treatment ●*Co-morbidities:* Down syndrome, esophageal atresia, VATER syndrome, rectovaginal fistula ●*Procedure results:* Abnormal physical exam; meconium particles in urine with high imperforate anus ●*Test findings:* High imperforate anus: abnormal cystogram/ultrasound

Impetigo ●*Onset:* Acute ●*Male:female ratio:* M=F ●*Ethnicity:* All ❶ *Character:* Skin burning, itching, slight pain ❷ *Location:* Face, extremities ❸ *Pattern:* Extending honey-colored crusts, occasional bullae ●*Precipitating factors:* Skin breakdown, poor hygiene ●*Relieving factors:* Antibiotics ●*Clinical course:* Resolves in weeks, may recur ●*Co-morbidities:* Eczema ●*Procedure results:* No relevant procedures ●*Test findings:* Skin culture

Images of ❶ *Character,* ❷ *Location,* ❸ *Pattern on page 523*

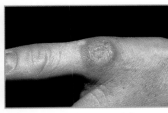

❶ *Character* A solitary crusted plaque

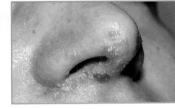

❷ *Location* Impetigo nares, yellow crust, pinkness and scale about the nose

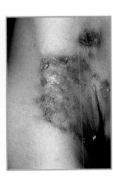

❸ *Pattern* Impetigo is common in the flexures. Crusting and erosions shown

Impingement syndrome ●*Onset:* Subacute ●*Male:female ratio:* M=F ●*Ethnicity:* All ●*Character:* Dull ache ●*Location:* Affected shoulder, upper arm ●*Pattern:* Worse with activity ●*Precipitating factors:* Activity above head ●*Relieving factors:* NSAIDs, corticosteroid injection, physical therapy ●*Clinical course:* Chronic if not treated ●*Co-morbidities:* None ●*Procedure results:* MRI shows degeneration of rotator cuff ●*Test findings:* No relevant tests

Inappropriate secretion of antidiuretic hormone ●*Onset:* Insidious ●*Male:female ratio:* M=F ●*Ethnicity:* All ●*Character:* Polydipsia ●*Location:* Fluid overload without edema ●*Pattern:* Irritability, lethargy, and possible seizures ●*Precipitating factors:* Water intoxication ●*Relieving factors:* Fluid restriction ●*Clinical course:* Dependent on etiology ●*Co-morbidities:* Brain tumor, pulmonary disease ●*Procedure results:* Head MRI to assess CNS pathology ●*Test findings:* Low serum sodium and osmolality with elevated urine sodium and osmolality

Incarcerated hernia ●*Onset:* Acute ●*Male:female ratio:* M(9):F(1) inguinal, M(1):F(3) femoral, variable depending on hernia type ●*Ethnicity:* African-Americans>white (3:1) for groin hernias ●*Character:* Painful, palpable, nonreducible ●*Location:* Groin or abdomen ●*Pattern:* Palpable nonreducible mass apparent when relaxed and supine ●*Precipitating factors:* Chronic cough, obesity, malnutrition, smoking, steroid use, prior surgery, increased abdominal pressure ●*Relieving factors:* Noninvasive manual reduction, surgical reduction ●*Clinical course:* May lead to strangulation and necrosis ●*Co-morbidities:* Prostatism, obesity, chronic cough, colon cancer, hepatomegaly.acites ●*Procedure results:* None relevant ●*Test findings:* CT abdomen or ultrasound showing incarceration, small bowel obstruction, or ischemia

Indirect neonatal hyperbilirubinemia ●*Onset:* Acute ●*Male:female ratio:* M=F ●*Ethnicity:* All ●*Character:* Jaundice ●*Location:* Eyes, skin ●*Pattern:* Jaundice beyond 2 weeks ●*Precipitating factors:* Hemolysis, hereditary glucuronyl transferase deficiency, breast milk, hypothyroidism, pyloric stenosis ●*Relieving factors:* Treatment of underlying disease process, feeding frequently and IV fluids, phototherapy, exchange transfusion ●*Clinical course:* Variable ●*Co-morbidities:* Isoimmunization with hemolysis, abnormal RBC morphology, Gilbert syndrome, G6PD deficiency, hypothyroidism, Crigler-Najjar syndrome, breast feeding, infection ●*Procedure results:* No relevant procedures ●*Test findings:* Elevated indirect or unconjugated bilirubin > than 2 weeks with a normal direct bilirubin, elevated reticulocyte count, Coombs' positive and low hemoglobin with hemolysis on smear; viral studies for hepatitis A, B, C and CMV and other infectious disease; metabolic screen

Infectious myringitis ●*Onset:* Acute ●*Male:female ratio:* M=F ●*Ethnicity:* All ●*Character:* Moderate to severe ear pain with or without hearing loss ●*Location:* Affected ear ●*Pattern:* Persistent pain ●*Precipitating factors:* None relevant ●*Relieving factors:* None relevant ●*Clinical course:* May be self-limited ●*Co-morbidities:* None relevant ●*Procedure results:* Otoscopy reveals inflamed tympanic membrane, possibly with granulation tissue ●*Test findings:* No relevant tests

Infective endocarditis ●*Onset:* Acute, subacute ●*Male:female ratio:* M>F (slightly) ●*Ethnicity:* All ●*Character:* Gradual onset of fever, fatigue, and anorexia without localizing symptoms, in patient with heart murmur ●*Location:* Systemic (fever), heart valves, valve rings, heart muscle, small blood vessels, skin, eye retina and subconjunctiva, kidney, joints, brain, spleen, other ●*Pattern:* Roth's spots (oval retinal hemorrhages with pale center), splinter hemorrhages (linear ungual dark streaks), Ostler nodes (small, painful nodules on finger/toe pads), Janeway lesions (painless nodular hemorrhages on palms and soles), polyarticular arthralgia, clubbing, progressive anorexia and weight loss, embolic events (bowel ischemia, pulmonary emboli in injection drug users, splenic infarct, renal infarct) ●*Precipitating factors:* Prosthetic heart valve, valvular heart disease, congenital heart disease, injection drug use, dental care, invasive medical procedure ●*Relieving factors:* None relevant ●*Clinical course:* Acute or gradual onset, progressive over days-to-months, fatal if untreated ●*Co-morbidities:* Valvular heart disease, congenital heart disease, prosthetic heart valve, injection drug use, stroke, renal failure, pulmonary emboli, pulmonary abscesses, endophthalmitis ●*Procedure results:* Vegetation, valve ring abscess, myocardial abscess, or dehiscence of prosthetic valve seen on Echo, multiple septic emboli/abscesses on chest X-ray, mycotic aneurysm/embolic cardiovascular accident (CVA) on contrast CT or MRI/magnetic resonance angiography (MRA) of head, splenic infarct on abdominal CT, isolation of organism from two blood cultures ●*Test findings:* High-grade bacteremia (persistently positive blood cultures), normocytic normochromic anemia, elevated ESR, microscopic hematuria, proteinuria, normal to elevated WBC

Influenza ●*Onset:* Acute ●*Male:female ratio:* M=F ●*Ethnicity:* All ●*Character:* Abrupt onset of systemic (fever, chills, myalgia, headache) followed by respiratory symptoms ●*Location:* Systemic (blood), upper respiratory (nasopharynx), muscles, head, joints (arthralgia) - common; less common: lungs, heart muscle, CNS, other ●*Pattern:* Rapid temperature rise in the first 24h with slow defervescence over several days, respiratory symptoms increase as fever trending down ●*Precipitating factors:* Annual outbreaks, sick contacts, chronic care facilities, winter months ●*Relieving factors:* Rest, acetaminophen ●*Clinical course:* Self-limiting ●*Co-morbidities:* Reye's syndrome, Guillain-Barré syndrome, bacterial pneumonia (pneumococcus, staphylococcus) ●*Procedure results:* Detection by rapid testing or isolation of virus from throat swabs, nasopharyngeal washes; interstitial pneumonitis on chest X-ray (uncommon) ●*Test findings:* Low, normal, or mildly elevated leukocyte count, elevated creatine phosphokinase (CPK)

Ingrown nail ●*Onset:* Subacute ●*Male:female ratio:* M=F ●*Ethnicity:* All ❶*Character:*

Pain ●*Location:* Toe ●*Pattern:* Redness, toe swelling, may have purulent discharge ●*Precipitating factors:* Trauma, onychomycosis ●*Relieving factors:* Soaks, surgery, antibiotics ●*Clinical course:* Remissions, exacerbations ●*Co-morbidities:* Onychomycosis ●*Procedure results:* No relevant procedures ●*Test findings:* No relevant tests

Inguinal hernia ●*Onset:* Insidious ●*Male:female ratio:* M=F ●*Ethnicity:* All ●*Character:*

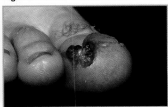

❶ *Character* *The lateral edge of the nail digs into the skin*

Often presents as a mass in the inguinal area that appears with increased intra-abdominal pressure (standing, straining); often uncomfortable, but may become painful if incarcerated; in strangulation - irreducible swelling in the groin, more severe pain, and signs of bowel obstruction may be seen ●*Location:* Left or right groin ●*Pattern:* Uncomfortable throughout the day, with relief when lying supine at night ●*Precipitating factors:* Straining the abdominal muscles ●*Relieving factors:* Lying supine, reducing the hernia manually ●*Clinical course:* Waxing and waning symptoms - if incarcerated, pain worsens, hernia may not reduce; strangulation is much more severe, with accompanying bowel obstruction ●*Co-morbidities:* None relevant ●*Procedure results:* Usually diagnosed clinically, but may be seen on U/S or CT scan ●*Test findings:* No relevant tests

Insect and spider bites and stings ●*Onset:* Acute ●*Male:female ratio:* M=F ●*Ethnicity:* All ●*Character:* Bee stings: anaphylaxis, airway edema; black widow spider: muscle pain, abdominal cramping, diaphoresis, hypertension; brown recluse spider: local tissue necrosis; tick bites: Lyme disease, paralysis ●*Location:* Bite location and systemic ●*Pattern:* Nonspecific ●*Precipitating factors:* Exposure to biting or stinging insects ●*Relieving factors:* Local wound care, antibiotics for brown recluse spider bites; narcotics, benzodiazepines, antivenin for black widow spider bites; ice, antihistamines for bee stings ●*Clinical course:* Variable ●*Co-morbidities:* None relevant ●*Procedure results:* No relevant procedures ●*Test findings:* Lyme test if suspected after tick bites

Insomnia ●*Onset:* Onset usually sudden, at time of psychological, social, or medical stress ●*Male:female ratio:* M=F ●*Ethnicity:* All ●*Character:* Difficulty initiating or maintaining sleep, or persistent experience of nonrestorative sleep, lasting at least a month ●*Location:* Nonspecific ●*Pattern:* Worsens with age ●*Precipitating factors:* Onset usually at time of psychological/social/medical stress, but perpetuating factors include negative associations and increased arousal ●*Relieving factors:* 'Sleep hygiene' education; use of sedatives may lead to dependancy and tolerance ●*Clinical course:* Young adults experience more difficulty falling asleep; with age, more problems maintaining sleep ●*Co-morbidities:* Increased incidence of stress-related psychophysiologic problems (e.g. tension headaches) ●*Procedure results:* Supporting polysomnography ●*Test findings:* High arousal in psychophysiologic tests

Insulinoma ●*Onset:* Insidious ●*Male:female ratio:* M(3):F(2) ●*Ethnicity:* All ●*Character:* Headache, slurred speech, confusion, coma, psychiatric alteration, tremulousness, diaphoresis, pallor, irritability ●*Location:* Nonspecific ●*Pattern:* Nonspecific ●*Precipitating factors:* Prolonged fasting ●*Relieving factors:* Oral intake, glucose, diazoxide, beta-blockers, octreotide, chemotherapy ●*Clinical course:* Variable ●*Co-morbidities:* MEN1 - multiple endocrine neoplasia type 1 (pituitary adenomas, islet cell tumors of pancreas, parathyroid tumors) ●*Procedure results:* Angiography - tumor flush ●*Test findings:* CT scan finding pancreatic mass, increased insulin C-peptide, hypoglycemia

Interdigital neuroma ●*Onset:* Adult ●*Male:female ratio:* M=F ●*Ethnicity:* All ●*Character:* Burning pain and cramping in third and fourth toes ●*Location:* Compression and irritation of branches of medial and lateral plantar nerves in fibro-osseous ring formed by metatarsal heads and deep transverse intermetatarsal ligaments ●*Pattern:* Chronic compression leading to neuroma formation ●*Precipitating factors:* Wearing closed tight-toed, high-heeled shoes; walking on hard surfaces ●*Relieving factors:* Wider shoes, metatarsal bar, soft insoles, orthotic devices, NSAIDs, local anesthetic/steroid injection; surgical excision ●*Clinical course:* Continued pain unless treated ●*Co-morbidities:* None relevant ●*Procedure results:* If needed, MRI most useful imaging study ●*Test findings:* Clinical exam most useful for diagnosis: tenderness in plantar aspect of distal foot over third and fourth metatarsals, compression of metatarsal heads together reproduces burning distally

Intestinal fistula ●*Onset:* Insidious ●*Male:female ratio:* M<F ●*Ethnicity:* For Crohn's disease: Middle European (Jewish) ●*Character:* Dependent on the site of fistula tract: cutaneous, vaginal, or urinary drainage of fecal material, diarrhea if bacterial overgrowth or small bowel to colon fistula ●*Location:* Dependent on site of fistula; commonly perianal in Crohn's disease ●*Pattern:* Nonspecific ●*Precipitating factors:* Intestinal inflammation precipitates fistula (Crohn's disease, diverticulitis, radiation injury) ●*Relieving factors:* Antibiotics, treatment of Crohn's disease (Infliximab for refractory fistulas), Seton placement in fistula tract, surgery ●*Clinical course:* In Crohn's, fistulas tend to be recurrent. Fistulas resulting from acute inflammatory process may be self-limited with treatment ●*Co-morbidities:* Crohn's, diverticulitis, radiation enteritis ●*Procedure results:* Fistulogram (contrast injected into fistula tract) ●*Test findings:* Elevated WBC if infection, if bacterial overgrowth, signs of malabsorption (low albumin, Ca, high PT), imaging contrast outling fistula tract

Intestinal obstruction ●*Onset:* Acute ●*Male:female ratio:* M=F ●*Ethnicity:* All ●*Character:* Episodes of crampy mid to lower abdominal pain that last 2-5 min, followed by short periods without pain. In proximal obstructions, episodes come every 4-5 min, with distal obstructions, every 10-15 min. Often accompanied by vomiting and abdominal distension; if pain becomes continuous, strangulation of bowel is a concern ●*Location:* Small bowel mid-abdomen; large bowel lower abdomen ●*Pattern:* Nonspecific ●*Precipitating factors:* None relevant ●*Relieving factors:* Patient needs to be nil by mouth with IV fluid replacement; a nasogastric tube is indicated to decrease intestinal distension; if obstruction is complete, surgical correction should be considered early; if partial obstruction, conservative therapy may be successful ●*Clinical course:* Progresses over hours to days; not typically self-limited ●*Co-morbidities:* Hernia; inflammatory diseases of the bowel (irritable bowel disease [IBD], diverticulitis); intussusception; intestinal masses; postoperative adhesions; volvulus; fecal impaction ●*Procedure results:* Imaging studies: upright abdominal X-ray or CT scan reveals the dilated bowel loops and may show the point of obstruction ●*Test findings:* Nonspecific: electrolyte panel may show signs of hypovolemia or dehydration

Intestinal parasites ●*Onset:* Subacute - common; acute and chronic - less common ●*Male:female ratio:* M=F ●*Ethnicity:* All ●*Character:* Diarrhea and abdominal pain lasting longer than one week, stool usually watery or loose, bowel obstruction - rare ●*Location:* Colon and small intestines - common, stomach and esophagus - less common, extraintestinal - less common (liver, lungs, CNS, muscles, other) ●*Pattern:* 1-2 weeks delay between exposure and symptoms ●*Precipitating factors:* Travel to/immigration from/residence in endemic areas (tropical, subtropical more common); drinking untreated water; eating undercooked fish, meat, or raw vegetables; pica in children ●*Relieving factors:* Hydration ●*Clinical course:* Incubation >1-2 weeks, prolonged diarrhea; self-limited in some, chronic, leading to malnutrition in others ●*Co-morbidities:* Anemia, iron deficiency, hypogammaglobulinemia, intussusception, bowel perforation, eosinophilic pneumonitis (Loeffler's syndrome), jaundice ●*Procedure results:* Ova, larvae, oocysts, cysts, trophozoites in direct wet mount form, or concentrated, or stained fresh stool, rarely material from string (duodenal sample) or 'scotch tape' (anus) tests; specific serology ●*Test findings:* Eosinophilia (common), elevated IgE (less common), positive stool for ova and parasites, positive serological tests

Intestinal perforation ●*Onset:* Acute, sometimes subacute ●*Male:female ratio:* M=F ●*Ethnicity:* All ●*Character:* Severe abdominal pain with peritoneal signs, fever, abdominal distention ●*Location:* Pain is diffuse ●*Pattern:* Depends on etiology ●*Precipitating factors:* Depends on etiology ●*Relieving factors:* Surgery, antibiotics, nasogastric suction ●*Clinical course:* Often fatal if not treated promptly, good outcome if surgically corrected ●*Co-morbidities:* Peptic ulcer disease, diverticulitis, intestinal ischemia, enteric infection, inflammatory bowel disease ●*Procedure results:* No relevant procedures ●*Test findings:* Abdominal film or CT scan - free air; contrast radiography - extravasation of contrast; elevated WBC, acidosis

Intracavernous carotid artery aneurysm ●*Onset:* Insidious ●*Male:female ratio:* M=F ●*Ethnicity:* All ●*Character:* Dilatation of the carotid artery ●*Location:* Aneurysm within the cavernous sinus, posterior to the superior orbital fissure ●*Pattern:* Pattern variable depending whether some or all nerves in cavernous sinus compressed by aneurysm; vertical diplopia: IV cranial nerve; horizontal diplopia, esotropia: VI cranial nerve; pain or numbness V cranial nerve ophthalmic branch; Horner syndrome oculosympathetic fibers ●*Precipitating factors:* Hereditary syndromes associated with intracranial aneurysms: Ehlers-Danlos, pseudoxanthoma elasticum, autosomal dominant polycystic kidney disease, familial aldosteronism type 1, and familial aneurysms, cigarette smoking, hypertension, estrogen deficiency, moderate to high alcohol intake ●*Relieving factors:* Surgical correction of aneurysm ●*Clinical course:* Progression to rupture in 5-10 years following onset of symptoms if not surgically corrected ●*Co-morbidities:* None relevant ●*Procedure results:* MR angiography capable of detection aneurysms 3-5mm; cerebral angiography required for definitive diagnosis ●*Test findings:* No relevant tests

Intracranial hemorrhage ●*Onset:* Acute ●*Male:female ratio:* M=F ●*Ethnicity:* All ●*Character:* Severe headache ●*Location:* Head, neck ●*Pattern:* Nonspecific ●*Precipitating factors:* Hypertension, AVM, aneurysm, trauma ●*Relieving factors:* Supportive care, management of increased intracranial pressure, surgical intervention ●*Clinical course:* Variable ●*Co-morbidities:* Hypertension, AVM, aneurysm, trauma ●*Procedure results:* No relevant procedures ●*Test findings:* MRI/MRA of the brain

Intraductal papilloma ●*Onset:* Insidious ●*Male:female ratio:* M<F ●*Ethnicity:* All ●*Character:* Bloody nipple discharge ●*Location:* Nipple ●*Pattern:* Nonspecific ●*Precipitating factors:* None relevant ●*Relieving factors:* Surgical excision ●*Clinical course:* Full recovery possible with treatment ●*Co-morbidities:* None relevant ●*Procedure results:* Mass of ductogram; normal mammogram ●*Test findings:* Intraductal papilloma on biopsy

Intrauterine growth retardation ●*Onset:* Insidious ●*Male:female ratio:* F ●*Ethnicity:* All ●*Character:* Ultrasound finding of poor fetal growth ●*Location:* Fetus ●*Pattern:* Nonspecific ●*Precipitating factors:* None relevant ●*Relieving factors:* Delivery ●*Clinical course:* Gradually worsens over the pregnancy ●*Co-morbidities:* Hypertension; diabetes; autoimmune disorders; TORCH infection ●*Procedure results:* No relevant procedures ●*Test findings:* Ultrasound demonstrating poor fetal growth

Intussusception ●*Onset:* Acute ●*Male:female ratio:* M(3):F(2) ●*Ethnicity:* All ●*Character:* Episodes of abdominal pain and distension, often with bloody stools; between episodes, patients feel generally well; abdominal exam during pain reveals abdominal distension and may reveal a firm mass at the site of obstruction ●*Location:* Small bowel intussusception - mid abdomen; large bowel intussusception - lower abdomen ●*Pattern:* Intermittent episodes with no distinct pattern ●*Precipitating factors:* None relevant ●*Relieving factors:* Each episode may resolve spontaneously, but surgical correction is curative ●*Clinical course:* Episodes occur intermittently, but the disorder is not self-limited ●*Co-morbidities:* Small and large bowel tumors (in children, usually benign - in adults, usually malignant); postoperative adhesions ●*Procedure results:* Barium studies and CT scan may reveal the intussusception, but laparotomy is definitive ●*Test findings:* No relevant tests

Iodine deficiency ● *Onset:* Subacute (days-months) to insiduous (may take years to manifest symptoms) ● *Male:female ratio:* M=F ● *Ethnicity:* All; poor socioeconomic status is principal risk factor ● *Character:* Goiter (palpably enlarged thyroid); mental retardation and cretinism (in neonates), reproductive failure can also occur ● *Location:* Thyroid; secondary effects on CNS ● *Pattern:* Diffuse goiter initially, may then become nodular; upregulation of TSH receptors, and TSH-independent thyroid hormone secretion may ensue; hyperthyroidism can be seen with iodine repletion or dye load ● *Precipitating factors:* Endemic regions; usually more inland and mountainous; poverty, other nutritional deficiencies increase risk ● *Relieving factors:* Improved diet (150mcg/d requirement in adult; 200mcg/d in pregnant or lactating female). iodization of salt; iodized water, oil, or iodine tablets/drops also therapeutic ● *Clinical course:* May be clinically silent in adults for significant time period, especially in areas of mild deficiency, but goiter ultimately develops; more acute recognition in neonates, where mental retardation and cretinism is seen ● *Co-morbidities:* Infertility; other nutritional deficiencies; hypothyroidism ● *Procedure results:* Ultrasound shows characteristic findings (diffuse enlargement early on, then nodular goiter); uptake scan should show low level of activity ● *Test findings:* Urine iodine reflective of current iodine nutritional status; thyroid size, serum thyroglobulin level (although nonspecific) indicative of iodine status over time

Iron deficiency anemia ● *Onset:* Insidious ● *Male:female ratio:* M<F ● *Ethnicity:* All ● *Character:* Fatigue, dyspnea on exertion, pica ● *Location:* Nonspecific ● *Pattern:* Nonspecific ● *Precipitating factors:* Blood loss (menorrhagia, GI bleeding), vegetarian diet, malabsorption, pregnancy, adolescent growth spurt, mild diet of infants ● *Relieving factors:* Blood transfusions, iron supplementation, treatment of bleeding source ● *Clinical course:* Progressive if untreated but can be self-limited depending on cause ● *Co-morbidities:* Blood loss (menorrhagia, GI blood loss, surgical blood loss), inadequate diet, malabsorption (celiac sprue, Crohn's disease) ● *Procedure results:* Low iron on bone marrow biopsy (though this test is usually not necessary for diagnosis) ● *Test findings:* Decreased MCV (microcytic, hypochromic anemia), decreased hemoglobin, decreased serum iron, ferritin and transferrin saturation

Irritable bowel syndrome ● *Onset:* Insidious ● *Male:female ratio:* M(1):F(2) ● *Ethnicity:* More common in developed countries ● *Character:* Abdominal pain, often in the lower abdomen, associated with change in stool frequency or consistency; pain is often worse after meals, relieved with defecation; patients may report abdominal distension and bloating, mucus in stools, and worsening of symptoms with stress; alternating constipation and diarrhea is common; patients do not have fever, weight loss, or bloody diarrhea ● *Location:* Pain is usually in the lower abdomen, with the left lower quadrant most frequently involved ● *Pattern:* Pain often worsens with meals; patients do not wake up at night with symptoms ● *Precipitating factors:* Meals; emotional stress ● *Relieving factors:* Defecation may relieve symptoms; bulk agents (psyllium) and antispasmodics may help, as may antidepressant medications (amitriptyline, nortriptyline); alosetron may be useful in patients with diarrhea-predominant IBS ● *Clinical course:* Symptoms wax and wane, but the disorder is not usually self-limited ● *Co-morbidities:* There is an increased incidence of depression or anxiety disorder in IBS patients ● *Procedure results:* Generally a clinical diagnosis; often, a sigmoidoscopy is performed which is normal; it is the absence of pathologic findings that characterizes IBS ● *Test findings:* No relevant tests

Ischemic bowel disease ● *Onset:* Acute (rarely subacute) ● *Male:female ratio:* M=F ● *Ethnicity:* All ● *Character:* Diffuse abdominal pain, often severe, with a relatively benign abdominal examination - often accompanied by loose, bloody stools; elderly patients may present with confusion, abdominal distension; when infarction occurs, patients develop acidosis, high amylase, diffuse peritonitis ● *Location:* Abdomen ● *Pattern:* Nonspecific ● *Precipitating factors:* Hypovolemia; poor oral intake or diarrhea are often precipitating factors ● *Relieving factors:* Hydration may be sufficient if there is no vascular occlusion; if there is a thrombus or embolus, surgery is definitive treatment (embolectomy or bypass); angiography with papaverine infusion may ameliorate symptoms prior to surgery ● *Clinical course:* May be self-limited, but often progresses to bowel infarction, with a 70-100% mortality

●*Co-morbidities:* Congestive heart failure (CHF), atrial fibrillation, history of myocardial infarction (MI), peripheral vascular disease, stroke; hypercoagulable states ●*Procedure results:* Angiography is definitive in embolic or thromotic occlusions ●*Test findings:* Upright abdominal X-ray or CT may show thumbprinting, bowel wall thickening, pneumatosis; WBC usually elevated to >15,000; when infarction occurs, metabolic acidosis and high amylase are seen

Ischemic encephalopathy
●*Onset:* Acute ●*Male:female ratio:* M=F ●*Ethnicity:* All ●*Character:* Loss of oxygen supply to central nervous system due to loss of circulation and/or impairment of respiration ●*Location:* Dysfunction of reticular activating system above level of mid-pons or bilateral cerebral hemispheric dysfunction ●*Pattern:* Variable depending on duration of anoxia; coma: state of pathologic unconsciousness; loss of ciliospinal, oculovestibular, and papillary reflexes indicating loss of brainstem function, movement disorders including myoclonus, choreoathetosis cerebellar ataxia, seizures ●*Precipitating factors:* Cardiac arrest, respiratory insufficiency, vascular catastrophe, poisoning (carbon monoxide or drug), trauma ●*Relieving factors:* Restoration of oxygenation early in course of acute event maximizes potential for recovery ●*Clinical course:* Variable determined by duration of anoxia: may vary from near complete recovery to brain death ●*Co-morbidities:* MI, seizures with aspiration, trauma e.g. drowning, strangulation, or foreign body in trachea ●*Procedure results:* CT and MRI of value only to eliminate other causes; EEG abnormal ●*Test findings:* Glasgow coma scale testing assesses level of severity and predicts outcome

Ischemic stroke
●*Onset:* Acute ●*Male:female ratio:* M=F ●*Ethnicity:* All ●*Character:* Weakness, numbness, confusion, ataxia, dysrhria, loss of vision all depending which section of the brain is involved ●*Location:* Nonspecific ●*Pattern:* Weakness, numbness, confusion, ataxia, dysarthria, loss of vision, all depending which section of the brain is involved ●*Precipitating factors:* Risk factors include: hypertention, diabetes, elevated cholesterol, tobacco use, heart disease, atrial fibrillation, heavy alcohol use, sedentary lifestyle, obesity ●*Relieving factors:* Treatment with intravenous or intra-arterial thrombolysis if time permits ●*Clinical course:* Variable ●*Co-morbidities:* Hypertention, diabetes, elevated cholesterol, tobacco use, heart disease, atrial fibrillation, heavy alcohol use, sedentary lifestyle, obesity ●*Procedure results:* MRI/MRA of the brain shows infarction or hemorrhage ●*Test findings:* No relevant tests

Ischiorectal abscess
●*Onset:* Insidious, acute ●*Male:female ratio:* M=F ●*Ethnicity:* All ●*Character:* Constant perineal/back pain exacerbated by sitting or walking, pain on defecation, fever ●*Location:* Ischiorectal fossa ●*Pattern:* Pain is throbbing, and exacerbated by defecation, erythema appears later ●*Precipitating factors:* Anal fissure, prolapsed hemorrhoids, anal sex, trauma, Crohn's disease, hematologic disorders, immunodeficiency states ●*Relieving factors:* Drainage ●*Clinical course:* Slowly progressive, and requires surgical drainage; rarely may cause a rapidly progressive necrotizing infection (such as Fournier's gangrene) ●*Co-morbidities:* Anal fissure, prolapsed hemorrhoids, Crohn's disease, hematologic disorders, immunodeficiency states ●*Procedure results:* Tender mass on digital rectal examination, inflammatory mass on endorectal ultrasound, CT, or MRI ●*Test findings:* Leukocytosis, inflammatory mass on endorectal ultrasound, CT, or MRI

Juvenile idiopathic arthritis ●*Onset:* Acute ●*Male:female ratio:* M=F ●*Ethnicity:* All ●*Character:* Dull ache around multiple joint areas ●*Location:* Several different patterns including systemic, polyarticular, and oligoarticular ●*Pattern:* Rash, fever, anorexia, fatigue are all common; systemic juvenile rheumatoid arthritis (JRA) may manifest a rash and fever in the late afternoon ●*Precipitating factors:* Immobility ●*Relieving factors:* NSAIDs, methotrexate, and etanercept ●*Clinical course:* 50% of patients will have symptoms for <10 years ●*Co-morbidities:* None ●*Procedure results:* Synovial fluid analysis with WBC >5,000 ●*Test findings:* Rheumatoid factor and/or antinucleic antibodies positive; erosions on joint radiographs

Kawasaki disease ●*Onset:* Acute ●*Male:female ratio:* M=F ●*Ethnicity:* Asians at highest risk but seen in all ethnicities ●*Character:* Vasculitis with inflammation ●*Location:* Blood vessels ●*Pattern:* High spiking fevers up over 104F (40C) for greater than 5 days, not improved with antibiotics ●*Precipitating factors:* Unknown infectious agent and genetic predisposition ●*Relieving factors:* Intravenous immunoglobulin (IVIG) and high-dose aspirin ●*Clinical course:* Children without coronary artery disease have a full recovery; 50% of coronary artery aneurysms resolve in first 2 years; some patients require coronary bypass grafting and rarely transplant ●*Co-morbidities:* Bilateral nonpurulent conjunctivitis, infected throat, red cracked lips, and strawberry tongue, swollen feet and hands with peeling, adenopathy, arthritis, meningitis, hepatitis ●*Procedure results:* Two-dimensional Echo at onset and repeated at 2 and 6 weeks may reveal coronary artery aneurysms, pericardial effusion, myocarditis ●*Test findings:* Normal to elevated WBC, elevated ESR, C-reactive protein, and platelets, with negative antinucleic antibodies, rheumatoid factor, and strep screen; CSF fluid and urine reveal elevated WBCs without bacteria

Keratoconjunctivitis sicca ●*Onset:* Insidious ●*Male:female ratio:* M=F ●*Ethnicity:* All ●*Character:* Foreign body sensation; blurred vision ●*Location:* Both eyes ●*Pattern:* Symptoms worse on cold windy days; slightly improved in warm, humid weather ●*Precipitating factors:* None relevant ●*Relieving factors:* Application of artificial tears improves condition ●*Clinical course:* Tends to be chronic but not progressive ●*Co-morbidities:* Sjögren's syndrome; rarely vitamin A deficiency ●*Procedure results:* Anesthetized Schirmer's test; measurement of tear breakup time ●*Test findings:* <10mm of wetting on anesthesized Schirmer's test; tear breakup time <10s

Kernicterus ●*Onset:* Acute ●*Male:female ratio:* M=F ●*Ethnicity:* All ●*Character:* Jaundice in first 24 hours ●*Location:* CNS, skin ●*Pattern:* Lethargy, poor feeding and loss of Moro's reflex initially, then severe CNS findings of bulging fontanelle, high-pitch cry and muscle twitching and seizures in first week; death common ●*Precipitating factors:* Elevated indirect bilirublin secondary to erythroblastosis fetalis and prematurity ●*Relieving factors:* Phototherapy and exchange transfusion ●*Clinical course:* Progression of severe CNS abnormalities in one third of those with significantly elevated indirect hyperbilirubinimia >25mg/dL due to hemolytic disease, less common in physiological jaundice; 75% with severe CNS abnormalities will die ●*Co-morbidities:* Choreoathetosis, mental retardation, deafness, quadraplegia ●*Procedure results:* Elevated bilirubin by icterometer, or by observing progression of skin color ●*Test findings:* Elevated indirect bilirubin in the serum, Coombs' positive, anemia, isoimmunization

Klinefelter's syndrome ●*Onset:* Insidious ●*Male:female ratio:* M ●*Ethnicity:* All ●*Character:* Delayed sexual development and tall stature ●*Location:* Hypoplastic testes ●*Pattern:* Abnormalities noted rarely before puberty ●*Precipitating factors:* 1/500 newborn males have a 47XXY chromosomal abnormality ●*Relieving factors:* Replacement therapy with testosterone injection ●*Clinical course:* Chronic ●*Co-morbidities:* Emotional and academic difficulties, infertility, gynecomastia and breast cancer, pulmonary disease, and varicose veins ●*Procedure results:* Testicular biopsy reveals hyalinized seminiferous tubules, and clumping of Leydig's cells ●*Test findings:* Postpubertal low testosterone, elevated FSH/LH

Korsakoff's syndrome ●*Onset:* Chronic ●*Male:female ratio:* M=F ●*Ethnicity:* All ●*Character:* Thiamine deficiency ●*Location:* Irreversible structural changes in medial dorsal nuclei due to thiamine deficiency ●*Pattern:* Impaired short-term memory and confabulation with otherwise grossly normal cognition ●*Precipitating factors:* Chronic alcoholism ●*Relieving factors:* Thiamine supplementation ●*Clinical course:* Complete or partial recovery in only approximately half of patients ●*Co-morbidities:* Wernicke's encephalopathy ●*Procedure results:* None relevant ●*Test findings:* Mental status testing notable for normal level of consciousness, memory of new events severely impaired; and immediate recall digit span and attention within normal levels

Kyphoscoliosis ●*Onset:* Insidious ●*Male:female ratio:* M=F ●*Ethnicity:* All ●*Character:* Abnormal curvature(s) of the spine; dull back ache ●*Location:* Thoracic, lumbar, or cervical spine ●*Pattern:* Nonspecific ●*Precipitating factors:* None relevant ●*Relieving factors:* Bracing, physical therapy, orthopedic surgery ●*Clinical course:* Usually limited by early diagnosis and bracing or therapy; some cases progressive ●*Co-morbidities:* Neuromuscular dystrophies, neurofibromatoses, metabolic bone disease, failure of vertebral body formation ●*Procedure results:* Plain radiographs of the back ●*Test findings:* No relevant tests

Kyphosis ●*Onset:* Subacute ●*Male:female ratio:* M=F ●*Ethnicity:* Caucasian and Asian ●*Character:* Dull ache around kyphotic spine (hunched or stooped appearance) ●*Location:* Usually thoracic spine but can also present in the cervical spine ●*Pattern:* Pain due to kyphosis is worse with activity ●*Precipitating factors:* Osteoporotic compression fractures may be due to low bone density, low calcium intake, hypovitaminosis D, glucocorticoid ingestion ●*Relieving factors:* NSAIDs, calcitonin, narcotics ●*Clinical course:* If due to a compression fracture, acute ache is followed by a dull pain ●*Co-morbidities:* Osteoporosis is associated with estrogen or testosterone deficiency, inflammatory arthritis, inflammatory bowel disease ●*Procedure results:* No relevant procedures ●*Test findings:* Plain radiographs reveal kyphotic spine

L

Labyrinthine dysfunction ●*Onset:* Insidious ●*Male:female ratio:* M=F ●*Ethnicity:* None ●*Character:* Generalized sense of dizziness, imbalance, dysequilibrium, true vertigo ●*Location:* Nonspecific ●*Pattern:* Usually persistent, chronic ●*Precipitating factors:* Worse with sudden movements, motion ●*Relieving factors:* None relevant ●*Clinical course:* May be slowly progressive, then plateaus ●*Co-morbidities:* Hearing loss, autoimmune disease, temporal bone trauma, head trauma ●*Procedure results:* Romberg may be positive towards affected ear; nystagmus infrequently present ●*Test findings:* Abnormal electronystagmography findings

Labyrinthitis ●*Onset:* Acute ●*Male:female ratio:* M=F ●*Ethnicity:* All ●*Character:* Vertigo and nausea, worse on movement ●*Location:* Nonspecific ●*Pattern:* Often symptoms worsen when patient is tired or stressed ●*Precipitating factors:* Usually follows acute upper respiratory tract infection ●*Relieving factors:* Antihistamines, antiemetics may be helpful ●*Clinical course:* Usually resolves spontaneously after 2-3 weeks ●*Co-morbidities:* Ménière's syndrome ●*Procedure results:* MRI scan to exclude acoustic neuroma if symptoms atypical or persistant ●*Test findings:* Abnormal caloric test

Lactating mastitis ●*Onset:* Acute ●*Male:female ratio:* F ●*Ethnicity:* All ●*Character:* Fever and chills, breast pain ●*Location:* Unilateral breast pain, usually localized ●*Pattern:* Erythema, pain, induration of a segment of the breast ●*Precipitating factors:* Develops after 2-4 weeks of breast-feeding ●*Relieving factors:* Expression and discarding of infected breast milk ●*Clinical course:* Resolves with appropriate antibiotics ●*Co-morbidities:* Staph infection in nursing neonate ●*Procedure results:* Culture of breast milk ●*Test findings:* U/S can diagnose abscess

Lactose intolerance ●*Onset:* Insidious ●*Male:female ratio:* M=F ●*Ethnicity:* More common in Asians and African-Americans ●*Character:* Episodes of watery diarrhea, abdominal pain, distension, and flatulence after ingestion of lactose-containing foods ●*Location:* Midabdomen ●*Pattern:* Symptoms occur after ingestion of lactose ●*Precipitating factors:* Lactose ingestion ●*Relieving factors:* Avoidance of lactose; lactase supplements prior to lactose ingestion are also effective ●*Clinical course:* Not self-limited ●*Co-morbidities:* None relevant ●*Procedure results:* Best diagnostic test is a 2-week lactose-free diet; lactose-hydrogen breath test may also reveal lactose malabsorbtion ●*Test findings:* Lactose breath hydrogen test: a rise in breath hydrogen >20ppm within 90 min of ingestion of 50g of lactose is positive for lactase deficiency

Laryngeal cancer ●*Onset:* Insidious ●*Male:female ratio:* M(5):F(1) ●*Ethnicity:* All ●*Character:* Persistent hoarseness ●*Location:* Throat/voice ●*Pattern:* Hoarse voice or loss of voice without variation ●*Precipitating factors:* Smoking ●*Relieving factors:* None relevant ●*Clinical course:* Slow progression ●*Co-morbidities:* Cigarette smoking, alcohol intake ●*Procedure results:* Suggestive lesion on fiberoptic laryngoscopy ●*Test findings:* Cancer on biopsy of larynx

Laryngitis ●*Onset:* Acute ●*Male:female ratio:* M=F ●*Ethnicity:* All ●*Character:* New hoarseness or aphonia associated with nasal congestion, malaise, and fever ●*Location:* Larynx, vocal cords ●*Pattern:* Progressive deepening or loss of voice over several days, associated with rhinorrhea and occasional sore throat ●*Precipitating factors:* Sick contacts ●*Relieving factors:* Voice rest, humidification ●*Clinical course:* Usually mild and self-limiting ●*Co-morbidities:* Upper respiratory infection ●*Procedure results:* Hyperemic vocal folds on laryngoscopy ●*Test findings:* No relevant tests

Lassa fever ●*Onset:* Acute/subacute ●*Male:female ratio:* M=F ●*Ethnicity:* West African ●*Character:* Gradual onset of fever, retrosternal chest pain with sore throat, cough, GI symptoms ●*Location:* Systemic (fever), pharynx, lung, eighth cranial nerve, upper GI tract, coagulation cascade (15-30%), capillary leak, conjunctiva, myocardium, pericardium (in men), other ●*Pattern:* Gradual onset of fever, fatigue, sore throat, rarely complicated by bleeding and capillary leak (edema); permanent deafness and transient alopecia may appear during convalescence ●*Precipitating factors:* Residence in/travel to western Africa, particularly Sierra Leone, Guinea, Liberia, Nigeria, person-to-person, nosocomial transmission, more common during the dry season (January-April) ●*Relieving factors:* Rest, hydration ●*Clinical course:* Gradual onset of fever, self-limiting within 7-10 days, complications may be fetal, 20% develop permanent deafness ●*Co-morbidities:* Fetal loss and abortions, deafness, alopecia (transient) ●*Procedure results:* Isolation of virus from blood/clinical material ●*Test findings:* Normal to mildly elevated WBC, normal to low platelets, mildly elevated hepatic transaminases, proteinuria

Late onset congenital adrenal hyperplasia ●*Onset:* Subacute ●*Male:female ratio:* M=F ●*Ethnicity:* All ●*Character:* Hirsutism, oligomenorrhea, acne, occasional clitoromegaly in females; males usually asymptomatic ●*Location:* Skin: increased hair and acne; genitals: clitoromegaly in female ●*Pattern:* Nonspecific ●*Precipitating factors:* >90% of cases genetic: most common 21-hydroxylase deficiency ●*Relieving factors:* Glucocorticoid single low dose at bedtime; alternative birth control pill ●*Clinical course:* Ongoing ●*Co-morbidities:* Infertility; hypertension if 11-hydroxylase deficiency ●*Procedure results:* Cortrosyn stimulation result: elevated 17 hydroxyprogesterone if 21-hydroxylase deficiency ●*Test findings:* 21-hydroxylase: basal 17 OH progesterone may be elevated but often normal; may have high DHEAS and testosterone

Laurence-Moon syndrome ●*Onset:* Insidious ●*Male:female ratio:* M=F ●*Ethnicity:* All ●*Character:* Retinal degeneration with vision loss and obesity ●*Location:* Eyes and body habitus ●*Pattern:* Loss of night vision by age 3 and 75% blind by age 20, obesity present by infancy ●*Precipitating factors:* Autosomal recessive disorder with retinal pigmentation ●*Relieving factors:* None relevant ●*Clinical course:* Most patients are obese, have low IQ and are blind by age 20 ●*Co-morbidities:* Polydactyly, syndactyly, hypogonadism, glomerulonephritis, hypertension, cardiac defects, hirsuitism, short stature, diabetes insipidus ●*Procedure results:* Ophthalmology examination reveals loss of night vision, then central with eventual blindness secondary to pigmental changes of the retina ●*Test findings:* Normal chromosome analysis; urine analysis with red blood cells and protein, low IQ on standard testing

Laxative abuse ●*Onset:* Acute ●*Male:female ratio:* M<F ●*Ethnicity:* All ●*Character:* In the more benign form of this disorder, a patient admits to using laxatives for constipation, but becomes dependent upon them for bowel movements; discontinuing medications leads to severe constipation; over time, increasing doses of medication are needed to avoid constipation; in the pathologic form of the disorder, a patient surreptitiously uses laxatives, then presents with a complaint of diarrhea, usually leading to an exhaustive and invasive workup; patients may become hypokalemic and alkalemic from the copious diarrhea ●*Location:* Chief symptom is diarrhea ●*Pattern:* No pattern ●*Precipitating factors:* None relevant ●*Relieving factors:* Benign form - patients may be able to wean off laxatives, but may still require occasional laxatives; pathologic form - psychiatric help is needed when the ruse is discovered ●*Clinical course:* Not self-limited ●*Co-morbidities:* Any constipating condition can lead to laxative use and overuse; the pathologic abuse syndrome may be associated with other psychiatric disorders ●*Procedure results:* Stool osmolarity tests reveal the presence of an osmotic gap (when osmotic laxatives are used); treating the stool with sodium hydroxide may show a pink color if phenolphthalein laxatives are used; colonoscopy may show melanosis (black color to the mucosa) if anthracycline laxatives are used (e.g. senna) ●*Test findings:* Hypokalemia, alkalemia

Legionnaires' disease ●*Onset:* Acute, subacute ●*Male:female ratio:* M>F ●*Ethnicity:* All ●*Character:* High fever, mild cough, chest pain, shortness of breath, pronounced GI symptoms ●*Location:* Lungs (most common); extrapulmonary (less common): blood, myocardium, pericardium, sinuses, liver, spleen, kidney, other ●*Pattern:* Fever is very high, pneumonia may involve several lobes, GI symptoms are common (nausea, diarrhea) ●*Precipitating factors:* Exposure to water aerosols (such as cooling towers), nosocomial transmission, chronic lung disease and smoking, AIDS, alcohol, SCID (severe combined immunodeficiency), chronic granulomatous disease, organ transplant, corticosteroid therapy ●*Relieving factors:* None relevant ●*Clinical course:* Incubation 2-10 days followed by fever and progressive cough. Improvement within 3-5 days of appropriate antibiotic therapy ●*Co-morbidities:* AIDS, COPD (chronic obstructive pulmonary disease), smoking, liver disease, diarrhea, immunosuppression, chronic granulomatous disease, SCID (severe combined immunodeficiency) ●*Procedure results:* Many neutrophils but no organisms on Gram-stained sputum, Legionella antigen detection in urine, infiltrates (commonly multilobar) with or without pleural effusion on chest X-ray, growth of Legionella or positive Legionella direct fluorescent antigen of sputum ●*Test findings:* Hyponatremia, mildly elevated hepatic transaminases, hypophosphatemia, hematuria, thrombocytopenia

Leprosy ●*Onset:* Chronic ●*Male:female ratio:* M(2):F(1) ●*Ethnicity:* Rare in developed nations ●*Character:* Tuberculoid: one or more hypopigmented skin patches with gradual loss of sensation; lepromatous: multiple symmetric skin and nasal mucosa nodules and plaques with hypesthesia ●*Location:* Skin of face, ears, wrists, elbows, buttocks, knees, other, peripheral nerves, mucous membranes (nasal), muscles (atrophy), cornea and iris, lymph nodes, testes, other ●*Pattern:* Tuberculoid: one or few skin lesions, progressive hypesthesia, late contractures, skin ulcerations, resorption of bone; lepromatous: numerous bilateral skin lesions, later hypesthesia, thickening of the skin, mucosal ulcerations ●*Precipitating factors:* Close contacts with untreated patients, residence in endemic areas ●*Relieving factors:* None relevant ●*Clinical course:* Chronic, slowly progressive, mutilating: hand crippling, bone resorption, blindness ●*Co-morbidities:* Gynecomastia, infertility in men, erythema nodosum leprosum, chronic skin ulcers ●*Procedure results:* Acid-fast bacilli in skin smears, detection of M. leprae by PCR (polymerase chain reaction) from skin scrapings/biopsy, granulomatous inflammation and foam cells on histopathology ●*Test findings:* Lepromatous: mild anemia, elevated ESR, hypergammaglobulinemia

Leptospirosis ●*Onset:* Abrupt ●*Male:female ratio:* M>F ●*Ethnicity:* All ●*Character:* Abrupt onset of fever, rigors, myalgias and headache, conjunctival suffusion without discharge, severe muscle tenderness in the lower extremities and lower back, in severe cases Weil's syndrome: biphasic illness - 1-3 days of improvement followed by jaundice, liver failure, renal failure, cardiac collapse, and hemorrhagic complications ●*Location:* Systemic - all organ systems involved (multi organ systems); more common: blood, CNS, eyes (conjunctivae, uveae), muscle, liver, kidney, heart, lungs (hemorrhagic pneumonitis), blood vessels (vasculitis) ●*Pattern:* Febrile illness is biphasic in severe cases, conjunctival suffusion common and without eye discharge, muscle ache is more pronounced in calves and lower back, jaundice and renal failure are in the second phase, initial fever is accompanied by severe headache, bilirubin is much more elevated than alkaline phosphatase ●*Precipitating factors:* Occupational exposure: loggers, hunters, animal trappers, farmers, livestock workers, abattoir workers, veterinarians, sewer workers, military personnel; recreational exposure: fresh water swimming, canoeing, kayaking, trail biking; worldwide distribution but more in the Caribbean, Central and South America, and Hawaii ●*Relieving factors:* Specific antimicrobial therapy ●*Clinical course:* Onset is abrupt; most cases are mild to moderate and respond to antibiotics; rarely complicated by Weil's syndrome which may lead to death (4-50%) ●*Co-morbidities:* Zoonosis ●*Procedure results:* Isolation of the organism from the blood or CSF during the first 10 days and from the urine for up to 30 days after symptoms; positive serology by microscopic agglutination test (MAT), macroscopic agglutination test, indirect hemagglutination, or ELISA; bilirubin is much more elevated than alkaline phosphatase, infiltrates on chest X-ray ●*Test findings:* Leukocytosis with a left shift, proteinuria, pyuria, granular casts, microscopic hematuria, elevated creatine kinase, elevated hepatic transaminases, bilirubin more elevated than alkaline phosphatase, isolation of Leptospira from blood or CSF during the first 10 days of illness or from the urine for up to 30 days, positive serology by microscopic agglutination test (MAT), macroscopic agglutination test, indirect hemagglutination, or ELISA

Lichen planus ● *Onset:* Subacute ● *Male:female ratio:* M<F ● *Ethnicity:* All ● *Character:* Itching ❷ *Location:* Wrists, ankles, lumbar, mucosa ❸ *Pattern:* Flat-topped purple papules ● *Precipitating factors:* Medications ● *Relieving factors:* Topical steroids ● *Clinical course:* Frequently resolves in 6 months ● *Co-morbidities:* Hepatitis ● *Procedure results:* No relevant procedures ● *Test findings:* Positive skin biopsy

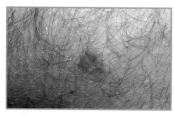

❶ *Character A solitary, violaceous plaque*

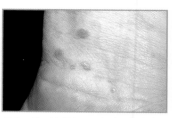

❷ *Location Multiple papules in a typical location*

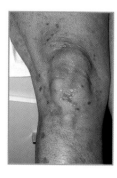

❸ *Pattern Multiple papules scattered widely*

Lichen sclerosis ● *Onset:* Insidious, chronic ● *Male:female ratio:* M<F ● *Ethnicity:* All ● *Character:* Vulvar itching and vulvodynia; pruritus is most common symptom; later, scarring can cause pain during intercourse and inability to have intercourse; in men, urethral strictures can result ● *Location:* Vulvar and penile (balanitis xerotica obliterans) ❸ *Pattern:* Begins as nonspecific erythema, and progresses to develop into whitish-gray, woody scarred mucosa or skin, with a peripheral zone of erythema or hyperpigmentation ● *Precipitating factors:* Borrelia burgdorferi infection has been implicated in Europe; possible hereditary predisposition ● *Relieving factors:* Potent topical steroid therapy; antipruritic agents at bedtime; treatment of superimposed bacterial infection ● *Clinical course:* Childhood disease with better prognosis than adult variant, at least from symptomatology point of view; local squamous cell carcinoma can occur in 5% ● *Co-morbidities:* Lichen planus, collagen vascular disease such as lupus erythematosus, graft-versus-host disease ● *Procedure results:* Early biopsy reveals a lichenoid infiltrate hugging the dermoepidermal junction; later, more classic findings reveal a sclerotic, pale, superficial dermis, atrophic epidermis and inflammatory infiltrate present at the junction of the sclerotic and normal dermis ● *Test findings:* No specific tests

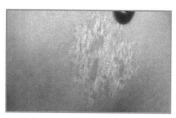

❸ *Pattern White papules coalescing into plaques in a child*

Lichen simplex chronicus ●*Onset:* Subacute, insidious ●*Male:female ratio:* M=F ●*Ethnicity:* All ●*Character:* Itchy plaque ●*Location:* Posterior neck, ankles, genitals, extensor forearms ●*Pattern:* Thick scaly red brown plaque ●*Precipitating factors:* Stress, eczema ●*Relieving factors:* Steroids - topical, intralesional; antihistamines ●*Clinical course:* Frequently chronic ●*Co-morbidities:* Eczema ●*Procedure results:* No relevant procedures ●*Test findings:* Skin biopsy

Lipemia retinalis ●*Onset:* Insidious ●*Male:female ratio:* M=F ●*Ethnicity:* All ●*Character:* Milky appearence to retinal vessels ●*Location:* Nonspecific ●*Pattern:* No eye symptoms ●*Precipitating factors:* Made worse by alcohol intake, uncontrolled diabetes ●*Relieving factors:* Reduce fat and cholesterol intake; maintain ideal body weight ●*Clinical course:* Slowly progressive if left untreated ●*Co-morbidities:* Xanthomas; pancreatitis; hepatosplenomegaly ●*Procedure results:* Evident on retinal exam ●*Test findings:* High serum and triglyceride and cholesterol levels

Lipoma ●*Onset:* Insidious ●*Male:female ratio:* M=F ●*Ethnicity:* All ●*Character:* Soft, mobile tissue mass ●*Location:* Subcutaneous, usually on back, shoulders, neck, rarely in the anterior mediastinum, retroperitoneum, GI tract ●*Pattern:* Nonspecific ●*Precipitating factors:* None relevant ●*Relieving factors:* Removal, often not necessary to treat ●*Clinical course:* Benign ●*Co-morbidities:* None relevant ●*Procedure results:* Biopsy - normal fat cells ●*Test findings:* No relevant tests

Liver cirrhosis ●*Onset:* Insidious ●*Male:female ratio:* Etiology dependent ●*Ethnicity:* All ●*Character:* Initially assymptomatic; jaundice, (encephalopathy), ascites, esophageal or gastric varices, coagulopathy; gynecomastia and testicular atrophy may occur in men ●*Location:* Abdomen and legs (swelling), skin (jaundice), CNS (confusion) ●*Pattern:* Nonspecific ●*Precipitating factors:* High protein meals may precipitate encephalopathy, salt intake may worsen edema/ascites ●*Relieving factors:* Lactulose relieves encephalopathy, diuretics treat edema and ascites, beta-blockers prevent variceal hemorrhage ●*Clinical course:* Progressive decline over months to years until death or liver transplantation ●*Co-morbidities:* Viral hepatitis, hemochromatosis, autoimmune hepatitis, alcoholic liver disease, nonalcoholic steatohepatitis, Wilson's disease, alpha-1 antitrypsin deficiency, drug-induced hepatitis ●*Procedure results:* Liver biopsy diagnositic, showing fibrous bands separating areas of normal liver cells (nodules); U/S may show a shrunken, nodular liver, with splenomegaly or perhepatic varices ●*Test findings:* Albumin decreased, PT elevated, bilirubin variably elevated, AST and ALT elevated, or normal; glucose may be low only in end stages

Liver failure ●*Onset:* Acute, subacute, chronic ●*Male:female ratio:* Etiology dependent ●*Ethnicity:* All ●*Character:* Fatigue, weight loss, diarrhea, edema, ascites, jaundice, encephalopathy ●*Location:* Systemic ●*Pattern:* Nonspecific ●*Precipitating factors:* Chronic hepatitis B, other viral hepatitis, alcohol abuse, poisoning, malignancy, primary biliary cirrhosis ●*Relieving factors:* Treatment depends on cause ●*Clinical course:* Varies depending on cause ●*Co-morbidities:* Hepatitis B, hepatitis C, HIV infection, esophogeal varices ●*Procedure results:* No relevant procedures ●*Test findings:* Abnormal liver function test; abnormal coagulation profile; infectious hepatitis screen may be positive depending on cause

Lower GI bleeding ●*Onset:* Insidious if low volume source such as a tumor, acute if high volume source such as diverticular bleeding ●*Male:female ratio:* M=F ●*Ethnicity:* All ●*Character:* Bloody stools - color usually correlates with site of bleeding: melena only if cecal source, maroon if R sided or proximal source, bright red if rectal source; change in bowel habits, lightheadedness, syncope, abdominal cramping ●*Location:* Nonspecific ●*Pattern:* Nonspecific ●*Precipitating factors:* Diverticulosis, inflammatory disorders, colitis, infectious gastroenteritis, radiation therapy, malignancy, nonsteroidal anti-inflammatory drugs ●*Relieving factors:* Supportive care including volume replacement or blood transfusions, correction of any coagulopathy, endoscopic therapy, angiography, surgery for severe, refractory cases ●*Clinical course:* Usually self-limited, and treatable, morbidity is fairly high but mortality is low (<4%) ●*Co-morbidities:* None relevant ●*Procedure results:* Colonoscopy or sigmoidoscopy - blood in colon, sometimes a source is visualized such as colitis, bleeding diverticula; angiography - vascular bluish at site of bleeding ●*Test findings:* Tagged red blood cell scan - localization of bleeding; anemia, increased RDW, MCV and reticulocytes

Lumbar disc disorders ●*Onset:* Acute ●*Male:female ratio:* M=F ●*Ethnicity:* All ●*Character:* Sharp or numbing pain ●*Location:* Midline or paraspinal in low back region; radiation into buttocks or posterior thigh ●*Pattern:* Pain worsens with straight leg raising, Valsalva ●*Precipitating factors:* Lifting or twisting motions involving the low back ●*Relieving factors:* NSAIDs, acetaminophen, corticosteroids, heat or cold, gentle stretching exercises ●*Clinical course:* Usually spontaneously resolves over 8-12 weeks ●*Co-morbidities:* Tobacco use ●*Procedure results:* Positive straight leg raise test ●*Test findings:* MRI with disc herniation

Lunate dislocation ●*Onset:* Acute ●*Male:female ratio:* M=F ●*Ethnicity:* All ●*Character:* Dull ache ●*Location:* Wrist ●*Pattern:* Worse with motion ●*Precipitating factors:* Trauma to wrist ●*Relieving factors:* Surgery ●*Clinical course:* Chronic with accelerated osteoarthritis ●*Co-morbidities:* Inflammatory arthritis of the wrist ●*Procedure results:* No relevant procedures ●*Test findings:* Radiographs of the wrist show dislocation of the lunate

Lung abscess ●*Onset:* Subacute ●*Male:female ratio:* M(4):F(1) ●*Ethnicity:* All ●*Character:* Cough often productive of fetid-smelling sputum, dyspnea, fatigue, weight loss, fever ●*Location:* Chest ●*Pattern:* Focal inspiratory rales, bronchial breath sounds, egophony ●*Precipitating factors:* Poor dentition, aspiration, tuberculosis, obstructing airway tumor or foreign body, substance abuse ●*Relieving factors:* Prolonged course of antibiotics (e.g. clindamycin 600mg po tid x 6 weeks for an anaerobic lung abscess), chest physiotherapy, restoring airway patency if needed ●*Clinical course:* Weeks-months ●*Co-morbidities:* Gingivitis, epilepsy, syncope, dysphagia secondary to stroke, esophageal or systemic disorder, substance abuse, cancer ●*Procedure results:* No relevant procedures ●*Test findings:* Chest X-ray: focal, cavitary infiltrate with thick, irregular border and air-fluid level, purulent sputum with definitive pathogen identified by Gram stain or culture (note: anaerobic pathogens may not grow secondary to difficulty culturing these organisms), may have positive blood cultures, leukocytosis, anemia, elevated ESR and lactate dehydrogenase

Lyme disease ●*Onset:* Acute, subacute ●*Male:female ratio:* M=F ●*Ethnicity:* All ●*Character:* Enlarging red macule with central clearing - common, migrating skin macules - less common, unilateral facial palsy/radiculopathy, fluctuating AV-blocks, intermittent joint swelling and pain ●*Location:* Skin of thigh, groin, axilla - most common; less common: other skin, systemic (fever, muscle), meninges, 7th cranial nerve, other cranial nerves, peripheral nerves, meninges, heart conduction system, knee(s), other large joints, lymph nodes; rare: eyes, bones, lungs, liver, other ●*Pattern:* Macular rash begins at tick bite site and has central clearing; it may be followed by migrating macules; joint pain is migratory, 1-2 joints at one time; cranial neuropathy is unilateral ●*Precipitating factors:* Tick bite in endemic areas: temperate (northeastern and midwestern USA, California,

Oregon, Europe, former Soviet Union, China, Japan) ●*Relieving factors:* None relevant ●*Clinical course:* Three stages: early localized (days-several weeks), early disseminated (several weeks), and late/persistent (months); most patients respond to antibiotic therapy, but rare chronic neurologic and rheumatologic sequela may be seen ●*Co-morbidities:* Babesia, Ehrlichia, tick-borne encephalitis, Bell's palsy, acrodermatitis chronica atrophicans, AV blocks ●*Procedure results:* CSF: lymphocytic pleocytosis (c.100 cells/mL), elevated protein, normal glucose; joint fluid: neutrophilic pleocytosis (500-100,000 cells/mL) and B. burgdorferi DNA by PCR (polymerase chain reaction), specific serology ●*Test findings:* Elevated ESR, elevated SGOT (>SGPT), elevated LDH, hematuria, proteinuria, normal to low HCT, normal to high WBC

Lymphadenopathy ●*Onset:* Insidious, acute ●*Male:female ratio:* M=F ●*Ethnicity:* All ●*Character:* Enlargement of a mass ●*Location:* Lymph nodes ●*Pattern:* Soft rubbery mass consistent with infection; hard adherent mass consistent with malignancy ●*Precipitating factors:* Proliferation of lymphoid tissue to greater than 1cm from infection such as Staphylococcus aureus, group A streptococcus, cat scratch or viral process such as CMV, EBV, or HIV, tuberculosis, and malignancy ●*Relieving factors:* Treatment of underlying infection with antibiotics, surgical drainage of an abcess, and biopsy for persistent mass ●*Clinical course:* Resolution in most cases but treatment for bacterial infection and malignant disease ●*Co-morbidities:* Malignancy including leukemias, lymphomas, teratoma, Kawasaki disease, tuberculosis ●*Procedure results:* Tuberculosis skin testing that is positive and biopsy positive for malignancy or infectious etiology ●*Test findings:* CBC with elevated WBC in bacterial infection or atypical lymphs in mononucleosis, positive CMV, EBV, toxoplasmosis, Bartonella henselae, STDs; chest film indicates adenopathy in the chest

Lymphangitis ●*Onset:* Acute ●*Male:female ratio:* M=F ●*Ethnicity:* All ●*Character:* Red streak from wound or area of cellulitis, chill, fever, malaise, tender and enlarged regional lymph nodes, tachycardia ●*Location:* Nonspecific ●*Pattern:* Nonspecific ●*Precipitating factors:* Bacterial skin infection, usually hemolytic strep or staph ●*Relieving factors:* Antibiotics (antistrep/staph such as penicillin), hot compresses, elevation of affected extremity, drainage of abscess ●*Clinical course:* With proper treatment, generally resolves in days. If not treated, can lead to septicemia ●*Co-morbidities:* None relevant ●*Procedure results:* No relevant procedures ●*Test findings:* Leukocytosis with a left shift, possibly positive blood cultures

Lymphatic obstruction ●*Onset:* Usually insidious, rarely subacute ●*Male:female ratio:* M=F ●*Ethnicity:* All ●*Character:* Swelling in affected extremity, painless edema, limb hypertrophy, skin induration, and pigmentation in later stages ●*Location:* Often involves an extremity ●*Pattern:* Nonspecific ●*Precipitating factors:* Trauma, congenital lymphatic abnormalities, irradiation, lymph node dissection, surgery, infection (filariasis) ●*Relieving factors:* Treatment is often not very satisfactory; treatment of the underlying disorder if it exists, elevation of involved body part, use of compression stockings, good hygiene, diuretics, rarely operative treatment ●*Clinical course:* Usually slowly progressive, but not life-threatening ●*Co-morbidities:* None relevant ●*Procedure results:* Lymphangiography or radioactive isotope studies can define lymphatic defect ●*Test findings:* No relevant tests

Lymphedema ●*Onset:* Insidious ●*Male:female ratio:* M<F ●*Ethnicity:* All ●*Character:* Early stages - soft, pitting edema; late stages - woody texture of limb with loss of normal contour ●*Location:* Extremities ●*Pattern:* Begins in distal extremity and progresses proximally ●*Precipitating factors:* Disruption of lymphatic channels (recurrent lymphangitis, filariasis, tuberculosis, neoplasm, surgery, radiation therapy) ●*Relieving factors:* Skin hygiene and emollients, prophylactic antibiotics, compression stockings, leg elevation (diuretics are not recommended) ●*Clinical course:* Lifelong, tends to progress but slow progression with appropriate care ●*Co-morbidities:* None relevant ●*Procedure results:* Lymphangiography or scintigraphy: dilated lymphatic channels +/- obstruction ●*Test findings:* No relevant tests

Lymphogranuloma venereum ●*Onset:* Acute/subacute ●*Male:female ratio:* M(5):F(1) ●*Ethnicity:* Africa, India, southeast Asia, South America, Caribbean ●*Character:* Acute genital ulcer; progressive suppurative lymphadenopathy ●*Location:* Vulva, vagina, penis, urethra, anus, rectum, inguinal lymph nodes, deep iliac lymph nodes, conjunctivae (neonates), meninges (rare) ●*Pattern:* Genital papule ulcerates then heals; lymphadenitis is progressive, painful, with purulent drainage/sinus tract formation ●*Precipitating factors:* Unprotected sexual contact; endemic in Africa, India, southeast Asia, South America ●*Relieving factors:* None relevant ●*Clinical course:* Ulcers resolve spontaneously; lymphadenopathy is progressive, may result in elephantiasis or hypertrophic genitalia ●*Co-morbidities:* Syphilis, HIV, elephantiasis, lymphatic obstruction ●*Procedure results:* Lymph node biopsy shows granulomas with central abscesses, serology for Chlamydia trachomatis L1-L3 (IgM>1:32; IgG>1:512) ●*Test findings:* C. trachomatis L1-L3 IgM>1:32 or IgG>1:512

Macroglossia ●*Onset:* Congenital/indolent ●*Male:female ratio:* M=F ●*Ethnicity:* All ●*Character:* Asymptomatic enlargement of the tongue; may impart subtle dysarthria or dysphagia ●*Location:* Oral cavity ●*Pattern:* Nonspecific ●*Precipitating factors:* None relevant ●*Relieving factors:* None relevant ●*Clinical course:* Usually persistent; may slowly enlarge ●*Co-morbidities:* Hypothyroidism; endocrine abnormalities; rare syndromes; amyloidosis ●*Procedure results:* Deep muscle biopsy may yield the etiology, especially for amyloidosis ●*Test findings:* MRI will differentiate between true macroglossia and tongue tumors; endocrine panel to rule out endocrinopathy

Macular degeneration ●*Onset:* Insidious/subacute/acute ●*Male:female ratio:* M<F ●*Ethnicity:* All ●*Character:* Blurred vision; central scotoma ●*Location:* Macular region of retina ●*Pattern:* Typically bilateral ●*Precipitating factors:* None relevant ●*Relieving factors:* None relevant ●*Clinical course:* Slowly progressive ●*Co-morbidities:* None relevant ●*Procedure results:* No relevant procedures ●*Test findings:* Drusen, retinal pigment epithelial change, hemorrhage in the macula on fundus examination

Malabsorption ●*Onset:* Usually insiduous ●*Male:female ratio:* M=F ●*Ethnicity:* All ●*Character:* Asymptomatic or mild GI distress (distention, flatulence), watery diarrhea; weight loss; edema possible. Symptoms/signs of specific vitamin and nutrient deficiencies (anemia due to B12, folate, iron deficiency; metabolic bone disease (vitamin D); coagulopathy (vitamin K); cheilosis (vitamin B); etc). Milk intolerance in lactase deficient patients. Abdominal pain rare unless chronic pancreatitis, Crohn's disease ●*Location:* Can be global (sprue) or regional (pernicious anemia) ●*Pattern:* Greasy, foul-smelling, pale, voluminous stool; chronic diarrhea common ●*Precipitating factors:* Independent risk factors for underlying causes: i.e. ethyl alcohol or bile stones and pancreatic insufficiency, gastrectomy or small bowel disease/resection, milk product consumption in patient with lactose intolerance; can also be caused by celiac disease, irritable bowel syndrome, or infections (tropical sprue or giardiasis) ●*Relieving factors:* Depends on underlying cause; nutritional restrictions (i.e. gluten in sprue patients), nutrient and vitamin supplementation (iron, folate, fat-soluble vitamins), antibiotics in tropical sprue ●*Clinical course:* Symptoms persist, possibly worsen as long as underlying disorder exists; weight loss more likely with long-standing malabsorption ●*Co-morbidities:* Metabolic bone disease, vitamin deficiencies; dermatitis herpetiformis and/or autoimmune disease in sprue ●*Procedure results:* 72 h (quantitative) fecal fat measurement or (qualitative) sudan stain. D-xylose test for carbohydrate malabsorption. Other tests include empiric gluten-free diet trial, antiendomysial or antigliadin Abs (for sprue), small bowel biopsy, endoscopy (cobblestoning/other characteristic findings in Crohns), upper gastrointestinal/small bowel follow-through to identify diverticula or other anatomic abnormalities predisposing to bacterial overgrowth ●*Test findings:* Different findings for each of multiple etiologies causing malabsorption; positive fecal fat is suggestive

Malaria ●*Onset:* Acute, relapsing (Plasmodium vivax and P. ovale); persistent (P. malaria) ●*Male:female ratio:* M=F ●*Ethnicity:* All ●*Character:* Acute onset of fever and chills, certain types are relapsing ●*Location:* Systemic (RBCs, fever, chills), metabolic (lactic acidosis, hypoglycemia), CNS (coma), liver, spleen, kidneys, lungs (noncardiogenic pulmonary edema), other ●*Pattern:* Daily paroxysmal fever initially, cyclic paroxysmal fever later in course (48 or 72h), fever accompanied by shaking chills and approximately 2-6h later, sweats ●*Precipitating factors:* Mosquito (Anopheles) bite (i.e. travel to/residence in endemic areas), blood transfusion, previous untreated malaria, congenital ●*Relieving factors:* None relevant ●*Clinical course:* Acute onset, paroxysmal illness; may be rapidly fatal in nonimmune individuals. P. ovale and P. vivax may relapse; chronic asymptomatic persistence seen in untreated P. malaria; complications: coma, hypoglycemia, nephrotic syndrome, hemolytic anemia, noncardiogenic pulmonary edema, splenomegaly, splenic rupture ●*Co-morbidities:* None relevant ●*Procedure results:* Intraerythrocytic parasite on thin blood smears, parasites on thick blood smears ●*Test findings:* Anemia, low haptoglobin, elevated hepatic transaminases, lactate dehydrogenase, and reticulocytes, thrombocytopenia, proteinuria, hemoglobinuria, elevated serum creatinine

Male pattern baldness ●*Onset:* Insidious ●*Male:female ratio:* M ●*Ethnicity:* All ●*Character:* Hair loss ●*Location:* Scalp ●*Pattern:* Loss of scalp hair: vertex, frontal ●*Precipitating factors:* None relevant ●*Relieving factors:* Minoxidil, finasteride ●*Clinical course:* Progressive ●*Co-morbidities:* None relevant ●*Procedure results:* No relevant procedures ●*Test findings:* Skin biopsy helpful

Malignant hypertension ●*Onset:* Acute, subacute ●*Male:female ratio:* M>F ●*Ethnicity:* Young African-American men are particularly prone ●*Character:* Encephalopathy (e.g. headache, irritability, alterations in mental status) with or without nephropathy, with or without heart failure, with or without papilledema ●*Location:* Vision changes/loss, chest pain, congestive heart failure, stroke, kidney failure ●*Pattern:* Diastolic pressures >120-130mm Hg (or even lower when associated symptoms are present); systolic pressures >200mm Hg (if symptomatic) or >230-240mm Hg (if a symptomatic) ●*Precipitating factors:* Unknown ●*Relieving factors:* Parenteral agents recommended, such as beta-blockers, nitroprusside, nitroglycerin, others ●*Clinical course:* If untreated, less than 25% 1-year survival; 1% 5-year survival; complications: brain damage, heart failure, renal failure, visual loss, dissections ●*Co-morbidities:* Underlying hypertension (either essential or secondary) ●*Procedure results:* No relevant procedures ●*Test findings:* Fundoscopic examination may reveal papilledema; evidence of long-standing hypertension such as ECG/Echo may reveal hypertrophy; decreased renal function/proteinuria also likely

Malignant lymphadenopathy ●*Onset:* Insidious ●*Male:female ratio:* M=F ●*Ethnicity:* All ●*Character:* Hard, fixed, nontender lymph nodes generally larger than 1-2cm.; other signs of underlying malignancy such as fatigue and weight loss ●*Location:* Can be generalized or localized; if localized usually follows lymphatic drainage of the primary tumor ●*Pattern:* Nonspecific ●*Precipitating factors:* Underlying malignancy ●*Relieving factors:* Treatment of underlying malignancy ●*Clinical course:* Depends on the underlying malignancy ●*Co-morbidities:* None relevant ●*Procedure results:* Lymph node biopsy revealing tumor ●*Test findings:* Depends on underlying malignancy and lymph node location

Malignant salivary gland tumor ●*Onset:* Insidious ●*Male:female ratio:* M=F ●*Ethnicity:* All ●*Character:* Asymptomatic enlargement of salivary gland ●*Location:* Affected salivary gland ●*Pattern:* May have local nerve paralysis ●*Precipitating factors:* None relevant ●*Relieving factors:* None relevant ●*Clinical course:* Slow progressive enlargement ●*Co-morbidities:* Radiation therapy to head and neck ●*Procedure results:* CT or MRI with contrast demonstrates mass or tumor ●*Test findings:* No relevant tests

Malignant thymoma ●*Onset:* Insidious ●*Male:female ratio:* M=F ●*Ethnicity:* All ●*Character:* Asymptomatic, cough, dyspnea, dysphagia, venacaval compression with plethoric facies, swollen upper extremity ●*Location:* Anterior mediastinum ●*Pattern:* Nonspecific ●*Precipitating factors:* None relevant ●*Relieving factors:* Surgical removal, postoperative radiation, chemotherapy for metastatic disease ●*Clinical course:* Related to aggressiveness of disease (with metastatic disease 5-10 year survival) and presence of associated systemic disorder, poor prognosis in children ●*Co-morbidities:* Myasthenia gravis, cytopenias, collagen vascular disease, other carcinoma, hypogammaglobulinemia ●*Procedure results:* Biopsy: usually no cytologic atypia, the diagnosis of cancer is made on invasion of the capsule ●*Test findings:* Cytopenias, elevated ESR, hypogammoglobulinemia

Mallet finger ●*Onset:* Acute/chronic (if untreated) ●*Male:female ratio:* M=F ●*Ethnicity:* All ●*Character:* Flexion deformity of a finger, limited extension ●*Location:* Distal interphalangeal joint ●*Pattern:* Nonspecific ●*Precipitating factors:* Any disruption of the terminal extensor tendon, e.g. via sudden force on tip of finger or hyperextension, laceration, crush injury, fracture of the distal phalanx ●*Relieving factors:* Splinting, surgery ●*Clinical course:* Some permanent loss of function is common ●*Co-morbidities:* None relevant ●*Procedure results:* No relevant procedures ●*Test findings:* X-ray shows fracture if present

Mallory-Weiss tear ●*Onset:* Acute ●*Male:female ratio:* M=F ●*Ethnicity:* All ●*Character:* Vomiting of blood or 'coffee ground' material, usually after repeated episodes of vomiting (nonbloody at first); may have midchest or epigastric pain; no history of prior vomiting in <10% ●*Location:* Chest, epigastrium ●*Pattern:* Occurs after repeated vomiting/retching ●*Precipitating factors:* Repeated vomiting ●*Relieving factors:* Antiemetics will relieve vomiting; GI bleeding may require endoscopy and sclerotherapy of esophageal tear ●*Clinical course:* Lasts hours-to-days; usually self-limited ●*Co-morbidities:* Any disorder causing vomiting ●*Procedure results:* Esophagogastroduodenoscopy reveals tear in distal esophagus, usually at gastroesophageal junction ●*Test findings:* Anemia if bleeding is significant

Malnutrition ●*Onset:* Subacute/chronic ●*Male:female ratio:* M=F ●*Ethnicity:* All ●*Character:* Weight loss, muscle wasting, subcutaneous fat loss, pallor, weakness, alopecia, skin rash, glossitis/stomatitis, edema ●*Location:* Temporal muscle wasting is a common indicator ●*Pattern:* Nonspecific ●*Precipitating factors:* Poor intake, malabsorption/maldigestion, gastrointestinal losses, increased nutritional needs ●*Relieving factors:* Replacement of specific vitamins, oral or parenteral feedings (oral are preferred if the gastrointestinal tract is intact), if severe malnutrition must refeed slowly ●*Clinical course:* Gradual improvement with replacement if underlying cause (e.g. malabsorption) can be corrected but more difficult if malnutrition is a reflection of poor underlying state of health ●*Co-morbidities:* None relevant ●*Procedure results:* Triceps skin fold decreased ●*Test findings:* Low albumin, prealbumin, transferrin, creatine, aspartate transaminase

Mammary duct ectasia ●*Onset:* Subacute/recurrent ●*Male:female ratio:* M<F ●*Ethnicity:* All ●*Character:* Gray-to-green, thick nipple discharge, nipple retraction, mastalgia, possible subareolar abscess, rare fistula to periareolar skin ●*Location:* Breasts, mostly unilateral ●*Pattern:* Nonspecific ●*Precipitating factors:* None relevant ●*Relieving factors:* Warm compresses, antibiotics, incision and drainage, surgical excision of ducts ●*Clinical course:* Recurrent/remitting ●*Co-morbidities:* Very rare hyperplasia and malignancy ●*Procedure results:* Biopsy distinguishes between benign duct ectasia and precancerous conditions ●*Test findings:* Mammography may not be able to distinguish from malignant lesion

Manic depression ●*Onset:* Variable ●*Male:female ratio:* M=F ●*Ethnicity:* Cultural sensitivity critical to expression of psychosis ●*Character:* Presence of both depressed and manic mood (abnormally and persistently elevated, expansive, or irritable mood) ●*Location:* Nonspecific ●*Pattern:* Variable combinations of depressive and manic (or hypomanic) episodes ●*Precipitating factors:* Often follows psychosocial stressor(s), especially loss; may be precipitated by antidepressant medication ●*Relieving factors:* Individuals frequently do not recognize they are ill and may resist efforts to be treated ●*Clinical course:* Extremely variable ●*Co-morbidities:* Substance abuse, anxiety disorders, gambling; antisocial acts; serious financial difficulties ●*Procedure results:* No relevant procedures ●*Test findings:* Sleep disturbance

Marfan's syndrome ●*Onset:* Insidious ●*Male:female ratio:* M=F ●*Ethnicity:* All ●*Character:* Tall stature with long limbs and lax joints ●*Location:* Musculoskeletal ●*Pattern:* Nonspecific ●*Precipitating factors:* Chromosomal abnormality with autosomal dominance with abnormal synthesis of fibrillin ●*Relieving factors:* Physical therapy to improve muscle tone, moderate exercise, endocarditis prophylaxis, beta-adrenergics to prevent aortic dilatation ●*Clinical course:* Decreased longevity secondary to aortic root dilitation and rupture ●*Co-morbidities:* Hypotonia and lax ligaments, long thin limbs, lens dislocation, arachnodactyly, pectus carinatum, mitral valve prolapse, aortic root dilatation ●*Procedure results:* Cardiac Echo: aortic root dilatation, mitral valve prolapse; slit lamp examination: lens abnormalities ●*Test findings:* Negative amino acid studies

Mastalgia ●*Onset:* Subacute, insidious ●*Male:female ratio:* F ●*Ethnicity:* All ●*Character:* Aching or sharp pain in one or both breasts ●*Location:* Diffuse, localized ●*Pattern:* Cyclic, noncyclic ●*Precipitating factors:* Cyclic mastalgia associated with normal hormonal changes; unproven: excess caffeine ●*Relieving factors:* NSAIDs; cyclic pain treated with danazol, bromocriptine, tamoxifen; noncyclic breast pain improves with removal of underlying lesion if present ●*Clinical course:* Variable ●*Co-morbidities:* Fibroadenomas, musculoskeletal chest wall pain ●*Procedure results:* Excisional biopsy confirms fibroadenoma ●*Test findings:* U/S distinguishes solid mass or cystic lesion, mammogram positive for nonspecific abnormality; cyclic mastalgia has no detectable abnormality

Mastoiditis ●*Onset:* Acute ●*Male:female ratio:* M=F ●*Ethnicity:* All ●*Character:* Severe ear pain with hearing loss and fever ●*Location:* Affected ear ●*Pattern:* Persistent or worsening pain ●*Precipitating factors:* Antecedent upper respiratory tract infection or history of ear disease ●*Relieving factors:* None relevant ●*Clinical course:* May progress to neurologic or serious otologic complications ●*Co-morbidities:* History of chronic ear disease ●*Procedure results:* Otoscopy reveals bulging red eardrum; mastoid region is swollen and or exquisitely tender; auricle may be reflected forward ●*Test findings:* No relevant tests

Measles ●*Onset:* Acute ●*Male:female ratio:* M=F ●*Ethnicity:* All ●*Character:* Upper respiratory symptoms and fever, followed by a nonpruritic maculopapular rash beginning on the face and spreading down the trunk and extremities ●*Location:* Upper respiratory, systemic, skin (behind the ears spreading to trunk and limbs, including palms and soles), oral mucosa, lungs, CNS, mesenteric lymph nodes, other ●*Pattern:* Rash begins after fever; Koplik's spots appear just before the rash; rash begins on face, spreads down the trunk and limbs, and includes the palms and soles ●*Precipitating factors:* Sick contact, winter and spring epidemics, lack of immunization ●*Relieving factors:* None relevant ●*Clinical course:* Incubation: 10 days; prodrome: 2-4 days; illness lasts about 10 days, self-limiting with 0.3-10% mortality from complications, more severe in adults ●*Co-morbidities:* None relevant ●*Procedure results:* Multinucleated giant cells/positive measles immunofluorescence assay in respiratory secretions, isolations of virus from culture, positive measles IgM ●*Test findings:* Leukopenia, lymphopenia, mildly elevated hepatic transaminases (less common)

Meatal stenosis ●*Onset:* Subacute ●*Male:female ratio:* M ●*Ethnicity:* All ●*Character:* Difficulty in directing the stream into the toilet; dysuria ●*Location:* Penis, distal meatus ●*Pattern:* Nonspecific ●*Precipitating factors:* Circumcision, hypospadias repair ●*Relieving factors:* Meatotomy, dilatation with a catheter (rarely successful) ●*Clinical course:* Progressive if untreated in severe stenosis ●*Co-morbidities:* Circumcision, hypospadias ●*Procedure results:* No relevant procedures ●*Test findings:* No relevant tests

Meckel's diverticulum ●*Onset:* Subacute/acute ●*Male:female ratio:* M=F ●*Ethnicity:* All ●*Character:* Intermittent painless bleeding ●*Location:* Rectal ●*Pattern:* Painless currant jelly or melanotic stools ●*Precipitating factors:* Acid-secreting mucosa causes ulceration of adjacent ileal mucosa ●*Relieving factors:* Surgery ●*Clinical course:* Recurrent until surgery ●*Co-morbidities:* Intussusception, volvulus, hypovolemia, anemia ●*Procedure results:* Positive uptake of technetium on a Meckel's radionuclide scan ●*Test findings:* Anemia

Meconium ileus ●*Onset:* Acute ●*Male:female ratio:* M=F ●*Ethnicity:* All ●*Character:* Abdominal distension/pain, bilious vomiting, failure to pass meconium ●*Location:* Abdomen/intestine (ileum) ●*Pattern:* Worsening symptoms ●*Precipitating factors:* None relevant ●*Relieving factors:* Disimpaction with water soluble enemas/IV antibiotics/surgery ●*Clinical course:* Progressive unless underlying cause treated: peritonitis/perforation ●*Co-morbidities:* Cystic fibrosis, Hirschsprung disease ●*Procedure results:* No relevant procedures ●*Test findings:* Plain films of abdomen show ground glass appearance in right lower quadrant, air/fluid levels, peritoneal calcification, pneumoperitoneum, abnormal contrast studies of intestine

Medial epicondylitis ●*Onset:* Subacute ●*Male:female ratio:* M=F ●*Ethnicity:* All ●*Character:* Dull ache ●*Location:* Medial elbow ●*Pattern:* Worse with use ●*Precipitating factors:* Wrist flexion ●*Relieving factors:* NSAIDs, ice, U/S treatment, cortisone injection ●*Clinical course:* Gradual improvement ●*Co-morbidities:* None relevant ●*Procedure results:* No relevant procedures ●*Test findings:* No relevant tests

Megaloblastic anemias ●*Onset:* Insidious ●*Male:female ratio:* M=F ●*Ethnicity:* All ●*Character:* Fatigue, weakness, dyspnea on exertion ●*Location:* Nonspecific ●*Pattern:* Nonspecific ●*Precipitating factors:* Drugs that impair DNA metabolism, pregnancy, excessive alcohol intake, inadequate intake of vitamin B12 or folate ●*Relieving factors:* Specific replacement therapy (vitamin B12, folate), blood transfusions, treatment of the underlying disorder if one exists ●*Clinical course:* Progressive unless treated ●*Co-morbidities:* Alcoholism, malabsorptive syndromes (sprue, Crohn's), pernicious anemia, gastrectomy, rare enzyme deficiencies ●*Procedure results:* Bone marrow biopsy: hypercellular, megaloblastic changes; nuclear: cytoplasmic asynchronism in erythroid cells ●*Test findings:* Anemia, elevated mean corpuscular volume (at least >100fL), anisocytosis, low reticulocyte count, hypersegmented neutrophils, misshapen platelets

Megaureter ●*Onset:* Chronic ●*Male:female ratio:* M(3):F(1) ●*Ethnicity:* All ●*Character:* Mostly identified on prenatal U/S; pain and discomfort in some individuals ●*Location:* Abdomen, flank and pelvis ●*Pattern:* Nonspecific ●*Precipitating factors:* Secondary megaureter precipitated by bladder neck obstruction, neurogenic bladder, or prior surgery ●*Relieving factors:* Surgical correction in primary megaureter; correction and treatment of all secondary causes of megaureter ●*Clinical course:* Progressive if untreated; need to differentiate between primary and secondary megaureters ●*Co-morbidities:* Bladder neck obstruction, neurogenic bladder, prior surgery ●*Procedure results:* Voiding cystourethrogram possibly showing vesicoureteral reflux; diuresis renal scan possibly showing obstruction ●*Test findings:* U/S, intravenous pyelogram and CT: hydroureteronephrosis

Meig's syndrome ●*Onset:* Insidious ●*Male:female ratio:* M=F ●*Ethnicity:* All ●*Character:* Weight loss, dyspnea, chest tightness ●*Location:* Pleural effusion: unilateral (80%) and rightsided (c. 90%) > leftsided ●*Pattern:* Dullness to percussion and decreased breath sounds, abdominal ascites ●*Precipitating factors:* Secretion of large amounts of fluid by ovarian or uterine tumors leads to ascites and, if pores in the diaphragm, pleural effusion ●*Relieving factors:* Removal or treatment of pelvic tumor ●*Clinical course:* Chronic and progressive without treatment ●*Co-morbidities:* Ascites associated with ovarian tumors (benign or malignant, cystic or solid), fibromyomas ●*Procedure results:* Chest X-ray, abdominal U/S: pleural effusion associated with ascites and pelvic mass ●*Test findings:* Pleural effusion: exudate with WBC <1000/mm³

Melanoma ●*Onset:* Subacute, insidious ●*Male:female ratio:* M=F ●*Ethnicity:* Fair skin ❶ *Character:* Bleeding, growing papule ❷ *Location:* Any skin site ❸ *Pattern:* Dark/multicolored, irregular shape ●*Precipitating factors:* None relevant ●*Relieving factors:* Excision ●*Clinical course:* Fatal if not treated ●*Co-morbidities:* None relevant ●*Procedure results:* No relevant procedures ●*Test findings:* Positive skin biopsy

Images of ❶ *Character,* ❷ *Location,* ❸ *Pattern on page 546*

Melanoma: Images *see text page 545*

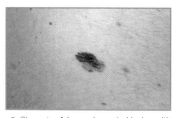

❶ *Character A large pigmented lesion with irregular edges and variegated color*

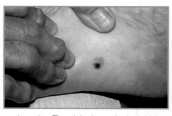

❷ *Location The pink plaque is the initial mole. The black lesion within is the melanoma*

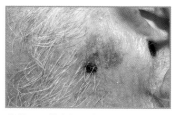

❸ *Pattern Nodular melanoma arising in lentigo maligna melanoma*

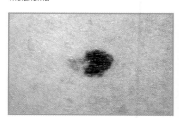

❸ *Pattern Growing black area with irregular edges and an adjacent pink macule*

Membranous glomerulonephritis ●*Onset:* Subacute ●*Male:female ratio:* M=F ●*Ethnicity:* All ●*Character:* Second most common cause of nephrotic syndrome in non-diabetic adults ●*Location:* IgG, other immunoglobulins and complement deposit in subepithelial space ●*Pattern:* Normal BP and peripheral edema present at onset ●*Precipitating factors:* Most often idiopathic; drugs: gold or penicillamine toxicity, NSAIDs, captopril; chronic renal transplant rejection ●*Relieving factors:* Cytotoxic drugs: cyclophosphamide or chlorambucil; cyclosporine for nonresponders; glucocorticosteroids used but rarely effecitve ●*Clinical course:* Spontaneous remission in 5-20% cases, partial remission in 25-40%; some progress to end-stage renal disease; prognosis worst in male patients and those with heavy proteinuria ●*Co-morbidities:* Other renal diseases: focal glomerulosclerosis, diabetic nephropathy, IgA nephropathy, crescentic glomerulonephritis; renal vein thrombosis; malignancy, especially solid tumors; systemic lupus erythematosus; hepatitis B and C; congenital or secondary syphillis; sarcoidosis; Sjogren's syndrome; schistosomiasis ●*Procedure results:* Renal biopsy, light microscopy: basement membrane thickening, no cellular infiltration; electron microscopy: electron-dense deposits across glomerular basement membrane in subepithelial space; immunofluorescence is positive ●*Test findings:* Urine sediment and plasma creatinine normal or minimally abnormal at onset

Ménière's disease ●*Onset:* Chronic recurrent/episodic ●*Male:female ratio:* M=F ●*Ethnicity:* None ●*Character:* Vertiginous episodes with fluctuating hearing loss, aural pressure, and tinnitus ●*Location:* Affected ear (infrequently bilateral) ●*Pattern:* Episodes last 2 to 24h ●*Precipitating factors:* None relevant ●*Relieving factors:* Patients usually are immobilized during acute attack ●*Clinical course:* Episodes spontaneously remit, with lingering sense of the imbalance for days; episodes can come at extremely variable frequencies ●*Co-morbidities:* Allergy or autoimmune disease ●*Procedure results:* During acute attack: normal otoscopy, pronounced nystagmus, emesis, imbalance; in between attacks: normal examination ●*Test findings:* Audiogram usually demonstrates sensorineural hearing loss in affected ear

Meningioma ●*Onset:* Subacute/insidious ●*Male:female ratio:* M=F ●*Ethnicity:* All ●*Character:* Asymptomatic, headache, seizures, mental status change ●*Location:* CNS ●*Pattern:* Nonspecific ●*Precipitating factors:* None relevant ●*Relieving factors:* Neurosurgical intervention ●*Clinical course:* Extremely slow in progression in most cases ●*Co-morbidities:* None relevant ●*Procedure results:* No relevant procedures ●*Test findings:* MRI of the brain

Meningococcemia ●*Onset:* Acute (common)/chronic (very rare) ●*Male:female ratio:* M=F ●*Ethnicity:* All ●*Character:* Sudden onset of fever, prostration, maculopapular-petechial rash, disseminated intravascular coagulation (DIC), rapidly progressive multiple organ failure ●*Location:* Systemic (septicemic) illness involving skin (including palms and soles), coagulation cascade (DIC), meninges, CNS, cardiovascular collapse, multiple organ failure ●*Pattern:* Fever is of sudden onset and very high (rarely hypothermia); rash develops over several hours, is maculopapular-petechial, rapidly becoming hemorrhagic, on the trunk and limbs (lower extremities > upper extremities); may involve palms, soles, conjunctivae, palate; fulminant meningitis is common ●*Precipitating factors:* Worldwide distribution, close sick contacts, outbreaks, epidemics in sub-Saharan Africa, China, South America, deficiency in a terminal complement component ●*Relieving factors:* None relevant ●*Clinical course:* Rapidly progressive over hours leading to multiple organ failure, shock, and death if untreated; some cases are mild; rarely, mild chronic infection over weeks-to-months ●*Co-morbidities:* Deficiency in a terminal complement component (C5-9), properdin deficiency, influenza A, seizures, hydrocephalus, DIC, herpes labialis ●*Procedure results:* Gram-negative diplococci in blood or CSF (rarely petechial aspirate, synovium, pleura, other), isolation of organism from blood, CSF, other, rapid immunoassay ●*Test findings:* Leukocytosis with bandemia (may be normal or low), thrombocytopenia, prolonged prothrombin time (PT) and partial thromboplastin time (PTT), increased fibrin split products, decreased fibrinogen (DIC), low CSF glucose, neutrophilic CSF pleocytosis (may be normal), Gram-negative diplococci in blood or CSF

Meniscal tear ●*Onset:* Acute ●*Male:female ratio:* M=F ●*Ethnicity:* All ●*Character:* Sharp pain with occasional locking of the knee ●*Location:* Knee joint line ●*Pattern:* Worse with flexion of the affected knee ●*Precipitating factors:* Sudden traumatic flexion ●*Relieving factors:* Anti-inflammatory agents, physical therapy to strengthen quadriceps and hamstring muscles, meniscectomy ●*Clinical course:* Symptoms of meniscal irritation often temporary unless meniscal tear is large ●*Co-morbidities:* Obesity ●*Procedure results:* Knee MRI with meniscal tear ●*Test findings:* Synovial fluid analysis: WBC <500 cells/mL

Menopause ●*Onset:* Subacute onset over months or abrupt onset ●*Male:female ratio:* F ●*Ethnicity:* All ●*Character:* Hiatus in menses progressing to cessation ●*Location:* Nonspecific ●*Pattern:* No menses for one year; vasomotor instability, insomnia, urogenital atrophy ●*Precipitating factors:* Can be induced by oophorectomy, chemotherapeutic agents, radiation therapy ●*Relieving factors:* Symptoms reduced/relieved by estrogen replacement therapy ●*Clinical course:* Symptoms last average of 6-24 months, up to 5 years ●*Co-morbidities:* Osteoporosis, myalgias/arthralgias, increased risk of cardiovascular disease ●*Procedure results:* No relevant procedures ●*Test findings:* Elevated follicle-stimulating hormone, estradiol <30pg/mL

Menstrual headache ●*Onset:* Acute, subacute ●*Male:female ratio:* F ●*Ethnicity:* All ●*Character:* Throbbing sensation in the bitemporal, bifrontal, or occipital area ●*Location:* Nonspecific ●*Pattern:* Usually associated with visual symptomatology, nausea, vomiting; may have ataxia, confusion, weakness or paresthesias ●*Precipitating factors:* Menstruation, stress, anxiety, fatigue, hunger ●*Relieving factors:* Analgesics, rest, sleep, stress reduction ●*Clinical course:* Self-limited and occurs only around the time of menstruation ●*Co-morbidities:* None relevant ●*Procedure results:* No relevant procedures ●*Test findings:* Normal neurological examination

Meralgia paresthetica ●*Onset:* Gradual ●*Male:female ratio:* M=F ●*Ethnicity:* All ●*Character:* Pain and/or dysesthesia in anterolateral thigh ●*Location:* Compression of lateral cutaneous nerve in course from lumbosacral plexus through abdomen under inguinal ligament to subcutaneous thigh ●*Pattern:* Abnormal pinprick/light touch on anterolateral thigh ●*Precipitating factors:* Obesity, tight garments around waist, scar tissue at inguinal ligament ●*Relieving factors:* Weight loss, avoidance of tight garments at waist ●*Clinical course:* Benign and self-limited ●*Co-morbidities:* Obesity, injury or prior surgery leading to scarring at inguinal ligament ●*Procedure results:* Electromyogram and nerve conduction velocity likely normal in mild cases ●*Test findings:* Abnormal pinprick and light touch testing along lateral thigh; remainder of neurological examination of lower extremities within normal levels

Mesenteric adenitis ●*Onset:* Acute ●*Male:female ratio:* M=F ●*Ethnicity:* All ●*Character:* Acute/sharp abdominal pain, diffuse localized; fever ●*Location:* Right lower quadrant abdominal pain ●*Pattern:* Worsening pain/symptoms ●*Precipitating factors:* Yersinia infection ●*Relieving factors:* Pain control, self-limited ●*Clinical course:* Self-limited unless bacteremia - then treat with antibiotics ●*Co-morbidities:* Yersinia pseudotuberculosis infection ●*Procedure results:* Possible positive culture of tissue/blood ●*Test findings:* Normal appendix on CT and U/S; enlarged mesenteric lymph nodes, thickened terminal ileum on U/S; culture positive lymph node for Yersinia pseudotuberculosis

Mesothelioma ●*Onset:* Insidious ●*Male:female ratio:* M>F ●*Ethnicity:* All ●*Character:* Nonpleuritic chest wall pain, dyspnea, fever/chills, less commonly: asymptomatic pleural effusion, dysphagia, lower extremity weakness, Horner's syndrome, facial plethora and upper extremity swelling ●*Location:* Right lung involved more commonly than the left ●*Pattern:* Nonspecific ●*Precipitating factors:* Asbestos exposure, less commonly previous radiation therapy and Thorotrast (contrast agent) exposure ●*Relieving factors:* Surgery, radiation, chemotherapy or a combination ●*Clinical course:* Depends on several prognostic factors. Median survival 4-18 months ●*Co-morbidities:* None relevant ●*Procedure results:* Pleural biopsy confirming mesothelioma; thoracentesis: exudative, hemorrhagic fluid ●*Test findings:* Chest X-ray: unilateral pleural effusion, pleural plaques, interstitial fibrosis

Metabolic acidosis ●*Onset:* Acute or subacute varying with underlying disorder ●*Male:female ratio:* M=F ●*Ethnicity:* All ●*Character:* Low serum pH and low bicarbonate concentration ●*Location:* Nonspecific symptoms: diarrhea, hyperventilation, hypotension, anorexia, or coma ●*Pattern:* Nonspecific ●*Precipitating factors:* Ketoacidosis, starvation, alcohol, lactic acidosis, diarrhea and enterostomy, ingestions of salicylates, ethylene glycol; administration of acetazolamide, ammonium chloride, lysine hydrochloride, arginine hydrochloride ●*Relieving factors:* Administration of serum bicarbonate controversial; correction of volume status; IV insulin for diabetic ketoacidosis; initiation of hemodialysis for uremia; oral sodium citrate/sodium bicarbonate for chronic nonemergent acidosis ●*Clinical course:* Varies with underlying disorder and severity; can be rapidly fatal if treatment not initiated emergently in cases of ingestion or diabetic ketoacidosis ●*Co-morbidities:* Diabetes, alcoholism, endstage renal disease, diarrhea ●*Procedure results:* No relevant procedures ●*Test findings:* Etiology determined by: blood urea nitrogen, creatinine, glucose, lactate, serum ketones, serum osmolality and toxic screen; anion gap suggests underlying disorder: normal in type 1 and type 2 renal tubular acidosis; elevated anion gap associated with uremia in chronic renal failure

Metabolic encephalopathy ●*Onset:* Usually subacute ●*Male:female ratio:* M=F ●*Ethnicity:* All ●*Character:* Character depends on the specific etiology; hepatic encephalopathy is episodic, with ataxia, action tremor, asterixis ('flapping tremor'), sensorial clouding and dysarthria; uremic encephalopathy is characterized by dysarthria, gait instability, asterixis and multifocal myoclonus (uremic twitching) ●*Location:* Pseudolaminar necrosis in the cerebral and cerebellar cortex and neuronal loss in the basal ganglia and cerebellum ●*Pattern:* Can develop as acute delirium, but usually begin with mental dullness and drowsiness, patients drift in and out of sleep, but remain easily arousable; stretch reflexes become brisk, and patients can develop a positive babinski reflex; deeper stages of coma can manifest with decerebrate and decorticate posturing ●*Precipitating factors:* Chronic liver disease (high protein diet), chronic renal disease, anticonvulsants, cimetidine, steroids, hemodialysis, radiation therapy, methotrexate and sudden hydration ●*Relieving factors:* Hepatic or renal transplant, discontinuation of inciting drug or procedure ●*Clinical course:* Without definitive therapy, patients usually progress to a stage of reduced cognition and frequent episodes of delirium ●*Co-morbidities:* Chronic liver disease and chronic renal disease; excessive alcohol intake ●*Procedure results:* If hepatic or renal transplant prior to permanent neuronal damage, recovery can occur ●*Test findings:* Early on, CT scans can show cortical atrophy, cerebral edema, and MRI may show increased signal in the globus pallidus in T1 weighted studies

Metastatic cancer ●*Onset:* Subacute/insidious ●*Male:female ratio:* M=F ●*Ethnicity:* All ●*Character:* Varies with location; weight loss, pain, and anemia common accompanying symptoms ●*Location:* Bone, lung, liver, brain, breast, skin, other ●*Pattern:* Nonspecific ●*Precipitating factors:* Prior history of cancer ●*Relieving factors:* Varies with histology and location; chemotherapy, surgery and radiotherapy are potential options ●*Clinical course:* Varies with histolgy, location; overall prognosis is poor with few cures ●*Co-morbidities:* None relevant ●*Procedure results:* Imaging and/or biopsy depending on location and primary tumor ●*Test findings:* Anemia, raised ESR frequently found

Metastatic neoplasm of the liver ●*Onset:* Subacute/insidious ●*Male:female ratio:* M=F ●*Ethnicity:* All ●*Character:* Malaise, weight loss, right upper quadrant pain, abdominal swelling, jaundice ●*Location:* Nonspecific ●*Pattern:* Nonspecific ●*Precipitating factors:* Wide variety of malignancies, most commonly lung and breast ●*Relieving factors:* Treatment of underlying cancer, liver transplant if primary tumor removed and liver metastasis is solitary, directed therapies (ethanol injection, cryotherapy, laser therapy) ●*Clinical course:* Prognosis depends on extent of liver replacement; overall prognosis is poor with few cures ●*Co-morbidities:* Primary cancer of various types ●*Procedure results:* Hepatic lesion on U/S, CT, or MRI; guided liver biopsy: positive for metastatic tumor; paracentesis if ascites, can show malignant cells ●*Test findings:* Elevated transaminases, alkaline phosphatase (disproportionately high) and bilirubin; if advanced, elevated prothrombin time/partial thromboplastin time, decreased albumin

Metastatic neoplasm of the lung ●*Onset:* Acute/subacute/insidious ●*Male:female ratio:* M=F ●*Ethnicity:* All ●*Character:* Cough, shortness of breath, dyspnea on exertion, hemoptysis, wheezing ●*Location:* Chest ●*Pattern:* Nonspecific ●*Precipitating factors:* Metastatic cancer ●*Relieving factors:* Treatment of underlying cancer, including radiation and chemotherapy ●*Clinical course:* Progressive unless cured ●*Co-morbidities:* Dependent on underlying cause ●*Procedure results:* Lung biopsy shows malignant cells, sputum sample may show malignant cells ●*Test findings:* Chest X-ray may show mass, lymphadenopathy, or interstitial disease

Metatarsalgia ●*Onset:* Subacute ●*Male:female ratio:* M<F ●*Ethnicity:* All ●*Character:* Burning ache ●*Location:* Metatarsal heads ●*Pattern:* Pain worsens with weightbearing ●*Precipitating factors:* Worse at the end of the day ●*Relieving factors:* Orthotic devices, change in footwear ●*Clinical course:* Progressive ●*Co-morbidities:* Rheumatoid arthritis, degenerative arthritis, obesity ●*Procedure results:* No relevant procedures ●*Test findings:* No relevant tests

Methemoglobinemia ●*Onset:* Acute, subacute, chronic ●*Male:female ratio:* M=F ●*Ethnicity:* All ●*Character:* Blue skin color; in severe cases: headache, weakness, breathlessness, or death ●*Location:* Nonspecific ●*Pattern:* Nonspecific ●*Precipitating factors:* Hereditary or acquired; acquired form due to exposure to drugs: nitrates, nitrites, sulfonamides, lidocaine, aniline dyes ●*Relieving factors:* Oral methylene blue or ascorbic acid; IV methylene blue for severe cases ●*Clinical course:* Full recovery with treatment ●*Co-morbidities:* Rule out cyanosis due to heart or lung disease ●*Procedure results:* No relevant procedures ●*Test findings:* No relevant tests

Migraine headache ●*Onset:* Acute, subacute ●*Male:female ratio:* M(1):F(3) ●*Ethnicity:* All ●*Character:* Throbbing sensation in the bitemporal, bifrontal, or occipital area ●*Location:* Nonspecific ●*Pattern:* Usually associated with visual symptomatology, nausea, vomiting; may have ataxia, confusion, weakness, or paresthesias ●*Precipitating factors:* Menstruation, stress, anxiety, fatigue, hunger ●*Relieving factors:* Analgesics, rest, sleep, stress reduction ●*Clinical course:* Usually self-limited but can last hours, days, weeks or months ●*Co-morbidities:* None relevant ●*Procedure results:* No relevant procedures ●*Test findings:* Normal neurological examination

Milk-alkali syndrome ●*Onset:* Acute, subacute (Cope's), or chronic (Burnett's) forms ●*Male:female ratio:* M<F ●*Ethnicity:* All ●*Character:* Triad: hypercalcemia, metabolic alkalosis, renal insufficiency (hypercalcemia manifestations: nausea/vomiting, constipation, weakness, mental status changes, polyuria, polydipsia, muscle aches, pruritis, metastatic calcifications/nephrocalcinosis) ●*Location:* Nonspecific ●*Pattern:* Nonspecific ●*Precipitating factors:* Ingestion of excessive calcium and alkali (antacids/calcium carbonate) ●*Relieving factors:* Stop calcium/alkali ingestion, hydration, furosemide after IV fluid ●*Clinical course:* Resolves with conservative therapy; renal insufficiency may persist in subacute/chronic forms despite correction of hypercalcemia ●*Co-morbidities:* Renal insufficiency, metabolic bone disease possible due to hypercalcemia and secondary hypoparathryoidism ●*Procedure results:* Serology ●*Test findings:* Hypophosphatemia (precedes decreased glomerular filtration rate), increased creatinine, elevated bicarbonate (28-40mEq/L) and serum pH (7.47-7.62); decreased parathyroid hormone may be seen

Millard-Gubler syndrome ●*Onset:* Acute ●*Male:female ratio:* M=F ●*Ethnicity:* All ●*Character:* Nonspecific ●*Location:* Brainstem ●*Pattern:* Nonspecific ●*Precipitating factors:* Hypertension, diabetes ●*Relieving factors:* Supportive care ●*Clinical course:* Static ●*Co-morbidities:* Hypertension, diabetes, tobacco use, heavy alcohol, elevated cholesterol ●*Procedure results:* MRI of the brain ●*Test findings:* No relevant tests

Miscarriage ●*Onset:* Subacute ●*Male:female ratio:* F ●*Ethnicity:* All ●*Character:* Vaginal bleeding or cramping ●*Location:* Uterine cramping ●*Pattern:* Minor cramping and/or light bleeding gradually crescendos over hours to days ●*Precipitating factors:* Rare; usually spontaneous ●*Relieving factors:* Spontaneous passage of pregnancy tissue or a D&C ●*Clinical course:* Symptoms usually abate over 1-2 hours after passage of tissue ●*Co-morbidities:* Diabetes ●*Procedure results:* No relevant procedures ●*Test findings:* U/S shows fetal loss

Mitral regurgitation ●*Onset:* Insidious, acute ●*Male:female ratio:* M=F ●*Ethnicity:* All ●*Character:* Chronic disease: fatigue and dyspnea, progresses to orthopnea, paroxysmal nocturnal dyspnea, peripheral edema; acute disease: acute pulmonary edema ●*Location:* Lungs ●*Pattern:* Worse with exertion and lying down ●*Precipitating factors:* Rheumatic fever, mitral valve prolapse, infarction/ischemia, left ventricle dilatation, annular calcification, endocarditis, rupture of papillary muscles/chordae tendinae, connective tissue disease, increased afterload, prolonged PR interval ●*Relieving factors:* Diuretics, vasodilators (e.g. ACE inhibitors in chronic disease, nitroprusside/intra-aortic balloon pump in acute regurgitation); revascularization if ischemic in origin; mitral valve repair/replacement if severe symptoms and left ventricle end diastolic dimension >6cm or if acute and surgery not contraindicated; recommend endocarditis prophylaxis ●*Clinical course:* Chronic disease: may be asymptomatic for years; prognosis depends on etiology and left ventricle function; acute disease: rapid progression to severe symptoms and death ●*Co-morbidities:* Rheumatic fever, mitral valve prolapse, coronary artery disease, cardiomyopathy, endocarditis, congenital heart disease, connective tissue diseases, atrial fibrillation ●*Procedure results:* Echo determines mitral valve/papillary muscle/chordal anatomy and extent of blood going into left atrium in systole by Doppler; also allows assessment of left ventricle dimensions and ejection fraction; chest X-ray: large left ventricle and atrium ●*Test findings:* Examination with holosystolic apical murmur radiating to axilla, decreased S1, +S3; ECG with left atrial and left ventricular enlargement with or without atrial fibrillation

Mitral regurgitation secondary to papillary muscle dysfunction ●*Onset:* Usually acute, but can be insidious ●*Male:female ratio:* M=F ●*Ethnicity:* All ●*Character:* Shortness of breath, orthopnea, paroxysmal nocturnal dyspnea, chest pain, fatigue, congestive hepatomegaly, edema, ascites ●*Location:* Chest ●*Pattern:* Worse with exertion and lying down ●*Precipitating factors:* Coronary artery disease, severe anemia, shock, coronary arteritis, anomalous left coronary artery, left ventricle dilatation, papillary muscle infiltration by amyloid/sarcoid/granuloma/neoplasm, congenital malposition or absence of a papillary muscle, trauma ●*Relieving factors:* Diuretics, vasodilators (e.g. ACE inhibitors in chronic disease; nitroprusside/intra-aortic balloon pump in acute regurgitation); revascularization if ischemic in origin; mitral valve repair/replacement if acute and surgery not contraindicated; endocarditis prophylaxis recommended ●*Clinical course:* If chronic can have slow progression, ultimately leading to ventricular dysfunction; if acute can be fatal if not treated ●*Co-morbidities:* Coronary artery disease, dilated cardiomyopathy, amyloidosis, sarcoidosis, parachute mitral valve, trauma ●*Procedure results:* Echo of chronic mitral regurgitation (MR): dilated left atrium and ventricle and MR; acute MR: normal left atrial and ventricular size with severe MR; Swan-Ganz catheter with elevation of PA pressure ●*Test findings:* Examination in acute MR with +S3, +S4, soft systolic, decrescendo murmur at the apex radiating to the axilla; chest X-ray with pulmonary edema

Mitral stenosis ●*Onset:* Insidious ●*Male:female ratio:* M<F ●*Ethnicity:* All (more common in developing world) ●*Character:* Shortness of breath, orthopnea, paroxysmal nocturnal dyspnea, chest pain, hemoptysis, hoarseness, palpitations, stroke ●*Location:* Chest ●*Pattern:* Worse with exertion, stress, infection, fever, pregnancy, atrial fibrillation ●*Precipitating factors:* Rheumatic fever, carcinoid, systemic lupus erythematosus, rheumatoid arthritis, amyloid, obstruction due to left atrial thrombus, tumor or vegetation ●*Relieving factors:* Decreased salt intake, diuretics, and beta-blockers for mild symptoms; digoxin and coumadin in patients with atrial fibrillation; mitral balloon valvuloplasty or mitral valve surgery in moderate-to-severe symptoms, valve area of <1cm2, and/or pulmonary hypertension ●*Clinical course:* Asymptomatic for 15-20 yrs, then progress from mild to severe within 3 yrs ●*Co-morbidities:* Rheumatic fever, carcinoid, systemic lupus erythematosus, rheumatoid arthritis, amyloid, obstruction due to left atrial thrombus, tumor or vegetation ●*Procedure results:* Echo with reduced mitral valve area, increased transmitral gradient, evidence of left atrial enlargement ●*Test findings:* On examination, loud S1, opening snap followed by rumbling, low-pitched diastolic murmur at apex; opening snap and diastolic murmur reduced during inspiration and augmented during expiration

Mitral valve prolapse ●*Onset:* Insidious ●*Male:female ratio:* M(1):F(2) ●*Ethnicity:* All ●*Character:* Asymptomatic to nonspecific: atypical chest pain, fatigue, palpitations, postural orthostasis and other symptoms of autonomic dysfunction ●*Location:* Apical chest ●*Pattern:* Brief attacks of pain not related to exertion ●*Precipitating factors:* Myxomatous valvular disease ●*Relieving factors:* Asymptomatic with mitral regurgitation: endocarditis prophylaxis; symptomatic: beta-blockers; patients with cerebral embolic events: anticoagulation; significant mitral regurgitation: surgery ●*Clinical course:* Asymptomatic for several years with progressive development of mitral regurgitation; increased incidence of cerebrovascular embolic events in these patients; low but increased incidence of sudden death ●*Co-morbidities:* Marfan's syndrome, Ehlers-Danlos, osteogenesis imperfecta, pseudoxanthoma elasticum, periarteritis nodosa, myotonic dystrophy, von Willebrand's disease, hyperthyroidism, Ebstein's anomaly, Holt-Oram syndrome, ischemic heart disease ●*Procedure results:* Echo demonstrates valve prolapse; mitral regurgitation may or not be present ●*Test findings:* Examination: mid-systolic click with or without mid-late systolic murmur, loudest at the apex and radiating to the axilla

Mononucleosis ●*Onset:* Acute/subacute ●*Male:female ratio:* M=F ●*Ethnicity:* All ●*Character:* Malaise followed by fever, lymphadenopathy, sore throat ●*Location:* Systemic ●*Pattern:* A prodrome of fatigue, myalgia, and malaise lasts 1-2 weeks; lymphadenopathy and pharyngitis with exudates appear before splenomegaly and hepatitis; macular rash appears after ampicillin use ●*Precipitating factors:* Contact with oral secretions (kissing); less common: blood transfusion, transplantation ●*Relieving factors:* None relevant ●*Clinical course:* Incubation: 4-6 weeks, prodrome: 1-2 weeks, symptomatic illness: 2-4 weeks, convalescence: weeks-to-months; symptoms are uncommon in young children; most cases are self-limited ●*Co-morbidities:* Erythema nodosum, erythema multiforme, ampicillin rash, autoimmune hemolytic anemia, Guillain-Barré syndrome, splenic rupture, oral hairy leukoplakia (in HIV) ●*Procedure results:* Positive heterophile test, positive EBV-specific (anti-VCA) IgM ●*Test findings:* Common: elevated WBC, lymphocytosis (>10%), atypical lymphocytes (mildly), elevated hepatic transaminases, elevated bilirubin; less common: thrombocytopenia, anemia, neutropenia

Motion sickness ●*Onset:* Acute ●*Male:female ratio:* M=F ●*Ethnicity:* All ●*Character:* Nausea, sensation of imbalance and disorientation ●*Location:* Nonspecific ●*Pattern:* Nonspecific ●*Precipitating factors:* Occurs in moving vehicles, boats, amusement rides ●*Relieving factors:* Anticholinergics, antihistamines ●*Clinical course:* Self-limited ●*Co-morbidities:* None relevant ●*Procedure results:* No relevant procedures ●*Test findings:* No relevant tests

Mucocutaneous candidiasis ●*Onset:* Acute, subacute (common), chronic (CMC) is rare ●*Male:female ratio:* M<F ●*Ethnicity:* All ●*Character:* Creamy white patches on the tongue (thrush), odynophagia (esophagitis), vulvar pruritus, curdlike discharge (vaginitis) ●*Location:* Mouth (thrush), vagina, gluteal/neck/groin skin folds (intertrigo), nails (paronychia), perineum (diaper rash), penis (balanitis), esophagus, other GI, hair follicles, chronic mucocutaneous (skin, nails, hairs) ●*Pattern:* Creamy white patches on the tongue or palate (thrush), thick curdlike vaginal discharge and extreme pruritus (vaginitis) ●*Precipitating factors:* Antibacterial therapy, oral contraceptive pill, steroid and antimetabolite therapy, diabetes mellitus, HIV, AIDS, pregnancy, immersion of hands in water (paronychia), T cell dysfunction (CMC) ●*Relieving factors:* Discontinuation of antibacterials, topical nystatin or azole, oral azole, IV amphotericin (in severe cases) ●*Clinical course:* Resolution with therapy common, relapses common: especially if predisposing factor ongoing, CMC is chronic and progressive; patients often succumb to bacterial superinfections ●*Co-morbidities:* HIV and AIDS, diabetes mellitus, steroid therapy; CMC: hypothyroidism, Addison's, thymic dysfunction ●*Procedure results:* Irregular mucosa on barium esophagram, pseudomembranes on esophageal endoscopy ●*Test findings:* Yeast and pseudohyphae on potassium hydroxide-suspended/Gram-stained skin scrapings, growth of Candida in culture (rarely needed)

Mucopolysaccharidosis ●*Onset:* Variable depending on specific mutation; usually early childhood ●*Male:female ratio:* M=F (except in X-linked inheritance) ●*Ethnicity:* All ●*Character:* Phenotypic variance including mental retardation, visceromegaly, coarse facies, corneal clouding, joint stiffness, hernias, dysostosis multiplex; gigantism often occurs early; extent of neurologic vs somatic sequelae depends on specific enzyme defect; some forms allow adult survival with normal intelligence ●*Location:* Systemic condition; affected areas often reflective of storage sites of biochemical substrate with abnormal metabolism/inadequate degradation due to enzymatic defect (i.e. heparin sulfate, dermatan sulfate, and keratin sulfate) ●*Pattern:* Broad spectrum of diseases due to deficiencies of one of a group of enzymes which degrade heparin sulfate, dermatan sulfate, and keratin sulfate; pattern is variable depending on specific enzymatic defect ●*Precipitating factors:* Genetic; most mucopolysaccharidosis (MPS) diseases are autosomal recessive, with the exception of MPS II (i.e. Hunter's syndrome), which is X-linked; degree of phenotypic expression is variable ●*Relieving factors:* Specific therapy generally not effective; care is largely symptomatic/supportive; genetic counseling/prevention ●*Clinical course:* Ranges from lethal in childhood (i.e. MPS IH, Hurler's syndrome) to death in second/third decade (i.e. MPS III), to adult survival (ie.

MPS II/mild Hunters, MPS IS, and others); particularly severe or mild forms of any of the above can exist; prototype MPS (Hurler's, or MPS IH) marked by excessive growth during the first year of life followed by poor growth late in the course and death within the first decade ●*Co-morbidities:* Multiple congenital somatic abnormalities common; postmortem analysis in MPS prototype, Hurler's, often shows hydrocephalus, cardiovascular disease (occlusion of coronary arteries) ●*Procedure results:* Biopsy of skin, bone marrow, rectal mucosa, liver, peripheral nerve, conjunctiva, or other tissue for light and electron microscopy with or without chemical analysis of biopsy tissue ●*Test findings:* Spot urine for mucopolysaccharidosis; metachromatic staining of peripheral leukocytes and bone marrow; specific enzyme assays in serum, leukocytes, or cultured skin fibroblasts; X-ray findings can be characteristic in MPS IH (Hurler's): enlargement of sella turcica with a distinctive 'shoe-shaped' fossa, broadening and shortening of the long bones, vertebral hypoplasia and beaking in the lumbar region, resulting in accentuated kyphosis or gibbus deformity

Mullerian dysgenesis ●*Onset:* Insidious ●*Male:female ratio:* F ●*Ethnicity:* All ●*Character:* May be primary amenorrhea; may be incidental discovery ●*Location:* Nonspecific ●*Pattern:* May present with primary amenorrhea though not necessarily ●*Precipitating factors:* May be associated with inutero DES exposure ●*Relieving factors:* Surgical repair ●*Clinical course:* May have no clinical impact or may be associated with infertility, primary amenorrhea or primary dysmenorrhea ●*Co-morbidities:* Infertility ●*Procedure results:* Visualized anomaly on examination or laparoscopy ●*Test findings:* Hysterosalpingogram reveals anomaly; MRI may be useful

Multinodular goiter ●*Onset:* Insidious but may be acute ●*Male:female ratio:* M=F ●*Ethnicity:* All ●*Character:* Palpitations, sweating, tremor, weight loss ●*Location:* Irregular enlarged thyroid, brisk reflexes, hand tremor ●*Pattern:* Nonspecific ●*Precipitating factors:* Iodine load, e.g. IV contrast, angiography ●*Relieving factors:* Antithyroid medication and beta blockade, permanent treatment radioactive iodine or more rarely surgery ●*Clinical course:* Progressive, does not remit ●*Co-morbidities:* Systolic hypertension, atrial tachyarrhythmias ●*Procedure results:* Heterogenous thyroid scan ●*Test findings:* Suppressed thyroid-stimulating hormone, high T4 (T3)

Multiple myeloma ●*Onset:* Insidious ●*Male:female ratio:* M=F ●*Ethnicity:* All ●*Character:* Bone pain, fatigue, dyspnea on exertion, infection, pathologic fracture, mucosal bleeding, vertigo, visual disturbances, alterations in mental status, numbness/weakness of lower extremities ●*Location:* Pain often in back or ribs ●*Pattern:* Nonspecific ●*Precipitating factors:* None relevant ●*Relieving factors:* Palliation with combination chemotherapy, treatment for renal failure; for younger patients allogeneic bone marrow transplant, for others autologous ●*Clinical course:* Median survival is 3 years; prognosis is affected by a number of factors ●*Co-morbidities:* Renal failure is a result of the disease ●*Procedure results:* Bone marrow biopsy: infiltration with plasma cells, which commonly appear abnormal ●*Test findings:* Anemia, rouleau formation, paraprotein on serum protein electrophoresis or urinary protein electrophoresis, hypercalcemia, renal failure, elevated ESR, narrow anion gap; X-ray with lytic bone lesions often in axial skeleton

Multiple sclerosis ●*Onset:* Acute/subacute/insidious ●*Male:female ratio:* M<F ●*Ethnicity:* More common in those of northern European descent ●*Character:* Weakness, paresthesias, numbness, visual loss, vertigo, diplopia, bladder control problems ●*Location:* Brain, spinal cord ●*Pattern:* Waxing and waning signs and symptoms over time ●*Precipitating factors:* None relevant ●*Relieving factors:* Immunosuppression, methylprednisolone, interferon, cyclophosphamide, supportive care ●*Clinical course:* Slowly progressive ●*Co-morbidities:* None relevant ●*Procedure results:* No relevant procedures ●*Test findings:* MRI of the brain and spinal cord

Mumps ●*Onset:* Acute ●*Male:female ratio:* M=F ●*Ethnicity:* All ●*Character:* Fever and painful swelling of one or both parotid glands ●*Location:* Common: one or both parotid glands; less common: other salivary glands, testicles, pancreas, CNS (brain and meninges), VIIIth cranial nerve, myocardium, other ●*Pattern:* Parotid swelling is bilateral or unilateral, painful, and may cause earache, and difficulty swallowing, eating, or talking; meningismus is common; orchitis is common postpuberty, usually unilateral, and may result in atrophy ●*Precipitating factors:* None relevant ●*Relieving factors:* None relevant ●*Clinical course:* Incubation 12-25 days, prodrome 1-2 days (up to 7 days), clinical illness 7-10 days, self-limited in most; complications: sensorineural deafness, aseptic meningitis, sterility (rare), testicular atrophy, spontaneous abortions, diabetes ●*Co-morbidities:* None relevant ●*Procedure results:* CSF with lymphocytic pleocytosis (100-1000 cells, neutrophilic in first 24h), low glucose ●*Test findings:* Nonspecific, elevated amylase (common), elevated lipase (rare)

Munchausen syndrome ●*Onset:* Usually early adulthood ●*Male:female ratio:* M=F ●*Ethnicity:* All ●*Character:* Medical symptoms intentionally feigned/produced in order to assume the sick role ●*Location:* Nonspecific ●*Pattern:* Typically patients leave treatment setting when confronted with diagnosis of Munchausen ●*Precipitating factors:* Often follows hospitalization or personal experience with major medical condition ●*Relieving factors:* Behavioral therapy, psychotherapy may be beneficial in some patients ●*Clinical course:* Occasionally limited to brief episodes; more typically chronic course with multiple hospitalizations and medical procedures ●*Co-morbidities:* Substance abuse; iatrogenically induced medical conditions from unnecessary surgeries, procedures, medications ●*Procedure results:* Frequently new 'pathology' or 'complications' after initial workup negative ●*Test findings:* Specimens may reveal obvious contamination by the patient (e.g. feces in blood specimens)

Muscular back pain ●*Onset:* Acute, subacute ●*Male:female ratio:* M=F ●*Ethnicity:* All ●*Character:* Sharp or dull ●*Location:* Low back, can radiate into buttocks and posterior thighs ●*Pattern:* Worse with use ●*Precipitating factors:* Straining of back, lumbar flexion or extension ●*Relieving factors:* Laying supine often with knees flexed ●*Clinical course:* Usually remits within 4-8 weeks ●*Co-morbidities:* Degenerative arthritis, obesity ●*Procedure results:* No relevant procedures ●*Test findings:* Mild degenerative arthritis of lumbar spine on plain radiographs

Muscular dystrophy ●*Onset:* Insidious ●*Male:female ratio:* M=F ●*Ethnicity:* All ●*Character:* Developmental delay in standing and walking, weakness ●*Location:* Delayed walking; clumsy, waddling gait; pronounced lumbar lordosis ●*Pattern:* Proximal weakness vs distal weakness ●*Precipitating factors:* Inherited as a sex-linked recessive trait ●*Relieving factors:* Physical therapy may prolong function ●*Clinical course:* Progressive and eventually patient succumbs to respiratory infections ●*Co-morbidities:* None relevant ●*Procedure results:* No relevant procedures ●*Test findings:* Genetic testing, positive genetic defect

Muscular strain ●*Onset:* Acute ●*Male:female ratio:* M=F ●*Ethnicity:* All ●*Character:* Pain or tenderness in muscle, especially with movement; may see mild swelling ●*Location:* Any muscle may be strained, but extremities most common; also neck, back, abdominal or chest wall muscles ●*Pattern:* Nonspecific ●*Precipitating factors:* Pain in muscle following acute injury (stress) or overuse; worsens with movement or use of that muscle ●*Relieving factors:* Rest most important; ice, anti-inflammatories, analgesics; strengthening exercises when pain improved ●*Clinical course:* Resolves with rest and anti-inflammatories; healing depends on size of muscle injured and how often it is used ●*Co-morbidities:* None relevant ●*Procedure results:* No relevant procedures ●*Test findings:* Radiographs to rule out fractures if suspected

Myasthenia gravis ●*Onset:* Insidious, subacute ●*Male:female ratio:* M(2):F(3) ●*Ethnicity:* All ●*Character:* Periodic weakness, fatigue, ptosis, transient diplopia, difficulty in swallowing

● *Location:* Nonspecific ● *Pattern:* Symptoms worse after prolonged use/exercise or fatigue ● *Precipitating factors:* Prolonged use/exercise or fatigue ● *Relieving factors:* Rest; anticholinesterase drugs such as pyridostigmine bromide, corticosteroids, immunosuppressant drugs, thymectomy, plasmaphoresis ● *Clinical course:* Variable, can be self-limiting or life-long ● *Co-morbidities:* None relevant ● *Procedure results:* Positive for acetylcholine receptor antibodies in 85% ● *Test findings:* Electromyelogram with repetitive nerve stimulation with decreasing amplitudes

Mycoplasmal pneumonia ● *Onset:* Acute ● *Male:female ratio:* M>F ● *Ethnicity:* All ● *Character:* Pronounced cough with small amounts of whitish sputum, fever and chills, dyspnea, nausea and vomiting (less common) ● *Location:* Chest ● *Pattern:* Bronchial breath sounds, inspiratory rales, egophony ● *Precipitating factors:* None relevant ● *Relieving factors:* Antibiotics ● *Clinical course:* Illness last days-to-weeks, but weakness may last longer; low mortality ● *Co-morbidities:* Otitis ● *Procedure results:* No relevant procedures ● *Test findings:* Leukocytosis, focal or diffuse infiltrate(s) on chest X-ray, sputum with neutrophils yet no definitive organism

Myelodysplastic syndromes ● *Onset:* Insidious ● *Male:female ratio:* M=F ● *Ethnicity:* All ● *Character:* Symptoms of anemia (fatigue, headaches), easy bleeding and bruising, signs of infection ● *Location:* Nonspecific ● *Pattern:* Nonspecific ● *Precipitating factors:* Usually diopathic but can be associated with exposure to radiation, benzene, or alkylating chemotherapeutic agents ● *Relieving factors:* Supportive therapy (transfusions, antibiotics), hematopoietic growth factors, chemotherapy, bone marrow transplantation ● *Clinical course:* Depends on form of myelodysplasia and chromosomal abnormalities; overall, may have a prolonged course (10 years), but the disease is ultimately fatal without aggressive therapy ● *Co-morbidities:* Genetic or congenital factors (Down syndrome, Fanconi's anemia), aplastic anemia ● *Procedure results:* Bone marrow biopsy: hypercellular with signs of ineffective and disordered production (megaloblastic erythroid features, ringed sideroblasts, left-shifted myeloid series with deficient granules, dwarf megakaryocytes) ● *Test findings:* Anemia (normo- to macrocytic with reduced reticulocytes), neutropenia with or without Pelger-Huet cells (bilobed nuclei), thrombocytopenia with abnormal forms, cytogenetic abnormalities in two-thirds

Myeloproliferative disorders ● *Onset:* Insidious, except a rare form of acute myelofibrosis ● *Male:female ratio:* M=F ● *Ethnicity:* All ● *Character:* Fatigue, weakness, abdominal fullness, easy bleeding, pruritus, bone pain, paresthesias, weight loss ● *Location:* Bone pain is usually in the lower extremities, hemorrhage in the mucous membranes and intestinal tract ● *Pattern:* Nonspecific ● *Precipitating factors:* None relevant ● *Relieving factors:* Chemotherapy, radioactive phosphorus; myelofibrosis: transfusions, androgens, prednisone, splenectomy; essential thrombocytosis: plasmapheresis, antiplatelet drugs; polycythemia vera: phlebotomy ● *Clinical course:* Common to transform into acute leukemia, which is often fatal; polycythemia vera and essential thrombocytosis may have a prolonged course ● *Co-morbidities:* None relevant ● *Procedure results:* Bone marrow biopsy: hypercellular; myelofibrosis: dry tap in late disease and increased fibrosis ● *Test findings:* Myelofibrosis: anemia with abnormal RBCs (teardrop poikilocytosis), leukoerythroblastosis, giant abnormal platelets; essential thrombocytosis: platelet count >600,000, mild anemia, mild increase in WBC; polycythemia vera: RBCs increased

Myocardial infarction ● *Onset:* Acute ● *Male:female ratio:* M>F (M=F after age 70)

●*Ethnicity:* All groups ●*Character:* Sudden onset of chest pain, shortness of breath, hypotension with or without syncope; may be complicated by hemodynamic instability; examination may reveal crackles in the lungs, S3/S4 heart sounds, elevated neck veins, arrhythmias ●*Location:* Substernal chest pain with possible radiation to the jaw/left arm; pain not pleuritic in nature; associated symptoms of shortness of breath, nausea, diaphoresis may be present ●*Pattern:* More common early in the morning (6-9 a.m.); symptoms tend to be progressive unless therapy is initiated ●*Precipitating factors:* Exertion, stress, other cardiac stressors such as cocaine use; unknown what exactly precipitates plaque rupture resultant myocardial infarction ●*Relieving factors:* Therapy options: aspirin, nitrates, heparin, beta-blockers; for ST elevation myocardial infarction, lytic or invasive therapy ●*Clinical course:* Untreated acute myocardial infarction is associated with high morbidity/mortality; symptoms usually persistent unless therapy is undertaken or infarction is completed ●*Co-morbidities:* Risk factors for the development of coronary artery disease include old age, hypertension, hyperlipidemia, diabetes, family history of coronary artery disease, smoking, cocaine use ●*Procedure results:* Echo may reveal regional wall motion abnormalities; cardiac catheterization may reveal elevated right/left heart filling pressures, coronary artery disease ●*Test findings:* Chest X-ray may reveal heart failure; ECG with ST/T-wave abnormalities, blood work may reveal elevated creatine kinase-myocardial band fraction or high troponin/lactate dehydrogenase levels

Myopathy ●*Onset:* Variable ●*Male:female ratio:* M=F ●*Ethnicity:* All ●*Character:* Muscle weakness, pain, limpness, stiffness, spasm, cramping, twitching, loss of muscle mass or change in volume ●*Location:* Generalized; affects muscle fiber itself ●*Pattern:* Can be progressive with time; must be differentiated from CNS disorders or neuropathy ●*Precipitating factors:* Disorder that affects integrity of muscle fibers; rarely, toxic medications can result in lysis of muscle groups ●*Relieving factors:* None relevant ●*Clinical course:* Varies depending on disorder causing myopathy; difficult for destroyed muscle fibers to regenerate; can have compensatory hypertrophy if partial damage occurs ●*Co-morbidities:* Collagen vascular disease, myasthenia gravis, Guillain-Barré syndrome, AIDS, Lyme disease ●*Procedure results:* Muscle biopsy is usually helpful, especially if process is inflammatory ●*Test findings:* Electromyogram (EMG) can be performed

Myopia ●*Onset:* Insidious ●*Male:female ratio:* M=F ●*Ethnicity:* All ●*Character:* Blurred distance vision ●*Location:* Usually both eyes are involved ●*Pattern:* Slowly progressive over decades ●*Precipitating factors:* A variety of environmental and genetic factors are postulated to contribute to myopia ●*Relieving factors:* Corrective lens, contact lens, or refractive surgery improve vision ●*Clinical course:* Lasts a lifetime; slowly progressive but often stabilizes in the third or fourth decade of life ●*Co-morbidities:* Often no associated conditions but can be seen in Down syndrome, Marfan's syndrome, homocystinuria, and a host of very rare syndromes ●*Procedure results:* Assessment of refractive error ●*Test findings:* Myopic corrective lens improves vision

Myotonia congenita ●*Onset:* Subacute ●*Male:female ratio:* M=F ●*Ethnicity:* All ●*Character:* Myotonia of muscles; children resemble bodybuilders ●*Location:* Muscles ●*Pattern:* Stable and not progressive for many years ●*Precipitating factors:* Autosomal dominant (Thomsen disease) or autosomal recessive (Becker disease) at 7q35 gene locus: gene is important for integrity of chloride channels of sarcolemma ●*Relieving factors:* None relevant ●*Clinical course:* Stable for many years but can be progressive ●*Co-morbidities:* Myotonic dystrophy may coexist in same family ●*Procedure results:* Electomyelogram shows myotonia ●*Test findings:* Muscle biopsy shows minimal changes

Myotonic dystrophy ●*Onset:* Insidious ●*Male:female ratio:* M=F ●*Ethnicity:* All ●*Character:* Many neurologic symptoms including predominant muscle wasting, ptosis, also frontal baldness, nasal voice, cataracts, testicular atrophy; GI tract effects: constipation, megacolon, dysphagia ●*Location:* Nonspecific ●*Pattern:* Nonspecific ●*Precipitating factors:* Hereditary: autosomal dominant ●*Relieving factors:* Immunosuppression, testosterone, supportive care ●*Clinical course:* Progressive ●*Co-morbidities:* Diabetes ●*Procedure results:* Muscle biopsies with diagnostic findings; swallowing study: oropharyngeal dysphagia; esophageal manometry: decreased upper esophageal pressure, decreased contraction of pharynx and upper esophagus ●*Test findings:* Chromosome analysis: 19q abnormality

Myxedema ●*Onset:* Insidious ●*Male:female ratio:* M(1):F(6) ●*Ethnicity:* All ●*Character:* Fatigue, sluggishness, weight gain, dry skin, constipation ●*Location:* Enlarged symmetric thyroid, though may be normal size ●*Pattern:* Nonspecific ●*Precipitating factors:* Radioactive iodine, thyroid surgery, postpartum state, viral infection ●*Relieving factors:* None relevant ●*Clinical course:* Progressive though subacute thyroiditis and postpartum thyroiditis may spontaneously resolve ●*Co-morbidities:* Diastolic hypertension, hypercholesterolemia ●*Procedure results:* No relevant procedures ●*Test findings:* Elevated TSH, low T4 (T3 not indicated), thyroid peroxidase antibodies elevated in Hashimoto's disease

Narcolepsy ●*Onset:* Insidious ●*Male:female ratio:* M=F ●*Ethnicity:* All ●*Character:* Excessive daytime sleepiness which progresses over years, cataleptic attacks, sleep paralysis, and may have hypnagogic hallucinations ●*Location:* Nonspecific ●*Pattern:* Nonspecific ●*Precipitating factors:* Genetic predisposition ●*Relieving factors:* Ritalin, amphetamines, imipramine ●*Clinical course:* Increases slowly in severity until age 50 ●*Co-morbidities:* Sleep apnea in 20% ●*Procedure results:* EEG and multiple sleep latency test ●*Test findings:* Occurrence of rapid eye movement (REM) and complete loss of muscle tone within 15 min of the onset of stage 1 of sleep occurring during two or more of five test periods

Nasal polyp ●*Onset:* Insidious ●*Male:female ratio:* M=F ●*Ethnicity:* All ●*Character:* Nasal obstruction, congestion; recurrent sinus infections ●*Location:* Nasal cavity and sinuses ●*Pattern:* Constant symptoms ●*Precipitating factors:* May be genetically linked ●*Relieving factors:* Use or abuse of topical nasal decongestants, oral decongestants ●*Clinical course:* Usually slow progression of polyp growth ●*Co-morbidities:* Allergic rhinitis, chronic sinusitis ●*Procedure results:* Nasal endoscopy reveals translucent multiple polyps ●*Test findings:* CT scan usually reveals sinusitis and nasal cavity obliteration with polyps

Navicular fracture ●*Onset:* Acute ●*Male:female ratio:* M=F ●*Ethnicity:* All ●*Character:* Pain in wrist following injury; tenderness of anatomical snuff box is diagnostic; increased pain with longitudinal compression of thumb or supination of hand against resistance ●*Location:* Wrist ●*Pattern:* Nonspecific ●*Precipitating factors:* Fall on outstretched hand ●*Relieving factors:* Ice, immobilization in thumb spica cast or splint; displaced fractures require surgical repair ●*Clinical course:* Usually heal within 6 to 8 weeks but may take longer; may develop avascular necrosis, delayed or nonunion ●*Co-morbidities:* None relevant ●*Procedure results:* No relevant procedures ●*Test findings:* Radiographs of wrist and scaphoid bone reveal fracture but may not be evident on initial X-rays; repeat radiographs after 2 weeks or MRI may reveal fracture

Near drowning ●*Onset:* Acute ●*Male:female ratio:* M>F ●*Ethnicity:* All ●*Character:* Respiratory failure, ischemic neurologic injury, and hypothermia common; examine for trauma or spinal injuries ●*Location:* Nonspecific ●*Pattern:* Nonspecific ●*Precipitating factors:* None relevant ●*Relieving factors:* Supportive care ●*Clinical course:* Varies depending on patient age and time to resuscitation; up to 25% of children initially in coma requiring CPR survive with intact neurologic function ●*Co-morbidities:* Alcohol or drug use by victims often seen; also pre-existing seizure disorder ●*Procedure results:* No relevant procedures ●*Test findings:* Chest X-ray may reveal pulmonary edema

Neck injury ●*Onset:* Acute or subacute, depending on etiology ●*Male:female ratio:* M=F ●*Ethnicity:* All ●*Character:* Stiffness, pain with neck movement, headache, radicular symptoms ●*Location:* Cervical spine, trapezius, occipital area ●*Pattern:* Pain worse with movement, best when supine ●*Precipitating factors:* History of trauma, pre-existing arthritis, poor sleeping habits or ergonomics, poor posture, weak musculature ●*Relieving factors:* Lying supine with neck in neutral position, rest, ice, NSAIDs, muscle relaxants, physical therapy ●*Clinical course:* Variable, improvement over time depending on diagnosis ●*Co-morbidities:* None relevant ●*Procedure results:* No relevant procedures ●*Test findings:* X-ray of cervical spine may show fracture, herniation of disc, or straightening of cervical spine or reversal of lordotic curve

Necrotizing enterocolitis ●*Onset:* Subacute ●*Male:female ratio:* M=F ●*Ethnicity:* All ●*Character:* Poor feeding, abdominal distension, nausea, heme-positive stools, lethargy, hypothermia, abdominal tenderness, GI bleeding, septic physiology ●*Location:* Nonspecific ●*Pattern:* Nonspecific ●*Precipitating factors:* Premature birth, early and aggressive feedings, enteric infection ●*Relieving factors:* Hold oral feedings, IV fluids, nasogastric tube, antibiotics, surgery ●*Clinical course:* If minor symptoms, resolution; if more severe symptoms, surgery may be necessary ●*Co-morbidities:* Premature birth ●*Procedure results:* No relevant procedures ●*Test findings:* Elevated WBC, low platelets, elevated prothrombin time/partial thromboplastin time, electrolyte abnormalities, pneumatosis on abdominal X-ray

Neonatal acne ●*Onset:* Subacute ●*Male:female ratio:* M>F ●*Ethnicity:* All ●*Character:* Papulopustular, rarely comedones; (infantile acne: often with comedones, inflammatory lesions, papules/pustules, occasional nodules) ●*Location:* Face/chin/forehead ●*Pattern:* May worsen during course of rash ●*Precipitating factors:* Hormonal stimulation of sebaceous glands ●*Relieving factors:* Daily cleansing with soap/water, retin-A, benzoyl peroxide ●*Clinical course:* Self-limited, resolves within 3-4 months; (infantile acne can last for 2-3 years) ●*Co-morbidities:* None relevant ●*Procedure results:* No relevant procedure ●*Test findings:* None needed but if persistent/severe, possibly elevated 17-ketosteroids

Neonatal respiratory distress syndrome ●*Onset:* Acute ●*Male:female ratio:* M=F ●*Ethnicity:* More common in Caucasians ●*Character:* Respiratory distress ●*Location:* Lungs ●*Pattern:* Shortly after birth the infant has respiratory distress with tachypnea and cyanosis ●*Precipitating factors:* Prematurity, maternal diabetes, male sex, and increased risk with siblings with respiratory distress syndrome, perinatal asphyxia and delivery by Cesarean section ●*Relieving factors:* Prenatal administration of glucocorticoid for premature patient; surfactant replacement therapy through the endotracheal tube, administration of oxygen, respiratory support by continuous positive airway pressure or mechanical ventilation, IV fluids to maintain fluid volume; packed RBCs ●*Clinical course:* Prenatal administration of steroids and postnatal dosing of surfactant decreases mortality and severity of lung disease ●*Co-morbidities:* BPD (bronchopulmonary dysplasia), chronic lung disease, retinopathy of prematurity, intraventricular hemorrhage with development abnormalities ●*Procedure results:* Shake test on the gastric amniotic fluid after birth ●*Test findings:* Chest film indicates low lung volumes with a reticulogranular pattern and air bronchograms, low p02 and high pCO2 by blood gas

Nephritic syndrome ●*Onset:* Acute-subacute; laboratory and clinical manifestations can wax/wane over days-to-months ●*Male:female ratio:* M=F ●*Ethnicity:* All ●*Character:* Hematuria, hypertension, oliguria, azotemia; salt and water retention can lead to pulmonary vascular congestion and facial/peripheral edema; proteinuria and active urinary sediment (RBC casts are characteristic) are frequent; rapid renal failure can also occur ●*Location:* Inflammation involving renal tubules and glomerular damage ●*Pattern:* Hematuria is often gross; patient may describe smoky-, cola-, or coffee-colored urine; hypertension and peripheral edema (often initially in nondependent areas, like periorbital region) ensues as glomerular fitration rate (GFR) falls; with marked reduction in GFR, oligoanuria may be present ●*Precipitating factors:* Multiple potential causes including immune-mediated mechanisms, post-strep infection, vasculitides, endocarditis, hemolytic uremic syndrome/thrombotic thrombocytopenic purpura, drugs/toxins ●*Relieving factors:* Address underlying cause (antibiotics for endocarditis, high-dose steroids for vasculitis); in severe cases, cytotoxic therapy (i.e. cyclophosphamide for Wegener's) or plasmapheresis may be helpful ●*Clinical course:* Variable depending on cause and patient population; generally more favorable prognosis in children than in adults; hypertension and edema often resolve (as quickly as one week) before urinary abnormalities (which can persist for weeks); longterm renal sequelae/rapidly progressive renal failure occurs in a subset of patients ●*Co-morbidities:* Hypertension ●*Procedure results:* Renal biopsy showing active inflammation; glomerulonephritis with or without extracapillary crescents (in rapidly progressive disease) is common; specific patterns of immunoglobulins, immune complexes can influence prognosis and treatment ●*Test findings:* RBC casts, hematuria, proteinuria on urinalysis; rise in serum creatinine

Nephroblastoma (Wilms' tumor) ●*Onset:* Insidious ●*Male:female ratio:* M=F ●*Ethnicity:* All ●*Character:* Asymptomatic mass ●*Location:* Abdominal ●*Pattern:* Vomiting or pain in 50% ●*Precipitating factors:* Hypertension with compression of renal artery ●*Relieving factors:* Surgical removal by flank incision and chemotherapy with vincristine and actinomycin, and for advanced disease, additional radiation ●*Clinical course:* Survival-based histology and stage, favorable histology (FH)/1 has a 2-year survival of 98% and anaplastic II has only 56% ●*Co-morbidities:* Genital anomalies, hemihypertrophy, aniridia, organomegly, hypertension, hematuria, mental retardation ●*Procedure results:* CT scan of the abdomen reveals inhomogeneous mass with areas of necrosis ●*Test findings:* Chest film indicates pulmonary metastasis in 10-15%, blood on urinalysis, and deletion on chromosome 11

Nephrotic syndrome ●*Onset:* Usually subacute ●*Male:female ratio:* M=F ●*Ethnicity:* All ●*Character:* Facial and peripheral edema, hypercholesterolemia, renal insufficiency, hypoalbuminemia, proteinuria ●*Location:* Periorbital or pedal edema ●*Pattern:* Glomerular injury causing protein loss; abnormal liver metabolism of cholesterol ●*Precipitating factors:* Multiple possible underlying etiologies including: diabetes, multiple myeloma, infection (hepatitis B/C, syphilis, HIV), IgA nephropathy (rare), rheumatic disease (systemic lupus erythematosus, rheumatoid arthritis), Hodgkin's disease, drugs (heroin, gold salts, NSAIDs, high dose captopril); minimal change disease more common in children ●*Relieving factors:* Treatment of underlying condition; steroids sometimes helpful, depending on underlying etiology ●*Clinical course:* Increasing severity of proteinuria with increasing glomerular damage; progressive renal failure may ensue; rate of progression depends on pathophysiology of each underlying cause ●*Co-morbidities:* Hypercholesterolemia, hypoalbuminemia; acquired hypercoagulability ●*Procedure results:* Urinalysis, 24h urine collection ●*Test findings:* Urinalysis with protein; maltese crosses may be seen (lipiduria); 24h urine shows >3.5g of protein (by definition); hypercholesterolemia

Nerve root compression ●*Onset:* Acquired/acute/subacute ●*Male:female ratio:* M=F ●*Ethnicity:* All ●*Character:* Also called radicular syndromes; characterized by partial paralysis and incomplete sensory loss; the specific manifestations vary depending on the site of the compression ●*Location:* Nerve root compression can occur at the cervical (brachial plexus), thoracic, lumbar and sacral nerve roots ●*Pattern:* Cervical: C5 lesions cause pain in shoulder and atrophy of deltoid; C6 lesions depress the biceps reflex; C7 lesions affect triceps, wrist flexors and pectoral muscles; C8 lesions intrinsic hand muscles and can be disabling; C8 and T1 lesions can cause a partial Horner's syndrome. Cranial nerve lesions are specific and affect sensation and motor innervation. Brachial plexus root compression lesions can be less severe as single nerves receive innervation from more than one root and hence lead to partial motor and sensory loss. Lumbar and sacral nerve root compression cause referred paresthesias more commonly known as sciatica ●*Precipitating factors:* Disc herniation, edema of nerves and fibrosis, trauma to vertebrae ●*Relieving factors:* Temporary relief with anti-inflammatory agents (steroids and nonsteroidal), surgical decompression ●*Clinical course:* Usually symptoms progress from paresthesias, then partial sensory or motor loss, culminating in complete paralysis and sensory loss ●*Co-morbidities:* Vertebral column deformities (scoliosis, kyphosis), ankylosing spondylitis, autoimmune rheumatologic disease, space-occupying lesions (vascular or solid tumors) ●*Procedure results:* Decompression can relieve symptoms if timely ●*Test findings:* Magnetic resonance imaging and myelography can demonstrate specific structural problems

Neuroblastoma ●*Onset:* Childhood, subacute ●*Male:female ratio:* M=F ●*Ethnicity:* All ●*Character:* Raised intracranial pressure, abdominal mass, depending on site of lesion ●*Location:* Autonomic nervous system or adrenal medulla ●*Pattern:* Nonspecific ●*Precipitating factors:* Genetic link ●*Relieving factors:* Supportive, steroids ●*Clinical course:* Variable ●*Co-morbidities:* None relevant ●*Procedure results:* CT scan of body part depending on location of symptoms ●*Test findings:* Elevated urinary vanillylmandelic acid (VMA)

Neurofibroma ●*Onset:* Plexiform neurofibroma: birth; childhood/adolescence/pregnancy ●*Male:female ratio:* M=F ●*Ethnicity:* All ●*Character:* Smooth/polypoid, as they grow may become globular, pear-shaped/pedunculated, soft or firm, flesh colored or violaceus/pink/blue; 1-2mm to several cm; some painful; 'buttonholing' - invaginated into an underlying dermal defect with moderate digital pressure ●*Location:* Over entire body but not usually palms or soles ●*Pattern:* May be along course of nerves (plexiform), may cause extremity overgrowth or bone deformity ●*Precipitating factors:* Genetic predisposition; neurofibroma (NF)-1: chromosome 17q11.2, NF-2 chromosome 22q1.11 ●*Relieving factors:* Surgical excision ●*Clinical course:* Growth, increasing number of lesions; malignant degeneration with age (usually not before 40 years) into neurofibrosarcoma or malignant schwannoma ●*Co-morbidities:* Neurofibromatosis ●*Procedure results:* Pathology: connective tissue and nerve fibers ●*Test findings:* Genetic predisposition defined by fetal DNA analysis

Neurofibromatosis ●*Onset:* Varies, depending on the location of neurofibromas ●*Male:female ratio:* M=F ●*Ethnicity:* All ●*Character:* Varies, depending on location of neurofibromas ●*Location:* NF-1: cutaneous lesions of pigmentary nevi, café au lait spots, sessile or pedunculated neurofibromas; NF-2: development of a neurolemma, on the VIIIth cranial nerve ●*Pattern:* Varies, depending on location of neurofibromas ●*Precipitating factors:* Autosomal dominant trait on chromosome 17 for NF-1 and chromosome 22 for NF-2 ●*Relieving factors:* Surgical removal of neurofibromas are necessary, depending on location ●*Clinical course:* Majority of patients do not suffer any serious complications; lesions producing peripheral nerve or spinal cord compression require surgical removal ●*Co-morbidities:* None relevant ●*Procedure results:* MRI of the brain ●*Test findings:* Genetic testing

Neurogenic bladder ●*Onset:* Chronic ●*Male:female ratio:* M=F ●*Ethnicity:* All ●*Character:* Urgency, frequency and/or urge incontinence in hyper-reflexic neurogenic bladder; inability to void with suprapubic pain in areflexic neurogenic bladder ●*Location:* Abdomen and pelvis ●*Pattern:* Nonspecific ●*Precipitating factors:* None relevant ●*Relieving factors:* Medications containing anticholinergics in hyper-reflexic neurogenic bladder; catheterization in areflexic neurogenic bladder ●*Clinical course:* Progressive ●*Co-morbidities:* Neurologic diseases (stroke, Parkinson's, tumors, multiple sclerosis, myelodysplasia), infection, bladder outlet obstruction (benign prostatic hyperplasia, strictures), tumor, stone, diabetes, trauma, prior pelvic surgery ●*Procedure results:* No relevant procedures ●*Test findings:* Urodynamics helping differentiate different kinds of neurogenic bladder: intravenous pyelogram, U/S, CT or MRI ruling out upper tract damage (hydronephrosis). MRI ruling out neurologic etiology

Newborn jaundice ●*Onset:* Acute ●*Male:female ratio:* M=F ●*Ethnicity:* Chinese, Japanese, Koreans, native Americans ●*Character:* Yellow ●*Location:* Skin, eyes ●*Pattern:* Yellow skin and eyes present in a newborn between days 2 and 7 of life ●*Precipitating factors:* Maternal diabetes, prematurity, drugs, polycythemia, trisomy 21, bruising and cephalohematoma, breast-feeding, weight loss and dehydration, slow to pass meconium, and sibling with jaundice ●*Relieving factors:* None relevant ●*Clinical course:* Resolves on own but may need phototherapy ●*Co-morbidities:* Trisomy 21 ●*Procedure results:* No relevant procedures ●*Test findings:* Serum indirect between 10 and 12mg/dL and normal direct bilirubin, Coombs' negative, with no isoimmunization and normal hemoglobin

Night terrors ●*Onset:* Acute but may become chronic ●*Male:female ratio:* M>F ●*Ethnicity:* All ●*Character:* Child 3- to 8-years old (usually but can be adult) awakens from deep sleep, sits straight up in bed and screams for up to 30 min before relaxing and going back to sleep ●*Location:* Occurs about 90 minutes into sleep in stage 3 or 4 ●*Pattern:* May occur following stressful event or when unusually fatigued ●*Precipitating factors:* Scary story, stressful event; runs in some families ●*Relieving factors:* Gently restrain child until calm; reduce stress and insure adequate sleeptime; if this does not help then try diazepam ●*Clinical course:* Most children outgrow by time they start school ●*Co-morbidities:* Not usually ●*Procedure results:* Disorder of NREM sleep ●*Test findings:* No relevant tests

Non-diabetic hypoglycemia ●*Onset:* Acute ●*Male:female ratio:* M=F ●*Ethnicity:* All ●*Character:* Confusion, diaphoresis, lightheadedness, hunger, seizures ●*Location:* Nonspecific ●*Pattern:* Nonspecific ●*Precipitating factors:* Fasting, insulinoma, nonindicated administration of insulin or sulfonylurea, adrenal insufficiency, hypopituitarism ●*Relieving factors:* Eating, IV glucose, surgery for insulinoma, hormone replacement for adrenal insufficiency and hypopituitarism ●*Clinical course:* Progressive ●*Co-morbidities:* Insulinoma, sepsis, large sarcomas, adrenal insufficiency, hypopituitarism ●*Procedure results:* No relevant procedures ●*Test findings:* Low plasma glucose with or without nonsuppressed insulin level depending on etiology

Non-functioning chromophobe pituitary adenoma ●*Onset:* Insidious ●*Male:female ratio:* M=F ●*Ethnicity:* All ●*Character:* Visual field defects, headache, oculomotor palsies, hormone deficiencies (amenorrhea, short stature, hypothyroidism) ●*Location:* Visual field defects, usually bitemporal hemianopsia ●*Pattern:* Nonspecific ●*Precipitating factors:* None relevant ●*Relieving factors:* Surgery, or radiation therapy if surgery is insufficient ●*Clinical course:* If small, easily treated; larger tumors can be difficult to treat ●*Co-morbidities:* None relevant ●*Procedure results:* Biopsy: sparsely granulated chromophobes ●*Test findings:* Decreased hormone levels, visual field defects

Non-Hodgkin's lymphoma ●*Onset:* Acute/insidious ●*Male:female ratio:* M>F ●*Ethnicity:* All ●*Character:* Painless lymphadenopathy, constitutional symptoms (fever, night sweats, weight loss), abdominal fullness (Burkitt's), CNS symptoms (HIV-related), pruritus, bone pain ●*Location:* Head, neck and chest, abdomen, pelvis, extranodal sites, CNS ●*Pattern:* Nonspecific ●*Precipitating factors:* History of malignancy, previous radiation treatment or immunosuppression, organ transplantation ●*Relieving factors:* Indolent lymphoma: palliative chemotherapy, if progressive possibly bone marrow transplant; intermediate-high grade: radiation, chemotherapy, autologous bone marrow transplant ●*Clinical course:* Depends on prognostic score and type of lymphoma; indolent: median survival 5-8 years; high-grade: 50% cure ●*Co-morbidities:* HIV, EBV infection, connective tissue disease, Crohn's disease, Helicobacter pylori infection (gastric lymphoma) ●*Procedure results:* Lymph node biopsy: positive for lymphoma; bone marrow biopsy (for staging); paratrabecular lymphoid aggregates if advanced disease; spinal tap positive for malignant cells (if involvement) ●*Test findings:* Increased WBC with left shift (leukemic phase), increased lactate dehydrogenase, cytopenias, hypercalcemia, serum protein electrophoresis: monoclonal antibodies

Non-traumatic tympanic membrane rupture ●*Onset:* Acute ●*Male:female ratio:* M=F ●*Ethnicity:* All ●*Character:* Usually preceded by stabbing pain in the ear, followed by relief once rupture occurs with subsequent otorrhea ●*Location:* Affected ear ●*Pattern:* Pain relieved after tympanic membrane rupture ●*Precipitating factors:* Severe acute otitis media ●*Relieving factors:* Postrupture relief ●*Clinical course:* After perforation, otorrhea may subside spontaneously or may persist until treated; pain may or may not subside; hearing loss will generally persist; often, if a small perforation, spontaneous repair will occur over a course of weeks ●*Co-morbidities:* Adenoid enlargement; rule out nasopharyngeal mass in adults ●*Procedure results:* Otoscopy reveals perforation with otorrhea ●*Test findings:* Audiometry will usually document conductive hearing loss

Noonan syndrome ●*Onset:* Acute ●*Male:female ratio:* M=F ●*Ethnicity:* All ●*Character:* Short stature, mental retardation, epicanthal folds, webbed neck, pectus carinatum/ excavatum, cubitus valgus, cryptorchidism, pulmonary valve stenosis, atrial septal defect, hypertrophic cardiomyopathy, hypertelorism, downward slanted palpebral fissures, ptosis, micrognathia, sensorineural hearing loss ●*Location:* Face/neck/heart/chest/genitalia ●*Pattern:* Nonspecific ●*Precipitating factors:* Autosomal dominant gene with variable expression, mapped to chromosome 12q ●*Relieving factors:* Correction of congenital anomalies, human growth hormone treatment ●*Clinical course:* Lifelong ●*Co-morbidities:* ALL, CML, Noonan-like features can be part of NF-1 gene mutation ●*Procedure results:* Normal karyotype ●*Test findings:* No relevant tests

Nutritional deficiencies ●*Onset:* Subacute ●*Male:female ratio:* M=F ●*Ethnicity:* All ●*Character:* Reduced food intake resulting in loss of fat, muscle, skin, and ultimately bone and viscera ●*Location:* Physical signs of nutritional and metabolic deficiencies prominent in skin: ecchymosis, follicular keratosis; hair: alopecia, dryness; eyes: angular palpebritis; mouth: angular stomatitis and cheilosis; temporal muscle wasting, sunken supraclavicular fossae, decreased adipose stores ●*Pattern:* During acute illness hypercatabolism mediated by catecholamines results in shift to fat as major fuel source ●*Precipitating factors:* Hypermetabolism associated with critical illness leading to loss of adipose and skeletal reserves; pre-existing malnutrition exacerbated by social, medical history, e.g. depression, anorexia, low socioeconomic status ●*Relieving factors:* Enteral or parenteral alimentation ●*Clinical course:* High incidence of mortality in untreated patients: >60% 30-day mortality for hypoalbuminemic patients (serum albumin <2.0g/dL) ●*Co-morbidities:* Increased susceptibility to infection, poor wound healing, increased frequency of decubitus ulcers, overgrowth of bacteria in GI tract, malabsorption ●*Procedure results:* Measurement of upper arm muscle circumference and triceps skin fold standardized to assess nutritional status ●*Test findings:* Serum albumin, total lymphocyte count reduced; absent delayed hypersensitivity

Obsessive compulsive disorder ●*Onset:* Typically gradual, although occasionally acute ●*Male:female ratio:* M(1):F(1.5) ●*Ethnicity:* All ●*Character:* Obsessions (recurrent, persistent, intrusive thoughts or impulses) ●*Location:* Nonspecific ●*Pattern:* Obsessions and compulsions are recognized by the patient as unreasonable or excessive (not so in children) ●*Precipitating factors:* May be exacerbated by stress ●*Relieving factors:* Compulsions themselves are repetitive behaviors whose goal is to reduce anxiety or distress ●*Clinical course:* Majority experience stress-related waxing and waning course ●*Co-morbidities:* Major depression; other anxiety disorders; eating disorders; obsessive-compulsive personality disorder; Tourette's disorder ●*Procedure results:* No relevant procedures ●*Test findings:* No relevant tests

Obstructive sleep apnea ●*Onset:* Insidious ●*Male:female ratio:* M>F ●*Ethnicity:* All ●*Character:* Daytime somnolence, morning headaches and confusion, nocturnal snoring, gasping or grunting, impotence, intellectual impairment ●*Location:* Brain, upper airway ●*Pattern:* Short, thick neck; small, crowded oropharynx; retro- or micrognathia; obesity ●*Precipitating factors:* Sleep, alcohol, benzodiazepines, barbiturates, phenobarbital ●*Relieving factors:* Weight loss, avoidance of precipitating factors, nocturnal noninvasive ventilation (usually continuous positive airway pressure (CPAP)), dental appliances; if severe and refractory to treatment, uvulopalatopharyngostomy or tracheotomy ●*Clinical course:* Progressive without treatment ●*Co-morbidities:* Hypothyroidism, acromegaly, neuromuscular disease, vocal cord paralysis, amyloidosis; often associated with obesity, hypertension ●*Procedure results:* No relevant procedures ●*Test findings:* Polysomnography that reveals an apnea/hypopnea index >15 events/h

Occipital cortex lesion ●*Onset:* Acute ●*Male:female ratio:* M=F ●*Ethnicity:* All ●*Character:* Bilateral damage to the visual occipital cortex leads to cortical blindness; characterized by a normal fundoscopic examination, normal pupillary reflexes to light, and unawareness of blindness on the part of the patient ●*Location:* Occipital cortex involvement ●*Pattern:* Because of preservation of pupillary reflexes, visual loss may be associated with a conversion reaction (hysteria); transient visual loss from basilar artery insufficiency ●*Precipitating factors:* Migraine, hypertensive encephalopathy or postictal state ●*Relieving factors:* Treatment of inciting stimulus ●*Clinical course:* Can be reversible if basilar artery insufficiency, or hypertension ●*Co-morbidities:* Hypertension (malignant hypertensive crisis), migraine, seizure disorder ●*Procedure results:* No relevant procedures ●*Test findings:* MRI scans can delineate extent of cortical parenchyma involved

Ocular trauma ●*Onset:* Acute ●*Male:female ratio:* M=F ●*Ethnicity:* All ●*Character:* Corneal abrasions cause pain, foreign body sensation, tearing; iritis from trauma causes pain, photosensitivity; hyphema may be associated with blurred vision ●*Location:* Eye ●*Pattern:* Nonspecific ●*Precipitating factors:* Direct blow to eye or orbit; scratches to eye ●*Relieving factors:* Antibiotic ointment, cycloplegics, patching ●*Clinical course:* Small abrasions will heal within 24-48 hours ●*Co-morbidities:* None relevant ●*Procedure results:* Slit lamp examination will reveal abrasions on fluorescein staining as well as smaller hyphemas; evert eyelids to look for foreign bodies ●*Test findings:* Radiographs or CT scans can reveal orbital fractures

Oculopharyngeal muscular dystrophy ●*Onset:* Insidious ●*Male:female ratio:* M=F ●*Ethnicity:* All ●*Character:* Blepharoptosis, dysphagia ●*Location:* Eyelids and swallowing mechanism ●*Pattern:* Severe eyelid ptosis with progressive significant dysphagia ●*Precipitating factors:* None relevant ●*Relieving factors:* Modification of diet to small bolus ●*Clinical course:* Slowly progressive ●*Co-morbidities:* None relevant ●*Procedure results:* No relevant procedures ●*Test findings:* Video fluoroscopic swallowing examination reveals cervical dysphagia at the cricopharyngeus

Onychomycosis ●*Onset:* Insidious ●*Male:female ratio:* M<F ●*Ethnicity:* All ❶ *Character:* Pain, unsightly nails ❷ *Location:* Nails ❸ *Pattern:* Thick crumbling nails ●*Precipitating fac-*

tors: Diabetes, moisture ●*Relieving factors:* Antifungals ●*Clinical course:* Progressive ●*Co-morbidities:* Tinea pedis ●*Procedure results:* Positive potassium hydroxide ●*Test findings:* Nail culture positive

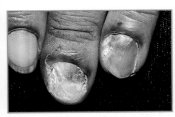

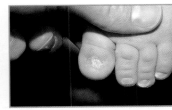

❶ *Character* Nail splitting, breakage, and nail bed involvement are prominent here

❷ *Location* Near total destruction of the nail in an infant with onychomycosis

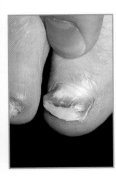

❸ *Pattern* Thickened and discolored nail, as fungus invades from below and creates debris

Optic atrophy ●*Onset:* Usually subacute/insidious ●*Male:female ratio:* M=F ●*Ethnicity:* All ●*Character:* Poor distance and near vision; poor color vision ●*Location:* Can involve one or both eyes ●*Pattern:* Persistent poor vision ●*Precipitating factors:* Depends on the cause ●*Relieving factors:* None; once symptoms secondary to optic atrophy develop there is little that can be done to relieve them ●*Clinical course:* Depends on the cause ●*Co-morbidities:* A variety of conditions can produce this sign, including compressive lesions, trauma, optic neuritis, ischemic optic neuropathy ●*Procedure results:* Inability to correct vision with glasses, poor color vision and fundus examination; other procedures performed depend on the differential diagnosis for this sign ●*Test findings:* Small pale optic nerve on fundus examination; other findings depend on the cause

Optic neuritis ●*Onset:* Acute ●*Male:female ratio:* M<F ●*Ethnicity:* All ●*Character:* Blurred vision, pain on eye movement; decreased color vision ●*Location:* Optic nerve ●*Pattern:* Typically unilateral. Afferent pupillary defect ●*Precipitating factors:* None relevant ●*Relieving factors:* None relevant ●*Clinical course:* Near complete resolution in 2 weeks; can recur ●*Co-morbidities:* Multiple sclerosis ●*Procedure results:* Disc edema on fundus examination (disc may appear normal) ●*Test findings:* No relevant tests

Oral cavity cancer ●*Onset:* Insidious ●*Male:female ratio:* M=F ●*Ethnicity:* Asian ●*Character:* Variable: oral cavity lesion, oral cavity pain, oral cavity bleeding ●*Location:* Oral cavity: tongue, gingiva, buccal mucosa, floor of mouth, hard palate ●*Pattern:* Lesion may range from ulcer to plaque-like leukoplakia to exophytic lesion ●*Precipitating factors:* Smoking, alcohol use, smokeless tobacco, betel nut use ●*Relieving factors:* Occasionally, topical anesthetic sprays or ointments for painful lesions ●*Clinical course:* Symptoms usually persist until diagnosis ●*Co-morbidities:* Chronic obstructive pulmonary disease; history of head and neck malignancy ●*Procedure results:* Oral cavity biopsy reveals carcinoma with invasion ●*Test findings:* No relevant tests

O

Oral leukoplakia • Orbital cellulitis • Orbital hemorrhage • Orbital tumor • Orchitis • Oro-facial dyskinesia • Orthostatic hypotension

Oral leukoplakia ●*Onset:* Insidious ●*Male:female ratio:* M>F ●*Ethnicity:* All ●*Character:* White patches along oral mucosa ●*Location:* Oral cavity, gums, tongue ●*Pattern:* Variable ●*Precipitating factors:* Cigarette smoking, chewing tobacco use, lichen planus, scalding hot tea ●*Relieving factors:* None relevant ●*Clinical course:* Chronic persistent ●*Co-morbidities:* None relevant ●*Procedure results:* White discoloration on oral cavity examination ●*Test findings:* Variable, depending on pathology

Orbital cellulitis ●*Onset:* Acute ●*Male:female ratio:* M=F ●*Ethnicity:* All ●*Character:* Blurred vision, diplopia, achy pain ●*Location:* Orbit/sinuses ●*Pattern:* Unilateral proptosis on external examination; lid edema, erythema ●*Precipitating factors:* Preceding sinus infection ●*Relieving factors:* None relevant ●*Clinical course:* Rapidly progressive, requires antibiotic therapy for resolution ●*Co-morbidities:* Sinusitis, upper respiratory illness, otitis media ●*Procedure results:* CT/MRI show sinus opacity and occasionally subperiosteal abscess ●*Test findings:* Positive blood and tissue cultures

Orbital hemorrhage ●*Onset:* Acute ●*Male:female ratio:* M>F ●*Ethnicity:* All ●*Character:* Lid erythema ●*Location:* Usually unilateral orbital and periorbital tissue ●*Pattern:* Nonspecific ●*Precipitating factors:* Cranial facial trauma; occasionally spontaneous orbital hemorrhage occurs with orbital tumors and leukemia ●*Relieving factors:* None relevant ●*Clinical course:* Rapidly progresses, self-limited ●*Co-morbidities:* Fractured orbital bones, retained orbital foreign body, intraocular pathology ●*Procedure results:* CT/MRI of the orbit show blood and possibly air in the orbit ●*Test findings:* No relevant tests

Orbital tumor ●*Onset:* Subacute/insidous; rarely acute (rhabdomyosarcoma) ●*Male:female ratio:* M=F ●*Ethnicity:* All ●*Character:* Proptosis ●*Location:* Usually unilateral ●*Pattern:* Nonspecific ●*Precipitating factors:* None relevant ●*Relieving factors:* None relevant ●*Clinical course:* Most tumors progress slowly; rhabdomyosarcoma progresses rapidly ●*Co-morbidities:* None relevant ●*Procedure results:* Asymmetric prominence of globes documented with an exophthalmometer ●*Test findings:* Mass lesion in orbit on CT or MRI

Orchitis ●*Onset:* Subacute ●*Male:female ratio:* M ●*Ethnicity:* All ●*Character:* Pain, swelling, induration ●*Location:* Scrotum, inguinal canal ●*Pattern:* Usually unilateral ●*Precipitating factors:* STD, UTI, indwelling Foley catheter, urethral stricture, urethral and transurethral surgery ●*Relieving factors:* Antibiotics; anti-inflammatory medications; scrotal elevation; surgical intervention (rarely used) ●*Clinical course:* Progressive if untreated, possibly leading to abscess formation, testicular necrosis or infertility ●*Co-morbidities:* STD, UTI, urethral strictures, benign prostatic hyperplasia, TB, prostatitis, hydrocele ●*Procedure results:* Doppler scrotal U/S or nuclear scan ruling out acute testicular torsion ●*Test findings:* Gram stain and culture of midstream urine or urethral swab: any or all possibly positive

Oro-facial dyskinesia ●*Onset:* Insidious ●*Male:female ratio:* M<F ●*Ethnicity:* All ●*Character:* Abnormal involuntary movements, usually occur when patients are at rest, frequently increased by movement and calm down during sleep; can be the drug-induced syndrome of tardive dyskinesia or oro-lingual-buccal dyskinesia; there are constant chewing movements of the jaw, writhing and protruding movements of the tongue, puckering movements of the mouth; intermittent tongue darting out of the mouth ('fly-catcher tongue') can occur ●*Location:* Can involve the lips, tongue, palate and facial muscles ●*Pattern:* For drug-induced syndromes, the dyskinesias can occur either during drug therapy or within 3 months of discontinuing antipsychotic medication ●*Precipitating factors:* Antipsychotic medications ●*Relieving factors:* Discontinuation of antipsychotic medication (especially dopamine blockers), or treat with dopamine-depleting drugs such as reserpine ●*Clinical course:* Prevalence increases with age ●*Co-morbidities:* Huntington's disease, Meige syndrome, schizophrenia ●*Procedure results:* No relevant procedures ●*Test findings:* No relevant tests

Orthostatic hypotension ●*Onset:* Acute ●*Male:female ratio:* M=F ●*Ethnicity:* All ●*Character:* Decline in blood pressure (>20mmHg) and a rise in heart rate immediately upon standing ●*Location:* Nonspecific ●*Pattern:* Lightheadedness, dizziness, syncope

566

●*Precipitating factors:* Dehydration, autonomic neuropathy (as seen in diabetics), medications ●*Relieving factors:* Change from sitting/lying position in most cases; rehydration if dehydrated. In autonomic dysfunction, beta-blockers/serotonin receptor antagonists may be helpful ●*Clinical course:* Usually benign once patient is rehydrated adequately ●*Co-morbidities:* Usually elderly patients taking diuretics or vasodilators. Diabetics with autonomic dysfunction. GI bleeding may present with orthostatic hypotension ●*Procedure results:* No relevant procedures ●*Test findings:* No relevant tests

Osgood-Schlatter disease ●*Onset:* Subacute ●*Male:female ratio:* M>F ●*Ethnicity:* All ●*Character:* Dull ache ●*Location:* Tibial tuberosity ●*Pattern:* Pain with overuse ●*Precipitating factors:* Rapid growth spurt ●*Relieving factors:* Ice, rest, tibial brace ●*Clinical course:* Self-limited ●*Co-morbidities:* None relevant ●*Procedure results:* No relevant procedures ●*Test findings:* Enlarged tibial tuberosity, loose ossicles over tibia

Osler-Weber-Rendu syndrome ●*Onset:* Acute ●*Male:female ratio:* M=F ●*Ethnicity:* All ●*Character:* Telangiectasias on the lips, and oral and nasopharyngeal membranes, recurrent epistaxis, gastrointestinal hemorrhage (hematemesis, melena, hematochezia), sometimes high-output cardiac failure due to shunting in the liver ●*Location:* Telangiectasias on the lips and mucous membranes ●*Pattern:* Nonspecific ●*Precipitating factors:* Antiplatelet or anticoagulant medications ●*Relieving factors:* Local ablation to bleeding lesions, estrogens, aminocaproic acid ●*Clinical course:* Recurrent episodes of bleeding beginning in early childhood. Patients often require large numbers of blood transfusions over a lifetime ●*Co-morbidities:* Possibly hepatitis C, hepatitis B or HIV acquired in blood products ●*Procedure results:* Tissue biopsy: ectatic venules and capillaries without elastic lamina or muscle tissue; bleeding or vascular malformations on angiography ●*Test findings:* Telangiectasias in the intestine (small bowel most common) seen on endoscopy; anemia

Osteoarthritis ●*Onset:* Insidious ●*Male:female ratio:* M<F ●*Ethnicity:* More frequent in Caucasians than African-Americans and Asians ●*Character:* Dull ache over affected joint areas ●*Location:* Knees, hips, base of thumb, spine, shoulders ●*Pattern:* Pain worse after use of joint; morning stiffness less than 30 min ●*Precipitating factors:* Repetitive motion or strain placed on joint ●*Relieving factors:* Acetaminophen, NSAIDs, physical therapy, assistive devices ●*Clinical course:* Progressive with intermittent flares ●*Co-morbidities:* Obesity, inflammatory arthritis, chondrocalcinosis, hemochromatosis, acromegaly ●*Procedure results:* Synovial fluid analysis with WBC <500 ●*Test findings:* Plain radiographs with joint-space narrowing, sclerosis, osteophytosis

Osteochondritis dissecans ●*Onset:* Acute, subacute ●*Male:female ratio:* M(3):F(1) ●*Ethnicity:* All ●*Character:* Pain, swelling ●*Location:* Ankle, knee, elbow joints ●*Pattern:* Worse with use ●*Precipitating factors:* Trauma ●*Relieving factors:* Reducing weightbearing, immobilization, internal fixation ●*Clinical course:* Heals spontaneously in many cases, some require invasive procedures ●*Co-morbidities:* None relevant ●*Procedure results:* MRI shows separated osteochondral lesion ●*Test findings:* Plain radiographs are positive

Osteochondrosis ●*Onset:* Subacute ●*Male:female ratio:* Depends on type of osteochondrosis ●*Ethnicity:* All ●*Character:* Persistent pain, local swelling, limitation of motion, antalgic gait or limp ●*Location:* Hip, knee, talus ●*Pattern:* Nonspecific ●*Precipitating factors:* Trauma, infection, congenital, idiopathic, chronic alcoholism, sickle cell disease, chronic steroid use, hip dislocation or femoral neck fracture, collagen vascular disease ●*Relieving factors:* Nonweightbearing, joint protection, range of motion exercises, surgery ●*Clinical course:* Without treatment, subchondral collapse and fracture; most lead to secondary destructive joint disorders anyway ●*Co-morbidities:* Steroid use, chronic alcoholism, gout, collagen vascular disease ●*Procedure results:* Joint aspiration: sterile fluid; arthroscopy to assess underlying cartilage ●*Test findings:* X-ray: necrosis of bone with subchondral bone fracture, periarticular swelling; MRI same but better defines articular surface

Osteogenesis imperfecta ●*Onset:* Acute/insidious ●*Male:female ratio:* M=F ●*Ethnicity:* All ●*Character:* Fractures ●*Location:* Bones ●*Pattern:* Multiple fractures with minimal trauma prenatally to adulthood ●*Precipitating factors:* Structural or quantitative defects in type I collagen, autosomal dominant in 1 in 20,000 ●*Relieving factors:* Active physical rehabilitation, orthopedic management with splinting, casting and rod placement, growth hormone and intravenous bisphosphate ●*Clinical course:* Chronic condition with early death in types II and III; types I and IV with normal life span; recurrent fractures, pneumonias, cardiac failure ●*Co-morbidities:* Scoliosis, blue sclera, easy bruising, joint laxity, deafness ●*Procedure results:* Skin biopsy reveals collagen abnormalities, and prenatally by U/S ●*Test findings:* X-ray indicates osteoporosis, bowing, flaring, and fractures

Osteoma ●*Onset:* Insidious ●*Male:female ratio:* M=F ●*Ethnicity:* All ●*Character:* Dull ache and swelling over skull ●*Location:* Skull and ethmoid sinuses ●*Pattern:* Nonspecific ●*Precipitating factors:* None relevant ●*Relieving factors:* Surgical excision ●*Clinical course:* Chronic, usually asymptomatic ●*Co-morbidities:* Familial colonic polyposis ●*Procedure results:* Radiopaque lobular mass on plain radiograph. Bone biopsy with characteristic pathology ●*Test findings:* No relevant tests

Osteomalacia ●*Onset:* Insidious ●*Male:female ratio:* M<F (slightly) ●*Ethnicity:* All ●*Character:* Bone aches. Pain from fractures ●*Location:* Bones ●*Pattern:* Nonspecific ●*Precipitating factors:* Vitamin D deficiency, tumor-induced oncogenic osteomalacia ●*Relieving factors:* Vitamin D repletion ●*Clinical course:* Progressive ●*Co-morbidities:* None relevant ●*Procedure results:* X-ray may show pseudofractures ●*Test findings:* Borderline low-to-normal serum calcium, low serum phosphorus with elevated parathyroid hormone and alkaline phosphatase, low 25-hydroxyvitamin D3 level

Osteomyelitis ●*Onset:* Subacute ●*Male:female ratio:* M>F ●*Ethnicity:* All ●*Character:* Dull ache ●*Location:* Long bones of leg, vertebral bodies, foot, sacrum ●*Pattern:* Pain progressive throughout the day ●*Precipitating factors:* Pain with weightbearing ●*Relieving factors:* Debridement of affected bone, antibiotics ●*Clinical course:* Progressive ●*Co-morbidities:* Diabetic foot ulcers, decubitus skin ulcers, prosthetic joints, sickle cell disease, intravenous drug use, immunosuppression ●*Procedure results:* Positive bone biopsy ●*Test findings:* Elevated ESR

Osteonecrosis ●*Onset:* Acute ●*Male:female ratio:* M>F ●*Ethnicity:* African-American ●*Character:* Dull ache ●*Location:* Hip, knee, shoulder, foot, wrist ●*Pattern:* Nonspecific ●*Precipitating factors:* Pain with weightbearing ●*Relieving factors:* Unloading joint with assistive device, total joint replacement ●*Clinical course:* Progressive in weightbearing joints such as the hips or knees, frequently self-limiting in shoulders ●*Co-morbidities:* Steroid use, alcohol abuse, systemic lupus erythematosus, sickle cell disease ●*Procedure results:* Synovial fluid analysis with WBC <500 ●*Test findings:* MRI with bone infarcts

Osteoporosis ●*Onset:* Insidious but fracture acute ●*Male:female ratio:* M<F ●*Ethnicity:* Caucasian, Asian ●*Character:* Localized pain when fracture occurs ●*Location:* Spine, hip, and wrist most common sites for fracture ●*Pattern:* Nonspecific ●*Precipitating factors:* Menopause, lean body habitus, smoking, inadequate calcium and vitamin D intake, steroids, excessive alcohol intake ●*Relieving factors:* Increase calcium intake, exercise, antiresorptive medication ●*Clinical course:* Progressive ●*Co-morbidities:* Cushing's disease or syndrome, hypogonadism, multiple myeloma ●*Procedure results:* None relevant ●*Test findings:* Low bone mineral density

Osteosarcoma ●*Onset:* Subacute ●*Male:female ratio:* M=F ●*Ethnicity:* All ●*Character:* Pain ●*Location:* Knee and proximal humerus ●*Pattern:* Worse with weightbearing ●*Precipitating factors:* None relevant ●*Relieving factors:* Surgical excision and chemotherapy ●*Clinical course:* Often fatal ●*Co-morbidities:* Paget's disease, bone irradiation, multiple hereditary exostoses ●*Procedure results:* Bone biopsy with characteristic pathology ●*Test findings:* Elevated alkaline phosphatase

Otitis externa ●*Onset:* Acute ●*Male:female ratio:* M=F ●*Ethnicity:* All ●*Character:* Moderate to severe ear pain and otorrhea ●*Location:* Ear ●*Pattern:* Persistent pain ●*Precipitating factors:* Swimming exposure or instrumentation of ear canal ●*Relieving factors:* Ice pack ●*Clinical course:* May progress with swelling of canal to complete occlusion of ear canal resulting in hearing loss ●*Co-morbidities:* Diabetes, eczema ●*Procedure results:* Otoscopy: swollen ear canal with otorrhea and tragal tenderness ●*Test findings:* Cultures of ear canal drainage usually positive for pseudomonas or Staphylococcus aureus

Otosclerosis ●*Onset:* Insidious ●*Male:female ratio:* M(1):F(2) ●*Ethnicity:* More commonly seen in Caucasians ●*Character:* Mild-to-moderate hearing loss in affected ear ●*Location:* Affected ear ●*Pattern:* Chronic nonfluctuating hearing loss ●*Precipitating factors:* None relevant ●*Relieving factors:* None relevant ●*Clinical course:* Generally very slow progression in hearing loss ●*Co-morbidities:* None relevant ●*Procedure results:* Otoscopy reveals a normal tympanic membrane ●*Test findings:* Audiogram reflects a conductive hearing loss in the affected ear with normal tympanogram

Ovarian torsion ●*Onset:* Acute ●*Male:female ratio:* F ●*Ethnicity:* All ●*Character:* Stabbing, lateralized abdominal pain, colicky in nature; often associated with nausea and vomiting ●*Location:* Lateralized ●*Pattern:* Acute, sharp abdominal pain often preceded by several days of crampy pain; often with nausea and vomiting. Pain increases with time ●*Precipitating factors:* Associated with adnexal masses, particularly dermoid cysts ●*Relieving factors:* Surgical removal or untorsing of ovary ●*Clinical course:* Acute onset with pain until complete ovarian necrosis; can be self-limiting if adnexa spontaneously untorses or over time as adnexa necroses ●*Co-morbidities:* Frequently associated with dermoid cysts ●*Procedure results:* Adnexal mass on U/S or CT scan; diminished or absent blood flow by Doppler ●*Test findings:* Slightly elevated WBC

Ovulatory bleeding ●*Onset:* Variable ●*Male:female ratio:* F ●*Ethnicity:* All ●*Character:* Cyclic bleeding in the middle of the menstrual cycle ●*Location:* Vagina ●*Pattern:* Repetitive, cyclic between midcycle ●*Precipitating factors:* None relevant ●*Relieving factors:* Birth control pills ●*Clinical course:* Bleeding is usually light and lasts 1-2 days ●*Co-morbidities:* None relevant ●*Procedure results:* No relevant procedures ●*Test findings:* Negative pregnancy test

Paget's disease ●*Onset:* Insidious ●*Male:female ratio:* M=F ●*Ethnicity:* Rare in African descent ●*Character:* Pain ●*Location:* Affected bones, usually pelvis, spine, skull, humerus, and tibia ●*Pattern:* Worse with weightbearing ●*Precipitating factors:* None relevant ●*Relieving factors:* Osteocalcin, bisphosphonates ●*Clinical course:* Waxing and waning, but often asymptomatic ●*Co-morbidities:* None relevant ●*Procedure results:* Plain radiographs: osteolysis. Bone scan: increased activity ●*Test findings:* Alkaline phosphatase elevated

Palmar-plantar warts ●*Onset:* Subacute/insidious ●*Male:female ratio:* M=F ●*Ethnicity:* All ●*Character:* Multiple painless, flesh-colored papules on hands. Painful, rough, indurated, flesh-colored papules on soles ●*Location:* Hands (mostly around nails), soles ●*Pattern:* Plantar papules are painful and hyperkeratotic. Hand papules are numerous, usually around the nails, and asymptomatic ●*Precipitating factors:* Contact, minor skin trauma, swimming in public pools (plantar), use of public showers (plantar) ●*Relieving factors:* None relevant ●*Clinical course:* Incubation over several months; some remit spontaneously; persistent warts, especially on soles, require ablative therapy ●*Co-morbidities:* Compromised cellular immunity ●*Procedure results:* Thrombosed capillaries are seen as black dots on plantar warts' surfaces ●*Test findings:* No relevant tests

Pancreatic cancer ●*Onset:* Insidious ●*Male:female ratio:* M(2):F(1) ●*Ethnicity:* More common in African-American population ●*Character:* Patients present with anorexia, weight loss, jaundice, pruritus. Abdominal pain occurs in many, and is a deep epigastric gnawing pain that can be quite severe. However, painless jaundice is also a clue to pancreatic malignancy. Symptoms progress over weeks-to-months with progressive weakness and weight loss. Diabetes is uncommon, and depression may occur prior to the diagnosis being made. Physical examination is notable for jaundice and cachexia ●*Location:* Pain is usually mid-epigastric ●*Pattern:* Progressive over weeks-to-months ●*Precipitating factors:* None relevant ●*Relieving factors:* Jaundice may be treated with bile duct stenting via endoscopic retrograde cholangio-pancreatography (ERCP), or with surgical resection of the tumor (usually a Whipple procedure). Pain is difficult to treat, and requires narcotic analgesia. Celiac axis injection may also provide pain relief ●*Clinical course:* Progresses over months, with mortality nearly inevitable: 5- year survival is <10% ●*Co-morbidities:* Chronic pancreatitis ●*Procedure results:* CT or endoscopic retrograde cholangio-pancreatography (ERCP) may show pancreatic mass lesion; biopsy can be diagnostic ●*Test findings:* Amylase and lipase may be elevated, but not universally

Pancreatic insufficiency ●*Onset:* Insidious ●*Male:female ratio:* M=F ●*Ethnicity:* All ●*Character:* Weight loss and diarrhea; usually steatorrhea, with light-colored stools that are foul-smelling and greasy, and which may be accompanied by oil droplets in the toilet bowl ●*Location:* If due to chronic pancreatitis, may have epigastric pain ●*Pattern:* Progressive diarrhea and weight loss over weeks-to-months ●*Precipitating factors:* Food intake, especially foods with high fat content ●*Relieving factors:* Pancreatic enzyme supplementation ●*Clinical course:* Progresses over weeks-to-months; not self-limited ●*Co-morbidities:* Chronic pancreatitis, pancreatic cancer, distal common bile-duct obstruction ●*Procedure results:* CT or endoscopic retrograde cholangio-pancreatography (ERCP) may show signs of chronic pancreatitis or pancreatic mass lesion ●*Test findings:* Fecal fat >7g per day (needs 72-hour collection while on diet containing 100g fat or more per day)

Pancreatic pseudocyst ●*Onset:* Insidious ●*Male:female ratio:* M=F ●*Ethnicity:* All ●*Character:* Persistent abdominal discomfort after acute pancreatitis, possibly early satiety and nausea. If the cyst is infected, fever, malaise. Note: many pseudocysts remain asymptomatic, and are diagnosed on imaging studies ●*Location:* Upper abdomen. Examination may reveal an abdominal mass ●*Pattern:* Nonspecific ●*Precipitating factors:* Usually a chronic problem, without precipitating factors ●*Relieving factors:* If the cyst is symptomatic, it can be drained via surgery, endoscopic techniques, or via interventional radiology. If there is associated pancreatic necrosis or if infection is suspected, surgical treatment is preferred ●*Clinical course:* May be self-limited over weeks-to-months, or may be unremitting, requiring treatment ●*Co-morbidities:* Acute pancreatitis of any cause ●*Procedure results:* Pseudocysts are best seen on CT or MRI scanning; aspiration of fluid is helpful if infection is suspected ●*Test findings:* Amylase and lipase may be persistently elevated

Panic disorder ●*Onset:* Often acute ●*Male:female ratio:* M=F ●*Ethnicity:* All ●*Character:* Discrete periods of intense fear or discomfort, accompanied by somatic signs and symptoms ●*Location:* Nonspecific ●*Pattern:* Frequency, pattern, and duration are extremely variable ●*Precipitating factors:* Some panic attacks are unexpected; others are situationally predisposed ●*Relieving factors:* Some report improvement with avoidance of certain provocative situations ●*Clinical course:* Variable, but often only partial improvement and long duration ●*Co-morbidities:* Major depression, substance-related disorders, other anxiety disorders, unclear association with mitral valve prolapse ●*Procedure results:* No relevant procedures ●*Test findings:* No relevant tests

Papilledema ●*Onset:* Acute/subacute/insidious ●*Male:female ratio:* M=F ●*Ethnicity:* All ●*Character:* Transient visual obscurations, headache, diplopia, nausea, vomiting, hemiparesis ●*Location:* Usually bilateral ●*Pattern:* Nonspecific ●*Precipitating factors:* Visual obscurations can be triggered by change in position ●*Relieving factors:* Maneuvers that lower intracranial pressure relieve the symptoms ●*Clinical course:* Slowly or rapidly progressive ●*Co-morbidities:* Intracranial or orbital mass lesions; systemic hypertension ●*Procedure results:* No relevant procedures ●*Test findings:* Ophthalmoscopic examination: early on swelling of nerve fiber layer, disc hyperemia associated with retention of the central cup; later splinter hemorrhage on disc margin, venous dilation/tortuosity, and nerve fiber layer infarcts

Paralytic ileus ●*Onset:* Acute or subacute ●*Male:female ratio:* M=F ●*Ethnicity:* All ●*Character:* Abdominal distention, nausea/vomiting, no passage of stool or flatus ●*Location:* Nonspecific ●*Pattern:* Nonspecific ●*Precipitating factors:* Abdominal surgery, certain medications (opiates), neurologic disorders, retroperitoneal process, electrolyte disturbances ●*Relieving factors:* Frequent turning or movement, correction of electrolytes, nasogastric and/or rectal tube ●*Clinical course:* Usually self-limited if postoperative, can be severe and require surgery if bowel dilation is extreme ●*Co-morbidities:* Parkinson's disease, dementia ●*Procedure results:* Endoscopy: dilated bowel often with area of transition to nondilated segment ●*Test findings:* Barium study: slow passage of barium but no obstruction; plain X-ray: dilated bowel but gas throughout; laboratory values: possible electrolyte abnormalities

Parkinson's disease ●*Onset:* Insidious ●*Male:female ratio:* M=F ●*Ethnicity:* All ●*Character:* Resting tremor, bradykinesia, rigidity of the extremities ●*Location:* Extremities ●*Pattern:* Nonspecific ●*Precipitating factors:* None relevant ●*Relieving factors:* Dopamine supplements or agonists, catechol-O-methyltransferase inhibitors ●*Clinical course:* Usually progressive ●*Co-morbidities:* None relevant ●*Procedure results:* Clinical diagnosis ●*Test findings:* No relevant tests

Paronychia ●*Onset:* Acute/subacute ●*Male:female ratio:* M(1):F(3) ●*Ethnicity:* All ❶ *Character:* Painful swelling by nail ❷ *Location:* Skin around nails ❸ *Pattern:* Red swelling around nail with loss of cuticle ●*Precipitating factors:* Moisture, cuticular damage ●*Relieving factors:* Antibiotics, antifungals, drainage ●*Clinical course:* Usually resolves with treatment ●*Co-morbidities:* None relevant ●*Procedure results:* No relevant procedures ●*Test findings:* No relevant tests

Images of ❶ *Character,* ❷ *Location,* ❸ *Pattern on page 572*

Paronychia: Images *see text page 571*

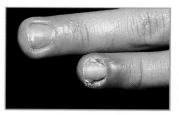

❶ *Character* Diffuse erythema is typical

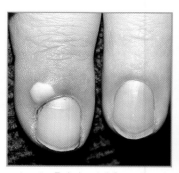

❷ *Location* Typical acute inflammation. A pocket of pus forms less commonly

Parotid calculus ●*Onset:* Subacute ●*Male:female ratio:* M=F ●*Ethnicity:* All ●*Character:* Recurring parotid gland swelling ●*Location:* Affected gland ●*Pattern:* Swelling more prominent after meals or citrus beverages ●*Precipitating factors:* Dehydration ●*Relieving factors:* Warm packs, avoidance of provocative foods ●*Clinical course:* Usually persistent chronic symptoms ●*Co-morbidities:* Possibly renal stones ●*Procedure results:* Obstruction of salivary flow in parotid duct on milking of gland; stone may be palpable (uncommon) ●*Test findings:* 15% radiopaque on mandibular plain films

Parotitis ●*Onset:* Acute ●*Male:female ratio:* M=F ●*Ethnicity:* All ●*Character:* Moderate-to-severe pain and swelling over parotid region, usually with fever ●*Location:* Affected gland ●*Pattern:* May be made worse by eating; pain gradually progresses with increased swelling ●*Precipitating factors:* Dehydration; inpatient hospitalization ●*Relieving factors:* Warm packs, avoidance of provocative foods (cheese, lemon, other) ●*Clinical course:* Usually progresses unless treated ●*Co-morbidities:* None relevant ●*Procedure results:* Pus emanating from parotid duct intraorally ●*Test findings:* Culture of parotid secretions usually positive for Staphylococcus aureus or other bacteria

Paroxysmal atrial tachycardia ●*Onset:* Acute ●*Male:female ratio:* M=F ●*Ethnicity:* All ●*Character:* Symptoms: palpitations, chest pressure, anxiety, dyspnea, lightheadedness, syncope ●*Location:* Nonspecific ●*Pattern:* Palpitations are common. Can be asymptomatic. Blood pressure normal or decreased ●*Precipitating factors:* Excessive caffeine, alcohol, cocaine, sympathomimetics ●*Relieving factors:* Depends on the nature of the arrhythmia. Re-entry pathways will break with vagal maneuvers. Atrial tachycardias do not break with vagal stimulation. Any underlying conditions should be treated ●*Clinical course:* Supraventricular tachycardias are usually self-limiting and easily controlled with vagal maneuvers or atrioventricular (AV)-nodal agents ●*Co-morbidities:* Hyperadrenergic states (e.g. fever), hyperthyroidism, possibly mitral valve prolapse ●*Procedure results:* Tachycardia is present. In cases of sinus node re-entry, AV-node re-entry (AVNRT), atrioventricular re-entry tachycardia (such as Wolff-Parkinson-White syndrome), atrial tachycardia, atrial flutter with constant block, the observed pulse is regular. In cases of atrial flutter with variable block, atrial fibrillation, multifocal atrial tachycardia, the observed pulse is irregular ●*Test findings:* Depending on type of arrhythmia, ECG can be diagnostic

Paroxysmal hemoglobinuria following exercise ●*Onset:* Acute ●*Male:female ratio:* M=F ●*Ethnicity:* All ●*Character:* Pain, hemoglobinuria ●*Location:* Back and thigh pain ●*Pattern:* Nonspecific ●*Precipitating factors:* Strenuous exercise (running, marching)

●*Relieving factors:* Cessation of exercise, thick-soled shoes ●*Clinical course:* Self-limited ●*Co-morbidities:* None relevant ●*Procedure results:* No relevant procedures ●*Test findings:* Urinalysis: positive for hemoglobin, occasionally myoglobinuria; hemoglobinemia, elevated LDH, decreased haptoglobin.

Paroxysmal nocturnal hemoglobinuria ●*Onset:* Subacute/insidious ●*Male:female ratio:* M=F ●*Ethnicity:* All ●*Character:* Hemoglobinuria; abdominal pain (due to mesenteric thrombosis); symptoms consistent with anemia (fatigue, dyspnea, weakness), aplastic anemia ●*Location:* Thrombosis tends to be in hepatic, mesenteric, or cerebral veins ●*Pattern:* Hematuria occurs predominantly in the first morning urine ●*Precipitating factors:* None relevant ●*Relieving factors:* Transfusions washed RBCs (not whole blood), iron and folate, androgens, prednisone, heparin for thromboses, antithymocyte globulin for marrow hypoplasia, bone marrow transplantation ●*Clinical course:* Prolonged, average survival 10 years; most have complications (40% venous thromboses); 15-30% aplastic anemia ●*Co-morbidities:* None relevant ●*Procedure results:* Bone marrow biopsy: variable morphology, hypoplasia or erythroid hyperplasia ●*Test findings:* Pancytopenia, Coomb's-negative hemolytic anemia, hemoglobinuria, urine hemosiderin, elevated lactate dehydrogenase, decreased leukocyte alkaline phosphatase

Partial apraxia ●*Onset:* Acute ●*Male:female ratio:* M=F ●*Ethnicity:* All ●*Character:* Inability to perform learned motor acts despite former ability and willingness to do so ●*Location:* Lesion of neural pathway, usually parietal lobe ●*Pattern:* Patient unable to conceptualize the needed movement patterns and translate them into necessary action; possible transient maturational lag ●*Precipitating factors:* Parietal lobe lesion ●*Relieving factors:* None relevant ●*Clinical course:* Lifelong or transient if normal lag ●*Co-morbidities:* Dementia in older patient ●*Procedure results:* No relevant procedures ●*Test findings:* Educational/neurologic testing

Parvovirus B19 infection ●*Onset:* Acute (fifth disease), acute and chronic (polyarthralgia), chronic (anemia) ●*Male:female ratio:* M=F ●*Ethnicity:* All ●*Character:* Erythema infectiosum: fever, cheek eruption, then a truncal rash in children. Fever and symmetric polyarthritis in adults. Aplastic anemia. Hydrops fetalis in neonates ●*Location:* Nonspecific ●*Pattern:* Facial rash after fever. Intensely red 'slapped cheek' appearance with circumoral pallor. Truncal rash (less common) is lacy maculopapular. Joint pain is symmetric. Can cause spontaneous abortion, idiopathic thrombocytopenic purpura (ITP) ●*Precipitating factors:* Sick contacts: outbreaks in schools, household transmission, transfusions (rare), sickle cell disease (aplastic crisis) ●*Relieving factors:* None relevant ●*Clinical course:* Fifth disease is acute, self-limiting within 7-10 days. Arthropathy in adults may persist for months. Aplastic crisis is usually transient (7-14 days) but may persist in immunosuppressed patients ●*Co-morbidities:* Sickle cell disease and hemolytic anemia (aplastic crisis), AIDS/other immunodeficiency (red cell aplasia), hemophagocytic syndrome, hydrops fetalis, spontaneous abortion, ITP, Henoch-Schonlein purpura ●*Procedure results:* DNA of parvovirus in plasma, joints, bone marrow, by polymerase chain reaction; giant pronormoblast with vacuoles in bone marrow. Parvo B19 specific serology (IgM and IgG) ●*Test findings:* Anemia, low reticulocyte count, positive B19 specific serology (IgM and IgG)

Patellar dislocation ●*Onset:* Acute ●*Male:female ratio:* M=F ●*Ethnicity:* All ●*Character:* Pain ●*Location:* Patella ●*Pattern:* Worse pain prior to reduction ●*Precipitating factors:* Traumatic force applied to patella ●*Relieving factors:* Reduction of patella ●*Clinical course:* Intermittent dislocation ●*Co-morbidities:* None relevant ●*Procedure results:* Plain radiograph shows dislocation ●*Test findings:* No relevant tests

Patent ductus arteriosus ●*Onset:* Acute ●*Male:female ratio:* M(1):F(2-3) ●*Ethnicity:* All ●*Character:* Apical pulse prominent, murmur ●*Location:* Heart ●*Pattern:* Continuous machinery-like murmur at second intercostal space or down left sternal border ●*Precipitating factors:* Female, maternal rubella, prematurity, congenital heart disease with failure of the patent ductus arteriosus (PDA) to close after birth ●*Relieving factors:* Surgical or catheter coil closing of PDA in a term infant >1 week ●*Clinical course:* Quick recovery after closure with resolution of cardiac failure, failure to thrive, risk of endocarditis. In premature infants, PDA will close spontaneously in most cases ●*Co-morbidities:* Complex congenital heart disease, aortic stenosis and ventricular septal defects, heart failure, Eisenmenger's syndrome with pulmonary hypertension, infective endocarditis ●*Procedure results:* Echo: PDA with left atrial and left ventricles enlarged. Catherization required only in atypical cases to demonstrate abnormality. ECG reveals left ventricular hypertrophy or biventricular enlargement. Chest X-ray indicates large pulmonary artery and normal or large heart ●*Test findings:* No relevant tests

Pellagra ●*Onset:* Gradual ●*Male:female ratio:* M=F ●*Ethnicity:* African ●*Character:* Deficiency of niacin leading to reduction of NAD and NADP coenzymes impairing tissue respiration, lipid metabolism and glycolysis ●*Location:* Skin: photosensitive pigmented dermatitis; neurologic: dementia, encephalopathy, peripheral neuropathy; GI: diarrhea, achlorhydria, glossitis, stomatitis ●*Pattern:* Dermatitis in sun-exposed areas. Neurologic symptoms nonspecific. Early: insomnia, fatigue, irritability, depression. Late: memory impairment, dementia, spastic spinal cord syndrome ●*Precipitating factors:* Low socioeconomic status leading to nutritional deficiency. Prolonged isoniazid therapy ●*Relieving factors:* Dietary sources: yeast, meat especially liver, cereals, legumes, seeds. Daily recommended intake = 15-20mg. High-dose replacement 1500-3000mg daily can cause flushing, liver function test abnormalities, myositis ●*Clinical course:* Replacement results in resolution of symptoms; untreated course is progressive over years with death due to secondary complications ●*Co-morbidities:* Alcoholism; Hartnup's disease: defect in tryptophan absorption; carcinoid syndrome ●*Procedure results:* Neuropathology: swelling, chromatolysis, loss of Nissl staining in large Betz cells of motor cortex ●*Test findings:* No specific testing for diagnosis (clinical suspicion and response to replacement). 24-hour urine excretion of metabolites: N-methylnicotinamide (NMN) and 2-pyridone reduced

Pelvic abscess ●*Onset:* Subacute ●*Male:female ratio:* M=F ●*Ethnicity:* All ●*Character:* Increasing pelvic pain associated with fever, sweats, chills ●*Location:* Nonspecific ●*Pattern:* Nonspecific ●*Precipitating factors:* Recent pelvic inflammatory disease (PID), gonorrhea, chlamydia, recent pelvic surgery ●*Relieving factors:* Antibiotics and almost always surgery ●*Clinical course:* Variable ●*Co-morbidities:* PID, gonorrhea, chlamydia ●*Procedure results:* U/S or CT scan ●*Test findings:* Elevated WBC

Pelvic inflammatory disease ●*Onset:* Subacute ●*Male:female ratio:* F ●*Ethnicity:* Nonspecific ●*Character:* Often within 7 days of menses; misdiagnosed up to 33% of the time ●*Location:* Lower abdomen ●*Pattern:* Mucopurulent vaginal discharge, pelvic pain, urethritis, cervical motion, adnexal tenderness indicating endometritis/salpingitis ●*Precipitating factors:* Gonorrhea, chlamydia, certain types of IUDs ●*Relieving factors:* Antibiotics ●*Clinical course:* Responds to antibiotic treatment ●*Co-morbidities:* Infertility, Fitz-Hugh-Curtis syndrome (perihepatic adhesions), chronic pelvic pain syndrome ●*Procedure results:* Pelvic examination to rule out abscess ●*Test findings:* Positive cultures for chlamydia, gonorrhea; elevated WBC and ESR; negative human chorionic gonadotropin

Pemphigus vulgaris ●*Onset:* Acute/subacute ●*Male:female ratio:* M=F ●*Ethnicity:* Jewish and Mediterranean descent ●*Character:* Tender, raw skin areas ●*Location:* Trunk, scalp, intertriginous, mucous membranes ●*Pattern:* Flaccid, weeping blisters; denuded skin ●*Precipitating factors:* None relevant ●*Relieving factors:* Steroids, immunosuppressives ●*Clinical course:* Chronic, potentially fatal ●*Co-morbidities:* None relevant ●*Procedure results:* No relevant procedures ●*Test findings:* Skin biopsy

Peptic ulcer ●*Onset:* Subacute ●*Male:female ratio:* M=F ●*Ethnicity:* All ●*Character:* Epigastric pain (may be relieved/worsened by food intake). Sometimes nausea and vomiting.

Complicated cases may have gastric outlet obstruction, upper GI bleeding, or perforation ●*Location:* Epigastrium ●*Pattern:* Pain may occur any time of day, and often occurs at night ●*Precipitating factors:* Food intake (fatty/spicy foods, coffee, alcohol), NSAIDs. Stress may worsen pain but is not a cause ●*Relieving factors:* Food intake helps some patients. Antacid use, H2-blockers, or proton pump inhibitors relieve symptoms and promote healing. Avoiding NSAIDs and treating Helicobacter pylori infection help prevent recurrences ●*Clinical course:* Symptoms wax and wane, but are generally not self-limited ●*Co-morbidities:* H. pylori infection, gastrinoma, multiple endocrine neoplastic disorder ●*Procedure results:* Upper endoscopy is diagnostic ●*Test findings:* H. pylori serology may be positive

Pericardial effusion ●*Onset:* Variable ●*Male:female ratio:* M=F ●*Ethnicity:* All ●*Character:* Shortness of breath, dull or achy chest pain. Effusion is usually associated with pericarditis ●*Location:* Substernal chest ●*Pattern:* Pain improved by sitting forward if associated with pericarditis ●*Precipitating factors:* Trauma, infection/irritation of the pericardium, rheumatologic diseases, medications (hydralazine, procainamide, isoniazid, doxorubicin), post-radiotherapy ●*Relieving factors:* Sitting forward, aspirin or anti-inflammatories if pericarditis is present. Sometimes effusion has to be drained for symptomatic relief (and diagnostic information) ●*Clinical course:* Depends on cause of effusion; can be slow accumulation with minimal signs or symptoms, vs rapid accumulation of fluid or blood with severe acute life-threatening signs or symptoms, including the possibility of tamponade ●*Co-morbidities:* Malignancy, infection (TB, viral, bacterial), rheumatologic diseases and other inflammatory disorders (sarcoid, irritable bowel disease, amyloid, temporal arteritis, systemic lupus erythematosus), aortic dissection, myxedema, myocardial infarction, uremia ●*Procedure results:* Echo demonstrating pericardial fluid. CT scan can also sometimes show effusion. Pericardiocentesis can be used diagnostically (test for fungal and bacterial Gram stain/culture, viral studies, acid-fast bacilli stain and mycobacterial culture, lactate dehydrogenase, complete blood count, protein), and therapeutically to drain large effusions for symptom relief. Diagnosis can be confirmed by cardiac catheterization or angiography, but this is rarely necessary ●*Test findings:* Diminished heart sounds, pericardial friction rub, cardiomegaly or 'water bottle' configuration of cardiac silhouette on chest X-ray, and global low voltage of QRS complex on ECG can be suggestive (global ST elevation and/or PR depression may also be seen if coexisting pericarditis). Echo is diagnostic (echo-free space). If effusion is large or hemodynamically compromising, distended jugular veins and hypotension can be seen. The heart swinging in the pericardial fluid can result in electrical alternans on ECG

Pericarditis ●*Onset:* Acute/subacute ●*Male:female ratio:* M>F ●*Ethnicity:* All ●*Character:* Chest pain often retrosternal (can be sharp, pleuritic, dull), worsened by lying supine, coughing, deep inspiration; dyspnea may also be present ●*Location:* Typically retrosternal or in left precordial regions and may radiate to trapezius ridge and neck; occasionally, midepigastrium ●*Pattern:* Pain can last for hours-to-days, typically no relation to effort ●*Precipitating factors:* Many possible causes for pericarditis exist including idiopathic, infectious (e.g. viral, TB, fungal, bacterial), acute myocardial infarction (e.g. Dressler's syndrome), uremia, autoimmune diseases (e.g. acute rheumatic fever, scleroderma, systemic lupus, rheumatoid arthritis), inflammatory disorders (e.g. sarcoidosis, amyloidosis, inflammatory bowel disease, Behcet's disease, temporal arteritis), drugs (e.g. hydralazine, procainamide, phenytoin, isoniazid), trauma, radiation, postcardiac surgery, myxedema ●*Relieving factors:* Pain relieved by leaning forward; nonspecific therapy may include bed rest and treatment with NSAIDs (e.g. aspirin or indomethicin). Also steroid therapy. Colchicine has been used effectively for recurrent cases ●*Clinical course:* Most cases of pericarditis are self-limiting with improvement noted in 2-6 weeks; minority may develop cardiac constriction and persistent symptoms ●*Co-morbidities:* Co-morbidities depend on the cause of the pericarditis (see precipitating factors) ●*Procedure results:* Friction rub on cardiac examination ●*Test findings:* ECG may reveal tachycardia with or without diffuse ST elevations with PR depressions; electrical alternans may be noted if large pericardial effusion is present; chest X-ray may reveal enlarged cardiac silhouette; Echo may reveal pericardial thickening with or without effusion; cardiac enzymes are usually normal but can be elevated (e.g. both creatine kinase/MB and troponin); blood work may reveal evidence of other underlying conditions

Perineal laceration ● *Onset:* Immediate due to trauma ● *Male:female ratio:* F ● *Ethnicity:* All ● *Character:* Nonspecific ● *Location:* Perineum ● *Pattern:* Trauma ● *Precipitating factors:* Frequently associated with straddle injuries (i.e. bicycle) or sexual abuse ● *Relieving factors:* Surgical repair where needed ● *Clinical course:* Variable ● *Co-morbidities:* Sexual abuse ● *Procedure results:* No relevant procedures ● *Test findings:* No relevant tests

Periorbital cellulitis ● *Onset:* Acute ● *Male:female ratio:* M=F ● *Ethnicity:* All ● *Character:* Blurred vision, mild achy pain ● *Location:* Periorbital tissue. Periorbital edema and erythema on external examination; proptosis is absent ● *Pattern:* Unilateral. Eye motility is full ● *Precipitating factors:* Preceding periocular trauma ● *Relieving factors:* None relevant ● *Clinical course:* Rapidly progressive; requires antibiotic therapy for resolution ● *Co-morbidities:* Sinusitis, upper respiratory illness, otitis media ● *Procedure results:* No relevant procedures ● *Test findings:* Positive blood and tissue cultures

Periosteal fibrosarcoma ● *Onset:* Subacute to chronic ● *Male:female ratio:* M=F ● *Ethnicity:* All ● *Character:* Pain in the affected bone with preserved range of motion. On examination, firm mass fixed to the underlying bone. Systemic symptoms are rare ● *Location:* Extremities, most often the tibial shaft. Rare in axial skeleton, hands, and feet ● *Pattern:* Nonspecific ● *Precipitating factors:* Paget's disease, irradiated bone, multiple hereditary exostosis, polyostotic fibrous dysplasia ● *Relieving factors:* Surgical resection (wide excision vs amputation), adjuvant chemotherapy, possibly radiation therapy ● *Clinical course:* 5-20% survival at 2 yrs, metastasis to other bones and lungs is common ● *Co-morbidities:* None relevant ● *Procedure results:* Biopsy: high-grade chondroblastic osteosarcoma arising from the bone cortex ● *Test findings:* Elevated alkaline phosphatase. Plain radiography: small, radiolucent lesion with bone spiculation; scooped-out appearance with Codman's triangle

Peripheral vascular disease ● *Onset:* Acute, subacute ● *Male:female ratio:* M>F ● *Ethnicity:* All ● *Character:* Pain, ache, cramp, numbness in the extremity involved with atherosclerosis. Typically, symptoms begin with exertion but can progress to symptoms at rest ● *Location:* Leg, calf, or may even involve buttock/hip, and thigh if aortoiliac vessels are involved ● *Pattern:* Symptoms tend to occur with exertion with mild-to-moderate vascular disease. Rest pain may eventually develop. Symptoms can also occur at night when the legs are in a 'neutral' position and improve when legs are in a dependent position ● *Precipitating factors:* With mild-to-moderate disease, exertion results in symptoms. With severe disease, rest symptoms can occur ● *Relieving factors:* Typically, rest relieves symptoms, antiplatelet agents such as aspirin, ticlopidine, or clopidogrel bisulfate. Worsening symptoms may require revascularization surgery ● *Clinical course:* Disease can progress from symptoms with extreme exertion to rest symptoms ● *Co-morbidities:* Diabetes mellitus, hypertension, hyperlipidemia, smoking, cocaine use, positive family history of coronary artery disease ● *Procedure results:* Decreased or absent pulses, bruits over main arteries, loss of distal hair with cold extremities, pallor, cyanosis. Elevation of the legs may result in worsening pallor. Findings vary depending on the extent of atherosclerosis ● *Test findings:* Doppler flow velocity or ankle-brachial index (ABI) can diagnose peripheral vascular disease (PVD). ABI <0.5 signifies severe PVD. Alternative means of diagnosis: magnetic resonance angiography or angiography

Peritonitis ● *Onset:* Acute ● *Male:female ratio:* M>F ● *Ethnicity:* All ● *Character:* Abdominal pain, usually severe ● *Location:* Varies depending on the etiology, but patient invariably lies still, as movement exacerbates pain ● *Pattern:* Pain severe and unremitting ● *Precipitating factors:* Movement exacerbates pain ● *Relieving factors:* Lying still minimizes pain; analgesics usually required. Intravenous fluids, antibiotics; evaluate rapidly for surgery ● *Clinical course:* Progresses over hours, not self-limited ● *Co-morbidities:* Inflammatory bowel disorders (irritable bowel disease, diverticulitis), intra-abdominal infections, perforated viscus, abdominal trauma ● *Procedure results:* CT scan may reveal the source of the peritonitis. Imaging may show free air in a perforation ● *Test findings:* WBC almost always elevated; hematocrit usually elevated from hemoconcentration; metabolic acidosis may be present. Examination: fever, tachycardia, often with hypotension. Abdomen tender to gentle palpation, with rebound tenderness. Bowel sounds may be absent; varying amounts of rigidity in the abdomen

Peritonsillar abscess ●*Onset:* Acute ●*Male:female ratio:* M=F ●*Ethnicity:* All ●*Character:* Severe sore throat, trismus, odynophagia, fever ●*Location:* Oral cavity/oropharynx ●*Pattern:* Nonspecific ●*Precipitating factors:* Antecedent tonsillitis or upper respiratory infection ●*Relieving factors:* Avoidance of swallowing; leaning forward ●*Clinical course:* Relatively rapid progression with increased swelling and pain ●*Co-morbidities:* None relevant ●*Procedure results:* Pus in peritonsillar space on needle aspiration ●*Test findings:* Bulging unilateral tonsil, uvular deviation, trismus, muffled voice

Perthes' disease ●*Onset:* Usually intermittent, subacute ●*Male:female ratio:* M(4):F(1) ●*Ethnicity:* All ●*Character:* Intermittent limp, ache or pain in hip, pain on movement ●*Location:* Hip ●*Pattern:* Age of onset typically 5 to 10 years, 85% unilateral ●*Precipitating factors:* None, symptoms are the result of compromised blood supply to femoral head ●*Relieving factors:* Management is conservative where possible (NSAIDs and rest), surgical intervention is sometimes required ●*Clinical course:* Spontaneous resolution usually occurs after months or sometimes years ●*Co-morbidities:* None relevant ●*Procedure results:* Hip X-ray: initial changes, widening of joint space with increased bone density at epiphysis; in more established disease, flattening and lateral subluxation of the femoral epiphysis may occur ●*Test findings:* No relevant tests

Pertussis ●*Onset:* Gradual ●*Male:female ratio:* M<F ●*Ethnicity:* All ●*Character:* Catarrhal stage: upper respiratory symptoms; paroxysmal stage: forceful cough spasms with neck-vein distension, bulging eyes, and post-tussive vomiting; convalescent stage: gradual waning in cough intensity. Apnea in infants. Persistent cough in adults ●*Location:* Ciliated respiratory cells of nose, and upper and lower airway common. Lungs, CNS (seizures, encephalopathy) - rare ●*Pattern:* Cough spasm begins acutely with 10 to 30 forceful coughs followed by vomiting. Cough is worst at night. Spasm intensity wanes gradually. Distinctive whoop in pediatric cases. Nonparoxysmal persistent cough in adults ●*Precipitating factors:* Sick contacts, outbreaks, lack of immunization, age-related waning, immunity ●*Relieving factors:* Specific antibiotic if given early, beta-adrenergic inhaler ●*Clinical course:* Incubation 7-10 days, average duration 6-10 weeks, catarrhal stage 1-2 weeks, paroxysmal stage 2-4 weeks, convalescent stage several weeks. Antibiotics will shorten course if given in catarrhal stage. Complications: subconjuctival hemorrhage, seizure, secondary bacterial pneumonia, encephalopathy ●*Co-morbidities:* Malnutrition in infants ●*Procedure results:* Culturing Bartonella pertussis from nasopharynx, B. pertussis PCR or direct fluorescent antigen ●*Test findings:* Elevated WBC with marked lymphocytosis; specific serology

Pes planus ●*Onset:* Insidious ●*Male:female ratio:* M=F ●*Ethnicity:* All ●*Character:* Pain ●*Location:* Midfoot ●*Pattern:* Worse with weightbearing ●*Precipitating factors:* Poorly fitting shoes ●*Relieving factors:* Orthotics, podiatric surgery ●*Clinical course:* Chronic pain ●*Co-morbidities:* None relevant ●*Procedure results:* No relevant procedures ●*Test findings:* Tarsal coalition is detectable on plain radiographs

Peutz-Jeghers syndrome ●*Onset:* Subacute, insidious ●*Male:female ratio:* M=F ●*Ethnicity:* All ●*Character:* Colicky abdominal pain, freckled gums/lips, hamartomas of small intestine/stomach, clubbing ●*Location:* Abdomen ●*Pattern:* Colicky abdominal pain, possible GI bleeding ●*Precipitating factors:* Genetic, autosomal dominant ●*Relieving factors:* Polyp removal ●*Clinical course:* Progressive, lifelong ●*Co-morbidities:* Intussusception, malignant polyps ●*Procedure results:* Polyps on abdomen CT scan or endoscopy ●*Test findings:* Iron-deficiency anemia

Pharyngitis ●*Onset:* Acute ●*Male:female ratio:* M=F ●*Ethnicity:* All ●*Character:* Sore throat, odynophagia, fever ●*Location:* Throat/pharynx ●*Pattern:* Exudate and erythema along posterior pharyngeal wall ●*Precipitating factors:* None relevant ●*Relieving factors:* Saltwater gargles, cold liquids ●*Clinical course:* Viral: self limited; otherwise, slow progression or plateau ●*Co-morbidities:* None relevant ●*Procedure results:* No relevant procedures ●*Test findings:* Throat culture may be positive in bacterial pharyngitis

Pheochromocytoma ● *Onset:* Acute spells, but may be insidious ● *Male:female ratio:* M=F ● *Ethnicity:* Less frequent in African-Americans ● *Character:* Headache, palpitations, diaphoresis ● *Location:* Most commonly adrenal ● *Pattern:* Characteristically episodic but may have sustained hypertension ● *Precipitating factors:* None relevant ● *Relieving factors:* Alpha-adrenergic blockade, volume expansion ● *Clinical course:* Progressive ● *Co-morbidities:* Catecholamine-induced cardiomyopathy and congestive heart failure, multiple endocrine neoplasia type 2, Von Hippel-Lindau disease, neurofibromatosis ● *Procedure results:* CT/MRI of adrenal shows adrenal mass ● *Test findings:* Elevated 24-hour urine for catecholamines, vanilllylmandelic acid, and metanephrines

Phimosis and paraphimosis ● *Onset:* Subacute and chronic for phimosis. Acute for paraphimosis ● *Male:female ratio:* M ● *Ethnicity:* All ● *Character:* Phimosis: unretractable foreskin, pain on erection. Paraphimosis: constriction of glans penis, pain, ulceration, drainage, swelling ● *Location:* Distal penis, foreskin ● *Pattern:* Symptom progression with disease progression ● *Precipitating factors:* Phimosis: poor hygiene, frequent diaper rash in infants. Paraphimosis: leaving foreskin retracted by inexperienced healthcare provider ● *Relieving factors:* Phimosis: treatment of coexisting balanitis when present, dorsal slit, circumcision. Paraphimosis: manual reduction, dorsal slit, circumcision ● *Clinical course:* Phimosis: progressive when untreated. Paraphimosis: when untreated, progressive to major infection and eventual ischemia and gangrene of the glans ● *Co-morbidities:* UTI, urethritis, balanitis ● *Procedure results:* No relevant procedures ● *Test findings:* No relevant tests

Phobia ● *Onset:* If associated with trauma or unexpected panic attacks, tends to be acute ● *Male:female ratio:* M=F ● *Ethnicity:* Content (and prevalence) of phobias varies with culture and ethnicity ● *Character:* Marked and persistent fear that is excessive or unreasonable, cued by presence or anticipation of a specific object or situation ● *Location:* Nonspecific ● *Pattern:* Feared objects/situations tend to involve things that may actually represent a threat or have previously done so ● *Precipitating factors:* Traumatic events, observing others traumatized, informational transmission ● *Relieving factors:* Avoidance of phobic situation ● *Clinical course:* Age of onset most typically childhood; if disorder persists into adulthood, remits only infrequently ● *Co-morbidities:* Panic disorder with agoraphobia, other anxiety disorders ● *Procedure results:* No relevant procedures ● *Test findings:* No relevant tests

Photodermatitis ● *Onset:* Acute, subacute ● *Male:female ratio:* M=F ● *Ethnicity:* All ❶ *Character:* Rash ❷ *Location:* Sun-exposed arms, face ❸ *Pattern:* Papules, plaques ● *Precipitating factors:* Sun exposure ● *Relieving factors:* Sunblock, steroids, antimalarials ● *Clinical course:* Persists ● *Co-morbidities:* None relevant ● *Procedure results:* No relevant procedures ● *Test findings:* No relevant tests

Images of ❶ *Character,* ❷ *Location,* ❸ *Pattern on page 579*

Phrenic nerve palsy ● *Onset:* Acute ● *Male:female ratio:* M=F ● *Ethnicity:* All ● *Character:* Unilateral or bilateral palsy can manifest differently; unilateral diaphragmatic paralysis is usually asymptomatic; bilateral palsy can lead to paradoxical respiration with the abdomen being drawn in with inspiration, decreased oxygenation and difficulty breathing in a supine position ● *Location:* Specific site of injury can occur at any site along path of phrenic nerves, in particular on the left side where the nerve loops around the aortic arch; mediastinal mass may entrap phrenic nerves bilaterally leading to diaphragmatic paralysis ● *Pattern:* Diaphragmatic paralysis ● *Precipitating factors:* Mediastinal or pulmonary tumors; cardiac 'cold cardioplegia' during surgery; herpes zoster ● *Relieving factors:* None relevant ● *Clinical course:* Unilateral palsy can be asymptomatic, with almost 75% of vital capacity preserved; abnormalities become more pronounced when supine ● *Co-morbidities:* For unilateral lesions, usually nerve injuries, postsurgical or postzoster; bilateral palsy usually due to a generalized neuropathy or myopathy or may be idiopathic ● *Procedure results:* No relevant procedures ● *Test findings:* Sniff maneuver with fluoroscopy demonstrates problem; nerve conduction studies

Photodermatitis: Images *see text page 578*

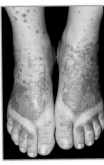

❶ *Character* Acute onset of red-brown plaques after sun-exposure

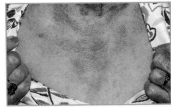

❷ *Location* Red scaly plaques on sun-exposed areas of the chest

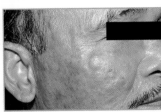

❸ *Pattern* Close-up showing coalescent red plaques

Phyllode tumor ●*Onset:* Subacute to chronic ●*Male:female ratio:* M<F ●*Ethnicity:* All ●*Character:* Breast mass (smooth, rounded, multinodular), possibly skin ulceration ●*Location:* Breast ●*Pattern:* Nonspecific ●*Precipitating factors:* None relevant ●*Relieving factors:* Wide surgical excision ●*Clinical course:* Depends on subtype (benign, borderline or malignant). Twenty to 50% are malignant and 5% of these metastasize. Twenty percent recur locally ●*Co-morbidities:* None relevant ●*Procedure results:* Biopsy: epithelial elements with connective stroma ●*Test findings:* No relevant tests

Pituitary basophilic adenoma (Cushing's disease, ACTH-producing adenoma) ●*Onset:* Gradual ●*Male:female ratio:* M(1):F(8) ●*Ethnicity:* All ●*Character:* Central obesity, weight gain, striae, moon facies, supraclavicular fat pad, easy bruisability, proximal muscle weakness, hyperpigmentation ●*Location:* Central fat, moon face, supraclavicular fat pad ●*Pattern:* Nonspecific ●*Precipitating factors:* None relevant ●*Relieving factors:* Pituitary surgery to remove adenoma ●*Clinical course:* May be progressive, often over long period of time ●*Co-morbidities:* Infection, osteoporosis, impaired wound healing ●*Procedure results:* MRI/CT may show pituitary tumor if large enough. If tumor not seen, petrosal sinus sampling may help lateralize tumor location ●*Test findings:* Elevated 24-hour free cortisol; failure to suppress cortisol in dexamethasone 1mg overnight suppression test but suppression with low dose (0.5mg every 6h for eight doses)

Pituitary eosinophilic adenoma (prolactinoma) ●*Onset:* Insidious unless present acutely with pituitary apoplexy ●*Male:female ratio:* M=F ●*Ethnicity:* All ●*Character:* Galactorrhea, oligomenorrhea, or amenorrhea in women; impotence in men ●*Location:* Pituitary ●*Pattern:* Nonspecific ●*Precipitating factors:* Pituitary tumor ●*Relieving factors:* Bromocriptine, cabergoline, pituitary surgery ●*Clinical course:* Progressive, but some tumors may spontaneously remit ●*Co-morbidities:* Multiple endocrine neoplasia (MEN type 1) ●*Procedure results:* Pituitary mass on CT or MRI ●*Test findings:* Elevated prolactin

Pituitary hypothyroidism ●*Onset:* Insidious ●*Male:female ratio:* M=F ●*Ethnicity:* All ●*Character:* Lethargy, fatigue, weight gain, constipation without goiter ●*Location:* Pituitary ●*Pattern:* Nonspecific ●*Precipitating factors:* Pituitary surgery, pituitary tumor, pituitary irradiation ●*Relieving factors:* Thyroid hormone replacement ●*Clinical course:* Progressive ●*Co-morbidities:* Hypercholesterolemia, obesity ●*Procedure results:* No relevant procedures ●*Test findings:* Low level of T4 in the face of low or inappropriately low thyroid-stimulating hormone (TSH) level

Pityriasis rosea ●*Onset:* Acute ●*Male:female ratio:* M=F ●*Ethnicity:* All ❶ *Character:* Itching, rash ●*Location:* Trunk, arms ❸ *Pattern:* Pink-tan scaly oval plaques along skin cleavage lines. Often starts with 'herald patch' ●*Precipitating factors:* None relevant ●*Relieving factors:* Erythromycin, UV light ●*Clinical course:* Resolves in 1-2 months ●*Co-morbidities:* None relevant ●*Procedure results:* No relevant procedures ●*Test findings:* No relevant tests

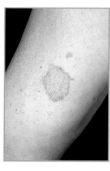

❶ *Character*
Solitary red
papulosquam
ous plaque on
the arm, a
first sign

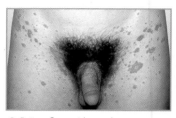

❸ *Pattern* Symmetric papulosquamous plaques in sun-protected areas e.g. groin are typical

Pityriasis versicolor ●*Onset:* Gradual ●*Male:female ratio:* M=F ●*Ethnicity:* All ❶ *Character:* Macular, hypopigmented or hyperpigmented, occasionally scaling, superficial, oval skin lesions ❷ *Location:* Upper trunk and waist, arms (proximal>distal), neck, face, other skin ❸ *Pattern:* Single or multiple skin lesions are oval, macular, or patchy. Lesions are lighter than surrounding skin in summer (fail to tan) and darker in winter (versicolor) ●*Precipitating factors:* Worldwide: more common in tropics and subtropics, more common in teens to thirties, person-to-person contact with scaling lesions ●*Relieving factors:* None relevant ●*Clinical course:* Incubation: unknown, gradual progression, some are self-limited, others require (topical) therapy ●*Co-morbidities:* None relevant ●*Procedure results:* Round yeast forms and short hyphae on potassium hydroxide (KOH) preparations from skin scrapings, yellow fluorescence under Wood's light ●*Test findings:* Round yeast forms and short hyphae on KOH preparations from skin scrapings

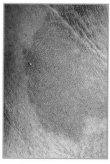

❶ *Character*
Hyperpigmented slightly
scaly plaques

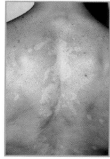

❷ *Location* Typical
hypopigmented areas on
the back.

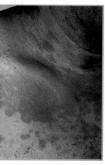

❸ *Pattern* Typical
hyperpigmented areas

Placenta previa ●*Onset:* Variable ●*Male:female ratio:* F ●*Ethnicity:* All ●*Character:* Painless bleeding ●*Location:* Placental ●*Pattern:* Varied from staining to copious vaginal bleeding ●*Precipitating factors:* Usually nothing though may be associated with intercourse ●*Relieving factors:* Bedrest; tocolysis if associated with contractions ●*Clinical course:* Variable: sometimes insignificant staining, sometimes uncontrollable bleeding ●*Co-morbidities:* Placenta accreta, vaso previa ●*Procedure results:* Placenta covering internal cervical os on U/S ●*Test findings:* No relevant tests

Plague ●*Onset:* Rapid, acute ●*Male:female ratio:* M=F ●*Ethnicity:* Developing nations ●*Character:* Rapid onset of fever and extremely painful regional lymphadenopathy (bubonic); dyspnea and cough (pneumonic); shock and coagulopathy (septicemic) ●*Location:* Common: lymph nodes (inguinal > axillary or cervical > other), skin (eschar), lungs, bloodstream (sepsis), coagulation cascade (disseminated intravasscular coagulation [DIC]). Less common: CNS and meninges, eye, pharynx, other ●*Pattern:* Fever is high, with chills and headache, bubo is extremely tender, eschar seen distal to bubo, cough is initially blood-tinged then frankly bloody, shock and DIC are common ●*Precipitating factors:* Flea bite, exposure to rodents, rural areas, outbreaks in urban areas, poor sanitation, person-to-person respiratory transmission, bioterrorism ●*Relieving factors:* None relevant ●*Clinical course:* Incubation: 2-6 days, rapidly progressive within 1-4 days, symptoms respond to antibiotics within 2-5 days, high case-fatality rate if untreated ●*Co-morbidities:* None relevant ●*Procedure results:* Bipolar-staining (safety-pin) Gram-negative coccobacilli in node aspirate/blood/sputum/CSF, massive growth of Yersinia pestis in culture (warn laboratory - biohazard), specific serologic tests, consolidation (patchy, and rarely cavitary) on chest X-ray ●*Test findings:* Elevated WBC (or leukemoid), granulocyte predominance, left shift, mild thrombocytopenia, DIC, mildly elevated hepatic transaminases

Plantar fasciitis ●*Onset:* Subacute ●*Male:female ratio:* M=F ●*Ethnicity:* All ●*Character:* Dull ache ●*Location:* Sole of foot ●*Pattern:* Pain worst with first step of the day ●*Precipitating factors:* Long periods of standing, long-distance running ●*Relieving factors:* Heel cushions, NSAIDs, physical therapy, night splints ●*Clinical course:* Self-limited ●*Co-morbidities:* Diabetes, obesity ●*Procedure results:* Bone scan may show inflammation at calcaneal tuberosity ●*Test findings:* Normal radiographs of the feet or calcaneal spurs

Pleural effusion ●*Onset:* Acute, insidious ●*Male:female ratio:* M=F ●*Ethnicity:* All ●*Character:* Dyspnea, chest discomfort ●*Location:* Chest ●*Pattern:* Dullness to percussion, decreased breath sounds ●*Precipitating factors:* Pneumonia, congestive heart failure (CHF), nephrosis, cirrhosis, tumor, pulmonary emboli, postoperative, pancreatic disease, pleurisy, mediastinal or hilar lymphatic obstruction, others ●*Relieving factors:* Physical removal of fluid by needle or chest tube; preventing fluid formation (e.g. treatment of CHF, renal or liver failure) ●*Clinical course:* Variable, depending on etiology ●*Co-morbidities:* None relevant ●*Procedure results:* Chest X-ray: blunting of costophrenic angle; decubitus chest X-ray: layering of fluid in pleural space ●*Test findings:* Pleural fluid cell counts plus differential, cytology, Gram stain and culture, pH and pleural fluid and serum total protein, lactate dehydrogenase, cholesterol, triglycerides, amylase may be helpful in distinguishing etiology

Pleurisy ●*Onset:* Acute ●*Male:female ratio:* M=F ●*Ethnicity:* All ●*Character:* Sharp chest pain upon deep inspiration or cough ●*Location:* Chest ●*Pattern:* Dullness to percussion, decreased breath sounds ●*Precipitating factors:* Viral infection ●*Relieving factors:* Symptomatic treatment - NSAID and antitussive - plus treatment of underlying disease ●*Clinical course:* Usually self-limiting over days-to-weeks ●*Co-morbidities:* Connective tissue disease (especially rheumatoid arthritis), drugs, pulmonary emboli, pneumonia, trauma, postoperative, Dressler's syndrome, tuberculosis, benign asbestos-related pleural effusions ●*Procedure results:* No relevant procedures ●*Test findings:* Chest X-ray: bilateral low lung volumes; plate-like atelectasis; unilateral, small pleural effusion; chest X-ray may be normal

Plummer-Vinson syndrome ●*Onset:* Infancy/toddler/adolescence/adult ●*Male:female ratio:* M=F ●*Ethnicity:* All ●*Character:* Dysphagia for solids ●*Location:* Mucosal membrane in esophagus lumen ●*Pattern:* Persistent symptoms ●*Precipitating factors:* Possibly iron-deficiency anemia ●*Relieving factors:* Some resolve with anemia treatment or surgery ●*Clinical course:* Persistent until treated ●*Co-morbidities:* Iron-deficiency anemia ●*Procedure results:* Abnormal barium swallow or esophagoscopy ●*Test findings:* Microcytic, hypochromic anemia if present

Pneumothorax ●*Onset:* Acute ●*Male:female ratio:* M>F ●*Ethnicity:* All ●*Character:* Dyspnea, chest discomfort, cough ●*Location:* Chest ●*Pattern:* Unilateral decreased breath sounds, tympanitic to percussion; hypotension and trachea deviated away from pneumothorax if under tension ●*Precipitating factors:* Spontaneous, extremes of barometric pressure (scuba diving or mountain climbing), trauma, underlying lung disease ●*Relieving factors:* Chest thoracostomy; supplemental oxygen and observation if small; consider pleurodesis if recurrent or slow to heal ●*Clinical course:* Resolution depends on the size of the pleural defect and the presence of comorbid illness; for spontaneous pneumothorax: 23-28% recurrence rate within 5 years (most within 1 year) ●*Co-morbidities:* Chronic obstructive pulmonary disease, pulmonary fibrosis, trauma or procedure, pneumonia, respiratory failure requiring positive pressure ventilation ●*Procedure results:* No relevant procedures ●*Test findings:* Chest X-ray: air in the pleural space

Poisoning ●*Onset:* Minutes to hours ●*Male:female ratio:* M=F ●*Ethnicity:* All ●*Character:* Nonspecific ●*Location:* Nonspecific ●*Pattern:* Nonspecific ●*Precipitating factors:* Ingestion of toxin, exposure to toxin ●*Relieving factors:* None relevant ●*Clinical course:* Variable ●*Co-morbidities:* None relevant ●*Procedure results:* No relevant procedures ●*Test findings:* Poison may appear on toxicologic screen

Poliomyelitis ●*Onset:* Subacute, insidious ●*Male:female ratio:* M=F ●*Ethnicity:* Disease not eradicated in Africa and India ●*Character:* Febrile illness followed by a progressive flaccid paralysis ●*Location:* Upper or lower extremities ●*Pattern:* Nonspecific ●*Precipitating factors:* Fecal-oral contamination of the patient, oral polio virus vaccination ●*Relieving factors:* Supportive ●*Clinical course:* Variable ●*Co-morbidities:* None relevant ●*Procedure results:* Electromyogram/nerve conduction studies ●*Test findings:* No relevant tests

Polyarteritis nodosa ●*Onset:* Subacute ●*Male:female ratio:* M(2.5):F(1) ●*Ethnicity:* All ●*Character:* Dull ache ●*Location:* Hands, proximal muscles, testes, abdomen ●*Pattern:* Nonspecific ●*Precipitating factors:* None relevant ●*Relieving factors:* Corticosteroids, cyclophosphamide ●*Clinical course:* Progressive ●*Co-morbidities:* None relevant ●*Procedure results:* Necrotizing vasculitis of medium-sized vessels, mesenteric angiogram with beading ●*Test findings:* Elevated erythrocyte sedimentation rate, decreased C3 and C4

Polycystic kidney disease ●*Onset:* Acute ●*Male:female ratio:* M=F ●*Ethnicity:* All ●*Character:* Bilateral flank masses from cystic kidneys ●*Location:* Abdomen ●*Pattern:* Worsening symptoms of hypertension, kidney failure ●*Precipitating factors:* Genetic, autosomal recessive ●*Relieving factors:* Supportive treatment of kidney function, hypertension ●*Clinical course:* Progressive ●*Co-morbidities:* Liver cysts, cirrhosis, hypertension, oligohydramnios, hematuria ●*Procedure results:* Abdominal ultrasound, intravenous pyelogram show myltiple cysts ●*Test findings:* Hematuria, abnormal renal function tests

Polycystic ovarian disease ●*Onset:* Subacute, insidious ●*Male:female ratio:* F ●*Ethnicity:* All ●*Character:* Irregular menses worsening since menarche ●*Location:* Nonspecific ●*Pattern:* Oligomenorrhea, amenorrhea ●*Precipitating factors:* Obesity (BMI>27), insulin resistance ●*Relieving factors:* Weight loss, oral contraceptives, antiandrogens, metformin ●*Clinical course:* Unrelenting. Long-term risk of endometrial hyperplasia and cancer, cardiovascular disease, diabetes, hirsuitism, acne ●*Co-morbidities:*

Infertility ●*Procedure results:* Positive menses withdrawal after medroxyprogesterone ●*Test findings:* Total testosterone elevated, follicle-stimulating hormone (FSH) and prolactin; hyperthecosis on pelvic U/S

Polycythemia vera ●*Onset:* Insidious ●*Male:female ratio:* M>F ●*Ethnicity:* All ●*Character:* Impaired oxygen delivery (headache, dizziness, angina). Venous thrombosis and thromboembolism, easy bleeding and bruising, pruritus, abdominal discomfort ●*Location:* Nonspecific ●*Pattern:* Nonspecific ●*Precipitating factors:* None relevant ●*Relieving factors:* Phlebotomy, myelosuppressive therapy, treatment of complications ●*Clinical course:* Prolonged survival with treatment (median 10 years); can transform into acute leukemia ●*Co-morbidities:* None relevant ●*Procedure results:* Bone marrow biopsy: hypercellular with hyperplasia of erythroid lines and megakaryocytes, decreased iron stores, possibly fibrosis ●*Test findings:* Elevated red cell mass, mild leukocytosis and thrombocytosis, elevated leukocyte alkaline phosphatase (LAP) score, elevated vitamin B12, presence of chromosomal abnormality in 30%

Polymyalgia rheumatica ●*Onset:* Subacute ●*Male:female ratio:* M(1):F(2) ●*Ethnicity:* Caucasian ●*Character:* Dull ache with limitation in range of motion of affected joints ●*Location:* Shoulders or hips, occasionally in hands and wrists ●*Pattern:* Worse in the morning ●*Precipitating factors:* None relevant ●*Relieving factors:* Corticosteroids ●*Clinical course:* Progressive, rarely remits ●*Co-morbidities:* Giant cell arteritis ●*Procedure results:* No relevant procedures ●*Test findings:* Elevated ESR

Polymyositis/dermatomyositis ●*Onset:* Subacute ●*Male:female ratio:* M(1):F(2) ●*Ethnicity:* African descent slightly higher than Caucasian ●*Character:* Dull ache ●*Location:* Proximal muscles ●*Pattern:* Rash on hands ●*Precipitating factors:* None relevant ●*Relieving factors:* Corticosteroids, azathioprine, methotrexate, intravenous immunoglobulin ●*Clinical course:* Progressive ●*Co-morbidities:* None relevant ●*Procedure results:* Inflammation on muscle biopsy ●*Test findings:* Elevated muscle enzymes, positive antinuclear antibody, elevated ESR

Pontine hemorrhage ●*Onset:* Acute ●*Male:female ratio:* M=F ●*Ethnicity:* All ●*Character:* Characterized by vertigo, nystagmus, ataxia, Horner's syndrome, crossed face-and-body pain and temperature loss; there can be ipsilateral deafness and tinnitus; if the space-occupying hemorrhage affects medial pontine structures, facial weakness and ipsilateral gaze paresis may occur; larger lesions can cause contralateral hemiparesis; if VIIth cranial nerve nucleus involved, ipsilateral facial weakness can occur; palatal myoclonus can also occur ●*Location:* Medial or lateral pontine vascular lesions can be further subdivided into superior, mid and inferior pontine lesions respectively ●*Pattern:* Specifically (details related to pontine infarction but can resemble small hemorrhage), medial inferior lesion (ipsilateral abduction gaze paralysis), medial superior lesion (internuclear ophthalmoplegia), lateral inferior (ipsilateral facial paralysis) and lateral mid-pons lesion (ipsilateral facial numbness) ●*Precipitating factors:* Atrioventricular malformations, amyloid angiopathy, tumors; for infarction, anterior inferior cerebellar or superior cerebellar arteries (lateral pontine lesions); paramedian branches of the basilar artery (medial pontine lesion) ●*Relieving factors:* Intravascular embolization or surgical decompression (rare) ●*Clinical course:* Rapidly progressive ●*Co-morbidities:* None relevant ●*Procedure results:* No relevant procedures ●*Test findings:* MRI helps delineate extent of brainstem soft tissue involvement

Porphyria ●*Onset:* Subacute, acute ●*Male:female ratio:* M=F ●*Ethnicity:* Highest incidence of acute intermittent porphyria (AIP) occurs in Lapland, Scandinavia and UK: 1-2/100,000 ●*Character:* A group of genetic or acquired deficiencies of activity of enzymes in the heme biosynthetic pathway. Metabolic intermediates produced in excess accumulate ●*Location:* Neurovisceral symptoms associated with increased production of porphobilinogen (PBG) and/or delta aminolevulinic acid (ALA): abdominal pain, psychiatric disorders such as psychosis, delirium, coma, peripheral neuropathy, bulbar palsy. Photocutaneous symptoms: photosensitization and skin damage by UV light caused by porphyrins ●*Pattern:* Porphyrias now identified by individual mutations in the specific gene for the deficient enzymes; historically separated into hepatic and erythroid. Hepatic: acute intermittent porphyria (AIP), hereditary coproporphyria (HCP), variegate porphyria (VP), ALA dehydratase porphyria (ADP). Erythropoietic porphyrias: congenital erythropoietic porphyria (CEP), hepatoerythropoietic porphyria (HEP), erythropoietic porphyria (EPP). Photosensitive only: porphyria cutanea tarda (PCT). AIP most common ●*Precipitating factors:* Genetic heterogeneity present in all forms. Clinical severity related to environmental factors - drugs: sulfonamides, barbiturates; diet: decreased caloric intake; intercurrent illness, smoking, psychologic stress, alcohol excess ●*Relieving factors:* Photosensitive symptoms: sun avoidance, beta-carotene, cholestyramine. AIP: IV glucose, IV heme preparations, e.g. hemin, heme arginate. Supportive treatment, e.g. correct electrolyte disturbance due to syndrome of in appropriate secretion of antidiuretic hormone (SIADH), ventilatory support for respiratory failure due to bulbar paralysis. Stop exacerbating medications, treat intercurrent illness ●*Clinical course:* Severe AIP attacks especially if bulbar paralysis present, may be life-threatening ●*Co-morbidities:* Hemolytic anemia present in erythropoietic porphyrias ●*Procedure results:* No relevant procedures ●*Test findings:* Watson-Schwartz test used for emergency screening. Tests used to identify metabolites produced and/or excreted in RBCs, plasma, urine, feces. Aminolevulinic acid (ALA), porphobilinogen (PBG), uroporphyrin excreted in urine. Protoporphyrin in feces. Coproporphyrin in both

Portal hypertension ●*Onset:* Insidious ●*Male:female ratio:* M=F ●*Ethnicity:* All ●*Character:* Symptoms include increase in abdominal girth (ascites), pedal edema, upper GI bleeding from esophageal or gastric varices; renal failure. Examination may show ascites, vascular spider angiomata on the upper body, splenomegaly, edema ●*Location:* Increase in abdominal girth, lower extremity swelling ●*Pattern:* Nonspecific ●*Precipitating factors:* Salt intake may increase ascites and edema ●*Relieving factors:* Salt restriction; diuretics (spironolactone and furosemide are most effective). Definitive therapies include shunt procedure, surgical portosystemic shunt, and liver transplantation (if portal hypertension is due to cirrhosis) ●*Clinical course:* Usually progressive over months-toyears, not self-limited ●*Co-morbidities:* Cirrhosis of any cause, obstruction of hepatic vessels (hepatic veins, portal vein), congenital hepatic fibrosis, schistosomiasis ●*Procedure results:* Direct measurement of hepatic venous pressures is definitive. Presence of esophageal varices on endoscopy is very suggestive ●*Test findings:* Platelet count is usually low. If the portal hypertension is due to cirrhosis, international normalized ratio (INR) may be high, bilirubin may be elevated. Often hyponatremic if ascites is present

Portal vein thrombosis ●*Onset:* Subacute, acute ●*Male:female ratio:* M<F ●*Ethnicity:* All ●*Character:* Hematemesis from variceal hemorrhage, abdominal distension from ascites, upper abdominal tenderness from splenomegaly ●*Location:* Ruptured esophageal varices cause hematemesis, left upper quadrant pain over enlarged spleen, abdominal distension from ascites ●*Pattern:* Hematemesis of bright red blood may present acutely and be unrelenting; ascites may be early and transient or persistent ●*Precipitating factors:* Infection (local or systemic) especially in children, umbilical vein catheterization with sepsis, abdominal trauma, pancreatitis, intra-abdominal sepsis, cirrhosis ●*Relieving factors:* No home or medical therapies are effective - mechanical problem requires mechanical solution; endoscopy needed for bleeding varix banding/sclerosis, portal-systemic shunt needed to bypass thrombosed portal vein ●*Clinical course:* Progressive problem until surgically or mechanically addressed (i.e. shunt procedure) ●*Co-morbidities:* Cirrhosis, hypercoagulable states, pancreatitis,

splenectomy, hepatocellular carcinoma, Budd-Chiari syndrome (hepatic vein thrombosis) ●*Procedure results:* Venous-phase angiography reveals thrombosed portal vein ●*Test findings:* CT or MRI may show thrombosis of portal vein

Post-concussive syndrome ●*Onset:* Acute ●*Male:female ratio:* M=F ●*Ethnicity:* All ●*Character:* Headaches, dizziness, insomnia, restlessness, anxiety, depression and inability to concentrate can occur in about 40% of patients with a history of head trauma ●*Location:* No specific lesions identified; psychogenic vs organic etiology ●*Pattern:* No direct correlation between extent of trauma and symptoms; some improvement in symptoms is to be expected ●*Precipitating factors:* Minor or major head trauma ●*Relieving factors:* Somewhat self-limiting; mainly psychotherapy, but anticonvulsants and physiotherapy help ●*Clinical course:* In 2-6 months, major symptoms such as dizziness and headache can subside; psychoneurotic symptoms can persist (may be correlated to litigation procedings) ●*Co-morbidities:* Patients with previous history of neurotic symptoms are at higher risk of developing post-traumatic symptoms, although they can also develop in patients with previously good adjustment ●*Procedure results:* No relevant procedures ●*Test findings:* No correlation with specific MRI or CT scan findings

Post-traumatic stress disorder ●*Onset:* Variable; symptoms typically begin within 3 months of trauma, although delay of months to years is possible ●*Male:female ratio:* M=F ●*Ethnicity:* Recent emigrants from areas of major social unrest and civil conflict at risk ●*Character:* Trauma; avoidance of stimuli associated with trauma; numbing; hyperarousal ●*Location:* Nonspecific ●*Pattern:* Person's response to trauma involved intense fear, helplessness, or horror ●*Precipitating factors:* Person experienced or witnessed major trauma with actual or threatened death, injury, or harm; may occur after childhood sexual or physical abuse ●*Relieving factors:* Avoidance of stimuli associated with the trauma; numbing; detachment ●*Clinical course:* Variable duration and course, with complete recovery in about 50% cases, others with persisting symptoms for year or more ●*Co-morbidities:* Major depression; substance-related disorders; panic disorder; agoraphobia; specific phobias ●*Procedure results:* No relevant procedures ●*Test findings:* Increased arousal in autonomic function (e.g. heart rate, respiratory rate, sweating)

Posterior communicating artery aneurysm ●*Onset:* Acute if bleeding occurs, insidious prior to bleed unless aneurysm enlarges ●*Male:female ratio:* M=F ●*Ethnicity:* All ●*Character:* Aneurysms compress the oculomotor nerve and almost always affect the size of the pupil and/or optic tract; oculomotor palsy in an otherwise awake patient (absence of transtentorial herniation) should raise suspicion for this aneurysm ●*Location:* Most common site is the junction of the internal carotid and posterior communicating arteries ●*Pattern:* Without bleeding: oculomotor palsy in an awake patient; with bleeding: 'thunderclap headache' or 'worst headache ever' is described, some may remain lucid while others lose consciousness (grave prognosis); a number of patients will complain of a stiff neck, nausea or vomiting a few days prior to manifesting major symptoms, probably from a leak in the aneurysm ●*Precipitating factors:* Hypertension, atherosclerosis ●*Relieving factors:* Surgical clipping or intravascular embolization, decompression of the hemorrhage ●*Clinical course:* 30% patients rebleed in first month after primary bleed; cause of death is directly related to bleeding in about 40% patients ●*Co-morbidities:* Risk increased in smokers and in alcohol dependence ●*Procedure results:* Good prognosis if aneurysm clipped successfully ●*Test findings:* MRI or CT scans help delineate site of hemorrhage; CSF is grossly bloody; cerebral arteriography is the definitive diagnostic procedure

Posterior fossa tumor ●*Onset:* Insidious ●*Male:female ratio:* M=F ●*Ethnicity:* All ●*Character:* Lesions may produce hydrocephalus, signs of raised intracranial pressure, cerebellar dysfunction, contralateral hemianopia; tumors arising from the petrous bone can affect cranial nerves, and cerebellopontine tumors can mimic acoustic nerve tumors ●*Location:* Tumors are mainly meningiomas, arising from posterior petrous bone, clivus, undersurface of tentorium, foramen magnum or convexity of cerebellar hemispheres ●*Pattern:* May go unrecognized for years; can develop acute hemifacial spasm, cerebellopontine angle syndrome and disorders of the midbrain ●*Precipitating factors:* Meningiomas ●*Relieving factors:* Decompression via a transtentorial approach ●*Clinical course:* Specific lesions cause specific manifestations e.g. clivus lesions can cause cervical-occipital pain and signs of high spinal cord involvement, related to symptoms of lower cranial nerve involvement ●*Co-morbidities:* None relevant ●*Procedure results:* Surgical removal via transtentorial approach ●*Test findings:* Imaging studies with CT and MRI scans can delineate the space-occupying lesions

Posterior urethral valves ●*Onset:* Subacute ●*Male:female ratio:* M=F ●*Ethnicity:* All ●*Character:* Distended bladder, weak urinary stream, urinary tract infection (UTI); if severe: failure to thrive ●*Location:* Kidneys/urethra ●*Pattern:* Worsening symptoms ●*Precipitating factors:* None relevant ●*Relieving factors:* Surgery: transurethral ablation of valve leaflets or vesicotomy if needed ●*Clinical course:* Progressive unless treated ●*Co-morbidities:* End-stage renal disease/chronic renal insufficiency unless treated, vesicoureteral reflux; prenatal: oligohydramnios, pulmonary hypoplasia ●*Procedure results:* Prenatal ultrasound: bilateral hydronephrosis, distended bladder, oligohydramnios. Renal ultrasound. Voiding cystourethrogram. ●*Test findings:* Elevated serum creatinine

Postictal/postseizure phase ●*Onset:* Acute ●*Male:female ratio:* M=F ●*Ethnicity:* All ●*Character:* Terminal phase of seizure; all movements have ended if a tonic clonic seizure, the body lies still; pupils are reactive to light, breathing may be labored ●*Location:* Varies with seizure focus ●*Pattern:* Persists for a few minutes; patient then opens eyes and may seem disoriented/confused for first few minutes; may be some amnesia, speech may be slurred or confused; often the patient will fall into deep sleep ●*Precipitating factors:* Factors that precipitate a seizure will precipitate a postical state, most commonly after a generalized tonic-clonic seizure ●*Relieving factors:* Treatment of seizures will prevent postical states ●*Clinical course:* Most patients will recall the aura prior to succumbing to the seizure, but nothing after that until the postical phase has resolved ●*Co-morbidities:* Patients may sustain injuries such as a bitten tongue, vertebral fracture, periorbital hemorrhage, subdural hematoma and other injuries depending on their situation prior to the seizure ●*Procedure results:* No relevant procedures ●*Test findings:* EEG can be flat, with brain waves resuming preseizure pattern after a while

Postpartum hair loss ●*Onset:* Acute ●*Male:female ratio:* F ●*Ethnicity:* All ●*Character:* Rapid shedding of hair ●*Location:* Scalp ●*Pattern:* Hair loss 3-6 months postpartum ●*Precipitating factors:* Postpartum ●*Relieving factors:* None relevant ●*Clinical course:* Self-limited - months ●*Co-morbidities:* None relevant ●*Procedure results:* No relevant procedures ●*Test findings:* No relevant tests

Postphlebitic syndrome ●*Onset:* Insidious ●*Male:female ratio:* M<F ●*Ethnicity:* All ●*Character:* Dull ache ●*Location:* Over affected limb ●*Pattern:* Pain worsens as the day goes on ●*Precipitating factors:* Worse with activity ●*Relieving factors:* Heat, elevation, compression stockings ●*Clinical course:* Often progressive ●*Co-morbidities:* All risk factors for deep vein thrombosis (immobility, cancer, hypertension, family history) ●*Procedure results:* No relevant procedures ●*Test findings:* Ultrasound ruling out acute deep vein thrombosis

Prader-Willi syndrome ●*Onset:* Subacute ●*Male:female ratio:* M=F ●*Ethnicity:* All ●*Character:* Binge-eating, obesity ●*Location:* Nonspecific ●*Pattern:* Almond-shaped palpebral fissures, small hands/feet, hypotonia at birth, voracious appetite, obesity ●*Precipitating factors:* Genetic, deletion of 15q11-13 - paternal chromosome ●*Relieving factors:*

Behavioral modification ●*Clinical course:* Progressive ●*Co-morbidities:* Obesity, short stature, hypogonadism, mental retardation ●*Procedure results:* Deletion at chromosome 15q11-13 ●*Test findings:* Deletion at chromosome 15q11-13

Precocious puberty ●*Onset:* Subacute ●*Male:female ratio:* M<F (idiopathic) ●*Ethnicity:* All ●*Character:* Girls <8 years; boys <9 years: secondary sex characteristics, increased growth ●*Location:* Axillae, genitalia ●*Pattern:* Progressive pubertal development ●*Precipitating factors:* 90% idiopathic or possible CNS abnormality ●*Relieving factors:* Gonadotropn-releasing hormone (GnRH) agonist; correction of CNS abnormality ●*Clinical course:* Progressive until treated ●*Co-morbidities:* None relevant ●*Procedure results:* Abnormal head CT/MRI, advanced bone age ●*Test findings:* Elevated luteinizing hormone (LH), abnormal GnRH stimulation test

Pregnancy-induced hypertension ●*Onset:* Insidious, subacute, acute ●*Male:female ratio:* F ●*Ethnicity:* All ●*Character:* Swelling, headaches, right upper quadrant abdominal pain in pregnant women ●*Location:* Nonspecific ●*Pattern:* Nonspecific ●*Precipitating factors:* None relevant ●*Relieving factors:* Delivery ●*Clinical course:* Variable - sometimes indolent sometimes rapidly progressive; rarely can appear up to 2 weeks postpartum ●*Co-morbidities:* Hypertension, renal disease, lupus ●*Procedure results:* No relevant procedures ●*Test findings:* Proteinuria, thrombocytopenia, elevated transaminases, elevated uric acid

Premature atrial contraction ●*Onset:* Acute, chronic ●*Male:female ratio:* M=F ●*Ethnicity:* All groups ●*Character:* Typically asymptomatic. Some patients may feel palpitations, 'extra heart beat' or 'skipped' beat ●*Location:* Substernal ●*Pattern:* Episodic ●*Precipitating factors:* Alcohol, caffeine, electrolyte imbalance, infection, inflammation, drug toxicity, catecholamine excess, electrolyte disorders ●*Relieving factors:* Most cases are asymptomatic. If symptomatic, therapy of underlying disorder is indicated. Beta blocker therapy or calcium channel blocker therapy may be useful but rarely needed in this condition ●*Clinical course:* Typically not a life-threatening condition, self-limiting, most cases need no specific therapy ●*Co-morbidities:* Hyperthyroidism, myocardial ischemia, drug toxicity. Premature atrial contractions (PACs) can occur in the presence or absence of structural heart disease ●*Procedure results:* No relevant procedures ●*Test findings:* EKG, Holter or event monitoring may reveal premature atrial contractions

Premature ventricular contraction ●*Onset:* Acute, chronic ●*Male:female ratio:* M=F ●*Ethnicity:* All ●*Character:* Typically asymptomatic. Some patients may feel palpitations, 'extra heart beat' or 'skipped' beat ●*Location:* Substernal, typically no radiation. Frequent premature ventricular contractions may result in lightheadedness or dizziness in rare cases ●*Pattern:* Episodic ●*Precipitating factors:* Alcohol, caffeine, electrolyte imbalance, infection, inflammation, hyperthyroidism, myocardial ischemia, drug toxicity, catecholamine excess, electrolyte disorders. Structural heart disease may or may not be present ●*Relieving factors:* No specific therapy if premature ventricular contractions occur rarely. Address underlying disorders. Medical treatment sometimes indicated: beta blockers ●*Clinical course:* Typically not a life-threatening condition if premature ventricular contractions occur occasionally. With more frequent premature ventricular contractions, especially of different morphologies, or if runs of ventricular tachycardia occurs or if 'R-on-T phenomenon' occurs, referral to cardiology recommended, especially if structural heart disease ●*Co-morbidities:* None relevant ●*Procedure results:* No relevant procedures ●*Test findings:* EKG, Holter or event monitoring may reveal premature ventricular contractions

Premenstrual syndrome ●*Onset:* Subacute ●*Male:female ratio:* F ●*Ethnicity:* All ●*Character:* Emotional lability, irritability, anxiety, depression; food cravings, breast tenderness/swelling, headache, bloating, weight gain, myalgias, arthralgias ●*Location:* Nonspecific ●*Pattern:* Symptoms occur exclusively or significantly worsen in luteal phase resolving with end of menses ●*Precipitating factors:* Poor nutrition, lack of exercise, excess alcohol ●*Relieving factors:* NSAIDs, behavioral therapy, lifestyle interventions, bromocriptine or spironolactone for breast tenderness/bloating, SSRIs during luteal phase, daily calcium supplementation 1000mg, evening primrose oil, gonadotropin-releasing hormone (GnRH) agonist for severe refractory cases ●*Clinical course:* Symptoms recur if treatment stopped. Symptoms resolve after menopause ●*Co-morbidities:* Personal and family history of alcoholism, mood disorders, schizophrenia, eating disorders, postpartum depression ●*Procedure results:* No relevant procedures ● *Test findings:* 30% increase in symptoms documented on symptom charting during luteal phase (progesterone >5ng/mL)

Prepubescent vulvovaginitis ●*Onset:* Insidious, subacute ●*Male:female ratio:* F ●*Ethnicity:* All ●*Character:* Vulvar pruritus, vaginal discharge ●*Location:* Labia minora, majora, vaginal introitus ●*Pattern:* Vulvar exanthematous, thin, or white vaginal discharge ●*Precipitating factors:* Retained foreign body in vagina, poor hygiene ●*Relieving factors:* Sitz baths, meticulous hygiene, antifungal topical agents ●*Clinical course:* Progresses over 2-3 days ●*Co-morbidities:* Diabetes mellitus, sexual abuse ●*Procedure results:* Wet preparation of vaginal secretion with potassium hydroxide solution to visualize hyphae ● *Test findings:* Exclude gonorrhea/chlamydia/syphilis

Presbycusis ●*Onset:* Insidious ●*Male:female ratio:* M=F ●*Ethnicity:* All ●*Character:* Bilaterally symmetric, slowly progressive hearing loss ●*Location:* Both ears ●*Pattern:* Often worse in high frequencies ●*Precipitating factors:* Family history ●*Relieving factors:* None relevant ●*Clinical course:* Usually slowly progressive symmetric hearing loss over years ●*Co-morbidities:* None relevant ●*Procedure results:* No relevant procedures ● *Test findings:* Audiometry reveals symmetric sensorineural hearing loss

Pressure ulcer ●*Onset:* Acute, subacute ●*Male:female ratio:* M<F ●*Ethnicity:* All ●*Character:* Skin lesion ●*Location:* Bony prominences - sacrum, trochanter ●*Pattern:* Ulcer border noninflamed ●*Precipitating factors:* Prolonged bedrest ●*Relieving factors:* Debridement, antibiotics, pressure relief ●*Clinical course:* Can resolve in months, frequently chronic ●*Co-morbidities:* Vascular or neurological problems ●*Procedure results:* No relevant procedures ● *Test findings:* No relevant tests

Primary biliary cirrhosis ●*Onset:* Insidious ●*Male:female ratio:* M(1):F(10) ●*Ethnicity:* No predisposition ●*Character:* Fatigue; generalized pruritus without rash ●*Location:* Pruritus over whole body ●*Pattern:* Fatigue and pruritus may increase over time ●*Precipitating factors:* None relevant ●*Relieving factors:* Antihistamines, cholestyramine, ursodiol, rifampin, opioid antagonists ●*Clinical course:* Slow progression to liver failure over 15-20 years ●*Co-morbidities:* Autoimmune thyroid disease, Sjögren's syndrome, other collagen-vascular disorders ●*Procedure results:* Liver biopsy with inflammation of the small bile ducts ● *Test findings:* Elevated alkaline phosphatase, positive antimitochondrial antibody (AMA)

Primary ciliary dysplasia ●*Onset:* Acute or subacute ●*Male:female ratio:* M=F ●*Ethnicity:* All ●*Character:* Cough, sinusitis, infertility ●*Location:* Chest, sinus ●*Pattern:* Nonspecific ●*Precipitating factors:* Genetic disorder ●*Relieving factors:* Symptomatic treatment: antibiotics ●*Clinical course:* Progessive ●*Co-morbidities:* Sinusitis, infertility, rhinitis, bronchiectasis, some have situs inversus ●*Procedure results:* Biopsy shows absence of dynein arms of cilia ● *Test findings:* Absence/near absence of mucociliary transport

Primary HIV infection ●*Onset:* Acute, subacute, chronic ●*Male:female ratio:* M>F ●*Ethnicity:* All ●*Character:* Primary infection: fever, severe sore throat, rash, lymphadenopathy, oral lesions, polyarthralgia. Symptomatic chronic infection: progressive weight loss, persistent generalized lymphadenopathy, intermittent diarrhea, oral thrush, frequent vaginal yeast infections, other. Advanced infection: opportunistic infections (see AIDS), dementia, wasting, other ●*Location:* Systemic (fever, weight loss), lymphoid organs, lymph nodes, skin and oral mucosa, GI tract from mouth to anus, CNS, peripheral nerves, muscle, any other organ ●*Pattern:* Primary infection: disseminated maculopapular rash, oral ulcers, severe sore throat, generalized or cervical lymphadenopathy, 'aseptic' meningoencephalitis. Symptomatic chronic infection: progressive weight loss, recurrent or persistent oral thrush, persistent nontender generalized lymphadenopathy, progressive wasting, chronic diarrhea, polyneuropathy ●*Precipitating factors:* Men who have sex with men, intravenous drug users, multiple sex partners, unprotected vaginal, anal, or oral sex; exposure to blood products before the mid-1980s; exposure to contaminated blood or body fluids, born to HIV-infected mother, residence in highly endemic/epidemic areas ●*Relieving factors:* None relevant ●*Clinical course:* Chronic progressive infection, incurable. Acute HIV syndrome begins 2-6 weeks after infection and lasts days-weeks. In untreated individuals, asymptomatic latent infection and early symptomatic disease last 10 years (highly variable), and late complications (AIDS) begin with CD4 <200, death within 1-2 years. Treatment reduces morbidity, mortality, prolongs survival ●*Co-morbidities:* Syphilis, STD, idiopathic thrombocytopenic purpura (ITP), recurrent herpes zoster, seborrheic dermatitis, oral thrush, oral hairy leukoplakia, aphthous ulcers, molluscum contagiosum, recurrent genital herpes simplex virus, condyloma acuminata, frequent vaginal candidiasis, cervical dysplasia, tuberculosis, non-Hodgkin's lymphoma, peripheral neuropathy, aseptic meningitis, dementia, recurrent bacterial infections, chronic diarrhea, chronic hepatitis C, chronic hepatitis B, giardiasis, salmonellosis, other ●*Procedure results:* No relevant procedures ●*Test findings:* Thrombocytopenia, anemia, leukopenia, low CD4 cell count, elevated gammaglobulins, low albumin, low cholesterol (untreated), mildly elevated hepatic transaminases (in primary infection)

Primary intracerebral hemorrhage stroke ●*Onset:* Acute ●*Male:female ratio:* M<F ●*Ethnicity:* All ●*Character:* Sudden onset of headache, weakness, confusion, numbness, mental status change, seizures ●*Location:* Nonspecific ●*Pattern:* Nonspecific ●*Precipitating factors:* Hypertension, diabetes mellitus, increasing age, heavy alcohol or drug usage ●*Relieving factors:* Surgical removal of hemorrhage, pending location or supportive care and control of intracranial pressure ●*Clinical course:* Variable ●*Co-morbidities:* Hypertension, diabetes mellitus, elevated cholesterol, increasing age, tobacco usage, atrial fibrillation, heavy alcohol usage ●*Procedure results:* MRI/CT of the brain shows hemorrhage ●*Test findings:* No relevant tests

Primary lung malignancy ●*Onset:* Subacute ●*Male:female ratio:* M>F ●*Ethnicity:* All ●*Character:* Cough, chest discomfort, dyspnea, hemoptysis, focal wheezing ●*Location:* Chest with potential for metastasis to any organ (most commonly adrenal, liver, brain, lung, bone) ●*Pattern:* Focal inspiratory rales, expiratory monophonic wheeze or rhonchi, or findings consistent with pleural effusion ●*Precipitating factors:* Smoking (80-90%), asbestos or other environmental carcinogen, HIV ●*Relieving factors:* Chemotherapy, radiotherapy with or without surgical excision for limited stage (<3b) non-small cell lung cancer (NSCLC), chemotherapy, radiotherapy for small cell lung cancer (SCLC) ●*Clinical course:* Overall 5-year survival rate is 10-12%. If NSCLC with stage 1, 60-80%; stage 2, 25-50% 5-year survival. If SCLC with limited stage disease treated with chemotherapy and radiotherapy, 18-24 month median survival; with extensive disease, palliative treatment, 10-12 month median survival ●*Co-morbidities:* Chronic obstructive pulmonary disease (COPD), coronary artery disease (CAD) other smoking-related illnesses ●*Procedure results:* Sputum or bronchoalveolar lavage fluid cytology, lung biopsy with histological evidence for malignancy ●*Test findings:* Chest X-ray or high resolution computed tomography with evidence for focal nodule or mass, lymphangitic spread, pleural effusion or focal atelectasis; may be normal

Proctitis ●*Onset:* Subacute ●*Male:female ratio:* M=F ●*Ethnicity:* All ●*Character:* Rectal inflammation can manifest either as diarrhea or constipation - accompanied by rectal pain, tenesmus, often with bloody stools ●*Location:* Rectum and perianal area ●*Pattern:* No pattern ●*Precipitating factors:* None relevant ●*Relieving factors:* If due to infection, antibiotic treatment may shorten the period of symptoms. If due to irritable bowel disease, mesalamine, or steroids in suppository or enema form may relieve inflammation. In more refractory cases, systemic steroids may be needed ●*Clinical course:* May be self-limited if due to infection, but usually requires treatment for relief of symptoms if due to irritable bowel disease ●*Co-morbidities:* Ulcerative colitis, herpes simplex infection, bacterial gastroenteritis ●*Procedure results:* Flexible sigmoidoscopy shows rectal inflammation, biopsies may be diagnostic of infection or irritable bowel disease ●*Test findings:* Stool cultures may be diagnostic of bacterial infection. WBC may be elevated

Prostate calculus ●*Onset:* Chronic ●*Male:female ratio:* M ●*Ethnicity:* All ●*Character:* Majority asymptomatic. Rare presentation with terminal hematuria, hematospermia, pain ●*Location:* Perineal/pelvic ●*Pattern:* Nonspecific ●*Precipitating factors:* None relevant ●*Relieving factors:* Surgery: open or endoscopic resection of prostate is curative and indicated in the few symptomatic patients ●*Clinical course:* Benign ●*Co-morbidities:* Benign prostatic hyperplasia, prostatitism, urethritis, urethral stricture ●*Procedure results:* Calcification seen on radiographic or ultrasound study ●*Test findings:* No relevant tests

Prostatic abscess ●*Onset:* Acute/subacute ●*Male:female ratio:* M ●*Ethnicity:* All ●*Character:* Urine retention (34%), fever (33%), dysuria (27%), frequency (23%), pain (23%), urethral discharge (7%) ●*Location:* Perineal/pelvic ●*Pattern:* Mostly perineal pain (23%); radiating to lower back (1%) only ●*Precipitating factors:* Urinary tract infection, prostatitis, urethritis ●*Relieving factors:* Pathogen-specific antimicrobial. Incision and drainage of abscess ●*Clinical course:* Progressive to sepsis if untreated ●*Co-morbidities:* Diabetes, dialysis, immunocompromised patients, urethral instrumentation ●*Procedure results:* Diagnosis of abscess by transrectal untrasound or CT ●*Test findings:* Escherichia coli on culture in 70% of patients. Other less likely causative agents: Pseudomonas, Staphylococci, Neisseria gonorrhea and obligate anaerobic bacteria

Prostatic cancer ●*Onset:* Subacute ●*Male:female ratio:* M ●*Ethnicity:* Most common in African-Americans. Low incidence in Asians ●*Character:* Usually asymptomatic. Obstructive voiding symptoms, bone pain, and/or renal failure in advanced disease ●*Location:* Prostate ●*Pattern:* Localized to prostate when detected early by prostate cancer screen (prostate-specific antigen [PSA], digital rectal examination) ●*Precipitating factors:* None relevant ●*Relieving factors:* Surgery, radiation therapy, hormonal treatment ●*Clinical course:* Slow to progress. 80% will progress within 10 years if left untreated ●*Co-morbidities:* None relevant ●*Procedure results:* Surgery and radiation therapy (external beam or brachytherapy): potentially curable in confined disease ●*Test findings:* PSA >4 (lower PSA will not exclude cancer). confirmation of diagnosis by biopsy, bone scan ruling out metastasis

Prostatitis ●*Onset:* Abrupt for acute prostatitis. Subacute for all other ●*Male:female ratio:* M ●*Ethnicity:* All ●*Character:* Acute prostatitis: fever, chills, pain, irritative and obstructive voiding symptoms. Chronic prostatitis: irritative voiding symptoms and pain ●*Location:* Prostate, pelvis and genitalia/perineal area ●*Pattern:* Recurrent urinary tract infection (UTI) with chronic bacterial prostatitis ●*Precipitating factors:* UTI, sexual intercourse ●*Relieving factors:* Sitz bath, antibiotics, alpha blockers ●*Clinical course:* Acute bacterial prostatitis: complete resolution with treatment. Recurrent UTI in chronic bacterial prostatitis ●*Co-morbidities:* Urethral stricture ●*Procedure results:* Expressed prostatic fluid and/or urine after prostatic massage. For bacterial prostatitis: positive WBC, positive bacteria or positive culture and sensitivity. For nonbacterial prostatitis: positive WBC, negative bacteria and negative culture and sensitivity ●*Test findings:* Urine culture and sensitivity: positive in acute and chronic bacterial prostatitis, negative in nonbacterial prostatitis

Protein-losing enteropathy ●*Onset:* Usually insidious, can be subacute particularly, in the setting of graft-versus-host disease ●*Male:female ratio:* M=F ●*Ethnicity:* All ●*Character:*

Given the diverse etiologies, signs and symptoms vary but often include diarrhea, peripheral edema, weight loss ●*Location:* Nonspecific ●*Pattern:* Nonspecific ●*Precipitating factors:* Whipple's disease (Tropheryma whippelii), Crohn's disease, celiac sprue, constrictive pericarditis, graft versus host disease, congenital or acquired intestinal lymphangiectasia, tumors of the small intestine, alpha heavy chain disease, giant hypertophic gastritis, allergic gastroenteropathy ●*Relieving factors:* Depend on underlying etiology: Whipple's disease, antibiotics; Crohn's disease, intravenous fluids, nutritional supplementation with medium-chain triglycerides ●*Clinical course:* Depends on etiology. Whipple's is easily treated, other etiologies can be more chronic such as Crohn's disease ●*Co-morbidities:* None relevant ●*Procedure results:* Small bowel biopsy: depends on etiology. Small bowel X-ray: may show mucosal abnormalities; strictures if Crohn's disease ●*Test findings:* Low albumin, immunoglobulins, and lymphocyte count; elevated stool alpha-antitrypsin

Pseudobulbar palsy ●*Onset:* Acute ●*Male:female ratio:* M=F ●*Ethnicity:* All ●*Character:* Follows at least two major cerebral infarcts on contralateral sides of the brain, or multiple lacunar infarcts, can occur at different times ●*Location:* Cerebral cortex ●*Pattern:* Bilateral corticospinal reflex signs with or without bilateral hemiparesis, dysphagia, dysarthria, and emotional incontinence due to release of limbic functions ●*Precipitating factors:* Amyotrophic lateral sclerosis, infarction, multiple sclerosis ●*Relieving factors:* None relevant ●*Clinical course:* Progressive dysarthria and dysphagia; fasciculations can develop in arms and legs ●*Co-morbidities:* Amyotrophic lateral sclerosis ●*Procedure results:* No relevant procedures ●*Test findings:* MRI or CT scans can show evidence of previous strokes

Pseudogout ●*Onset:* Acute ●*Male:female ratio:* M=F ●*Ethnicity:* All ●*Character:* Stiffness and pain in affected joints ●*Location:* Knee, wrist, ankle, shoulder ●*Pattern:* Nonspecific ●*Precipitating factors:* Trauma to joint, intercurrent medical illness ●*Relieving factors:* Nonsteroidal anti-inflammatory drugs (NSAIDs), corticosteroids, colchicine ●*Clinical course:* Spontaneously remits ●*Co-morbidities:* Hyperparathyroidism, hypothyroidism, hypophosphatasia, hemochromatosis, Wilson's disease ●*Procedure results:* Calcium pyrophosphate dihydrate crystals in synovial fluid ●*Test findings:* Chondrocalcinosis on radiograph

Pseudomembranous colitis ●*Onset:* Acute ●*Male:female ratio:* M=F ●*Ethnicity:* All ●*Character:* Watery diarrhea, lower abdominal cramps, low-grade fever in a patient recently taking antibiotics. May be more severe, with colonic dilation, sepsis, significant mortality ●*Location:* Lower abdomen ●*Pattern:* Begins 1-6 weeks after antibiotic use, lasts 3-7 days with treatment ●*Precipitating factors:* Antibiotic use ●*Relieving factors:* Cessation of offending antibiotic; oral metronidazole or vancomycin to treat infection ●*Clinical course:* With treatment, lasts 3-7 days ●*Co-morbidities:* None relevant ●*Procedure results:* Sigmoidoscopy shows pseudomembranes in rectum and sigmoid colon - biopsy is characteristic ●*Test findings:* Stool positive for the Clostridium difficile toxin

Pseudotumor cerebri ●*Onset:* Onset in childhood, increasing in adolescence ●*Male:female ratio:* M<F 20% or more above ideal body weight ●*Ethnicity:* All ●*Character:* Increased intracranial presuure with normal CSF content ●*Location:* Low conductance of CSF outflow pathways and rise in sagittal sinus pressure causing partial compression of major venous sinuses ●*Pattern:* Absence of neurologic signs except cranial nerve 6 palsy, papilledema, pulsatile headache, nausea/vomiting, neck or retro-ocular pain worse with eye movement ●*Precipitating factors:* No known cause; exacerbated by many medications, anemia, endocrine disorders and nutritional disorders ●*Relieving factors:* Diuretics, corticosteroids, repeated lumbar punctures and treatment of underlying conditions such as obesity, anemia; surgery reserved for severe visual function impairment and incapacitating headache ●*Clinical course:* Visual loss including diminished visual acuity and visual field deficits may occur after several years ●*Co-morbidities:* 70% patients have empty sella on MRI ●*Procedure results:* Neuroimaging negative for deformity, displacement or obstruction of ventricular system ●*Test findings:* Normal CSF fluid except for increased pressure >200mm H2O in nonobese and >250 in obese patients

Psittacosis ●*Onset:* Acute, gradual ●*Male:female ratio:* M=F ●*Ethnicity:* All ●*Character:* Fever and severe headache followed by nonproductive hacking cough and, less commonly, pleuritic chest pain (atypical pneumonia) ●*Location:* Lungs, upper airway, cervical lymph nodes, nasal mucosa (epistaxis), pleural space, muscles, myocardium, pericardium, less commonly endocardium, CNS, skin (Horder's spots), spleen, liver, other ●*Pattern:* Cough is dry and hacking, epistaxis is common, X-ray findings more prominent than symptoms suggest; headache and photophobia are common; lethargy and delirium less common; a faint rash may appear ●*Precipitating factors:* Exposure to psittacine (or other) birds; birds may appear ill with ruffled feathers and diarrhea, or be asymptomatic ●*Relieving factors:* None relevant ●*Clinical course:* Incubation: 7-14 days, illness begins acutely or gradually and lasts 1-3 weeks, longer duration and relapses may occur ●*Co-morbidities:* None relevant ●*Procedure results:* Pulmonary infiltrates (interstitial, other) on chest X-ray, specific serologic tests ●*Test findings:* WBC: normal-low and then elevated; transient proteinuria, specific serologic tests

Psoas abscess ●*Onset:* Acute or insidious (depending on etiology) ●*Male:female ratio:* M=F ●*Ethnicity:* All ●*Character:* Unilateral or bilateral lower back pain which may be associated with neurologic deficits or constitutional symptoms (fever, weight loss, night sweats, or fatigue) ●*Location:* One or both iliopsoas muscles; may be extending from adjacent bowel, abdominal cavity, perinephric area, or spinal cord (vertebrae or discs) ●*Pattern:* Pain is constant but increases with extension of the leg at the hip (stretching the psoas muscle - psoas sign) ●*Precipitating factors:* Tuberculosis or bacterial infection of the spine, trauma, perinephric infection, bowel perforation or infection, retroperitoneal hematoma, bacteremia ●*Relieving factors:* Flexion of the leg at the hip (contracting the psoas muscle) ●*Clinical course:* Usually requires drainage for cure, otherwise may spread to adjacent structures ●*Co-morbidities:* Diverticulitis, appendicitis, Crohn's disease, perinephric abscess, tuberculosis, osteomyelitis, bacteremia, endocarditis, trauma, diabetes ●*Procedure results:* Positive psoas sign on physical examination, mass or phlegmon on abdominal CT or MRI ●*Test findings:* Elevated white blood cells (WBC), erythrocyte sedimentation rate (ESR), and C-reactive protein (CRP)

Psoriasis ●*Onset:* Subacute, insidious ●*Male:female ratio:* M=F ●*Ethnicity:* Higher incidence in Caucasians ❶ *Character:* Skin lesions ❷ *Location:* Scalp, elbows, knees, nails, any location ❸ *Pattern:* Demarcated red scaly plaques ●*Precipitating factors:* Infection (especially streptococcus), medications ●*Relieving factors:* Topical steroids, vitamin D analogs, retinoids, phototherapy ●*Clinical course:* Persistent ●*Co-morbidities:* Psoriatic arthritis ●*Procedure results:* No relevant procedures ●*Test findings:* No relevant tests

Images of ❶ *Character,* ❷ *Location,* ❸ *Pattern on page 593*

Psoriatic arthritis ●*Onset:* Insidious ●*Male:female ratio:* M<F (slightly) ●*Ethnicity:* Caucasians most commonly ●*Character:* Dull ache with stiffness ●*Location:* Large joints, small joints, hip, sacroiliac joints; pitting of nails ●*Pattern:* Oligoarticular, symmetric polyarticular, axial ●*Precipitating factors:* Inactivity or worsening of skin disease ●*Relieving factors:* Non-steroidal anti-inflammatory drugs (NSAIDs), methotrexate, sulfasalazine, etanercept ●*Clinical course:* Chronic with intermittent flares ●*Co-morbidities:* Psoriasis of the skin ●*Procedure results:* No relevant procedures ●*Test findings:* Erosions of the distal interphalangeal joints on plain radiographs

Pubic lice ●*Onset:* Acute, subacute, insidious ●*Male:female ratio:* M=F ●*Ethnicity:* All ●*Character:* Marked pruritus, nits, adult lice in pubic hair (rarely other body hair) ●*Location:* Pubic hair, eyebrows, eyelashes, axillary hair, back and chest hair in men, adjacent skin ●*Pattern:* Extreme pruritus. Macules, papules, excoriations may be seen. Rarely blue macules in adjacent skin ●*Precipitating factors:* Sexual contact, close body contact ●*Relieving factors:* Washing with pediculicide, combing eggs and lice out of the hair, hot-cycle (130°F) machine washing of all clothing and bedlinens, petroleum to eyelid ●*Clinical course:* Acute, persistent, good response to therapy, relapse may occur; retreatment recommended at day

Psoriasis: Images *see text page 592*

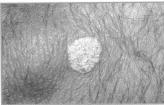

❶ *Character A typical papulosquamous plaque on the elbow*

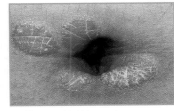

❶ *Character Multiple papulosquamous plaques around the umbilicus*

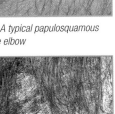

❷ *Location Diffuse scale on the scalp*

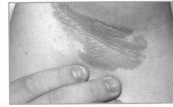

❷ *Location Axillary psoriasis often lacks scale. Nail pits also affected*

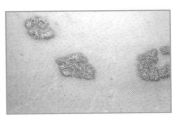

❸ *Pattern Multiple well-defined papulosquamous plaques*

7-10 ●*Co-morbidities:* Syphilis, gonorrhea, Chlamydia trachomatis, hepatitis B, HIV infection ●*Procedure results:* Finding nits (eggs), live nymphs, adult lice in pubic, eye, axillary, chest, back hair ●*Test findings:* No relevant tests

Puerperal infection (endometritis) ●*Onset:* Subacute ●*Male:female ratio:* F ●*Ethnicity:* Nonspecific ●*Character:* Uterine tenderness; fevers; chills ●*Location:* Uterine ●*Pattern:* Gradually progressive ●*Precipitating factors:* Recent delivery ●*Relieving factors:* Antibiotics ●*Clinical course:* Slowly progressive; rarely self-limiting ●*Co-morbidities:* Recent delivery; group B streptococcus ●*Procedure results:* No relevant procedures ●*Test findings:* Elevated white blood cells (WBC)

Pulmonary hamartoma ●*Onset:* Insidious ●*Male:female ratio:* M=F ●*Ethnicity:* All ●*Character:* Asymptomatic, nonproductive cough ●*Location:* Chest ●*Pattern:* Nonspecific ●*Precipitating factors:* None relevant ●*Relieving factors:* Excision ●*Clinical course:* Slow growth over years ●*Co-morbidities:* Differential diagnosis of solitary pulmonary nodule ●*Procedure results:* Lung biopsy, usually surgical; 'popcorn' pattern of calcification on chest CT ●*Test findings:* No relevant tests

Pulmonary hemosiderosis ●*Onset:* Subacute, insidious ●*Male:female ratio:* M=F ●*Ethnicity:* All ●*Character:* Cough, fever, dyspnea (hemoptysis is absent in >50% of patients) ●*Location:* Chest ●*Pattern:* Bilateral inspiratory rales ●*Precipitating factors:* Idiopathic ●*Relieving factors:* Steroid therapy ●*Clinical course:* Repeated episodes of bleeding lead to pulmonary fibrosis and early mortality ●*Co-morbidities:* Exclude drug reaction, systemic vasculitis, mitral valve disease, coagulopathy; in pediatric patients, associated with celiac disease, elevated IgA ●*Procedure results:* Bland pulmonary hemorrhage without capillaritis on lung biopsy ●*Test findings:* Hemosiderin-laden macrophages in sputum, elevated diffusing capacity of the lungs for carbon monoxide (DLCO) or evidence for alveolar hemorrhage by bronchoscopy, anemia, elevated lactate dehydrogenase (LDH)

Pulmonary hypertension ●*Onset:* Insidious ●*Male:female ratio:* M=F ●*Ethnicity:* All ●*Character:* Exertional dyspnea, chest pain, syncope ●*Location:* Heart, chest ●*Pattern:* Loud P2, murmur of tricuspid insufficiency ●*Precipitating factors:* Parenchymal lung disease, chronic thromboembolic disease, connective tissue disease (especially scleroderma, lupus, rheumatoid arthritis), left-sided valvular or myocardial disease, congenital heart disease, cirrhosis, HIV, chronic cocaine use, diet-suppressive medications ●*Relieving factors:* Anticoagulation, vasodilators (once determined to be safe), such as calcium channel blockers (nifedipine or diltiazem) and epoprostenol; consider lung transplantation ●*Clinical course:* Progressive with high mortality, median survival approximately 3 years after diagnosis ●*Co-morbidities:* Cor pulmonale ●*Procedure results:* Mean pulmonary arterial pressure >25mm Hg at rest or >30mmHg with exercise ●*Test findings:* Echocardiogram: enlargement of right-heart chambers, paradoxical motion of the interventricular septum, tricuspid insufficiency; electrocardiogram: right axis deviation (RAD) and right ventricular (RV) strain; chest X-ray: enlarged central pulmonary arteries, right heart dilation

Pulmonary infarction ●*Onset:* Acute ●*Male:female ratio:* M<F ●*Ethnicity:* All ●*Character:* Pleuritic chest pain, dyspnea, cough ●*Location:* Chest ●*Pattern:* Inspiratory rales, dullness to percussion or a normal examination ●*Precipitating factors:* Venous thrombosis ●*Relieving factors:* Oxygen, anticoagulation with low molecular weight or unfractionated heparin followed by warfarin, consider thrombolysis in select cases ●*Clinical course:* Weeks-to-months to resolution, radiographic appearance may evolve to a cavitary nodule prior to resolution ●*Co-morbidities:* Deep vein thrombosis (DVT), right heart failure with massive pulmonary embolus, pleural effusion ●*Procedure results:* High probability ventilation/perfusion ratio (V/Q) scan or pulmonary angiogram or chest CT consistent with an arterial clot ●*Test findings:* No relevant tests

Pulmonary thromboembolism ●*Onset:* Acute ●*Male:female ratio:* M<F ●*Ethnicity:* All ●*Character:* Chest discomfort, dyspnea, cough, presyncope, palpitations, fever, wheezing ●*Location:* Chest, may be associated with calf deep vein thrombosis ●*Pattern:* Examination may be misleadingly normal, tachycardia, tachypnea, elevated jugular venous pressure (JVP), focal inspiratory rales or signs of a pleural effusion, right-sided S3, lower extremity cord, warmth, tenderness or edema ●*Precipitating factors:* Inactivity (e.g. long plane flight, car trip), surgery, lower extremity injury, pregnancy, estrogen therapy, hypercoagulable state ●*Relieving factors:* Anticoagulation, thrombolysis, thrombectomy ●*Clinical course:* Weeks-to-months ●*Co-morbidities:* Hypercoagulable state, malignancy, lupus ●*Procedure results:* No relevant procedures ●*Test findings:* Evidence of a vascular occlusion by pulmonary arteriogram, IV bolus contrast chest CT, venogram or ultrasound

Pulmonary valve stenosis ●*Onset:* Congenital onset acute to insidious, depending on degree of stenosis; acquired onset insidious ●*Male:female ratio:* M=F ●*Ethnicity:* All ●*Character:* Presence and severity of symptoms depends on degree of stenosis: in neonate, may see cyanosis; later in life, may see gradual right heart failure symptoms; may be asymptomatic; may see cyanosis later in life if concurrent atrial septal defect or patent foramen ovale ●*Location:* Right heart failure symptoms include abdominal distension (liver enlargement, ascites), dependent edema ●*Pattern:* Nonspecific ●*Precipitating factors:* Disease gradually progressive, so do not see daily variations in symptoms (other than leg edema worsening with being upright) ●*Relieving factors:* Prostaglandin E1 can maintain ductus arteriosus patency in newborn, reducing cyanosis; leg elevation can reduce edema in adults ●*Clinical course:* Chronic and insidiously progressive if severe pulmonic stenosis until balloon valvuloplasty performed or surgical modification/replacement of valve ●*Co-morbidities:* Congenital: can see with right ventricle and/or pulmonary artery hypoplasia, Noonan's syndrome, seen in tetralogy of Fallot; acquired: carcinoid syndrome, rheumatic valve disease ●*Procedure results:* Right heart catheterization reveals elevated RV pressure, pressure gradient across pulmonic valve; angiocardiography outlines stenotic valve and shows poststenotic dilation of PA; Echo reveals elevated RV systolic pressures, thickened pulmonic cusps, increased velocity across pulmonic valve ●*Test findings:* ECG in infant shows predominant leftward forces, but later in life, see RV strain/overload pattern

Pulmonic valve insufficiency (pulmonic regurgitation) ●*Onset:* Typically insidious, rarely subacute ●*Male:female ratio:* M=F ●*Ethnicity:* All ●*Character:* Symptoms depend on primary disorder that led to pulmonic regurgitation (PR); PR itself may worsen right-sided heart failure symptoms ●*Location:* Ankle/leg swelling, right upper abdominal discomfort ●*Pattern:* If present, heart failure symptoms worsen with increased salt/fluid intake; leg edema worse with standing ●*Precipitating factors:* Pulmonary hypertension; pulmonic valve endocarditis may be related to IV drug use ●*Relieving factors:* Heart failure management with diuretics, salt/fluid restriction, compression stockings; treatment of underlying problem that led to PR ●*Clinical course:* Depends on precipitating diagnosis; causes of pulmonary hypertension may be progressive (especiallly primary) or slowly reversible with treatment (especially secondary); endocarditis is treatable with antibiotics and occasionally with valve surgery ●*Co-morbidities:* Primary pulmonary hypertension, secondary pulmonary hypertension (pulmonary embolism, all causes of left-sided heart failure), pulmonic valve endocarditis, Marfan's syndrome, congenital, trauma, carcinoid syndrome ●*Procedure results:* With right-heart catheterization, IV contrast injected into pulmonary artery (PA) will reflux back to right ventricle (RV); electrocardiogram (ECG) may show right-sided volume and/or pressure overload (e.g. right ventricular hypertrophy [RVH], P pulmonale); echocardiogram may show RV enlargement and may see jet of PR on Doppler evaluation ●*Test findings:* No relevant tests

Pyelonephritis ●*Onset:* Acute; chronic or complicated may be subacute or chronic over weeks-months ●*Male:female ratio:* M<F ●*Ethnicity:* Vesicoureteral reflux (VUR) much less common in African-American children ●*Character:* Infection of upper urinary tract ●*Location:* Acute presentation flank pain, nausea/vomiting, fever >38C; dysuria and urinary frequency may be absent; sepsis with shock and renal failure rare ●*Pattern:* Acute or chronic; uncomplicated (occurring in healthy, young, nonpregnant female) vs complicated (occurring in all others) ●*Precipitating factors:* Chronic associated with chronically obstructing stone disease, VUR ●*Relieving factors:* Oral fluoroquinolones indicated for acute uncomplicated cases; hospitalization indicated for patients unable to maintain oral hydration ●*Clinical course:* Acute uncomplicated pyelonephritis does not progress to chronic renal failure; chronic pyelonephritis can lead to progressive renal scarring ●*Co-morbidities:* Pregnancy; presence of chronic indwelling urinary catheters ●*Procedure results:* Technetium DMSA renal scan and voiding cystourethrogram detects presence and severity of VUR and renal scarring in chronic condition ●*Test findings:* Urinalysis: pyuria, hematuria, white blood cell (WBC) casts indicate renal origin, Gram stain to identify bacteria, urine culture positive; blood: leukocytosis, raised erythrocyte sedimentation rate (ESR), C-reactive protein (CRP)

Pyloric stenosis ●*Onset:* Subacute in infants or in adults ●*Male:female ratio:* M=F ●*Ethnicity:* Infantile syndrome seen more commonly in Caucasians ●*Character:* Infants: age 1 week to 5 months - nonbilious vomiting, with weight loss and dehydration; jaundice in 2-5%. Adults: epigastric pain, bloating and distension, nausea and vomiting after meals; usually due to pyloric or duodenal ulcer disease, so peptic ulcer disease (PUD) symptoms may occur prior to outlet obstruction ●*Location:* Adults: epigastrium and upper abdomen ●*Pattern:* Symptoms occur after food intake ●*Precipitating factors:* Food intake ●*Relieving factors:* Infants: IV fluids to correct dehydration, and surgical pyloromyotomy (recurrence rate is 1-3% after surgical repair). Adults: nasogastric suction and IV fluids acutely; if due to edema from PUD, treatment with IV acid suppression may relieve symptoms; if due to stricturing, endoscopic dilation or surgery is needed ●*Clinical course:* Not self-limited - symptoms usually lead to medical attention within days (infants) to weeks (adults) ●*Co-morbidities:* Infants: congenital disorder; adults: PUD, gastric malignancy ●*Procedure results:* Infants - sonography can confirm the diagnosis; adults - esophagogastroduodenosocpy (EGD) confirms the diagnosis ●*Test findings:* Dehydration and hypochloremic alkalosis are common; in infants, bilirubin may be elevated in up to 50% of cases

Pyogenic infection ●*Onset:* Acute ●*Male:female ratio:* M=F ●*Ethnicity:* All ●*Character:* Pus-forming process, fever, chills, yellow discharge or drainage, white exudates ●*Location:* Any organ: skin, throat, eye, tooth, liver, muscle, abscess in any organ ●*Pattern:* Infected area is tender, warm, erythematous, and fluctuant; discharge or exudate is thick and yellow ●*Precipitating factors:* Surgical procedure, trauma, injury ●*Relieving factors:* Drainage, specific antibiotic therapy ●*Clinical course:* Most pyogenic infections are mild to moderate and resolve with adequate therapy (antibiotic and drainage when necessary). Some can be severe, persistent, or even fatal ●*Co-morbidities:* Diabetes, congenital immunodeficiency, injection drug use, dermatosis, rheumatic fever, HIV, Job's syndrome, hyper-IgE ●*Procedure results:* Abscess on imaging studies, leukocytes and bacteria on Gram stain or pathology specimen, purulent drainage ●*Test findings:* Leukocytosis, leukocytes and bacteria on Gram stain or pathology specimen, growth of bacteria on culture

Pyogenic liver abscess ●*Onset:* Insidious ●*Male:female ratio:* M=F ●*Ethnicity:* No predisposition ●*Character:* Malaise, fever, dull abdominal pain, often in right upper quadrant (RUQ); weight loss usually occurs ●*Location:* RUQ of abdomen ●*Pattern:* Slowly progressive symptoms over weeks-to-months ●*Precipitating factors:* None relevant ●*Relieving factors:* Antibiotic therapy and drainage of abscess cavity ●*Clinical course:* Progressive over weeks-to-months ●*Co-morbidities:* History of recent cholangitis, cholecystitis, diverticulitis, recent dental work ●*Procedure results:* Aspiration of purulent material from the abscess is diagnostic ●*Test findings:* Fluid-filled cavity on ultrasound or CT; usually white blood cell (WBC) elevated, alkaline phosphatase elevated

Pyridoxin deficiency ●*Onset:* Subacute to insidious ●*Male:female ratio:* M=F ●*Ethnicity:* All; poor socioeconomic status is principal risk factor ●*Character:* (Neonatal) seizures; neuropathy ●*Location:* Peripheral neuropathy ●*Pattern:* Sensory changes ●*Precipitating factors:* B6 (pyridoxin) deficiency can result in neuropathy especially in the setting of isonicotinic acid hydrazide (INH), penicillamine, or cycloserine administration ●*Relieving factors:* Pyridoxine can be given as part of treatment plan in hydralazine overdose, toxicity from INH, cycloserine, penicillamine, or as prophylaxis with INH therapy ●*Clinical course:* Slowly progressive neuropathy (until deficiency is corrected); seizures can be acute in neonates ●*Co-morbidities:* Neuropathy; coexisting vitamin deficiencies ●*Procedure results:* No relevant procedures ●*Test findings:* Peripheral neuropathy in susceptible patients

Radiation sickness ●*Onset:* Acute, subacute ●*Male:female ratio:* M=F ●*Ethnicity:* All ●*Character:* Nausea, vomiting, diarrhea, seizures, erythema of skin, hair loss, anemia; earlier onset GI symptoms implies higher exposure dose and more systemic effects ●*Location:* Nonspecific ●*Pattern:* Nonspecific ●*Precipitating factors:* Exposure to any source of ionizing radiation ●*Relieving factors:* Clean and cover open wounds, remove any contaminated material or clothing; chelating agents may be useful ●*Clinical course:* Low-dose exposure may be asymptomatic; higher doses may cause transient abnormalities or lead to more serious systemic complications or death ●*Co-morbidities:* None relevant ●*Procedure results:* No relevant procedures ●*Test findings:* Bone marrow depression seen on complete blood count 20-30 days after exposure

Raised intracranial pressure ●*Onset:* Gradual (malignancy) or abrupt (trauma) depending on underlying etiology ●*Male:female ratio:* M=F ●*Ethnicity:* All ●*Character:* Decreased cerebral blood flow due to expanding lesions within the cranial cavity ●*Location:* Raised intracranial pressure above 15mm Hg with intermittent plateau waves of 25-60mm Hg due to diminished intracranial compliance ●*Pattern:* Coma, marked hypertension, papilledema, decorticate and decerebrate posturing, Kussmaul or Cheyne-Stokes breathing ●*Precipitating factors:* Cerebral hemorrhage, encephalitis, brain edema after stroke, head trauma with intracerebral, subdural or epidural hemorrhage, brain malignancy ●*Relieving factors:* Fluid restiction, osmotic agents such as mannitol, hyperventilation via intubation and mechanical ventilation, corticosteroids ●*Clinical course:* Variable with etiology - usually long-term deficits persist ●*Co-morbidities:* Venous thromboembolism, seizures, complications of corticosteroids including opportunistic infections ●*Procedure results:* Continuous intracranial pressure monitoring in ICU setting to guide therapy ●*Test findings:* Emergent head CT without contrast is test of choice to assess intracerebral hemorrhage or tumor

Ramsay Hunt syndrome ●*Onset:* Acute ●*Male:female ratio:* M=F ●*Ethnicity:* All ●*Character:* Unilateral pain and vesicular eruption in external ear, with loss of taste in anterior two-thirds of tongue, and facial palsy ●*Location:* Geniculate ganglion of the VIIth cranial nerve (ear canal, anterior two thirds of tongue) ●*Pattern:* Rash is vesicular, pain is severe, and may precede appearance of vesicles, findings are unilateral, facial palsy ipsilateral ●*Precipitating factors:* Immunosuppression, HIV or none ●*Relieving factors:* None relevant ●*Clinical course:* Vesicles resolve after 3-5 days in the normal host and >7 days in the immunocompromised. Pain and neurologic deficits gradually resolve over weeks-to-months ●*Co-morbidities:* HIV/AIDS, immunosuppression, chemotherapy, meningoencephalitis, disseminated zoster ●*Procedure results:* Positive varicella direct fluorescent antigen of vesicular material, multinucleated cells on Tzanck smear of lesion-base scrapings ●*Test findings:* No relevant tests

Recreational drug abuse ●*Onset:* Acute, subacute ●*Male:female ratio:* M>F ●*Ethnicity:* All ●*Character:* Vary with each drug. Agitation, hallucinations, confusion, anxiety most commonly seen: cocaine can cause cardiac ischemia, dysrhythmias, seizures; opiates cause respiratory depression ●*Location:* Nonspecific ●*Pattern:* Nonspecific ●*Precipitating factors:* None relevant ●*Relieving factors:* Treatment mainly supportive. Benzodiazepines useful in treating amphetamines and cocaine effects; nalaxone reverses opiate effects ●*Clinical course:* Not applicable ●*Co-morbidities:* None relevant ●*Procedure results:* No relevant procedures ●*Test findings:* Toxicologic screens may indicate a particular drug

Recurrent laryngeal nerve injury ●*Onset:* Usually acute in onset ●*Male:female ratio:* M=F ●*Ethnicity:* All ●*Character:* Hoarseness often with dysphagia ●*Location:* Larynx/voice ●*Pattern:* Persisted hoarseness, often worse at the end of the day ●*Precipitating factors:* Usually history of thyroid surgery, thoracic surgery, blunt or penetrating trauma to the neck, or recent intubation for surgery ●*Relieving factors:* None relevant ●*Clinical course:* Symptoms may be permanent, especially if nerve has been transected; blunt or partial injury to the nerve has a reasonable chance for spontaneous recovery ●*Co-morbidities:* None relevant ●*Procedure results:* Fiberoptic laryngoscopy reveals vocal cord paralysis/paresis ●*Test findings:* No relevant tests

Recurrent laryngeal nerve palsy ●*Onset:* Acute, insidious ●*Male:female ratio:* M=F ●*Ethnicity:* All ●*Character:* Persistent hoarseness ●*Location:* Larynx/voice ●*Pattern:* Hoarseness is constant, but may be worse after long periods of voice use, or at the end of the day ●*Precipitating factors:* Viral prodrome may be present; history of recent neck or thoracic surgery ●*Relieving factors:* Voice rest ●*Clinical course:* Usually persistent hoarseness ●*Co-morbidities:* Check for other cranial nerve palsies ●*Procedure results:* Fiberoptic laryngoscopy reveals unilateral vocal cord immobility; laryngeal electromyogram (EMG) reveals denervation ●*Test findings:* No relevant tests

Reflex sympathetic dystrophy ●*Onset:* Subacute ●*Male:female ratio:* M=F ●*Ethnicity:* All ●*Character:* Burning pain, hypersthesia, vasomotor and dystrophic changes, swelling ●*Location:* Usually in limb ●*Pattern:* Nonspecific ●*Precipitating factors:* Typically begins after trauma to limb and/or hemiplegia ●*Relieving factors:* Physical therapy, NSAIDs, corticosteroids, sympathetic blockade, sympathetic ganglionectomy ●*Clinical course:* May progress to atrophy if untreated ●*Co-morbidities:* Emotionally unstable, anxious, socially withdrawn ●*Procedure results:* Plain radiograph may show osteopenia. Bone scan may show increased or decreased uptake in affected limb ●*Test findings:* No relevant tests

Reflux laryngitis ●*Onset:* Subacute ●*Male:female ratio:* M=F ●*Ethnicity:* All ●*Character:* Hoarseness or loss of voice ●*Location:* Throat/voice ●*Pattern:* Worsening of voice quality with increasing use during the day; may be painful ●*Precipitating factors:* Heavy meal; supine position ●*Relieving factors:* Gargles, cough drops or lozenges ●*Clinical course:* May be persistent or intermittent ●*Co-morbidities:* Gastroesophageal reflux disease ●*Procedure results:* Inflamed, edematous vocal cords on fiberoptic laryngoscopy; inflammation of arytenoids ●*Test findings:* None relevant

Reiter's syndrome ●*Onset:* Acute ●*Male:female ratio:* M>F ●*Ethnicity:* Caucasians > African descent ●*Character:* Dull ache ●*Location:* Low back pain, lower extremity joints, hands ●*Pattern:* Worse in the morning ●*Precipitating factors:* Sexually transmitted diseases and gastroenteritis ●*Relieving factors:* Non-steroidal anti-inflammatory drugs (NSAIDs), sulfasalazine, hydroxychloroquine ●*Clinical course:* Self-limiting in most patients ●*Co-morbidities:* Venereal disease, gastroenteritis ●*Procedure results:* No relevant procedures ●*Test findings:* Elevated erythrocyte sedimentation rate (ESR), positive HLA-B27, anemia

Renal artery stenosis ●*Onset:* Subacute; embolic disease occurs acutely ●*Male:female ratio:* M=F ●*Ethnicity:* Fibromuscular dysplasia more common in Caucasians ●*Character:* Hypertension and/or ischemic nephropathy caused by narrowing of renal artery leading to activation of renin-angiotensin system (RAS) ●*Location:* Unilateral or bilateral stenosis of renal artery proximally, distally or renal artery branches ●*Pattern:* 70% cases due to atherosclerosis; 30% due to fibromuscular dysplasia: medial, perimedial, or intimal fibroplasia. Abrupt onset of hypertension, malignant hypertension, increased blood pressure (BP) in previously well-controlled patient indication of RAS ●*Precipitating factors:* Smoking; genetic predisposition ●*Relieving factors:* Medical treatment of hypertension; surgery indicated if refactory to medical therapy ●*Clinical course:* Progression to renal insufficiency frequent; accelerated retinopathy; refractory hypertension; hypertension may persist even if stenosis corrected due to injury to contralateral kidney ●*Co-morbidities:* Peripheral vascular disease, coronay artery disease (CAD), neurofibromatosis, polyarteritis nodosum, Takayasu's arteritis, cholesterol emboli, aortic dissection ●*Procedure results:* Percutaneous transluminal renal arteriography (PTRA) with or without stenting; duplex ultrasound with Doppler, MR angiography, demonstrate narrowing of artery ●*Test findings:* No relevant tests

Renal calculi ●*Onset:* Sudden ●*Male:female ratio:* M(4):F(1) ●*Ethnicity:* All ●*Character:* Severe agonizing pain; patient in constant motion; no comfortable position ●*Location:* Costovertebral angle ●*Pattern:* Waxes and wanes; typical acute episode occurring during the night or early morning ●*Precipitating factors:* Hot weather; dehydration; diet rich in purine and oxalate; low fluid intake; excessive milk intake; excessive vitamins; usage of medication: loop diuretics, corticosteroids, uricosuric agents, dyazide; chemotherapy; prolonged periods of immobilization; urinary tract infection (UTI) ●*Relieving factors:* Spontaneous unobstruction or passage of stone; surgical manipulation: endoscopic, percutaneous, extracorporeal shock-wave lithotripsy (ESWL), or open surgery; medication: analgesics, anti-inflammatory, narcotics, thiazides, orthophosphates, sodium cellulose phosphate, allopurinol, citrates, and magnesium ●*Clinical course:* Spontaneous passage of smaller stones (>80% chance for stones <5mm in size); otherwise, intermittent and progressive renal obstruction ●*Co-morbidities:* Gout; malignancy; renal tubular acidosis; medullary sponge kidney; sarcoidosis; cystinuria; UTI; urethral strictures; ureteropelvic junction obstruction; horseshoe kidney; benign prostatic hyperplasia (BPH); hypertension ●*Procedure results:* Plain abdominal film: 90% radiopaque stones; stone size, location, and degree of obstruction determined by intravenous pyelogram (IVP), ultrasound, or CT without contrast; >98% stone-free rate with surgical intervention ●*Test findings:* Urine analysis: positive RBC, possible WBC, possible crystals; urine pH <5.5 suspicious for uric acid stone

Renal cell adenocarcinoma ●*Onset:* Subacute, insidious ●*Male:female ratio:* M(2):F(1) ●*Ethnicity:* All ●*Character:* Majority asymptomatic; classic triad of hematuria, abdominal mass, flank pain ●*Location:* Abdomen, flank, retroperitoneum ●*Pattern:* Nonspecific ●*Precipitating factors:* Smoking, obesity, exposure to toxic occupational compounds, analgesic abuse ●*Relieving factors:* Surgery: radical or partial nephrectomy; immunotherapy for advanced disease ●*Clinical course:* Progressive to metastasis (lung, liver, bone, brain), local invasion of adjacent organs, vena cava invasion ●*Co-morbidities:* Von Hippel-Lindau disease; adult polycystic kidney disease; horseshoe kidney; acquired renal cystic disease from chronic renal failure ●*Procedure results:* IV pyelogram, CT, ultrasound, MRI; all helpful in differentiating a cyst from a solid tumor ●*Test findings:* Anemia (20-40%); polycythemia (3%); hematuria (36%); hypercalcemia (6%); possible elevation of alkaline phosphate or liver enzymes (20%)

Renal infarction ●*Onset:* Acute/abrupt ●*Male:female ratio:* M=F ●*Ethnicity:* All ●*Character:* Sharp and severe pain without radiation ●*Location:* Flank pain 61%; abdominal pain 28% ●*Pattern:* Mostly unilateral ●*Precipitating factors:* Embolic event, blunt trauma, angiographic manipulation ●*Relieving factors:* Intra-arterial fibrinolysis, systemic anticoagulation, surgery ●*Clinical course:* Progressive; loss of renal function; hypertension ●*Co-morbidities:* Cardiac disease, embolic events, hypertension, peripheral vascular disease ●*Procedure results:* Fibrinolysis: 100% renal salvage; anticoagulation: 30% renal savage; surgery: 20% renal salvage. Selective arteriography to locate thrombus ●*Test findings:* Urinalysis: hematuria 65%, pyuria 50%, proteinuria 70%; lactate dehydrogenase (LDH) always elevated

Renal tubular acidosis ●*Onset:* Subacute ●*Male:female ratio:* M=F ●*Ethnicity:* All ●*Character:* Non-anion gap (hyperchloremic) metabolic acidosis ●*Location:* 3 types: distal (type I), proximal (type II), and hypoaldosterone (type IV) ●*Pattern:* Type I: impaired hydrogen ion secretion; type II: decreased bicarbonate absorption; type IV: impaired renal ammoniagenesis ●*Precipitating factors:* Congenital/hereditary forms for each; other associations: type I (autoimmune disease, ifosfamide, amphotericin, cirrhosis, sickle cell anemia, lithium, renal transplant), type II (Fanconi's, ifosfamide, cysteinosis, multiple myeloma [light chain disease]), type IV (diabetes mellitus, heparin, non-steroidal anti-inflammatory drugs [NSAIDs], angiotensin-converting enzyme (ACE) inhibitors, adrenal insufficiency, HIV, congenital adrenal hyperplasia, renal failure) ●*Relieving factors:* Alkali (potassium citrate) to replace lost bicarbonate or neutralize retained acid in types I, II; potassium restriction with or without diuretics in type IV; fludrocortisone acetate used rarely in type IV ●*Clinical course:* May be mild or asymptomatic but can result in significant metabolic acidosis and associated electrolyte abnormalities (potassium [K+], phosphate [PO4-], calcium [Ca++], magnesium [Mg++]) ●*Co-morbidities:* Bone disease, hypophosphatemia (type II), hyperkalemia (type IV, II) or hypokalemia (type I). Hypercalciuria with associated nephrolithiasis or nephrocalcinosis common in type I ●*Procedure results:* Urine pH >7.5 and >15% filtered HCO3- in urine when serum HCO3- normal during bicarbonate infusion are hallmark findings for type II. Inability to acidify urine with acid load is characteristic of type I ●*Test findings:* Urine pH inappropriately high (>5.5); renin, aldosterone serum levels low in type IV (but rarely checked; usually treated empirically)

Renal vein thrombosis ●*Onset:* Acute or chronic ●*Male:female ratio:* M=F ●*Ethnicity:* All ●*Character:* Acute: flank pain, acute decline in glomerular filtration rate (GFR), hematuria, proteinuria; chronic: may be asymptomatic ●*Location:* Flank ●*Pattern:* Back pain, lower extremity thrombophlebitis or asymmetric edema, dilated abdominal veins may be present ●*Precipitating factors:* Nephrotic syndrome or other hypercoagulable state, GU malignancy, extrarenal compressing tumor. In infants: dehydration with severe gastroenteritis or sepsis may predispose ●*Relieving factors:* Anticoagulation ●*Clinical course:* May see spontaneous resolution of thrombus or recanalization. Renal function may decline acutely; usually improves with thrombus resolution ●*Co-morbidities:* Embolization causing pulmonary embolism (PE) or infarct. Abnormal Doppler flow or characteristic MRI, angiographic findings ●*Procedure results:* Renal ultrasound or venography ●*Test findings:* Lactate dehydrogenase (LDH), alkaline phosphatase (AP) may be elevated with associated infarct

Repetitive strain injury ●*Onset:* Insidious ●*Male:female ratio:* M=F ●*Ethnicity:* All ●*Character:* Dull ache ●*Location:* Upper extremities and low back ●*Pattern:* Worse with repetitive motion ●*Precipitating factors:* Motion related to repetitive strain ●*Relieving factors:* Altered ergonomics ●*Clinical course:* Progressive if not addressed ●*Co-morbidities:* Depression, prior trauma ●*Procedure results:* No relevant procedures ●*Test findings:* No relevant tests

Respiratory syncytial virus infection ●*Onset:* Subacute, acute ●*Male:female ratio:* M=F ●*Ethnicity:* All ●*Character:* Cough, wheeze, rhinorrhea, tachypnea ●*Location:* Chest wall, accessory respiratory muscles ●*Pattern:* Worsening respiratory status ●*Precipitating factors:* Exposed to/contracts respiratory syncytial virus (RSV) virus ●*Relieving factors:* Oxygen, IV fluids, bronchodilators, ribavirin in indicated cases ●*Clinical course:* Progresses until illness resolves ●*Co-morbidities:* Underlying coronary heart disease (CHD), bronchopulmonary dysplasia (BPD), severe immunodeficiency, prematurity ●*Procedure results:* Chest X-ray shows hyperinflation with air trapping, peribronchial thickening; RSV-antigen positive from nasopharyngeal swab ●*Test findings:* No relevant tests

Restless leg syndrome ●*Onset:* Chronic ●*Male:female ratio:* M=F ●*Ethnicity:* All ●*Character:* Stereotyped periodic movements of one or both legs, during sleep or wakefulness; in nocturnal myoclonus, movement occurs in non-REM sleep and is composed of foot dorsiflexion, big toe extension and knee/hip flexion (triple response); in restless leg syndrome, the patient feels an irresistable urge to move the legs, especially when sitting or lying, due to discomfort between knee and ankle, symptoms cause insomnia ●*Location:* Specific lesion unclear; disorder affects lower extremities ●*Pattern:* Usually legs most restless when lying down and early hours of the night; discomfort fades by the morning when the patient can get sleep ●*Precipitating factors:* Uremia, anemia, iron deficiency and drug withdrawal (benzodiazepines and barbiturates) ●*Relieving factors:* Treatment of choice is clonazepam, although levodopa plus benzerazide or carbidopa are effective ●*Clinical course:* Persistent problem ●*Co-morbidities:* Other sleep disorders such as sleep apnea, narcolepsy, cataplexy and drug dependency ●*Procedure results:* No relevant procedures ●*Test findings:* No relevant tests

Retained products of gestation ●*Onset:* Variable from minutes to weeks ●*Male:female ratio:* F ●*Ethnicity:* All ●*Character:* Irregular vaginal bleeding after a pregnancy ●*Location:* Uterus ●*Pattern:* Bleeding may be immediately after birth or up to weeks later ●*Precipitating factors:* Previous uterine surgeries (i.e. Cesarean sections) ●*Relieving factors:* D&C ●*Clinical course:* Bleeding may be immediately after birth or up to weeks later ●*Co-morbidities:* Placenta accreta ●*Procedure results:* Ultrasound ●*Test findings:* Positive human chorionic gonadotropin (HCG)

Retinal and vitreous hemorrhage ●*Onset:* Acute, subacute. insidious ●*Male:female ratio:* M=F ●*Ethnicity:* All ●*Character:* Blurred vision ●*Location:* Macula, peripheral retina, vitreous cavity ●*Pattern:* None ●*Precipitating factors:* Severe blunt trauma can precipitate retinal and vitreous hemorrhage ●*Relieving factors:* Vitrectomy can be performed to remove vitreous blood; management of retinal hemorrhage depends on the cause ●*Clinical course:*

Most conditions producing retinal and vitreous hemorrhage are progressive ●*Co-morbidities:* Diabetes ●*Procedure results:* Fundus examination reveals retinal or vitreous hemorrhage ●*Test findings:* No relevant tests

Retinal artery occlusion ●*Onset:* Acute ●*Male:female ratio:* M=F ●*Ethnicity:* All ●*Character:* Unilateral blurred vision ●*Location:* Retina ●*Pattern:* Typically affects one eye only; amaurosis fugax ●*Precipitating factors:* Emboli ●*Relieving factors:* None relevant ●*Clinical course:* Visual loss profound and complete within 90 min ●*Co-morbidities:* Atherosclerotic vascular disease; heart valvular disease ●*Procedure results:* No relevant procedures ●*Test findings:* Test for underlying conditions: giant cell arteritis; hypercoagulable state; emboli found on heart valve or in carotids

Retinal detachment ●*Onset:* Acute ●*Male:female ratio:* M=F ●*Ethnicity:* All ●*Character:* Painless loss of vision; shadow coming over visual field ●*Location:* Uniocular ●*Pattern:* Can happen any time ●*Precipitating factors:* Spontaneous or precipitated by trauma, inflammation, diabetic retinopathy or other causes ●*Relieving factors:* Usually requires surgical intervention ●*Clinical course:* Progressive retinal detachment occurs rapidly ●*Co-morbidities:* Myopia; lattice degeneration; Marfan's syndrome ●*Procedure results:* Indirect ophthalmoscopic examination ●*Test findings:* Separation of retina from the underlying tissue

Retinal exudates ●*Onset:* Usually subacute or insidious ●*Male:female ratio:* M=F ●*Ethnicity:* All ●*Character:* Blurred vision ●*Location:* Macula or peripheral retina ●*Pattern:* Many patterns exist, depending on underlying cause of retinal exudation ●*Precipitating factors:* None relevant ●*Relieving factors:* Treatment varies, depending on the cause of retinal exudate ●*Clinical course:* Most conditions producing retinal exudates are progressive ●*Co-morbidities:* Most common cause of retinal exudation is diabetic retinopathy ●*Procedure results:* Fundus examination: yellowish white lesions in the retina ●*Test findings:* No relevant tests

Retinal migraine ●*Onset:* Acute ●*Male:female ratio:* M=F ●*Ethnicity:* All ●*Character:* Acute headache, nausea, visual disturbance ●*Location:* Trigger sites in the V1 distribution ●*Pattern:* Monocular ●*Precipitating factors:* Triggered by certain foods or noxious stimuli ●*Relieving factors:* Abortive treatment with sumatriptan or dihydroergotamine ●*Clinical course:* Episodic; attacks typically last 10 min then usually clear ●*Co-morbidities:* Stroke, especially in young females; classic migraines ●*Procedure results:* No relevant procedures ●*Test findings:* No relevant tests

Retinal tear ●*Onset:* Acute ●*Male:female ratio:* M=F ●*Ethnicity:* All ●*Character:* Flashes of light; floaters; can progress to loss of vision (like a curtain coming up or down across the visual field) ●*Location:* Usually involves one eye ●*Pattern:* Flashes and floaters can remit or increase in frequency without relation to time ●*Precipitating factors:* Trauma can precipitate symptoms but they can occur spontaneously ●*Relieving factors:* Rarely bed rest can relieve symptoms, but usually only laser treatment or other surgical maneuvers to stabilize the retinal tear help ●*Clinical course:* Can progress rapidly to retinal detachment; small asymptomatic retinal breaks can be watched without treatment ●*Co-morbidities:* High myopia is the most common; also associated with many other conditions such as Marfan's syndrome and Stickler's syndrome ●*Procedure results:* Dilated fundus examination to find the location of the tear, usually in the peripheral retina; pigment cells in the vitreous may be present ●*Test findings:* No relevant tests

Retinal vein occlusion ●*Onset:* Acute, subacute ●*Male:female ratio:* M=F ●*Ethnicity:* All ●*Character:* Unilateral blurred vision ●*Location:* Retina ●*Pattern:* Retinal flame hemorrhages, cotton wool spots. Typically affects one eye only; amaurosis fugax ●*Precipitating factors:* None relevant ●*Relieving factors:* None relevant ●*Clinical course:* Initial visual loss profound and rapid in onset; subsequently, condition may completely resolve, partially resolve or progressively worsen over weeks-to-months ●*Co-morbidities:* Hypertension, glaucoma, hyperviscosity syndromes ●*Procedure results:* Serum electrophoresis and complete blood count (CBC) for bilateral simultaneous retinal venous disease ●*Test findings:* No relevant tests

Retinitis pigmentosa ●*Onset:* Insidious ●*Male:female ratio:* M>F ●*Ethnicity:* All ●*Character:* Nyctalopia (nightblindness), bilateral blurred vision, bone spicule change in retina, optic nerve pallor, attenuated retinal vessels ●*Location:* Retina. ●*Pattern:* Typically affects both eyes equally ●*Precipitating factors:* None relevant ●*Relieving factors:* None relevant ●*Clinical course:* Slowly progressive ●*Co-morbidities:* Cataract; several systemic conditions can be associated ●*Procedure results:* Electroretinogram confirms diagnosis ●*Test findings:* Extinguished retinal electrical responses to light stimuli

Retinoblastoma ●*Onset:* Acute, subacute ●*Male:female ratio:* M=F ●*Ethnicity:* All ❶ *Character:* Leukocoria (white pupil), strabismus, retinal mass ●*Location:* Eye ●*Pattern:* 75% unilateral ●*Precipitating factors:* None relevant ●*Relieving factors:* None relevant ●*Clinical course:* Rapidly progressive ●*Co-morbidities:* Osteogenic sarcoma; pineal tumor; other tumors ●*Procedure results:* Dilated fundus examination (may be under anesthesia); ultrasound B scan; neuroimaging shows white retinal-based lesion ●*Test findings:* No relevant tests

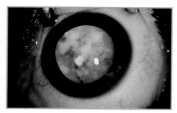

❶ *Character Mother noted a white pupillary reflex (leukokoria) in her child's eye*

Retinopathy of prematurity ●*Onset:* Insidious ●*Male:female ratio:* M=F ●*Ethnicity:* African-American infants less susceptible ●*Character:* Retinal vascular tortuosity, retinal detachment ●*Location:* Retina: demarcation line ●*Pattern:* Typically affects both eyes but asymmetrically ●*Precipitating factors:* Exposure to high oxygen levels ●*Relieving factors:* None relevant ●*Clinical course:* Progressive ●*Co-morbidities:* Hyaline membrane disease; myopia; amblyopia; early cataract formation; late-onset angle-closure glaucoma ●*Procedure results:* No relevant procedures ●*Test findings:* No relevant tests

Retroperitoneal hemorrhage ●*Onset:* Acute, subacute ●*Male:female ratio:* M=F ●*Ethnicity:* All ●*Character:* Abdominal or back pain, tender mass occasionally palpable, ecchymosis of flanks, psoas muscle irritation (increased pain with hip flexion against resistance), may see signs of shock but no obvious sources of hemorrhage ●*Location:* Retroperitoneum ●*Pattern:* Nonspecific ●*Precipitating factors:* Most common cause is traumatic pelvic fracture; may occur spontaneously or following strenuous activity in patients with increased bleeding risk (hemophilia or anticoagulation therapy) ●*Relieving factors:* Pelvic fractures may need fixation; treat shock and tranfuse blood; plasma or factor VIII in patients on anticoagulation therapy or with hemophilia ●*Clinical course:* Resuscitation and treatment of the cause usually results in full recovery ●*Co-morbidities:* Bleeding disorders ●*Procedure results:* Abdominal/pelvic CT scan diagnostic; loss of psoas shadow on abdominal radiographs ●*Test findings:* Hematuria, anemia

Retroperitonial fibrosis ●*Onset:* Insidious ●*Male:female ratio:* M=F ●*Ethnicity:* All ●*Character:* Dull flank pain, malaise, anorexia, weight loss ●*Location:* Flank, back, and abdominal pain ●*Pattern:* Nonspecific ●*Precipitating factors:* None relevant ●*Relieving factors:* Surgery to free up ureters and inferior vena cava ●*Clinical course:* Slowly progressive over years ●*Co-morbidities:* Crohn's disease, malignancy, psoriasis ●*Procedure results:* Open biopsy of retroperitoneum reveals fibrosis; CT or MRI are able to visualize the fibrosis ●*Test findings:* No relevant tests

Retrosternal goiter ●*Onset:* Insidious ●*Male:female ratio:* M(1):F(3) ●*Ethnicity:* All ●*Character:* Neck mass, dyspnea/dysphagia ●*Location:* Neck ●*Pattern:* Nonspecific ●*Precipitating factors:* More symptoms when prone or elevating arms above head

●*Relieving factors:* None relevant ●*Clinical course:* Usually progressive ●*Co-morbidities:* Hyperthyroidism; hypothyroidism ●*Procedure results:* I123 thyroid scan shows uptake under sternum ●*Test findings:* Widened mediastinum on chest X-ray. Thyroid-stimulating hormone (TSH) may be normal, low or high

Retroverted uterus in pregnancy ●*Onset:* Usually present around 10-12 weeks ●*Male:female ratio:* F ●*Ethnicity:* All ●*Character:* Vaginal/pelvic pain ●*Location:* Uterus ●*Pattern:* Worsening pain over several weeks ●*Precipitating factors:* Retroverted uterus ●*Relieving factors:* Manual uterine repositioning ●*Clinical course:* Extremely rare for uterus to become incarcerated; most retroverted gravid uteri will leave the pelvis spontaneously ●*Co-morbidities:* None relevant ●*Procedure results:* Pelvic examination demonstrates condition ●*Test findings:* No relevant tests

Reye's syndrome ●*Onset:* Acute ●*Male:female ratio:* M=F ●*Ethnicity:* All ●*Character:* Encephalopathy, fatty degeneration of liver, prodromal febrile illness - upper respiratory infection (URI)/chicken pox followed by improvement then protracted vomiting, delirium, stupor, seizures, coma, mild-to-moderate liver enlargement ●*Location:* Neurologic/gastrointestinal (GI) ●*Pattern:* Progressively worsening neurologic symptoms after apparent improvement from initial viral illness ●*Precipitating factors:* Aspirin ingestion while affected with influenza-like illness or varicella; loss of mitochondrial function leading to abnormal carnitine and fatty acid metabolism ●*Relieving factors:* Treatment of neurologic involvement - including increased intracranial pressure, coagulopathy ●*Clinical course:* Possibly fatal if not treated, but if treated early, outcome good ●*Co-morbidities:* Viral infection/varicella ●*Procedure results:* Liver pathology: yellow/white, fatty accumulation, altered mitochondrial morphology ●*Test findings:* Elevated liver enzymes: aspartate transaminase (AST), alanine transaminase (ALT), gamma glutamyl transpeptidase (GGT); lactate dehydrogenase (LDH), creatine kinase, serum ammonia, hypoglycemia, prolonged prothrombin time (PT)

Rh incompatibility ●*Onset:* Subacute ●*Male:female ratio:* M=F ●*Ethnicity:* More common in Caucasians ●*Character:* Fetal hydrops ●*Location:* Blood ●*Pattern:* Nonspecific ●*Precipitating factors:* Failure to prevent sensitization to Rh antibodies after previous pregnancy ●*Relieving factors:* Fetal blood transfusion ●*Clinical course:* Course variable: mild, to potential fetal death ●*Co-morbidities:* None relevant ●*Procedure results:* Amniocentesis: elevated bilirubin ●*Test findings:* Anti-D antibody on blood screening

Rhabdomyolysis ●*Onset:* Acute ●*Male:female ratio:* M=F ●*Ethnicity:* All ●*Character:* Muscle pain, dark urine ●*Location:* Diffuse or at site of focal (crush) injury ●*Pattern:* Nonspecific ●*Precipitating factors:* Alcohol abuse, muscle compression, seizures, metabolic derangements, drugs (cocaine, heroin, ecstasy, herbals, statins/gemfibrozil), metabolic myopathies ●*Relieving factors:* Avoid nephrotoxins; correct metabolic abnormalities; supportive care (intravenous fluids [IVF]); alkalinize urine to pH >6.5 to minimize pigment damage; monitor for hemodialysis requirement ●*Clinical course:* Self-limited once underlying etiology corrected ●*Co-morbidities:* Renal insufficiency; hyperkalemia, hyperuricemia, hyperphosphatemia, early hypocalcemia ●*Procedure results:* Urinalysis, serology ●*Test findings:* Positive blood but no red blood cells (RBCs) on urinalysis; positive myoglobin, elevated creatine kinase (CK) on serology

Rheumatic fever ●*Onset:* Acute, subacute ●*Male:female ratio:* M=F ●*Ethnicity:* All ●*Character:* Jones criteria and confirmation of streptococcal infection used for diagnosis (10% of cases lack the serologic evidence). For presumptive diagnosis, need two major, or one major and two minor criteria: Jones major criteria include carditis, erythema marginatum, subcutaneous nodules, Sydenham's chorea and arthritis. Jones minor criteria include fever, polyarthralgias, PR prolongation ●*Location:* Carditis is common and is manifested as sinus tachycardia, mitral regurgitation, S3, or friction rub. Migratory polyarthritis also occurs in 75% of cases. Sydenham's chorea, subcutaneous nodules and erythema marginatum occur less commonly (10% of cases) ●*Pattern:* Signs and symptoms of rheumatic fever usually occur within 2-3 weeks after infection; variability in clinical presentation is common ●*Precipitating factors:* The disorder is a systemic inflammatory process resulting from infection by hemolytic streptococcus. Exact mechanisms for its development in some infected patients is not fully understood ●*Relieving factors:* Bed rest; penicillin or other antibiotic therapy; salicylates for fever and joint pains ●*Clinical course:* Disease may last for months (immediate mortality <2%); persistent rheumatic fever may result in heart failure, valvular dysfunction (most commonly mitral and aortic) and pericarditis. Recurrent rheumatic fever has also been reported ●*Co-morbidities:* Initial attack due to streptoccocal infection, recurrent attacks may be more common in patients with carditis from prior event ●*Procedure results:* Examination findings are variable. Commonly, signs of heart failure, mitral regurgitation, S3-gallop and pericarditis. Raised, confluent macules +/- subcutaneous nodules may be present. Choreathetoid movements of the tongue, face, upper extremities may be present ●*Test findings:* Elevated sedimentation rate; positive titers for streptococcal infection in 90% of cases; PR prolongation; sinus tachycardia; abnormal valvular function/morphology on echocardiogram

Rheumatoid arthritis ●*Onset:* Subacute ●*Male:female ratio:* M(1):F(3) ●*Ethnicity:* All ●*Character:* Dull ache ●*Location:* Symmetric polyarthritis over small joints of hand or knees ●*Pattern:* Pain and stiffness are worse in the morning ●*Precipitating factors:* Concurrent infection, cessation of medications ●*Relieving factors:* Non-steroidal anti-inflammatory drugs (NSAIDs), corticosteroids, hydroxychloroquine, sulfasalazine, methotrexate, leflunomide, etanercept ●*Clinical course:* Progressive without treatment in most ●*Co-morbidities:* None relevant ●*Procedure results:* Synovial fluid analysis with white blood cells (WBC) >500 but less than 50,000 ●*Test findings:* Rheumatoid factor positive, elevated erythrocyte sedimemtation rate (ESR), anemia

Rheumatoid pneumoconiosis (Caplan's syndrome) ●*Onset:* Acute ●*Male:female ratio:* M<F ●*Ethnicity:* All ●*Character:* Shortness of breath and cough ●*Location:* Lungs ●*Pattern:* Nonspecific ●*Precipitating factors:* Coal dust ●*Relieving factors:* Inhaled corticosteroids ●*Clinical course:* If removed from coal dust, self-limited ●*Co-morbidities:* Rheumatoid arthritis ●*Procedure results:* Nodules on chest X-ray ●*Test findings:* No relevant tests

Rib fracture ●*Onset:* Acute ●*Male:female ratio:* M=F ●*Ethnicity:* All ●*Character:* Pain, tenderness over one or more ribs following trauma ●*Location:* Chest or abdomen ●*Pattern:* Nonspecific ●*Precipitating factors:* Most often follows direct trauma; pain may worsen with deep breathing or coughing ●*Relieving factors:* Analgesics (narcotics) for pain; may require intercostal nerve blocks if pain severe; strapping chest with elastic or adhesive tape may relieve pain in young, healthy patients ●*Clinical course:* Fractures usually heal by 4-6 weeks; complications - including pneumo- or hemothorax, liver or spleen injuries, pulmonary contusions or flail chest (multiple fractures) - may develop clinically several days after initial injury ●*Co-morbidities:* Elderly, alcohol abuse (frequent falls), osteoporosis ●*Procedure results:* Up to 50% of fractures may not be evident on initial radiographs ●*Test findings:* No relevant tests

Rickets in children ●*Onset:* Subacute ●*Male:female ratio:* M=F ●*Ethnicity:* All ●*Character:* Craniotabes (thin/soft skull), enlarged costochondral junction, thickened wrists/ankles, large anterior fontanelle/delayed closure, delayed teeth eruption, bowlegs ●*Location:* Skull, ribs, wrists, ankles, long bone shafts ●*Pattern:* Worsening symptoms without treatment ●*Precipitating factors:* Vitamin D deficiency: inadequate exposure to sunlight; inadequate intake of Vitamin D: breast fed ●*Relieving factors:* Dietary and supplementary sources of vitamin D ●*Clinical course:*

Variable ● *Co-morbidities:* Celiac disease, cystic fibrosis, anticonvulsant therapy: phenytoin/phe-nobarbital ● *Procedure results:* X-ray with epiphyseal enlargement at wrists/ankles; 'rachitic rosary' - beading of ribs at costochondral junction ● *Test findings:* Serum calcium - normal/low, decreased serum phosphorus, elevated serum alkaline phosphatase, decreased serum 25-hydroxycholecalciferol

Riedel's disease ● *Onset:* Insidious ● *Male:female ratio:* M=F ● *Ethnicity:* All ● *Character:* Anterior neck pressure, hard firm goiter fixed to surrounding structures, dysphasia, dyspnea ● *Location:* Anterior neck ● *Pattern:* Nonspecific ● *Precipitating factors:* None relevant ● *Relieving factors:* Thyroidectomy, thyroid hormone replacement, steroids may be helpful ● *Clinical course:* Progressive unless treated ● *Co-morbidities:* Retroperitoneal, retro-orbital and other organ fibrosis, rare hypoparathyroidism ● *Procedure results:* Thyroid biopsy reveals fibrosis ● *Test findings:* No relevant tests

Ringworm ● *Onset:* Gradual ● *Male:female ratio:* M=F (M>F for Tinea cruris) ● *Ethnicity:* All ❶ *Character:* Cutaneous fungal infection causing well-demarcated annular scaling skin patch(es) with an inflamed, pustular, or papular edge; scaling and erythema of scalp with areas of hair loss ❷ *Location:* Skin of scalp (capitis), neck and beard area (barbae), interdigital and under toes (pedis), groin or scrotum (cruris), other skin (corporis) ❸ *Pattern:* Annular scaly skin patches with an inflamed erythematous, pustular, or papular edge. Feet skin may be cracked, pruritus is common, hair loss is common with scalp involvement ● *Precipitating factors:* Animal exposure (corporis), military camps and male gender (cruris, pedis), children (capitis), moisture (cruris, pedis) ● *Relieving factors:* Topical antifungal therapy ● *Clinical course:* Incubation period unknown, slowly progressive, responding to topical antifungal therapy, rarely requires systemic therapy ● *Co-morbidities:* Cellulitis ● *Procedure results:* No relevant procedures ● *Test findings:* Chains of arthrospores visualized in potassium hydroxide preparations from skin scrapings; scalp infections with Microsporum spp. fluoresce green under Wood's light

Images of ❶ *Character,* ❷ *Location,* ❸ *Pattern on page 606*

Rocky Mountain spotted fever ● *Onset:* Acute ● *Male:female ratio:* M>F ● *Ethnicity:* US ● *Character:* Sudden onset of fever, headache, GI symptoms, followed by a generalized rash ● *Location:* Common: systemic (bloodstream), blood vessels, skin (generalized, may include palms and soles), muscles, gastrointestinal (GI) tract. Less common: brain and meninges, conjunctivae, lungs, myocardium, kidneys, liver, spleen, lymph nodes, other ● *Pattern:* Maculopapular-petechial rash begins days after fever, at wrists and ankles, spreads up, and involves palms and soles; 10% have no rash. Headache is severe ● *Precipitating factors:* Tick bite, occupational/recreational tick exposure in the US (south Atlantic, southeastern, south-central), Canada, Mexico, Central and South America ● *Relieving factors:* None relevant ● *Clinical course:* Incubation: 2-14 days, illness lasts 1-2 weeks, high case-fatality rate if untreated, responds within days to antibiotics therapy ● *Co-morbidities:* None relevant ● *Procedure results:* Specific serology ● *Test findings:* Common: thrombocytopenia, normal or mildly decreased white blood cells (WBC). Less common: anemia, mildly elevated transam-inases, coagulopathy (prolonged prothrombin time [PT] and partial thromboplastin time [PTT])

Rotator cuff syndrome ● *Onset:* Subacute ● *Male:female ratio:* M>F ● *Ethnicity:* All ● *Character:* Chronic dull ache with sharp pain during times of use ● *Location:* Around the shoulder joint ● *Pattern:* Worse with use ● *Precipitating factors:* Repetitive use of affected tendon ● *Relieving factors:* Ice, non-steroidal anti-inflammatory drugs (NSAIDs), rest, corti-sone injection, physical therapy ● *Clinical course:* Progressive unless patients change the motion of the affected joint area ● *Co-morbidities:* None relevant ● *Procedure results:* Normal plain radiographs and MRI ● *Test findings:* No relevant tests

Ringworm: Images *see text page 605*

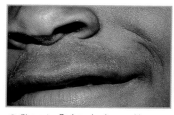

❶ *Character* Red, scaly plaque with an active border

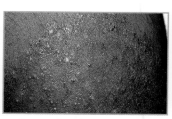

❶ *Character* Sometimes, tinea corporis may contain papules and pustules if the fungus invades the hair follicle

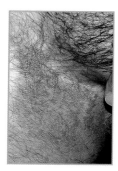

❷ *Location* Red, scaly plaque in the groin of a man

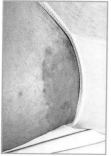

❸ *Pattern* Annular, red, scaly lesion in the groin of a woman

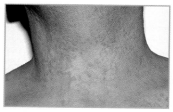

❸ *Pattern* Diffuse, coalescent, red, scaly and, at times, annular plaques

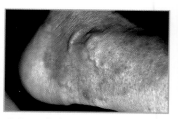

❸ *Pattern* Red, scaly plaque with an annular edge

Rotator cuff tear ●*Onset:* Acute or chronic ●*Male:female ratio:* M=F ●*Ethnicity:* All ●*Character:* Pain and tenderness in anterior aspect of the shoulder; weakness and pain with abduction or external rotation at shoulder ●*Location:* Shoulder joint ●*Pattern:* With chronic tears, pain initially worse at night, gradually worsens ●*Precipitating factors:* Fall on shoulder or outstretched arm, heavy lifting ●*Relieving factors:* Immobilizing with sling, analgesics; surgical repair in young active patients ●*Clinical course:* May develop chronic pain with or without surgical treatment ●*Co-morbidities:* Degenerative joint disease ●*Procedure results:* Radiographs usually show degenerative changes, may show superior displacement of humeral head; MRI is diagnostic ●*Test findings:* No relevant tests

Rotor syndrome ●*Onset:* Insidious ●*Male:female ratio:* M=F ●*Ethnicity:* All ●*Character:* Jaundice without other signs or symptoms ●*Location:* Nonspecific ●*Pattern:* Nonspecific ●*Precipitating factors:* Autosomal recessive inheritance; jaundice worse with physiologic stress ●*Relieving factors:* None relevant ●*Clinical course:* Normal health and life expectancy ●*Co-morbidities:* None relevant ●*Procedure results:* Liver biopsy - normal histology ●*Test findings:* Hyperbilirubinemia (<7mg/dL) 50% conjugated; characteristic urinary coproporphyrin pattern; normal transaminases and alkaline phosphatase

Rubella ●*Onset:* Acute ●*Male:female ratio:* M=F ●*Ethnicity:* All ●*Character:* Acute onset of fever, rash, posterior cervical lymphadenopathy ●*Location:* Skin. Posterior cervical, suboccipital, auricular lymphadenopathy. Symmetrical polyarthritis ●*Pattern:* Maculopapular rash begins on face and spreads down, petechiae on soft palate ●*Precipitating factors:* Lack of immunity (or immunization), sick contact, spring, school-aged children ●*Relieving factors:* None relevant ●*Clinical course:* Incubation 12-23 days, short or no prodrome, rash begins 14-17 days after exposure and lasts 3-5 days, lymphadenopathy lasts weeks, more severe in adults, self-limiting. Complications include encephalitis ●*Co-morbidities:* Congenital rubella syndrome, spontaneous abortion, stillbirth ●*Procedure results:* Specific serologic tests, isolation of Rubella in cell culture ●*Test findings:* Thrombocytopenia

Ruptured chordae tendinae ●*Onset:* Acute event that may cause acute or subacute symptoms ●*Male:female ratio:* M=F ●*Ethnicity:* All ●*Character:* May be asymptomatic or cause left-sided (mitral valve) or right-sided (tricuspid valve) heart failure symptoms ●*Location:* Nonspecific ●*Pattern:* Nonspecific ●*Precipitating factors:* May occur in setting of endocarditis, blunt chest trauma, or may be spontaneous with myxomatous valve apparatus ●*Relieving factors:* Heart failure symptoms are improved with diuretics ●*Clinical course:* Symptoms depend on degree of valvular regurgitation that ensues - may have no symptoms, symptoms that are stable with medical management, or progressive heart failure symptoms ●*Co-morbidities:* Myxomatous valves, connective tissue disorders, endocarditis, blunt trauma to chest ●*Procedure results:* Echo reveals flail chordal structure with dysfunctional valve leaflet (may partially prolapse) and valvular regurgitation ●*Test findings:* No relevant tests

Ruptured distal biceps tendon ●*Onset:* Acute ●*Male:female ratio:* M=F ●*Ethnicity:* All ●*Character:* Snapping sensation at time of rupture ●*Location:* Distal biceps ●*Pattern:* Weakness with elbow flexion ●*Precipitating factors:* Trauma ●*Relieving factors:* Surgery or physical therapy ●*Clinical course:* Complete resolution with surgical approach ●*Co-morbidities:* None relevant ●*Procedure results:* MRI shows ruptured tendon with swelling ●*Test findings:* No relevant tests

Ruptured mitral papillary muscle ●*Onset:* Acute ●*Male:female ratio:* M=F ●*Ethnicity:* All ●*Character:* Causes acute mitral regurgitation (MR) with sudden rise in left atrial pressure, resulting in acute pulmonary edema, dyspnea, and hypoxemia ●*Location:* Profound shortness of breath ●*Pattern:* Typically only a short MR murmur that may not even be audible ●*Precipitating factors:* Typically a complication of acute myocardial infarction (MI), but may be caused by severe chest trauma ●*Relieving factors:* Endotracheal intubation and intra-aortic balloon pump placement usually necessary to stabilize patient before surgery ●*Clinical course:* Acute presentation that requires surgical repair ●*Co-morbidities:* MI (typically of inferior wall), risk factors for coronary disease (hypertension, smoking, hypercholesterolemia, diabetes mellitus), rarely blunt trauma to the chest ●*Procedure results:* Elevated pulmonary capillary wedge pressure with tall v-waves on pulmonary artery catheter pressure tracing; flail mitral leaflet and MR on echocardiogram ●*Test findings:* No relevant tests

Ruptured/ hemorrhagic ovarian cyst ●*Onset:* Acute ●*Male:female ratio:* F ●*Ethnicity:* All ●*Character:* Stabbing pain or intermittent pain usually unilateral ●*Location:* Lateralized pelvic pain ●*Pattern:* Acute, sharp abdominal pain often preceded by several days of crampy pain; usually mid to late in the menstrual cycle ●*Precipitating factors:* Sometimes intercourse ●*Relieving factors:* Usually self-limiting though surgery occasionally necessary ●*Clinical course:* Acute onset of sharp pain with very gradual resolution over a few days to up to 2 weeks ●*Co-morbidities:* Need to rule out neoplasia ●*Procedure results:* Cyst or free fluid on ultrasound ●*Test findings:* Normal WBC; slight anemia; negative pregnancy test

Sacroiliitis ● *Onset:* Subacute ● *Male:female ratio:* M=F ● *Ethnicity:* All ● *Character:* Dull ache ● *Location:* Low back or upper buttock ● *Pattern:* Worse in the morning and improves with activity ● *Precipitating factors:* Inactivity ● *Relieving factors:* Physical therapy, NSAIDs, sulfasalazine ● *Clinical course:* Progressive ● *Co-morbidities:* Can be associated with ankylosing spondylitis, psoriasis, inflammatory bowel disease, or Reiter's syndrome; also part of juvenile chronic arthritis ● *Procedure results:* MRI shows inflammation of the sacroiliac joint ● *Test findings:* HLA-B27 positive

Salicylate poisoning ● *Onset:* Acute/chronic ● *Male:female ratio:* M=F ● *Ethnicity:* All ● *Character:* Mild/moderate: tinnitus, vertigo, vomiting, fever, abdominal pain. Severe: confusion, delirium, coma, seizures ● *Location:* Nonspecific ● *Pattern:* Nonspecific ● *Precipitating factors:* Chronic ingestions most common in the elderly ● *Relieving factors:* Gastric lavage if <60 min of ingestion; charcoal; urine alkalinization; hemodialysis for severe ingestions ● *Clinical course:* Full recovery with prompt treatment ● *Co-morbidities:* None relevant ● *Procedure results:* Chest X-ray may reveal pulmonary edema ● *Test findings:* Check aspirin level; arterial blood gas may reveal respiratory alkalosis with anion gap metabolic acidosis

Salivary gland calculi ● *Onset:* Chronic ● *Male:female ratio:* M>F (slightly) ● *Ethnicity:* All ● *Character:* Intermittent swelling of salivary glands with eating ● *Location:* Affected salivary gland ● *Pattern:* Worse with eating ● *Precipitating factors:* Eating ● *Relieving factors:* Warm compress, massage of gland ● *Clinical course:* Usually recurrent cyclical swelling of salivary gland ● *Co-morbidities:* Possibly renal stones ● *Procedure results:* Palpation of stone on examination; may see radiopaque stone on plain film (80% for submandibular gland) ● *Test findings:* No relevant tests

Salmonella infection ● *Onset:* Acute, chronic ● *Male:female ratio:* M=F ● *Ethnicity:* All ● *Character:* Diarrhea (sometimes bloody), fever, abdominal cramps ● *Location:* Small intestines, colon, Peyer's patches, bloodstream, atherosclerotic plaques, aortic, other arterial aneurysms ● *Pattern:* Diarrhea may be bloody, associated with abdominal cramps. Blood infection may localize in diseased arteries, aneurysms, prosthetic valves, joints ● *Precipitating factors:* Ingesting undercooked beef, poultry, eggs, foods contaminated with animal feces, unpasteurized milk; unwashed hands of infected food handler, handling reptiles; AIDS, sickle cell disease, lymphoma, steroid therapy, arteriosclerosis ● *Relieving factors:* Hydration ● *Clinical course:* Enteritis begins 12-72 hours after infection, lasts 4-7 days, resolves without therapy. Less common: long-term carriage (more with antibiotics). Immunocompromised, infants, or elderly persons may develop life-threatening blood or vascular infection and require antibiotics ● *Co-morbidities:* HIV, AIDS, sickle cell anemia, lymphoma, steroid or immunosuppressive therapy, arterial aneurysm, prosthetic valve, prosthetic joint, reactive arthritis (Reiter's syndrome) ● *Procedure results:* Isolation of Salmonella from stool, blood, other; RBC in stool ● *Test findings:* Elevated WBC, left shift, RBC in stool, Gram-negative rods in blood, Salmonella in blood or stool

Sarcoidosis ● *Onset:* Subacute ● *Male:female ratio:* M<F ● *Ethnicity:* Higher prevalence in Scandinavians, Irish females, African-American females, and Japanese ❶ *Character:* Dull ache ● *Location:* Joints, lungs ● *Pattern:* Worse in the morning ● *Precipitating factors:* None relevant ● *Relieving factors:* Corticosteroids ● *Clinical course:* Chronic with intermittent flares ● *Co-morbidities:* None relevant ● *Procedure results:* Noncaseating granulomas on synovial biopsy ● *Test findings:* Elevated ESR

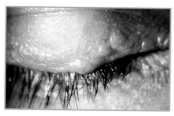

❶ *Character Biopsy of the nodules showed a typical sarcoidal granulomatous inflammatory reaction*

Scabies ● *Onset:* Subacute, insidious ● *Male:female ratio:* M=F ● *Ethnicity:* All ❶ *Character:* Severely pruritic skin papule and borrows, more pronounced in skin folds and between fingers ❷ *Location:* Hands (between fingers), folds of wrists, elbows or knees, penis, breasts, shoulder blades, other skin, generalized skin ● *Pattern:* Pruritus more intense at night and after showering, borrows may be seen, papules are small, secondary excoriations common ● *Precipitating factors:* Close person-to-person contact, sharing bedding or clothing, healthcare personnel, chronic care facilities ● *Relieving factors:* None relevant ● *Clinical course:* Asymptomatic for 4-6 weeks then rapid progression within days; more severe (Norwegian or crusted scabies) in immunocompromised persons; requires specific therapy ● *Co-morbidities:* AIDS, immunosuppression (more severe), secondary bacterial skin infections ● *Procedure results:* Demonstration of mite, ova, or feces in microscopic examination of skin scrapings ● *Test findings:* Washing clothes, bedding, towels in hot water and drying in a hot dryer, scabicide lotions, treating contacts

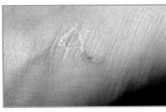

❶ *Character* Triangular scale with the thread of a burrow

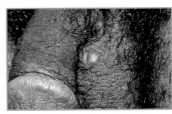

❷ *Location* Characteristic multiple inflammatory papules on the penis and scrotum

Scarlet fever ● *Onset:* Acute ● *Male:female ratio:* M=F ● *Ethnicity:* All ● *Character:* Pharyngitis and high fever followed by a generalized maculopapular rash ● *Location:* Systemic, skin (beginning in axillae, groin, and neck, spreading to torso and limbs, sparing palms and soles), pharynx, tonsils, tongue, cervical lymph nodes, other ● *Pattern:* Rash begins in axillae, groin, neck, generalizes, spares palms, soles, ace, papular (sandpaper), prominent in folds (Pastia lines). Tongue papillae enlarge (strawberry tongue), circumoral pallor, desquamation ● *Precipitating factors:* Surgical wound infection (rare), person-to-person contact, school-age children, crowding ● *Relieving factors:* None relevant ● *Clinical course:* Incubation: 1-7 days, rash appears 12-48 hours after fever, generalizes within 24 hours, lasts 6-9 days, fades with desquamation of tongue, palms, soles. Rapidly responds to antibiotic therapy ● *Co-morbidities:* Glomerulonephritis, rheumatic fever (rare) ● *Procedure results:* None relevant ● *Test findings:* Rapid streptococcal antigen detection from pharynx, group-A streptococci from throat, elevated antistreptolysin (ASLO)

Schatzki's ring ● *Onset:* Acute ● *Male:female ratio:* M=F ● *Ethnicity:* All ● *Character:* Intermittent difficulty swallowing solids; sensation of food sticking in mid-chest, resolves with drinking liquids or regurgitation. After episode, eating resumes normally ● *Location:* Midchest ● *Pattern:* Occurs more frequently with meat or bread; alcohol ingestion may induce episodes ● *Precipitating factors:* Alcohol use, eating large pieces of meat or bread, improper chewing ● *Relieving factors:* Drinking large amounts of liquid, regurgitation. Use of esophageal dilators to break the ring may eliminate symptoms ● *Clinical course:* Slowly progressive, with episodes increasing in frequency over time ● *Co-morbidities:* None relevant ● *Procedure results:* Barium swallow or upper endoscopy will demonstrate a ring of tissue near the gastroesophageal junction ● *Test findings:* No relevant tests

Schistosomiasis ●*Onset:* Acute, chronic ●*Male:female ratio:* M=F ●*Ethnicity:* Tropics, subtropics ●*Character:* Localized itch 24 hours after swimming; fever, chills, cough, hives, hepatosplenomegaly (Katayama fever: Schistosoma mansoni and S. japonicum),or dysuria/hematuria (S. haematobium) 4-8 weeks after swimming; end-organ vascular or tissue fibrosis 10-15 years after freshwater swimming ●*Location:* Skin (acute), portal vein, superior or inferior mesenteric veins, liver, spleen, urinary bladder, perivesical venules, ureters, colon, GI tract, right heart ventricle, pulmonary vessels (cor pulmonale), kidneys, brain, spinal cord, other ●*Pattern:* Fibrosis in affected organs: bloody stools (S. mansoni), portal hypertension/hematemesis (S. mansoni and S. japonicum), hematuria (S. haematobium), pulmonary hypertension (S. mansoni and S. japonicum), other ●*Precipitating factors:* Freshwater exposure/swimming in endemic areas ●*Relieving factors:* None relevant ●*Clinical course:* Swimmer's itch at 24 hours, Katayama fever or dysuria/hematuria at 4-8 weeks, fibrosis and end-organ disease at 10-15 years. May lead to cancer, renal, liver, heart failure ●*Co-morbidities:* Salmonellosis, chronic cystitis, bladder cancer, glomerulonephritis, portal hypertension, pulmonary hypertension, cor pulmonale, colonic polyps, esophageal varices ●*Procedure results:* Ova in stool, urine, or biopsy material (rectum, bladder, spine, brain, other), friable masses on cystoscopy/colonoscopy, periportal fibrosis on abdominal ultrasound, calcified eggs on CT of abdomen, pelvis, spine, brain, other, specific serology ●*Test findings:* Eosinophilia (swimmer's itch, Katayama fever), hematuria, RBC casts in urine, proteinuria, ova in stool/urine, periportal fibrosis

Schizophrenia ●*Onset:* Variable, although usually there is a prodromal period ●*Male:female ratio:* M=F ●*Ethnicity:* Cultural sensitivity critical (e.g. in some cultures, hallucinations with religious content may be considered normal part of religious experience) ●*Character:* Subtypes defined by most prominent symptoms: paranoid, catatonic, disorganized, undifferentiated, residual ●*Location:* Nonspecific ●*Pattern:* Episodic or continuous; residual, negative, or no symptoms between acute episodes ●*Precipitating factors:* Acute episodes may be precipitated by stressful events ●*Relieving factors:* Antipsychotic therapy ●*Clinical course:* Typically lifelong ●*Co-morbidities:* Substance abuse disorders (especially nicotine abuse and dependence); personality disorders may precede onset ●*Procedure results:* Brain imaging studies often reveal structural abnormalities; functional imaging techniques often reveal abnormal cerebral blood flow or glucose metabolism ●*Test findings:* Neuropsychological test findings often reveal broad range of dysfunction; motor abnormalities frequently noted upon examination

Scleritis ●*Onset:* Acute ●*Male:female ratio:* M<F (slightly) ●*Ethnicity:* All ❶ *Character:* Severe achy pain, blurred vision ●*Location:* Sclera. Purplish hue to ocular surface injection appreciated with ambient light ●*Pattern:* Usually unilateral ●*Precipitating factors:* None relevant ●*Relieving factors:* None relevant ●*Clinical course:* Progressive; requires treatment directed at the underlying cause ●*Co-morbidities:* Rheumatoid arthritis, Wegener's granulomatosis ●*Procedure results:* No relevant procedures ●*Test findings:* ANCA+ in Wegener's; RA+ in rheumatoid arthritis

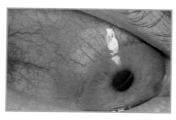

❶ *Character Deep, red, painful area of scleral inflammation*

Scleroderma ●*Onset:* Subacute ●*Male:female ratio:* M(1):F(4) ●*Ethnicity:* All ●*Character:* Dull ache, finger pain and thickening, telangiectasias ●*Location:* Hands, face ●*Pattern:* Worse in the morning; indurated stiff smooth skin ●*Precipitating factors:* Cold exacerbates Raynaud's symptoms ●*Relieving factors:* Corticosteroids, cyclophosphamide for lung disease, vasodilators for Raynaud's phenomenon, promotility agents for esophageal dysmotility ●*Clinical course:* Progressive ●*Co-morbidities:* Raynaud's phenomenon ●*Procedure results:* Skin biopsy: fibrosis with lymphocytic infiltrate in early skin lesions ●*Test findings:* Positive ANA, positive anti-Scl-70 antibody, positive anticentromere antibody

Scoliosis ●*Onset:* Insidious ●*Male:female ratio:* M(1):F(7) ●*Ethnicity:* All ●*Character:* Dull ache ●*Location:* Low back, ribs ●*Pattern:* Worse with use ●*Precipitating factors:* Lifting or twisting motions involving the low back ●*Relieving factors:* NSAIDs, acetaminophen, corticosteroids, heat or cold, gentle stretching exercises ●*Clinical course:* Progressive ●*Co-morbidities:* Muscular dystrophies, rheumatoid arthritis, infection of the spine, tumor of the spine ●*Procedure results:* Radiographs of the spine show curvature with degenerative changes ●*Test findings:* Normal laboratory studies

Seasonal affective disorder ●*Onset:* Typically develops as days shorten in fall, improving in spring ●*Male:female ratio:* M=F ●*Ethnicity:* All ●*Character:* Onset and remission of major depressive episodes at various times of the year ●*Location:* Nonspecific ●*Pattern:* Typically develops as the days shorten in fall improving in spring ●*Precipitating factors:* Day length ●*Relieving factors:* Bright visible-spectrum light ●*Clinical course:* Younger persons at risk for winter episodes ●*Co-morbidities:* Hypersomnia; carbohydrate craving; weight gain ●*Procedure results:* No relevant procedures ●*Test findings:* Abnormal thyroid function should be excluded

Sebaceous cyst ●*Onset:* Insidious ●*Male:female ratio:* M=F ●*Ethnicity:* All ●*Character:* Skin lesion ●*Location:* Trunk, neck, face, scalp ●*Pattern:* Light-colored, firm, circumscribed, movable nodule ●*Precipitating factors:* None relevant ●*Relieving factors:* Surgery, laser ●*Clinical course:* Persists or resolves with treatment ●*Co-morbidities:* None relevant ●*Procedure results:* No relevant procedures ●*Test findings:* Positive skin biopsy

Seborrheic dermatitis ●*Onset:* Subacute ●*Male:female ratio:* M=F ●*Ethnicity:* All ❶ *Character:* Flaky skin ❷ *Location:* Scalp, eyebrows, ears, paranasal, chest ❸ *Pattern:* Greasy yellow scale ●*Precipitating factors:* Stress ●*Relieving factors:* Mild topical corticosteroids ●*Clinical course:* Persistent ●*Co-morbidities:* Parkinson's disease ●*Procedure results:* No relevant procedures ●*Test findings:* No relevant tests

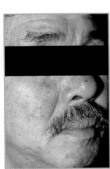

❶ *Character* Confluent erythema with scale of the nose, nasolabial folds, eyebrows and glabella

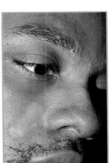

❶ *Character* Redness and scale symmetrically along the glabella, eyebrows, nose and cheeks

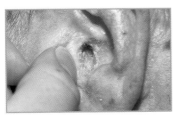

❷ *Location* Redness and scale in the ear is typical

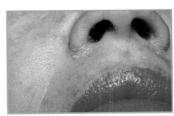

❸ *Pattern* Redness and scale along the base of the nose is typical

Seborrheic keratosis ●*Onset:* Insidious ●*Male:female ratio:* M=F ●*Ethnicity:* All ●*Character:* Skin lesion ●*Location:* Torso, face, scalp ●*Pattern:* Stuck on light brown/tan verrucous plaque ●*Precipitating factors:* None relevant ●*Relieving factors:* Cryosurgery or electrosurgery ●*Clinical course:* Persists or resolves with treatment ●*Co-morbidities:* None relevant ●*Procedure results:* No relevant procedures ●*Test findings:* Positive skin biopsy

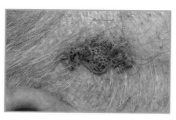

❸ *Pattern A stuck on wart plaque with horn cysts is shown*

Secondary amenorrhea (hypothalmic dysfunction) ●*Onset:* Abrupt or gradual cessation of menses ●*Male:female ratio:* F ●*Ethnicity:* All ●*Character:* Cessation of menses after menarche ●*Location:* Nonspecific ●*Pattern:* Oligomenorrhea, amenorrhea ●*Precipitating factors:* Decreased caloric intake, vigorous exercise, eating disorders, stress ●*Relieving factors:* Oral contraceptives, HRT, vitamin D, calcium supplementation ●*Clinical course:* Leads to conditions associated with estrogen deficiency if untreated, e.g. development of osteoporosis ●*Co-morbidities:* Sarcoidosis, hypothalmic cysts, lymphoma, histiocytosis X, eating disorders ●*Procedure results:* No withdrawal bleeding after progestin indicative of severe estrogen deficiency ●*Test findings:* Negative HCG, normal FSH and prolactin

Secondary amenorrhea (premature ovarian failure) ●*Onset:* Abrupt or gradual cessation of menses ●*Male:female ratio:* F ●*Ethnicity:* All ●*Character:* Cessation of menses prior to expected age menopause. vasomotor symptoms, vaginal dryness ●*Location:* Nonspecific ●*Pattern:* Oligomenorrhea, amenorrhea ●*Precipitating factors:* Autoimmune diseases, pelvic radiation, chemotherapy ●*Relieving factors:* HRT, oral contraceptives ●*Clinical course:* Irreversible, symptomatically treated ●*Co-morbidities:* Associated with diabetes mellitus, hypothyroidism, hypoadrenal. Infertility ●*Procedure results:* Progestin withdrawal bleeding may occur in early stages ●*Test findings:* Elevated FSH, normal TSH and prolactin. Negative HCG

Secretory villous adenoma ●*Onset:* Subacute ●*Male:female ratio:* M>F ●*Ethnicity:* All ●*Character:* Copious watery diarrhea with hypokalemia, hypochloremia, metabolic acidosis ●*Location:* Villous adenoma is usually in rectum or rectosigmoid ●*Pattern:* Diarrhea is progressive, with no daily pattern ●*Precipitating factors:* None relevant ●*Relieving factors:* Indomethacin may decrease diarrheal output; resection of the adenoma is definitive therapy ●*Clinical course:* Not self-limited ●*Co-morbidities:* None - villous adenomas do, however, have a higher rate of transformation to colon cancer ●*Procedure results:* Colonoscopy reveals the adenoma ●*Test findings:* Low potassium and chloride, metabolic acidosis

Senile purpura ●*Onset:* Gradual ●*Male:female ratio:* M=F ●*Ethnicity:* All ●*Character:* Skin lesions ●*Location:* Dorsal hands and forearms ●*Pattern:* Purpura, bullae, fragile skin ●*Precipitating factors:* Chronic sun exposure, minor trauma ●*Relieving factors:* Sunblock, moisturizers ●*Clinical course:* Usually worsens over time ●*Co-morbidities:* Lesions may get infected ●*Procedure results:* No relevant procedures ●*Test findings:* No relevant tests

Sepsis ●*Onset:* Acute ●*Male:female ratio:* M=F ●*Ethnicity:* All ●*Character:* Acute onset of fever or hypothermia, leukocytosis or leukopenia, tachycardia, tachypnea, later multiple-organ involvement or collapse ●*Location:* Systemic ●*Pattern:* Rapidly progressive. Disseminated intravascular coagulation (DIC) in severe cases ●*Precipitating factors:* Bacterial seeding from vasular catheters, indwelling catheters, invasive procedures, burns, perforated viscus, localized bacterial infection ●*Relieving factors:* Antibiotics, fluids, supportive therapy ●*Clinical course:* Acute onset, may rapidly lead to shock, multiple organ dysfunction, death. High mortality ●*Co-morbidities:* Neutropenia, cancer, diabetes, cirrhosis, immunosuppression, prosthetic devices ●*Procedure results:* Isolation of microbes from blood (or local site of infection) ●*Test findings:* Leukocytosis (less commonly leukopenia), left shift, respiratory alkalosis (early), lactic (metabolic) acidosis, elevated C-reactive protein, hypoalbuminemia, thrombocytopenia, hyperbilirubinemia, toxic granulation and Dohle bodies in WBC, disseminated intravascular coagulation (high fibrin[ogen] split products, low fibrinogen, prolonged prothrombin time and partial thromboplastin time), azotemia, elevated transaminases (shock)

Septal ulceration ●*Onset:* Subacute ●*Male:female ratio:* M=F ●*Ethnicity:* All ●*Character:* Nasal bleeding and pain ●*Location:* Anterior nasal cavity ●*Pattern:* Persistent pain and sensitivity within the nose, often with intermittent epistaxis ●*Precipitating factors:* Digital manipulation of the nose, use of topical nasal steroid sprays ●*Relieving factors:* Petroleum jelly ●*Clinical course:* May be self-limited with avoidance of provocative features ●*Co-morbidities:* Rarely: Wegener's granulomatosis, autoimmune disease ●*Procedure results:* Nasal ulcer on anterior rhinoscopy or nasal endoscopy ●*Test findings:* No relevant tests

Septic arthritis ●*Onset:* Acute ●*Male:female ratio:* M(1):F(4) (Neisseria infection); M(2):F(1) (other) ●*Ethnicity:* All ●*Character:* Pain, swelling and heat, and stiffness and loss of movement of affected joint(s) ●*Location:* Any joint can be involved; usually knee, hip, shoulder, wrist, ankle ●*Pattern:* Fever and pain around the affected joint areas are constant ●*Precipitating factors:* None relevant ●*Relieving factors:* Antibiotics with or without lavage or debridement of the affected joint area ●*Clinical course:* Progressive unless recognized and treated; if untreated, will lead to joint destruction, osteomyelitis, possible sepsis ●*Co-morbidities:* Joint prosthesis, diabetes mellitus, immunosuppression, intravenous drug use ●*Procedure results:* Synovial fluid analysis reveals WBC >50,000/mm^3 and a positive Gram stain ●*Test findings:* Elevated ESR

Septic bursitis ●*Onset:* Acute ●*Male:female ratio:* M=F ●*Ethnicity:* All ●*Character:* Pain on extremes of range of motion of affected joint - bursal region ●*Location:* Olecranon and prepatellar bursae most frequently become septic ●*Pattern:* Worse with motion of the joint area ●*Precipitating factors:* Sepsis is usually due to direct innoculation ●*Relieving factors:* Antibiotics, needle aspiration, and joint splinting ●*Clinical course:* After antibiotics are started, pain usually dissipates after 72 hours ●*Co-morbidities:* Immunosuppression, chronic trauma to bursal region, diabetes, alcohol abuse ●*Procedure results:* Bursal aspiration shows positive Gram stain and culture, extra-articular effusion by radiograph ●*Test findings:* No relevant tests

Serum sickness ●*Onset:* Subacute or less commonly acute ●*Male:female ratio:* M=F ●*Ethnicity:* All ●*Character:* Arthralgias, rash (morbilliform sometimes with urticaria), fever, lymphadenopathy, cerebritis, glomerulonephritis ●*Location:* Nonspecific ●*Pattern:* Occurs approximately 10 days after the precipitant ●*Precipitating factors:* Drugs, particularly antibiotics (penicillin is the most common); antiserums (e.g. horse antitetanus) ●*Relieving factors:* Antihistamines, pain relievers (aspirin), rarely corticosteroids ●*Clinical course:* Self-limited unless continued exposure to the antigen ●*Co-morbidities:* None relevant ●*Procedure results:* Skin biopsy - acute, necrotizing vasculitis; renal biopsy - hypercellular glomeruli with neutrophillic and monocytic infiltrate; immunofluorescence or electron microscopy - immunoglobulin deposits ●*Test findings:* No relevant tests

Sex cord/stromal ovarian cancer ●*Onset:* Insidious ●*Male:female ratio:* F ●*Ethnicity:* Nonspecific ●*Character:* Endocrinologic abnormalities - feminizing with granulosa cell tumors; masculinizing with Sertoli-Leydig cell tumors ●*Location:* Nonspecific ●*Pattern:* Estrogen-producing tumors, often present with vaginal bleeding or isosexual precocious puberty; androgen-producing tumors, virilization ●*Precipitating factors:* None relevant ●*Relieving factors:* None relevant ●*Clinical course:* Progression to invasion and distant metastases ●*Co-morbidities:* Granulosa cell tumors - endometrial hyperplasia, carcinoma; isosexual precocious puberty ●*Procedure results:* Granulosa cell tumors - Call-Exner bodies on histology ●*Test findings:* Leydig cell tumors - elevated testosterone:androstenedione ratio

Sexual abuse ●*Onset:* Acute ●*Male:female ratio:* M<F ●*Ethnicity:* All ●*Character:* Activity with child before age of legal consent that is for sexual gratification of adult or older child; symptoms can be: vaginal/rectal/penile pain/discharge/bleeding, chronic dysuria, enuresis, constipation, encopresis ●*Location:* Oral-genital, genital-genital, genital-rectal, hand-genital, hand-rectal, hand-breast; sexual anatomy/pornography exposure ●*Pattern:* Touching/intercourse/penetration into orifice; victim may show abnormal behaviors - sexualized activity/seductive behavior/age-inappropriate sexual knowledge/behavior/sleep disorders/low-self esteem/depression ●*Precipitating factors:* Most common form of incest - abuse of daughter by fathers/stepfathers and/or brother-sister incest; vulnerable/available victim - leading to innocent physical contact and then seduction/abuse ●*Relieving factors:* Victim reports behavior ●*Clinical course:* Interrupted if reported/diagnosed ●*Co-morbidities:* Sleep disorders, depression ●*Procedure results:* Abnormal physical examination consistent with sexual abuse ●*Test findings:* Laboratory findings of pregnancy, sperm, semen, non-pregnancy/delivery-related syphilis, gonorrhea, chlamydia, HSV II, HIV may be diagnostic

Sexual assault ●*Onset:* Acute ●*Male:female ratio:* M<F ●*Ethnicity:* All ●*Character:* Multiple traumatic injuries may occur; penetration and/or injury to sexual organs, anus, and mouth most common ●*Location:* Nonspecific ●*Pattern:* Nonspecific ●*Precipitating factors:* None relevant ●*Relieving factors:* Victims should be evaluated as soon as possible by a professional experienced in rape counseling; traumatic injuries need to be noted and treated; prophylactic treatment for sexually transmitted diseases and pregnancy prevention should be offered ●*Clinical course:* Variable ●*Co-morbidities:* None relevant ●*Procedure results:* Meticulous documentation of physical examination and evidence collection required ●*Test findings:* Culture for sexually transmitted diseases, pregnancy test, consider HIV and hepatitis testing

Sexual dysfunction in men ●*Onset:* Subacute. Acute in cases of major trauma leading to sexual dysfunction ●*Male:female ratio:* M ●*Ethnicity:* All ●*Character:* Dissatisfaction with the size, rigidity or duration of erection, and/or decreased libido ●*Location:* Genitalia/perineal area ●*Pattern:* Nonspecific ●*Precipitating factors:* Psychological instability (depression, performance anxiety); medications (beta-blockers, thiazides, other); illegal drugs, alcohol, nicotine ●*Relieving factors:* Sex therapy, oral medication (sildenafil), injection therapy (alprostadil), vacuum erectile devices, androgen replacement, penile prosthesis, revascularization surgery ●*Clinical course:* Progressive ●*Co-morbidities:* Hypertension, diabetes, spinal cord injury, depression, psychosis, hypothyrodism, coronary artery disease, peripheral vascular disease, Peyronie's disease, hypogonadism, renal failure ●*Procedure results:* Nocturnal penile tumescence: positive with psychogenic impotence. High satisfaction rate with penile prosthesis implantation ●*Test findings:* Low testosterone serum level: need to distinguish between primary and secondary hypogonadism

Sexual dysfunction in women ●*Onset:* Gradual, insidious ●*Male:female ratio:* F ●*Ethnicity:* All ●*Character:* Excitement phase dysfunction is inability to respond to sexual stimulation. Orgasmic phase dysfunction is inability to achieve orgasm despite normal sexual desire ●*Location:* Dyspareunia, vaginismus may suggest underlying pelvic pathology ●*Pattern:* Nonspecific ●*Precipitating factors:* Drug-induced reduction in sexual desire caused by multiple antihypertensives and SSRIs, androgen deficiency in postmenopausal women ●*Relieving factors:* Orgasmic dysfunction may improve with maturity and increased sexual experience. Behavioral counseling for excitement phase dysfunction ●*Clinical course:* Fails to improve or gradually worsens ●*Co-morbidities:* Medical causes: diabetes, hypothyroidism, multiple sclerosis, hyperprolactinemia, hypopituitarism; psychological disorders: anxiety, depression, somatization disorder ●*Procedure results:* Pelvic examination to rule-out underlying pelvic pathology ●*Test findings:* Appropriate laboratory testing to rule-out underlying medical cause, e.g. glucose, TSH, prolactin level

Shellfish poisoning ●*Onset:* Acute ●*Male:female ratio:* M=F ●*Ethnicity:* All ●*Character:* Symptoms occur within 2 hours of ingesting contaminated shellfish: paresthesias, ataxia, nausea, vomiting, diarrhea. May develop muscle weakness requiring mechanical ventilation

● *Location:* Nonspecific ● *Pattern:* Nonspecific ● *Precipitating factors:* Ingestion of contaminated mollusks containing neurotoxins. Most common in temperate waters between May and October. Associated with 'red tide'. Toxin is heat stable and not inactivated by cooking ● *Relieving factors:* Treatment is supportive ● *Clinical course:* Symptoms usually resolve over several days ● *Co-morbidities:* None relevant ● *Procedure results:* No relevant procedures ● *Test findings:* No relevant tests

Shigellosis ● *Onset:* Acute ● *Male:female ratio:* M=F ● *Ethnicity:* All ● *Character:* Abrupt onset of abdominal pain, diarrhea, often bloody, fever (dysentery) ● *Location:* Common: colon, systemic (fever, toxin effect). Rare: joints (reactive arthritis), brain (convulsions), kidneys and vessels (hemolytic-uremic syndrome) ● *Pattern:* Frequent small volume stools containing blood and pus, associated with abdominal cramps, and tenesmus. Fever in children may lead to seizures ● *Precipitating factors:* Person-to-person spread by the fecal-oral route, child care centers, chronic care facilities, ingestion of contaminated food/water in endemic areas ● *Relieving factors:* Hydration, specific antibiotics ● *Clinical course:* Incubation: 24-48 hours. Diarrhea in 50%, dysentery in approximately 25%, lasting 5-7 days without therapy, less with antibiotic therapy, rarely fatal ● *Co-morbidities:* Reiter's syndrome ● *Procedure results:* WBC and RBC in stool, isolation of Shigella from stool (rarely from blood), hemorrhagic mucosa and mucopurulent discharge on colonoscopy ● *Test findings:* Leukocytosis, anemia (less common), azotemia (rare), hyperchloremic acidosis (rare), severe anemia, azotemia

Shoulder injury ● *Onset:* Acute, subacute, chronic ● *Male:female ratio:* M=F ● *Ethnicity:* All ● *Character:* Pain in shoulder joint following an injury. Diminished range of motion. Anterior deformity implies dislocation. Swelling, tenderness over acromioclavicular joint implies joint separation. Fractures more common in elderly ● *Location:* Shoulder ● *Pattern:* Nonspecific ● *Precipitating factors:* Direct falls on shoulder or fall on outstretched arm ● *Relieving factors:* Use of sling or shoulder immobilizer. Dislocations require reduction ● *Clinical course:* Permanent decreased range of movement is common after injury ● *Co-morbidities:* None relevant ● *Procedure results:* Radiographs usually required to rule out fractures. Most common: clavicle and proximal humerus ● *Test findings:* No relevant tests

Sialadenitis ● *Onset:* Acute ● *Male:female ratio:* M=F ● *Ethnicity:* All ● *Character:* Persistent pain over affected gland with swelling ● *Location:* Affected salivary gland ● *Pattern:* May be worse with eating ● *Precipitating factors:* Dehydration; formation of salivary calculus ● *Relieving factors:* Warm compress; massage of gland ● *Clinical course:* May be self-limited ● *Co-morbidities:* Salivary gland calculus; debilitated state; history of radiation therapy ● *Procedure results:* Express material from duct of affected salivary gland ● *Test findings:* Culture of ductal drainage for bacteria

Sickle cell anemia ● *Onset:* Acute ● *Male:female ratio:* M=F ● *Ethnicity:* African (tropical) and African-American populations ● *Character:* Painful symmetric swelling of hands/feet; pain in chest, abdomen, back; hemolytic anemia, vaso-occlusive episodes ● *Location:* Bone pain; hemolytic anemia ● *Pattern:* Painful crises with infection, stress, dehydration ● *Precipitating factors:* Valine substitution for glutamic acid at the sixth position of betapolypeptide chain ● *Relieving factors:* Acetaminophen, codeine, NSAIDs, IV fluid ● *Clinical course:* Lifelong but bone marrow transplant may be curative ● *Co-morbidities:* Splenic enlargement, splenic sequestration, stroke, pulmonary/splenic infarct, kidney damage, priapism, susceptibility to meningitis/sepsis, cardiomegaly, gallstones ● *Procedure results:* No relevant procedures ● *Test findings:* Hemoglobin electrophoresis: Hb SS, low hemoglobin, smear with target cells, sickled cells, nucleated RBCs, Howell-Jolly bodies, positive sickle preparation

Sickle cell trait ●*Onset:* Insidious ●*Male:female ratio:* M=F ●*Ethnicity:* African-American, African, Middle Eastern ●*Character:* Usually asymptomatic; inability to concentrate urine; hematuria; under extreme conditions can have painful episodes and hemolytic anemia ●*Location:* Pain in back and long bones ●*Pattern:* Nonspecific ●*Precipitating factors:* Very low blood oxygen concentration (vigorous exertion at high altitude, unpressurized aircraft) ●*Relieving factors:* Increased ambient oxygen, hydration ●*Clinical course:* Patients have a normal life expectancy and typically never experience symptoms ●*Comorbidities:* None relevant ●*Procedure results:* No relevant procedures ●*Test findings:* Positive screening test for sickle cell hemoglobin, hemoglobin electrophoresis - 40% hemoglobin S, high-normal serum sodium

Sideroblastic anemia ●*Onset:* Insidious ●*Male:female ratio:* M=F ●*Ethnicity:* All ●*Character:* Fatigue, dyspnea on exertion, headache ●*Location:* Nonspecific ●*Pattern:* Nonspecific ●*Precipitating factors:* Alcohol abuse, medications (antituberculosis, chloramphenicol), lead, myelodysplasia ●*Relieving factors:* Remove precipitant (lead exposure, medication, alcohol); treat underlying myelodysplasia ●*Clinical course:* Resolves if precipitant can be removed ●*Co-morbidities:* None relevant ●*Procedure results:* Bone marrow biopsy - ringed sideroblasts, erythroid hyperplasia, increased iron stores ●*Test findings:* Moderate anemia, variable mean corpuscular volume, dimorphic RBC population, increased iron and total iron-binding capacity (TIBC)

Sinoatrial arrest or block ●*Onset:* Insidious, subacute ●*Male:female ratio:* M=F ●*Ethnicity:* All ●*Character:* If hemodynamically significant, causes syncope or presyncope ●*Location:* Nonspecific ●*Pattern:* Nonspecific ●*Precipitating factors:* Can be spontaneous, related to medications that inhibit the sinoatrial node (e.g. beta-blockers), or precipitated by situations that increase vagal tone ●*Relieving factors:* Atropine, pacemaker ●*Clinical course:* Sinus node dysfunction is typically insidiously progressive ●*Co-morbidities:* Other conduction system abnormalities, such as AV node disease or bundle branch block; atrial tachyarrhythmias also associated in 'tachy-brady' syndrome ●*Procedure results:* EKG reveals absence of P-waves, with resultant asystole or junctional rhythm ●*Test findings:* No relevant tests

Sinus bradycardia ●*Onset:* Insidious, subacute ●*Male:female ratio:* M=F ●*Ethnicity:* All ●*Character:* Typically asymptomatic, but may cause lightheadedness or presyncope ●*Location:* Nonspecific ●*Pattern:* Nonspecific ●*Precipitating factors:* May be physiologic from cardiovascular training (e.g. in athletes), may be precipitated by medications that slow sinoatrial node (e.g. beta blockers, amiodarone), may result from increased vagal tone (e.g. fright, heat, urination, coughing, gagging) ●*Relieving factors:* Lying down may relieve lightheadedness from low blood pressure; atropine ●*Clinical course:* Depends on etiology: self-limited (e.g. increased vagal tone lasting a few minutes); resolves with dose reduction or discontinuation of offending medication; a more chronic normal variant (e.g. athlete) ●*Co-morbidities:* History of situational syncope (sight of blood, fright, coughing, urination), cardiac conditions (such as coronary artery disease, valvular disease, tachyarrhythmias) that are treated with medications that slow sinoatrial activity (e.g. beta blockers) ●*Procedure results:* EKG reveals bradycardia with P-wave before each QRS complex; 1:1 ratio of P-waves to QRS complexes ●*Test findings:* No relevant tests

Sinus tachycardia ●*Onset:* Subacute ●*Male:female ratio:* M=F ●*Ethnicity:* All ●*Character:* Not a primary cardiac condition, may be associated with a host of medical conditions with various symptoms ●*Location:* Nonspecific ●*Pattern:* Worsens in association with exacerbation of the primary medical process that has precipitated the tachycardic response ●*Precipitating factors:* Any physiologic or medical condition that warrants or stimulates a faster heart rate ●*Relieving factors:* Treatment of the underlying condition ●*Clinical course:* Sinus tachycardia, being a reactive response, lasts as long as the underlying condition that precipitated it ●*Co-morbidities:* Any medical condition that stimulates sinoatrial node directly or necessitates faster heart rate to increase or maintain cardiac output

● *Procedure results:* EKG reveals preserved P-wave/QRS relationship (with 1:1 ratio); heart rate >100bpm ● *Test findings:* No relevant tests

Sjögren's syndrome ● *Onset:* Insidious ● *Male:female ratio:* M<F ● *Ethnicity:* All ● *Character:* Dry mouth, dry eyes ● *Location:* Mouth, eyes ● *Pattern:* Nonspecific ● *Precipitating factors:* Most noticeable while eating or outside ● *Relieving factors:* Salivary substitutes, pilocarpine, hydroxychloroquine, corticosteroids ● *Clinical course:* Progressive ● *Co-morbidities:* Rheumatoid arthritis, systemic lupus erythematosus ● *Procedure results:* Positive Shirmer's tear test, salivary gland biopsy with lymphocytic infiltrates ● *Test findings:* Elevated ESR, positive antinuclear antibody panel, positive rheumatoid factor

Skin abscess ● *Onset:* Acute ● *Male:female ratio:* M=F ● *Ethnicity:* All ● *Character:* Usually localized infection of skin and sometimes underlying soft tissue, absent systemic findings early on; characterized by redness, swelling that is fluctuant, pain and nonresponse to oral antibiotics ● *Location:* Can occur anywhere; especially prone areas include hairbearing areas, or sites of repetitive trauma/maceration such as skin folds ● *Pattern:* Begins as an erythematous papule which progresses to become a nodule; if untreated, lesion becomes a larger nodule that contains a central pus-filled cavity ● *Precipitating factors:* Trauma, skin folds, intravenous drug use, foreign body implantation, site of intravenous catheter ● *Relieving factors:* Oral antibiotics and incision and drainage of the abscess ● *Clinical course:* If treated early, no systemic manifestations, such as fever, occur ● *Co-morbidities:* Immunesuppression (diabetes mellitus, HIV/AIDS, organ transplant, carcinoma) ● *Procedure results:* Incision and drainage usually yields pus; biopsy would reveal a predominantly neutrophilic infiltrate with necrosis and debris ● *Test findings:* Culture from the abscess often shows Staphylococcus aureus although Gram-negative bacteria have been shown to cause abscesses in patients on longterm antibiotics

Sleep walking ● *Onset:* Acute ● *Male:female ratio:* M=F ● *Ethnicity:* All ● *Character:* Body movement - possibly open eyes - clumsy walking movements, event not remembered ● *Location:* Stage IV NREM sleep ● *Pattern:* Lasts 5-30 minutes, possibly 1-4 episodes weekly ● *Precipitating factors:* Immature CNS system, fatigue, stress, family history of sleep disturbances ● *Relieving factors:* Diminishing frequency with age, diazepam for severe cases ● *Clinical course:* Diminishing frequency with age ● *Co-morbidities:* Nocturnal enuresis, sleep talking ● *Procedure results:* No relevant procedure ● *Test findings:* Abnormal sleep study, normal EEG to rule out temporal lobe epilepsy

Sleeping sickness (African trypanosomiasis) ● *Onset:* Acute febrile illness; insidious, progressive CNS disease ● *Male:female ratio:* M=F ● *Ethnicity:* Africans ● *Character:* Skin chancre followed by fever, lymphadenopathy, pruritus. Weeks (east Africa) to year (west Africa) later: progressive headaches, indifference, somnolence, coma ● *Location:* Circinate skin rash, pruritus, fever, lymph nodes (posterior cervical triangle, other), CNS ● *Pattern:* Painful chancre at bite site. Bouts of high fever separated by afebrile episodes. Lymphadenopathy is tender. Progressive indifference and daytime somnolence over weeks to months ● *Precipitating factors:* Travel to/residence in endemic areas (Trypanosoma gambiense: west and central Africa; T. rhodesiense: east and southeast Africa) and tsetse fly bite (painful) ● *Relieving factors:* None relevant ● *Clinical course:* T. rhodesiense (east African) is more acute than T. gambiense (west African). Skin chancre within days, febrile illness days-weeks (self-limiting), CNS illness leads to death within week-months in east, months to years in west. Treatment is limited and potentially toxic ● *Co-morbidities:* None relevant ● *Procedure results:* Visualization of trypanosomes in wet preparation or Giemsa-stained blood; aspirate from chancre, lymph node, bone marrow, CSF ● *Test findings:* Leukocytosis, thrombocytopenia, anemia, hypergammaglobulinemia, rheumatoid factor, anti-DNA antibodies, positive heterophile

Slipped femoral epiphysis ●*Onset:* Acute, chronic ●*Male:female ratio:* M(2-3):F(1) ●*Ethnicity:* African descent slightly higher than Caucasian ●*Character:* Dull ache ●*Location:* Hip, thigh, knee ●*Pattern:* Worse with use ●*Precipitating factors:* None relevant ●*Relieving factors:* Surgical pinning ●*Clinical course:* Progressive pain, disability ●*Co-morbidities:* None relevant ●*Procedure results:* Plain radiograph with pathognomonic finding ●*Test findings:* No relevant tests

Smoke inhalation injury ●*Onset:* Acute ●*Male:female ratio:* M=F ●*Ethnicity:* All ●*Character:* Shortness of breath, cough, airway edema ●*Location:* Airways, lungs ●*Pattern:* Edema develops 12-24 hours after injury ●*Precipitating factors:* Exposure to smoke ●*Relieving factors:* Removal from environment ●*Clinical course:* Airway edema, respiratory failure, hypoxemia ●*Co-morbidities:* Burns, hypovolemia, carbon monoxide poisoning, cyanide poisoning ●*Procedure results:* Bronchoscopy shows location and degree of airway injury ●*Test findings:* Chest X-ray shows signs of pulmonary edema; arterial blood gases shows oxygen, carbon dioxide, and carbon monoxide levels

Snake and reptile bites ●*Onset:* Acute ●*Male:female ratio:* M=F ●*Ethnicity:* All ●*Character:* Range from local pain and swelling at bite to marked swelling, shock, coagulation abnormalities. Effects vary depending on species ●*Location:* Most common on extremities ●*Pattern:* Nonspecific ●*Precipitating factors:* None relevant ●*Relieving factors:* Tourniquets proximal to bite may be helpful. Keep victim calm. Antivenin is main therapy for poisonous snakebite. Treat shock and observe for compartment syndrome ●*Clinical course:* Most victims recover well if treated early and antivenin is used ●*Co-morbidities:* None relevant ●*Procedure results:* No relevant procedures ●*Test findings:* Abnormal coagulation studies and platelet counts

Soft tissue sarcoma ●*Onset:* Subacute to insidious ●*Male:female ratio:* M=F ●*Ethnicity:* All ●*Character:* Soft tissue mass, possibly with pain and swelling; weight loss and fatigue if metastatic disease ●*Location:* Depends on site of primary tumor; most common location is the lower extremity ●*Pattern:* Nonspecific ●*Precipitating factors:* Many possible predisposing factors though not conclusive such as prior radiation therapy, trauma, toxic exposure ●*Relieving factors:* Aggressive surgical resection, chemotherapy, high-dose radiation therapy ●*Clinical course:* Over 50% eventually die of this disease despite therapy, recurrences are common; poor prognostic factors include: older age, high-grade tumor, large size and positive lymph nodes ●*Co-morbidities:* None relevant ●*Procedure results:* Biopsy revealing sarcoma of tissue of origin (e.g. rhabdomyosarcoma, fibrosarcoma) ●*Test findings:* MRI or CT scan revealing a soft tissue mass

Solar retinopathy ●*Onset:* Acute ●*Male:female ratio:* M=F ●*Ethnicity:* All ●*Character:* Blurred vision; central scotoma; erythropsia ●*Location:* Both eyes ●*Pattern:* Yellow-white lesion in the macular region ●*Precipitating factors:* Excess photic exposure such as solar gazing, viewing an eclipse, or observing through a telescope ●*Relieving factors:* None relevant ●*Clinical course:* Immediate reduction in vision followed by a slow recovery over 6 months ●*Co-morbidities:* None relevant ●*Procedure results:* Yellow-white lesion in the center of the macula ●*Test findings:* No relevant tests

Somatization disorder ●*Onset:* Insidious; multiple somatic symptoms developing over several years; begins before age 30 ●*Male:female ratio:* M=F ●*Ethnicity:* Cultural differences influence the symptoms described ●*Character:* Symptoms not explained by organic disease or are out of proportion to the disease present ●*Location:* Nonspecific ●*Pattern:* Involvement of multiple organ systems ●*Precipitating factors:* Psychosocial stress ●*Relieving factors:* Explanation and reassurance may benefit the patient ●*Clinical course:* Chronic, but fluctuating; rarely remits completely; ●*Co-morbidities:* Major depressive disorder; panic disorder; substance-related disorder; histrionic, borderline, and antisocial personality disorders ●*Procedure results:* Absence of findings to support subjective complaints ●*Test findings:* Absence of findings to support subjective complaints

Spina bifida ●*Onset:* Fetus/newborn ●*Male:female ratio:* M=F ●*Ethnicity:* Possible increase in Ireland/Wales, Egyptians, Sikh Indians ●*Character:* Defective closure of spinal column ●*Location:* Spinal column; commonly lumbosacral area ●*Pattern:* Occulta: most without symptoms, midline defect of vertebra without protrusion of spinal cord/meninges - maybe with overlying hairy patch, lipoma, dermal sinus; meningocele: herniated meninges through vertebral defect; myelocele: herniated spinal cord myelomeningocele: herniated spinal cord and meninges ●*Precipitating factors:* Multifactorial: radiation, drugs, malnutrition, genetic, folate deficiency ●*Relieving factors:* Surgical correction for meningocele, myelomeningocele ●*Clinical course:* Occulta usually asymptomatic unless sinus present, surgical correction for other types, mortality rate 10-15% for meningomyelocele ●*Co-morbidities:* Hydrocephalus, Arnold-Chiari II formation, dysfunction of nervous/skeletal system - subluxation of hips/club feet, bowel/bladder incontinence (meningomyelocele), genitourinary anomalies (meningocele/myelocele/meningomyelocele), trisomy 18, triploidy, Meckel's syndrome, recurrent meningits: spina bifida occulta with dermal sinus tract ●*Procedure results:* Abnormal prenatal ultrasound, X-rays of spine, MRI/CT ●*Test findings:* Abnormal prenatal screening tests: elevated maternal serum/amniotic fluid alfa-fetoprotein

Spinal cord compression ●*Onset:* Subacute, acute, insidious ●*Male:female ratio:* M=F ●*Ethnicity:* All ●*Character:* Back/neck pain, weakness, sensory level, poor bowel/bladder control ●*Location:* Nonspecific ●*Pattern:* Nonspecific ●*Precipitating factors:* Trauma with vertebral fracture or subluxation, metastatic cancer, rheumatological disorders, infectious process - abscess ●*Relieving factors:* High-dose steroids, surgical intervention, radiation ●*Clinical course:* Variable ●*Co-morbidities:* None relevant ●*Procedure results:* MRI of the spine ●*Test findings:* No relevant tests

Spinal cord lesion ●*Onset:* Usually acute ●*Male:female ratio:* M=F ●*Ethnicity:* All ●*Character:* Manifests first with spinal shock/areflexia (depending on level of injury, quadriplegia with atonic bladder, bowel, gastric atony, muscular flaccidity, loss of sensation); next comes the phase of heightened reflex activity after a few weeks (positive Babinski, retention of urine, exaggerated tendon and withdrawal reflexes) ●*Location:* Injury can occur at any level of the spinal cord; often the central gray matter gets necrosed first as it is more vascular ●*Pattern:* After spinal shock with areflexia, within 6 weeks or so, the patient becomes hyper-reflexic; some patients complain of overactivity of one segment of the spinal cord below the level of the injury ●*Precipitating factors:* Trauma, especially to the cervical spine due to high velocity injury, or at any level due to a projectile transecting the cord or from a fall; hemorrhage and lack of blood supply to a segment; spaceoccupying lesion such as an abscess ●*Relieving factors:* Cord compression is an emergency; drainage of an abscess or removal of impacting bone fragments from a vertebral fracture can be lifesaving ●*Clinical course:* Patients with spinal cord injuries need supportive measures in place for adequate rehabilitation: assisted care facilities, allowing use of wheelchairs, and skin care to prevent skin breakdown and use of catheters for drainage of urine are necessary measures ●*Co-morbidities:* Depression, psychosis; phantom limb syndrome; a number of complications occur as a result of loss of motor and sensory function of spinal cord segments affected below level of injury, e.g. bowel and bladder dysfunction, pulmonary embolism ●*Procedure results:* No relevant procedures ●*Test findings:* Spinal radiographs may be of no help if there is no bony injury; soft-tissue lesions are best visualized with MRI scan

Spinal muscular atrophy ●*Onset:* Insidious ●*Male:female ratio:* M=F ●*Ethnicity:* All ●*Character:* Acute infantile spinal muscular atrophy (SMA): severe hypotonia, weakness with respiratory and bulbar muscle involvement. Late onset SMA: weakness and wasting of face, tongue, and proximal muscles ●*Location:* Generalized motor ●*Pattern:* Age of onset depends on subtype. Acute infantile SMA is progressive and death usually occurs before 2 years of age. Late onset SMA is variable, normal life span is unusual ●*Precipitating factors:* Genetic: autosomal dominant, recessive, and X-linked forms ●*Relieving factors:* Physical therapy, occupational therapy ●*Clinical course:* Progressive ●*Co-morbidities:* None relevant ●*Procedure results:* Acute infantile SMA: abnormalities of the long arm of chromosome 5 may be demonstrated ●*Test findings:* No relevant tests

Spinal stenosis and neurogenic claudication ●*Onset:* Subacute, acute, insidious ●*Male:female ratio:* M=F ●*Ethnicity:* All ●*Character:* Back/neck pain, leg pain during activity ●*Location:* Nonspecific ●*Pattern:* Made worse with activity ●*Precipitating factors:* Exercise ●*Relieving factors:* Leaning forward at the waist, bending over forward, rest, sitting ●*Clinical course:* Variable ●*Co-morbidities:* Degenerative joint disease ●*Procedure results:* Narrowed spinal lumen on MRI ●*Test findings:* No relevant tests

Splenic infarct ●*Onset:* Acute ●*Male:female ratio:* M=F ●*Ethnicity:* All ●*Character:* Left upper quadrant pain, fever ●*Location:* Nonspecific ●*Pattern:* Nonspecific ●*Precipitating factors:* Infective endocarditis, cardiac vegetation/clot, myeloproliferative syndromes, sickle cell anemia, polyarteritis nodosa, Hodgkin's lymphoma, bacteremia ●*Relieving factors:* Supportive measures, treatment of underlying disorder ●*Clinical course:* The infarct generally heals leading to an area of fibrosis. If multiple infarcts, the entire spleen can become fibrotic and dysfunctional ●*Co-morbidities:* None relevant ●*Procedure results:* Abdominal CT - wedge-shaped lesion in the spleen ●*Test findings:* No relevant tests

Splenomegaly ●*Onset:* Insidious, sometimes subacute ●*Male:female ratio:* M=F ●*Ethnicity:* All ●*Character:* Pain and sense of fullness in the left upper quadrant (LUQ), left shoulder pain, early satiety, signs and symptoms of the underlying process such as cirrhosis or malignancy ●*Location:* Pain is generally in the LUQ and sometimes in the left shoulder ●*Pattern:* Nonspecific ●*Precipitating factors:* Liver disease, infection (AIDS, brucellosis), hematologic malignancy (lymphoma, myelofibrosis), congestive heart failure, splenic vein thrombosis, storage diseases (Gaucher's), extramedullary hematopoiesis ●*Relieving factors:* Treatment of the underlying disease, treatment of any portal hypertension with non-selective beta blockers, in some cases splenectomy ●*Clinical course:* Depends on underlying etiology ●*Co-morbidities:* Liver disease, infection (AIDS, brucellosis), hematologic malignancy (lymphoma, myelofibrosis), congestive heart failure, splenic vein thrombosis, storage diseases (Gaucher's), extramedullary hematopoiesis ●*Procedure results:* Rarely a splenic biopsy is indicated and reveals underlying cause such as infection or malignancy ●*Test findings:* Radiographic findings of a large spleen (e.g. ultrasound length >13cm, visible spleen on plain X-ray), mild pancytopenia (due to sequestration), evidence of extravascular hemolysis, other tests are more dependent on underlying etiology

Squamous cell carcinoma ●*Onset:* Subacute ●*Male:female ratio:* M(2):F(1) ●*Ethnicity:* Fair skin ●*Character:* Skin lesion ●*Location:* Sun-exposed face, hands ❸ *Pattern:* Red, firm, crusted nodule ●*Precipitating factors:* Radiation, arsenic, scars, sun exposure ●*Relieving factors:* Excision ●*Clinical course:* Persists, resolves with treatment ●*Co-morbidities:* Actinic keratosis ●*Procedure results:* No relevant procedures ●*Test findings:* Positive skin biopsy

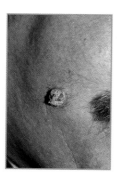

❸ *Pattern A rapidly growing inflammatory nodule with a central hyperkeratotic core*

Staphylococcal infection ●*Onset:* Acute (in most Staphylococcal aureus cases), acute or insidious (with other Staphylococci) ●*Male:female ratio:* M=F ●*Ethnicity:* All ●*Character:* Acute pyogenic infections or abscesses in any organ; skin eruptions; scalded skin syndromes; bacteremia, sepsis, toxic shock, or endocarditis, osteomyelitis, arthritis, eye infections, pneumonia, food poisoning; other ●*Location:* Skin, skin folds, eyes, lymph nodes, joints, bones, soft tissue, heart, lungs, surgical sites, bloodstream, urinary tract, any other organ ●*Pattern:* Acute or insidious infections that may affect any site. Pyogenic, may be associated with shock ●*Precipitating factors:* Trauma, surgery, lactation, dermatitis, immunosuppression, diabetes, tampon use, indwelling catheters or devices, injection drug use, heart valves, influenza (for pneumonia), ingestion of preformed toxin in contaminated food (cream) ●*Relieving factors:* None relevant ●*Clinical course:* Acute, progressive, may be catastrophic, although some are self limiting ●*Co-morbidities:* Trauma, burns, chronic skin disorders, surgery, newborns, nursing, influenza, cystic fibrosis, bronchiectasis, leukemia, cancer, diabetes mellitus, prosthetic valves, pacemakers, indwelling catheters, steroid therapy, immunosuppression, chemotherapy ●*Procedure results:* Isolation of Staphylococcus on culture or visualization of Gram-positive cocci in clusters on Gram stain of specimen from infected site, visualization of enhancing mass on contrast CT ●*Test findings:* Leukocytosis

Stasis dermatitis ●*Onset:* Acute, subacute ●*Male:female ratio:* M<F ●*Ethnicity:* All ●*Character:* Pain, itching ❷ *Location:* Legs ●*Pattern:* Skin erythema, edema, oozing, crusts ●*Precipitating factors:* Venous disease ●*Relieving factors:* Topical steroids relieve swelling ●*Clinical course:* Progressive when not treated ●*Co-morbidities:* Venous disease ●*Procedure results:* No relevant procedures ●*Test findings:* No relevant tests

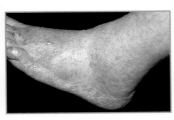

❷ *Location Redness and scale along with edema*

Stevens-Johnson syndrome ●*Onset:* Acute ●*Male:female ratio:* M(2):F(1) ●*Ethnicity:* All ❶ *Character:* Pain, burning ●*Location:* Acral, oral mucosa, conjuctiva, generalized ●*Pattern:* Bullae, erosions, crusts ●*Precipitating factors:* Infection, drugs ●*Relieving factors:* Symptomatic relief ●*Clinical course:* Resolves in a few weeks, can be fatal ●*Co-morbidities:* None relevant ●*Procedure results:* Positive skin biopsy ●*Test findings:* No relevant tests

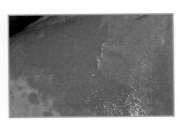

❶ *Character Epidermal detachment. Diffuse erythema with bulla formation and large erosions*

Stokes-Adams attacks ●*Onset:* Insidious underlying process that presents acutely ●*Male:female ratio:* M=F ●*Ethnicity:* All ●*Character:* Sudden loss of consciousness without warning ●*Location:* Nonspecific ●*Pattern:* Unpredictable sudden loss of consciousness may occur once or repeatedly ●*Precipitating factors:* Spontaneous, without any precipitant ●*Relieving factors:* Attack usually self-terminates with spontaneous improvement in AV node conduction, but might require emergent electrical pacing if high-grade AV block persists ●*Clinical course:* Underlying insidious process of AV node dysfunction is typically progressive, which, if not treated with pacemaker implantation, may result in recurrent Stokes-Adams attacks ●*Co-morbidities:* Other conduction system abnormalities, such as sinoatrial dysfunction and bundle branch block; infiltrative cardiac diseases (e.g. amyloidosis, sarcoidosis); mitral valve endocarditis with abscess formation; Lyme disease ●*Procedure results:* ECG might reveal AV node conduction problem, although intermittent nature of AV block might result in normal-appearing ECG ●*Test findings:* No relevant tests

Stomatitis ●*Onset:* Variable ●*Male:female ratio:* M=F ●*Ethnicity:* All ●*Character:* Irritation, burning, bleeding of oral cavity mucosa ●*Location:* Oral cavity, lips ●*Pattern:* Variable: ulceration, hemorrhagic, exudate of oral cavity mucosa ●*Precipitating factors:* Radiation therapy, chemotherapy, vitamin deficiency, malnutrition, poor dental hygiene ●*Relieving factors:* Anesthetic oral gargles ●*Clinical course:* May be self-limited ●*Co-morbidities:* Immunocompromised state; HIV infection; radiation therapy ●*Procedure results:* Scraping of oral cavity mucosa may reveal offending organism, if present; oral cavity biopsy reveals severe inflammation and possibly organisms ●*Test findings:* No relevant tests

Strabismus ●*Onset:* Insidious ●*Male:female ratio:* M=F ●*Ethnicity:* All ●*Character:* Diplopia ●*Location:* Nonspecific ●*Pattern:* Nonspecific ●*Precipitating factors:* None relevant ●*Relieving factors:* Closing one eye relieves diplopia ●*Clinical course:* Persistent if left untreated ●*Co-morbidities:* Rarely associated with other neurological conditions; amblyopia ●*Procedure results:* Neuroimaging only if there are associated neurological findings ●*Test findings:* No relevant tests

Streptococcal throat infection ●*Onset:* Acute ●*Male:female ratio:* M=F ●*Ethnicity:* All ●*Character:* Abrupt onset of sore throat, tender cervical adenopathy, fever ●*Location:* Posterior pharynx, tonsils, cervical (mandibular) lymph nodes. Uncommon: skin (scarlet fever, peritonsillar cellulitis), peritonsillar or retropharyngeal area, other ●*Pattern:* Enlarged erythematous tonsils with gray-white exudate ●*Precipitating factors:* Person-to-person contact, school-aged children, crowding ●*Relieving factors:* Throat lozenges ●*Clinical course:* Incubation: 2-4 days, self-limited within 3-7 days, scarlet fever, suppurative (abscess, cellulitis) and nonsuppurative (acute renal failure, poststreptococal glomerulonephritis) complications may occur ●*Co-morbidities:* Erythema nodosum ●*Procedure results:* Positive rapid streptococcal antigen detection, beta-hemolytic streptococci from throat culture, positive antistreptolysin-O ●*Test findings:* Mild-to-moderate leukocytosis, increased C-reactive protein

Stress ●*Onset:* Acute but may become chronic ●*Male:female ratio:* M>F ●*Ethnicity:* All ●*Character:* Not so much a discrete disorder as a combination of various physiologic (muscle tension, facial tics, fatigue, headaches, GI complaints), psychologic (forgetfulness, irritability, insomnia, anxiety), and behavioral symptoms ●*Location:* Physiologic and/or psychologic in response to an actual or perceived threat ●*Pattern:* In response to perceived danger body initiates protective adrenaline response with multiple possible effects depending on individual's coping skills ●*Precipitating factors:* Work pressures, traffic, holidays, caregiving responsibilities ●*Relieving factors:* Aerobic exercise, yoga/meditation, massage, support network ●*Clinical course:* Can be acute or chronic; chronic can lead to aggravation of asthma, hypertension, depression and reduced immune response ●*Co-morbidities:* Stress is a symptom but is associated with increased smoking, hypertension, other illnessess associated with sustained high cortisol levels ●*Procedure results:* No relevant procedures ●*Test findings:* No relevant tests

Sturge-Weber disease ●*Onset:* Subacute ●*Male:female ratio:* M=F ●*Ethnicity:* All ●*Character:* Facial nevus, usually unilateral; seizures; mental retardation ●*Location:* Vascular calcification, atrophy of leptomeninges and underlying brain ●*Pattern:* Facial nevus present at birth, seizures start within first year ●*Precipitating factors:* None relevant ●*Relieving factors:* Laser treatment for nevus, anitconvulsant therapy, possible hemispherectomy/lobectomy ●*Clinical course:* Lifelong ●*Co-morbidities:* Glaucoma, mental retardation ●*Procedure results:* Skull X-ray: intracranial calcification 'train track' pattern. Head CT: calcification, unilateral cortical atrophy, ipsilateral dilated lateral ventricle ●*Test findings:* No relevant tests

Subacute sclerosing panencephalitis ●*Onset:* Childhood and adolescence ●*Male:female ratio:* M=F ●*Ethnicity:* All ●*Character:* Decline in proficiency at school, personality changes, temper outbursts, language difficulty; then intellectual deterioration occurs with seizures, ataxia or myoclonus; as disease progresses, rigidity, hyper-reflexia and positive Babinski's reflexes are noted; end result is 'decortication' ●*Location:* Cerebral cortex and white matter and brainstem as well ●*Pattern:* Progressive intellectual impairment ●*Precipitating factors:* History of primary measles at a very young age; probable defective synthesis of M-protein required for viral membrane synthesis ●*Relieving factors:* No effective treatment available; need supportive care

- *Clinical course:* Usually progressive course within 1-3 years; in a few the course can be fulminant or very slow to progress ● *Co-morbidities:* Genodermatoses with defective cell-mediated immunity can make children more susceptible ● *Procedure results:* Biopsy reveals eosinophilic inclusions in cytoplasm and nuclei of neuronal and glial cells; other findings include destruction of neuronal cells, white matter fibrous gliosis ● *Test findings:* EEG reveals periodic bursts of high voltage waves, followed by relatively flat pattern; increased protein in CSF with oligoclonal bands on immunoelectrophoresis; degeneration of white matter on MRI

Subarachnoid hemorrhage and cerebral aneurysm stroke
● *Onset:* Acute ● *Male:female ratio:* M<F ● *Ethnicity:* All ● *Character:* Sudden onset of headache, weakness, confusion, numbness, mental status change, seizures ● *Location:* Nonspecific ● *Pattern:* Nonspecific ● *Precipitating factors:* Hypertension, tobacco usage ● *Relieving factors:* Surgical intervention and control of seizures or intracranial pressure ● *Clinical course:* Variable ● *Co-morbidities:* None relevant ● *Procedure results:* MRI/MRA or conventional angiogram showing the aneurysm ● *Test findings:* No relevant tests

Subclavian steal syndrome
● *Onset:* Acute ● *Male:female ratio:* M(2):F(1) ● *Ethnicity:* All ● *Character:* Syncope associated with arms above head or exercise of the upper extremities ● *Location:* Nonspecific ● *Pattern:* Nonspecific ● *Precipitating factors:* Elevated cholesterol, atherosclerosis ● *Relieving factors:* Supportive ● *Clinical course:* Variable ● *Co-morbidities:* None relevant ● *Procedure results:* Reversal of flow in the vertebral arteries and basilar artery with transcranial Dopplers ● *Test findings:* No relevant tests

Subdiaphragmatic abscess
● *Onset:* Subacute ● *Male:female ratio:* M=F ● *Ethnicity:* All ● *Character:* Fever, anorexia, malaise, usually with abdominal pain, but may be relatively painless. If persistent, there is often weight loss. Pain is usually in the right upper quadrant (RUQ) or left upper quadrant (LUQ), but may be referred to the shoulder. Patients may have dyspnea and pleuritic chest pain due to diaphragmatic irritation. Examination may show upper quadrant tenderness; crackles at lung base due to atelectasis ● *Location:* Upper abdomen, but may be referred to shoulder ● *Pattern:* Nonspecific ● *Precipitating factors:* Deep breathing may heighten discomfort ● *Relieving factors:* Both antibiotic therapy and drainage of the abscess are required; drainage may be via percutaneous catheter or surgical. Antibiotics should cover anaerobes, Gram-negative bacteria, and Enterococcus ● *Clinical course:* Usually progresses over days to weeks - not self-limited ● *Co-morbidities:* Abdominal trauma, inflammatory bowel disease, cholangitis or other biliary tract disease, postoperative complication ● *Procedure results:* Abdominal CT scan usually reveals the abscess - diagnosis is confirmed by sampling of the abscess contents (Gram stain and culture) ● *Test findings:* WBC, ESR usually elevated; liver function tests may be elevated if abscess is on the right

Subdural hematoma
● *Onset:* Acute and chronic subtypes ● *Male:female ratio:* M=F ● *Ethnicity:* All ● *Character:* Acute: almost 50% of patients were unconscious after injury and about 25% remained in a coma until arrival at a hospital, contralateral hemiparesis, unreliable eye signs including compression of the third cranial nerve or contralateral cerebral peduncle; chronic: take more than 3 weeks to manifest, occurs typically in age >50 yrs, many patients have history of epilepsy or alcoholism, subtle mental changes that can be mistaken for dementia ● *Location:* Subdural space, usually over the cerebral cortex convexity ● *Pattern:* Acute: rapid deterioration in level of consciousness, usually after trauma; chronic: gradual cognitive loss ● *Precipitating factors:* Acute: trauma, intracranial lesion; chronic: in up to 50% cases, no clear history of head trauma, history of alcoholism, epilepsy, history of shunts, bleeding disorders and anticoagulants ● *Relieving factors:* Surgical decompression ● *Clinical course:* Acute: although rapidly progressive and patients deteriorate quickly, surgical decompression can relieve symptoms, with the original state of the patient having a major impact on the outcome, i.e. Glasgow Coma Scale scores of 3-5 lead to a 75% mortality; chronic: good prognosis, mortality rate low at about 6% ● *Co-morbidities:* Dementia, alcoholism, shunt placement, low intracranial pressure, epilepsy ● *Procedure results:* Acute: good outcome if preprocedure Glasgow Coma Scale score closer to normal; chronic: generally, lower mortality and morbidity ● *Test findings:* CT or MRI scans demonstrate presence of spaceoccupying hemorrhage

Sun damage ●*Onset:* Subacute/acute ●*Male:female ratio:* M=F ●*Ethnicity:* All ●*Character:* Skin lesions ●*Location:* Any site, most commonly hands, feet, neck, back, face ●*Pattern:* Light-colored verrucous papules, frequently multiple ●*Precipitating factors:* Sun exposure, immunosuppression, atopy ●*Relieving factors:* Destruction: cryotherapy, electrosurgery, topical salicylic acid ●*Clinical course:* May resolve spontaneously, can persist for months/years ●*Co-morbidities:* None relevant ●*Procedure results:* No relevant procedures ●*Test findings:* No relevant tests

Sunburn ●*Onset:* Acute ●*Male:female ratio:* M=F ●*Ethnicity:* Fair skin ●*Character:* Pain, burning ❷ *Location:* Sun-exposed skin ●*Pattern:* Erythema, swelling, blisters ●*Precipitating factors:* Sun exposure ●*Relieving factors:* Antipruritic lotions ●*Clinical course:* Resolves in days ●*Co-morbidities:* None relevant ●*Procedure results:* No relevant procedures ●*Test findings:* No relevant tests

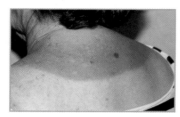

❷ *Location A painful, photodistributed erythema one day after significant sun exposure*

Superior vena cava syndrome ●*Onset:* Insidious ●*Male:female ratio:* M>F ●*Ethnicity:* All ●*Character:* Swelling and/or purplish discoloration of face, neck, arms ●*Location:* Face, head, arms, upper chest ●*Pattern:* Slowly progressive over weeks ●*Precipitating factors:* Unaffected by posture or activities ●*Relieving factors:* Surgical therapy, radiation therapy, or chemotherapy is needed to treat the offending mass that is compressing the superior vena cava (SVC) ●*Clinical course:* Progressive until SVC obstruction is relieved by debulking therapy ●*Co-morbidities:* Masses or tumors in region of SVC, especially right apical lung tumors and some mediastinal tumors; can result in venous thrombosis proximal to obstruction ●*Procedure results:* Imaging studies (chest X-ray, CT scan, MRI) reveal cause of compression of SVC, typically a tumor mass ●*Test findings:* No relevant tests

Syncope ●*Onset:* Acute ●*Male:female ratio:* M=F ●*Ethnicity:* All ●*Character:* Sudden loss of consciousness, sometimes preceded by a short prodrome (less than 1 min) ●*Location:* Nonspecific ●*Pattern:* Depends on etiology. Vagal syncope is situational (heat, fear, cough, urination), preceded by a prodrome, which may include warmth, nausea, fatigue, yawning, sweating. Cardiac arrhythmias (sinus arrest, heart block (Stokes-Adams attack), ventricular arrhythmia) are spontaneous and sudden. Cardiac outflow obstruction (aortic stenosis, hypertrophic cardiomyopathy) is typically sudden ●*Precipitating factors:* Depends on etiology. Vagal syncope (e.g. fright, heat, sight of blood). Syncope from hypertrophic cardiomyopathy precipitated by decreased left ventricular filling (e.g. dehydration). Aortic stenosis syncope typically spontaneous. Arrhythmic syncope is spontaneous ●*Relieving factors:* Loss of consciousness typically resolves spontaneously ●*Clinical course:* Syncope is, by definition, self-limited, but it may recur, depending on etiology ●*Co-morbidities:* May be in association with conduction system abnormalities, aortic stenosis, hypertrophic cardiomyopathy ●*Procedure results:* Depending on etiology, EKG might reveal bradyarrhythmia, heart block, tachyarrhythmia; echocardiography may reveal aortic stenosis, hypertrophic cardiomyopathy ●*Test findings:* No relevant tests

Syphilis ●*Onset:* Acute, subacute, chronic ●*Male:female ratio:* M>F ●*Ethnicity:* All ●*Character:* Primary: painless genital ulcer with raised firm borders; secondary: fever, genital lesions, generalized rash, generalized lymphadenopathy; tertiary: progressive dementia or aortic insufficiency ●*Location:* Primary: external genitalia, vagina, cervix, perianal area, mouth, regional lymph nodes; secondary: constitutional, skin (generalized including palms and soles), genital skin, generalized lymph nodes, oropharyngeal mucosa, meninges, eyes (uvea, retina, choroid), cranial nerves (II-VIII), kidneys, liver, other; tertiary: brain, spinal cord, aorta, eye, any organ (gumma) ●*Pattern:* Ulcer and lymphadenopathy painless. Secondary lesions generalized faint macular (skin, mucosa) or flat genital. Generalized paresis: personality, affect, reflexes (hyper), eye (Argyll-Robertson pupil), sensorium, intellect, speech; tabes ●*Precipitating factors:* Unprotected vaginal, anal, or oral sexual contact; direct contact with primary or secondary syphilitic rash, blood transfusion (if not tested) ●*Relieving factors:* None relevant ●*Clinical course:* Incubation 2-6 weeks. Ulcer heals spontaneously. Secondary begins 6-8 weeks after healing of primary, resolves in 2-6 weeks with 25% relapse in 2-4 years. Early latent = 1 year. Late latent >1 year. One-third of untreated develop tertiary syphilis years later, and 25% die from tertiary syphilis, cardiac or CNS complications ●*Co-morbidities:* Aortic insufficiency, gumma, general paresis, dementia, tabes dorsalis, chorioretinitis, optic neuritis, blindness, AIDS, gonorrhea, chlamydia, herpes, stillbirth, congenital syphilis ●*Procedure results:* Demonstration of spirochetes by dark-field microscopy or direct immunofluorescence in wet preparations from chancre, condylomata lata, skin rash, rapid plasma reagin (RPR), Venereal Disease Research Laboratory (VDRL) test, or specific treponemal serologic tests from plasma or CSF ●*Test findings:* Lymphocytic pleocytosis, increased protein in CSF (some of secondary), positive RPR or VDRL, positive specific treponemal serology

Syringomyelia ●*Onset:* Subacute, acute, insidious ●*Male:female ratio:* M=F ●*Ethnicity:* All ●*Character:* Weakness of the upper or lower extremities with disassociated sensory loss ●*Location:* Usually in the upper extremities/cervical area ●*Pattern:* Nonspecific ●*Precipitating factors:* Congenital abnormality, trauma ●*Relieving factors:* Surgical intervention ●*Clinical course:* Variable ●*Co-morbidities:* Hydrocephalus, dysraphic spinal cord ●*Procedure results:* MRI of the spine ●*Test findings:* No relevant tests

Systemic lupus erythematosus ●*Onset:* Subacute ●*Male:female ratio:* M(1):F(10) ●*Ethnicity:* African descent ●*Character:* Arthralgias, fatigue ●*Location:* Hands, knees ●*Pattern:* Rash on the cheeks sparing the nasolabial folds ●*Precipitating factors:* Sunlight, stress, infection ●*Relieving factors:* NSAIDs, glucocorticoids, hydroxychloroquine, azathioprine, methotrexate, cyclophosphamide ●*Clinical course:* Chronic with intermittent flares ●*Co-morbidities:* Complement deficiency ●*Procedure results:* Necrotizing lymph node biopsies, onion skinning on splenic biopsy, dermal-epidermal lymphocytic infiltrate on deep skin biopsy ●*Test findings:* Antinuclear antibody panel (ANA), dsDNA, anti-Sm antibody

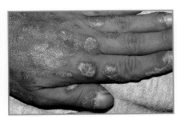

❷ *Location* Hyperkeratotic red plaques in photo-exposed areas

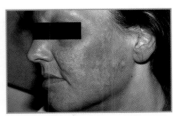

❸ *Pattern* Red scaly areas on the sun-exposed skin of the face

Tabes dorsalis ●*Onset:* Insidious ●*Male:female ratio:* M>F ●*Ethnicity:* All ●*Character:* Progressive ataxic gait, paresthesias, impotence, bladder disturbances, stool incontinence, areflexia ●*Location:* Posterior columns of spinal cord, dorsal roots, dorsal root ganglia. End organs: joints (ankles, knees), bladder, erectile function, bowel and bladder, eyes (optic nerve), skin ulcers, other ●*Pattern:* Wide-based gait, loss of sense of position with positive Romberg, loss of pain and temperature sensations, loss of deep tendon reflex with trophic joint degeneration (Charcot's), paresthesias, chronic skin ulcers ●*Precipitating factors:* Untreated syphilis, unprotected sexual contact, contact with syphilitic lesion, or blood transfusion decades prior ●*Relieving factors:* None relevant ●*Clinical course:* Begins years-to-decades after untreated syphilis, slowly progressive over months-to-years. Treatment may halt progression ●*Co-morbidities:* Charcot's joints, pressure and traumatic chronic skin ulcers, bowel and stool incontinence, impotence, falls and fractures, concentric visual field loss and blindness ●*Procedure results:* Positive CSF Veneral Disease Reserach Laboratory (VDRL) test, CSF pleocytosis and elevated protein ●*Test findings:* Positive rapid plasma reagin (RPR) or VDRL and specific treponemal serology in plasma, positive CSF VDRL, CSF pleocytosis and elevated protein

Takayasu's syndrome ●*Onset:* Fulminant, subacute ●*Male:female ratio:* M(1):F(8) ●*Ethnicity:* More common in Mexico and Far East ●*Character:* Malaise, fever, arthralgias, weight loss, loss of peripheral pulses, symptoms from organ ischemia ●*Location:* Affects the aorta and its large arterial branches, especially subclavian (93%), common carotid (58%), abdominal aorta (47%), renal (38%), aortic root/arch (35%), vertebral (35%) ●*Pattern:* Gradual progressive constitutional symptoms with eventual ischemic symptoms in limb or organ whose perfusion is affected ●*Precipitating factors:* Spontaneous and progressive ●*Relieving factors:* Symptoms not relieved without medical treatment ●*Clinical course:* Disease is progressive until treated with immunosuppressive therapy and possibly with mechanical intervention on stenosed vessels ●*Co-morbidities:* None relevant ●*Procedure results:* Arteriography reveals irregular vessel walls, focal or serial stenoses, possibly aneurysmal dilations in affected vessels ●*Test findings:* Elevated ESR, elevated immunoglobulin levels, mild anemia

Teething ●*Onset:* Subacute, acute ●*Male:female ratio:* M=F ●*Ethnicity:* All ●*Character:* Drooling, hands in mouth, irritability ❷ *Location:* Teeth/gums ❸ *Pattern:* Onset prior to and during teeth eruption ●*Precipitating factors:* Teeth eruption ●*Relieving factors:* Teething rings, oral analgesics, topical analgesics ●*Clinical course:* Resolves once teeth erupted ●*Co-morbidities:* None relevant ●*Procedure results:* No relevant procedures ●*Test findings:* No relevant tests

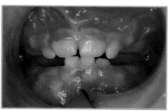

❷ *Location* Early primary dentition with central incisors first to erupt

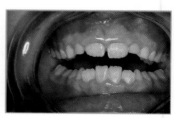

❷ *Location* Mixed dentition changes from primary to permanent dentition from 6 years

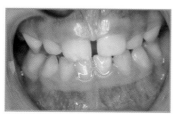

❸ *Pattern* Full primary dentition with all 20 teeth erupted by 3 years

Temporal arteritis ●*Onset:* Usually adulthood, after 50 years ●*Male:female ratio:* M=F ●*Ethnicity:* All ●*Character:* Headache: uni- or bilateral, throbbing in temporal area with redness, swelling, tenderness of temporal artery; also fever, malaise, anorexia, weakness, weight loss, polymyalgia of trunk muscles, neck, shoulders, hip/pelvis; synovitis ●*Location:* Aortic arch branches: temporal and occipital arteries, coronaries, and some peripheral arteries ●*Pattern:* Nonspecific ●*Precipitating factors:* Possible autoimmune reaction ●*Relieving factors:* Corticosteroids ●*Clinical course:* Worsening symptoms unless treated ●*Co-morbidities:* Ptosis, visual blurring, diplopia, transient/permanent blindness ●*Procedure results:* Artery biopsy: granulomatous inflammation of arteries; lymphocytic, epithelioid and giant cells; thickening of intimal layer with narrowing/occlusion of lumen; abnormal arteriogram ●*Test findings:* Elevated ESR and WBC

Temporal lobe epilepsy ●*Onset:* Adolescence and adulthood ●*Male:female ratio:* M=F ●*Ethnicity:* All ●*Character:* Can present with visceral symptoms (fear, anxiety, olfactory disturbances, and psychic phenomena), auditory hallucinations or complex visual phenomena, complex partial seizures characterized by behavioral arrest, staring, automatisms, and dystonic posturing of an extremity contralateral to the focus; seizures can last up to 2 min ●*Location:* Temporal lobe (symptoms may include language disturbances if dominant lobe involved) ●*Pattern:* Postictal confusion usually occurs, and change in language may occur, especially if the seizure focus is in the dominant temporal lobe; a large proportion of patients can develop generalized seizures ●*Precipitating factors:* CNS infection, trauma, febrile seizures; stress, menstruation and sleep deprivation are precipitants ●*Relieving factors:* Treatment with anticonvulsants is of benefit, with phenytoin and carbamazepine preferred ●*Clinical course:* Respond well to treatment, with relief of precipitating factors; postictal state after a seizure requires observation; duration of postictal state varies between individuals ●*Co-morbidities:* Spaceoccupying lesions in the temporal lobe ●*Procedure results:* Surgical ablation of seizure focus, if oral anticonvulsants do not work in 2 years ●*Test findings:* EEG, performed during interictal phase, shows spikes or sharp waves in the temporal area, enhanced during non-REM sleep; if performed during ictal phase, the EEG can be attenuated followed by a gradual buildup, intermixed with epileptic discharges

Temporomandibular joint syndrome ●*Onset:* Acute, chronic ●*Male:female ratio:* M(1):F(3) ●*Ethnicity:* All ●*Character:* Mild/severe pain over the temporomandibular joint (TMJ) ●*Location:* Temporomandibular joint possibly radiating to ear or face. Possible crepitus in TMJ area ●*Pattern:* Worse with chewing or jaw motion ●*Precipitating factors:* Night-time bruxism ●*Relieving factors:* Warm pack; NSAIDs ●*Clinical course:* Usually chronic ●*Co-morbidities:* None relevant ●*Procedure results:* Normal examination of the head and neck including larynx ●*Test findings:* Plain films of TMJ (relatively insensitive) may show degenerative disease

Tendinitis ●*Onset:* Subacute ●*Male:female ratio:* M>F (slightly) ●*Ethnicity:* All ●*Character:* Chronic dull ache with sharp pain during times of use ●*Location:* Single periarticular area ●*Pattern:* Worse with use ●*Precipitating factors:* Repetitive use of affected tendon ●*Relieving factors:* Ice, NSAIDs, rest, cortisone injection, physical therapy ●*Clinical course:* Progressive unless patients change the motion of the affected joint area ●*Co-morbidities:* Diabetes ●*Procedure results:* Normal radiographs ●*Test findings:* No relevant tests

Tension headache ●*Onset:* Subacute ●*Male:female ratio:* M<F ●*Ethnicity:* All ●*Character:* Nonthrobbing, vice-like tightness ●*Location:* Bitemporal, occipital, on top of the head ●*Pattern:* Nonspecific ●*Precipitating factors:* Stress, fatigue, anxiety, caffeine withdrawal ●*Relieving factors:* Stress management ●*Clinical course:* Overall prognosis is good but can progress to chronic daily headaches ●*Co-morbidities:* Anxiety, stress ●*Procedure results:* No relevant procedures ●*Test findings:* Normal neurological examination

Testicular malignancy ●*Onset:* Subacute ●*Male:female ratio:* M ●*Ethnicity:* Less frequent in African-Americans ●*Character:* Painless testicular nodule or swelling ●*Location:* Scrotum/testis ●*Pattern:* Unilateral (97%); bilateral (3%) ●*Precipitating factors:* None relevant ●*Relieving factors:* Surgical removal plus lymph node dissection, chemotherapy, or radiation ●*Clinical course:* Progressive; >90% cure with appropriate treatment ●*Co-morbidities:* Concomitant testicular events (trauma, epididymo-orchitis) bringing attention to testis ●*Procedure results:* Scrotal ultrasound: testicular mass. CT abdomen, pelvis, and chest: locates metastasis. Inguinal exploration with orchiectomy or biopsy = definite diagnosis ●*Test findings:* Alpha-fetoprotein: elevation in embryonal carcinoma, teratocarcinoma, and yolk sac tumors. Beta-HCG: elevation in choriocarcinoma, embryonal carcinoma, and pure seminoma

Testicular torsion ●*Onset:* Acute ●*Male:female ratio:* M ●*Ethnicity:* All ●*Character:* Pain, swelling ●*Location:* Scrotum/testis ●*Pattern:* Unilateral (98%); bilateral (2%) ●*Precipitating factors:* Minor trauma; vigorous activity ●*Relieving factors:* Manual reduction or surgical reduction and fixation ●*Clinical course:* Usually progressive except in cases of intermittent torsion; high salvage rate if treated within 6 hours of onset; high risk for testicular necrosis after 24 hours ●*Co-morbidities:* Scrotal trauma, Henoch-Schönlein purpura ●*Procedure results:* Absence or reduced blood flow on testicular Doppler ultrasound or nuclear scan ●*Test findings:* Urinalysis unremarkable

Tetanus ●*Onset:* Gradual, subacute ●*Male:female ratio:* M=F ●*Ethnicity:* All ●*Character:* Generalized: progressive trismus (locked jaw) and risus sardonicus followed by opisthotonus and generalized rigidity. Localized: local muscle spasms near wound site. Neonatal: generalized weakness followed by spasticity in a neonate ●*Location:* Nonspecific ●*Pattern:* Progressive muscle spasm begins near wound site or at masseter and orbicularis oris muscles, rarely only cephalic muscles (motor cranial nerves). Neonates present with flaccidity before spasm ●*Precipitating factors:* Contaminated wound/injury/laceration, animal bite, lack of or incomplete immunization, failure of aseptic technique during labor and delivery ●*Relieving factors:* Benzodiazepines, passive and/or active immunization with injury, decontamination of wounds ●*Clinical course:* Incubation: 2 days-2 months (average: 10 days); progression over 1-2 weeks; recovery over months; high case-fatality rate; requires immediate medical attention ●*Co-morbidities:* Infected wound, trauma, animal bite ●*Procedure results:* Characteristic EMG, lack of antitetanus antibodies (suggestive) ●*Test findings:* Elevated CPK (muscle), elevated creatinine, elevated phosphate, myoglobinuria

Tetralogy of Fallot ●*Onset:* Usually subacute, progressive ●*Male:female ratio:* M>F (slightly) ●*Ethnicity:* All ●*Character:* Cyanosis, dyspnea, 'blue'/'tet' spells, poor growth, pulmonary stenosis murmur ●*Location:* Cardiac/respiratory symptoms, color changes of skin ●*Pattern:* Worsening symptoms as disease progresses ●*Precipitating factors:* 'Tet' spells after crying or with pain ●*Relieving factors:* To relieve spell: knee to chest position, oxygen administration, prostaglandin E1, morphine; corrective surgery: Blalock-Taussig shunt ●*Clinical course:* 'Tet' spells usually resolve spontaneously or with treatment, disorder symptoms worsen without treatment ●*Co-morbidities:* Patent ductus arteriosus, atrioventricular defect (ASD), absent pulmonary artery or valve, congestive heart failure (CHF), cerebral thrombosis/ischemia, diabetes mellitus, splenomegaly/hepatomegaly, bacterial endocarditis, brain abscess, tracheoesophageal fistula, Down's syndrome, Noonan's syndrome, rubella syndrome ●*Procedure results:* Chest X-ray: 'coeur en sabot'/'boot-shaped heart', normal heart size, decreased pulmonary blood flow; ECG: right axis deviation, right ventricular hypertrophy (RVH); Echo: shows pulmonary stenosis, ventricular septal defect (VSD), dextroposition of aorta, RVH ●*Test findings:* Metabolic acidosis, hypoxemia, failed hyperoxia test

Thalassemia ●*Onset:* Subacute ●*Male:female ratio:* M=F ●*Ethnicity:* Mediterranean descent, African, Middle Eastern, Indian, Southeast Asian, Greek, Italian ●*Character:* Hypertrophy of erythropoietic tissue - face/skull bones, pallor, jaundice, enlarged spleen/liver, impaired growth ●*Location:* Hemolytic anemia, skin color changes, facial bones ●*Pattern:* Nonspecific ●*Precipitating factors:* Genetic defect - deletions of globin chain genes leads to absence/decreased production of hemoglobin chains ●*Relieving factors:* Transfusion, bone marrow transplantation ●*Clinical course:* Progressive, lifelong ●*Co-morbidities:* Impaired growth, diabetes mellitus, hemosiderosis, CHF, arrhythmias, delayed puberty ●*Procedure results:* No relevant procedures ●*Test findings:* Hypochromia, microcytosis, poikilocytes, target cells, anemia, high serum iron, saturated transferrin, elevated unconjugated bilirubin, elevated HbF, decreased HbA, increased HbA2

Thoracic aortic aneurysm ●*Onset:* Subacute, insidious ●*Male:female ratio:* M(3):F(1) ●*Ethnicity:* All ●*Character:* Asymptomatic, constant pain, shortness of breath ●*Location:* Chest, midscapular pain ●*Pattern:* Steady/boring ●*Precipitating factors:* Age, atherosclerosis, connective tissue disorders, infection, trauma ●*Relieving factors:* Beta-blockers ●*Clinical course:* Progressive: symptoms from either compression of adjacent structures, aortic insufficiency, rupture. Risk of rupture increased with size >6.0cm and rate of growth >0.5cm/year ●*Co-morbidities:* Hypertension, hyperlipidemia, atherosclerosis, Marfan's syndrome, Cogan's syndrome, Ehlers-Danlos syndrome, giant cell arteritis, syphilis, infective endocarditis, trauma ●*Procedure results:* Imaging studies show dilation of aorta 1.5x normal ●*Test findings:* No relevant tests

Thoracic aortic dissection ●*Onset:* Acute ●*Male:female ratio:* M(2):F(1) ●*Ethnicity:* All ●*Character:* Severe, sudden, sharp, tearing, or ripping pain ●*Location:* Anterior chest ●*Pattern:* Hypotension, pulse-deficit, neurologic signs/symptoms, aortic insufficiency mumur ●*Precipitating factors:* Prior cardiac surgery, trauma, connective tissue disease ●*Relieving factors:* Surgery ●*Clinical course:* Progressive; vascular compromise or rupture leads to death ●*Co-morbidities:* Hypertension, atherosclerosis, aortic aneurysm, Marfan's, Noonan's, Turner's, giant cell arteritis, trauma ●*Procedure results:* Chest X-ray: mediastinal widening. CT/MRI: double lumen and/or intimal flap ●*Test findings:* Hypotension, pulse-deficit, neurologic signs/symptoms, aortic insufficiency mumur

Thoracic outlet syndrome ●*Onset:* Insidious ●*Male:female ratio:* M=F ●*Ethnicity:* All ●*Character:* Decreased upper extremity pulses with tingling and numbness in medial aspect of arm secondary to compression of medial cord of brachial plexus and axillary artery by cervical rib or other structure ●*Location:* Upper extremity ●*Pattern:* Nonspecific ●*Precipitating factors:* Cervical rib ●*Relieving factors:* Surgical intervention ●*Clinical course:* Variable ●*Co-morbidities:* None relevant ●*Procedure results:* Chest X-ray and electromyogram (EMG)/nerve conduction studies ●*Test findings:* No relevant tests

Thrombocytopenia absent radius syndrome ●*Onset:* Acute ●*Male:female ratio:* M=F ●*Ethnicity:* All ●*Character:* Severe thrombocytopenia/absent/hypoplastic radii, defects of hands/legs and/or feet, congenital heart defect, small stature, mental retardation, hip dislocation ●*Location:* Hematologic/skeletal ●*Pattern:* Decreased severity of thrombocytopenia with advanced age ●*Precipitating factors:* Autosomal recessive ●*Relieving factors:* Treatment of thrombocytopenia ●*Clinical course:* Decreased severity of thrombocytopenia with advancing age ●*Co-morbidities:* Cow's milk allergy with eosinophilia, anemia ●*Procedure results:* Decreased platelets, with absence of hypoplasia of megakaryocytes, leukemoid granulocytosis, eosinophilia ●*Test findings:* Abnormal prenatal ultrasound, abnormal skeletal X-rays

Thrombophlebitis • Thrombotic thrombocytopenic purpura • Thyroglossal duct cyst • Thyroid carcinoma • Thyroid cyst • Thyroiditis

T

Thrombophlebitis ●*Onset:* Subacute, but may present with more acute symptoms ●*Male:female ratio:* Suppurative: M=F. Aseptic: F>M ●*Ethnicity:* All ●*Character:* Focal pain over superficial veins, tenderness to touch, possible local erythema and swelling ●*Location:* Superficial veins, typically in the lower extremities ●*Pattern:* Constant pain and tenderness over affected superficial vein(s) with tenderness to touch ●*Precipitating factors:* Superficial vein thrombosis is typically spontaneous ●*Relieving factors:* Local heat, NSAIDs, and extremity elevation typically improve symptoms; anticoagulation with heparin/warfarin occasionally hastens resolution ●*Clinical course:* If treated conservatively with local heat, NSAIDs and leg elevation, symptoms decrease in days, completely resolve in weeks ●*Co-morbidities:* Associated with IV catheters, varicose veins, hypercoagulable states, immobility, burns, malignancies ●*Procedure results:* Venous ultrasound reveals thrombus in superficial veins ●*Test findings:* No relevant tests

Thrombotic thrombocytopenic purpura ●*Onset:* Acute, subacute ●*Male:female ratio:* Predominantly females ●*Ethnicity:* All ●*Character:* Fever, nonfocal neurologic symptoms, weakness ●*Location:* Nonpalpable purpura seen on skin ●*Pattern:* Progressive nonfocal and/or focal neurologic symptoms, leading to confusion, coma, death ●*Precipitating factors:* Spontaneous, associated with some autoimmune conditions ●*Relieving factors:* Progressive and fatal unless plasmapheresis with plasma exchange is performed, which can cure ●*Clinical course:* Progressive and fatal over days-weeks without treatment ●*Co-morbidities:* Can be associated with lupus, scleroderma, Sjögren's syndrome, AIDS, pregnancy ●*Procedure results:* Biopsy of skin, muscle, lymph node, gingiva, bone marrow may show platelet and fibrin thrombi in arterioles +/- immunoglobulin and complement ●*Test findings:* Hemolytic anemia (MAHA), thrombocytopenia, elevated BUN and creatinine, elevated LDH, proteinuria

Thyroglossal duct cyst ●*Onset:* Subacute, acute ●*Male:female ratio:* M=F ●*Ethnicity:* All ●*Character:* Neck mass may present as infected mass, moves with swallowing and tongue protrusion ●*Location:* Neck ●*Pattern:* Nonspecific ●*Precipitating factors:* Embryologic development ●*Relieving factors:* Antibiotic treatment, surgical removal ●*Clinical course:* Presents as mass, resolves with treatment/removal ●*Co-morbidities:* Thyroglossal sinus ●*Procedure results:* Radionuclide scan will differentiate between this and undescended lingual thyroid ●*Test findings:* No relevant tests

Thyroid carcinoma ●*Onset:* Insidious but tracheal obstruction may present acutely ●*Male:female ratio:* M(1):F(3) ●*Ethnicity:* All ●*Character:* Usually asymptomatic but can cause local pressure symptoms and hoarseness ●*Location:* Neck ●*Pattern:* Nonspecific ●*Precipitating factors:* Prior history of head and/or neck irradiation, family history of thyroid cancer ●*Relieving factors:* Surgery ●*Clinical course:* Progressive enlargement of cancer locally; may metastasize ●*Co-morbidities:* Medullary carcinoma associated with MEN2 ●*Procedure results:* Thyroid nodule aspiration shows malignant cells or may show follicular cells with follicular neoplasm (either benign or malignant); thyroid scan: cold area on scan ●*Test findings:* Normal thyroid function tests

Thyroid cyst ●*Onset:* Gradual but can be acute if hemorrhage into cyst ●*Male:female ratio:* M<F ●*Ethnicity:* All ●*Character:* Thyroid nodule; may have neck discomfort and acute increase in nodule if hemorrhage ●*Location:* Neck ●*Pattern:* Nonspecific ●*Precipitating factors:* None relevant ●*Relieving factors:* Fine needle aspiration and drainage of cyst ●*Clinical course:* Usually asymptomatic and found on physical examination; may cause pain with acute enlargement ●*Co-morbidities:* None relevant ●*Procedure results:* Echogenic nodule on ultrasound of thyroid; fine needle aspirate yields fluid ●*Test findings:* Normal thyroid function tests

Thyroiditis ●*Onset:* Acute ●*Male:female ratio:* M<F ●*Ethnicity:* All ●*Character:* Neck and throat pain for subacute; palpitations/sweats/anxiety in hyperthyroid phase; fatigue, constipation in hypothyroid phase ●*Location:* Neck ●*Pattern:* Nonspecific ●*Precipitating factors:* Pregnancy, viral syndrome, radioactive iodine ●*Relieving factors:* Aspirin, steroids, beta-blockers during hyperthyroid phase, thyroxine replacement for hypothyroidism ●*Clinical course:* Usually resolves though may progress to permanent hypothyroidism ●*Co-morbidi-*

ties: None relevant ●*Procedure results:* No uptake on thyroid uptake or scan ●*Test findings:* During hyperthyroid phase high T4, low TSH and high ESR (subacute), then low T4 and elevated TSH in hypothyroid phase

Tinea versicolor ●*Onset:* Mostly adolescence, young adults, but can be from infancy to adulthood ●*Male:female ratio:* M=F ●*Ethnicity:* Often more apparent in darker-skinned people ●*Character:* Multiple, scaling oval macular, patchy lesions, hypopigmented/hyperpigmented ●*Location:* Usually upper trunk, proximal arms, face ●*Pattern:* Usually asymptomatic ●*Precipitating factors:* Fungus: Pityrosporum orbiculare (Malassezia furfur), possible genetic predisposition? ●*Relieving factors:* Selenium sulfide application, antifungal agents ●*Clinical course:* Chronic, more prominent in summer due to sunlight exposure ●*Co-morbidities:* None relevant ●*Procedure results:* No relevant procedures ●*Test findings:* Potassium hydroxide wet mount; blue white fluoresence under Wood's lamp

Tinnitus ●*Onset:* Usually chronic ●*Male:female ratio:* M=F ●*Ethnicity:* None ●*Character:* Usually constant ringing ●*Location:* Affected ear ●*Pattern:* Worse in quiet environments ●*Precipitating factors:* Heavy stress ●*Relieving factors:* White noise devices (masks sound) ●*Clinical course:* Usually chronic; most patients accommodate with time ●*Co-morbidities:* Sensorineural hearing loss ●*Procedure results:* Otoscopy reveals normal ear exam ●*Test findings:* Audiogram may be normal or show the hearing loss in the affected ear

Tongue tie ●*Onset:* Birth ●*Male:female ratio:* M=F ●*Ethnicity:* All ●*Character:* Short lingual frenulum ●*Location:* Short lingual frenulum ●*Pattern:* Usually stays relatively the same size as tongue grows ●*Precipitating factors:* None relevant ●*Relieving factors:* Surgery if needed - if very thick frenulum ●*Clinical course:* Remains present ●*Co-morbidities:* If very severe tongue tie, possible feeding/speech issues ●*Procedure results:* Surgical correction ●*Test findings:* No relevant tests

Tonsillar hypertrophy ●*Onset:* Insidious ●*Male:female ratio:* M=F ●*Ethnicity:* All ●*Character:* Frequent tonsillitis; muffled voice, halitosis, snoring ●*Location:* Oropharynx ●*Pattern:* Tonsils may swell with each infection ●*Precipitating factors:* None relevant ●*Relieving factors:* Saltwater gargles; cold liquids ●*Clinical course:* Chronic condition ●*Co-morbidities:* None relevant ●*Procedure results:* Symmetric tonsillar enlargement on examination; crypts may be present with purulent debris ●*Test findings:* No relevant tests

Tonsillitis ●*Onset:* Acute ●*Male:female ratio:* M=F ●*Ethnicity:* All ●*Character:* Acute sore throat, worse with swallowing ●*Location:* Oropharynx/tonsils ●*Pattern:* Persistent pain ●*Precipitating factors:* None relevant ●*Relieving factors:* Saltwater gargles; cold liquids ●*Clinical course:* Viral tonsillitis may be self-limited, lasting 3-7 days ●*Co-morbidities:* Tonsillar hypertrophy ●*Procedure results:* Throat swab: bacterial antigen or culture positive ●*Test findings:* No relevant tests

Torticollis ●*Onset:* Subacute, acute, insidious ●*Male:female ratio:* M=F ●*Ethnicity:* All ●*Character:* Pain and spasm in neck, resulting in decreased pain and movement ●*Location:* Neck ●*Pattern:* Nonspecific ●*Precipitating factors:* Unaccustomed exercise or posture, whiplash injury ●*Relieving factors:* NSAIDs, physical therapy ●*Clinical course:* Variable, often resolves spontaneously within 5-10 days ●*Co-morbidities:* None relevant ●*Procedure results:* No relevant procedures ●*Test findings:* No relevant tests

Tourette's syndrome ●*Onset:* Insidious ●*Male:female ratio:* (M)3:(F)1 ●*Ethnicity:* All ●*Character:* Onset before the age of 21, multiple motor tics, one or more vocal tics, fluctuating course and presence of tics for more than 1 year ●*Location:* Nonspecific ●*Pattern:* Nonspecific ●*Precipitating factors:* Excitement, extreme emotional states ●*Relieving factors:* Medication, relaxation ●*Clinical course:* Variable ●*Co-morbidities:* Learning disability, behavioral problems, ADHD ●*Procedure results:* Nonspecific abnormalities may be revealed in EEG studies ●*Test findings:* No relevant tests

Toxic epidermal necrolysis ●*Onset:* Acute ●*Male:female ratio:* M(1):F(2) ●*Ethnicity:* All ●*Character:* Lifethreatening disorder, requires specialist evaluation; heralding signs include sore and burning sensation of conjunctivae, lips and buccal mucosa ●*Location:* Mucous membrane lesions prominent; conjunctival erythema; macular eruption on the face progresses to trunk and extremities; epidermis becomes loose and easily detached with minimal friction; can shed fingernails and toenails ●*Pattern:* Begins as macular erythema progressing to violaceous papules ●*Precipitating factors:* Usually drug-induced, although can be idiopathic; Fas-Fas ligand-mediated apoptosis is a proposed mechanism ●*Relieving factors:* Discontinuation of precipitating drug; administration of systemic steroids early on; intravenous immunoglobulin proposed as anti-Fas modality ●*Clinical course:* Initially, nonspecific prodrome with fever, malaise, headaches and diarrhea; macular eruption progresses to become bullous, total body surface area involvement occurs rapidly; high mortality rate and patients usually need to be managed in a burn unit ●*Co-morbidities:* Other organ systems can be involved; sloughing of respiratory and gastrointestinal tracts can lead to breathing difficulty requiring intubation, and intestinal bleeding or occasionally even bowel perforation; renal failure and sepsis portend a poor prognosis ●*Procedure results:* Skin biopsy reveals complete epidermal necrosis, with minimal to absent inflam_matory infiltrate ●*Test findings:* Patients are usually managed in an ICU setting and are subjected to a wide variety of tests, including monitoring of CBC, liver function tests (LFTs), renal function, chest X-ray and blood cultures

Toxic shock syndrome ●*Onset:* Abrupt ●*Male:female ratio:* M(2):F(3) ●*Ethnicity:* All ●*Character:* Abrupt onset of fever, erythrodermic rash, hypotension, vomiting, and multi-organ system involvement ●*Location:* Systemic (fever, hypotension, tachycardia); entire skin, including palms and soles; mucous membranes (vagina, conjunctivae, oropharynx); entire GI tract (nausea, diarrhea); liver; muscles; kidneys; CNS; lungs (ARDS); other ●*Pattern:* Deep-red rash develops over hours, includes palms and soles, with subsequent desquamation (of palms and soles); patient confused and listless; mucous membranes (conjunctivae, vagina, oropharynx) are hyperemic; patient appears toxic; myalgia is severe, diarrhea profuse ●*Precipitating factors:* Tampon use, onset during menstruation, childbirth, vaginal manipulation, surgical or invasive medical procedure, focal infection with toxin-producing staphylococcus or streptococcus ●*Relieving factors:* ICU care ●*Clinical course:* Rapidly progressive, 5% are fatal, requires aggressive fluid management and ICU care; relapse common but milder ●*Co-morbidities:* Vaginal infection, surgery, diabetes (for strep TSS), alcoholism (for strep TSS) ●*Procedure results:* Isolation of strep or staph from clinical site (strep isolation required for diagnosis, staph isolation not required), production of toxin by isolated bacteria ●*Test findings:* Thrombocytopenia, hypocalcemia, azotemia; elevated creatinine, bilirubin, CPK (MM), hepatic transaminases; leukocytosis with a left shift; abnormal urinary sediment; isolation of strep or staph from clinical site

Toxoplasmosis ●*Onset:* Acute, persistent ●*Male:female ratio:* M=F ●*Ethnicity:* All ●*Character:* Nontender cervical lymphadenopathy in normal host; progressive focal neurologic deficits in immunocompromised host; progressive blurred vision or appearance of scotomas (ocular infection) ●*Location:* Cervical lymph nodes - most common. Occipital, supraclavicular, axillary, mediastinal, inguinal, or generalized lymph nodes - less common; CNS, lungs, myocardium, pericardium, skeletal muscles, posterior choroid and retina, other (systemic) ●*Pattern:* Asymptomatic infection most common; lymphadenopathy is nontender, focal, or generalized, +/- systemic symptoms; visual loss in congenital disease may present decades later and is either uni- or bilateral; CNS disease in AIDS is focal with possible meningoencephalitis ●*Precipitating factors:* Contact with soil frequented by cats or care for cat litterbox; consumption of undercooked or insufficiently frozen meat; acquisition of infection during pregnancy then transplacental transmission ●*Relieving factors:* None relevant ●*Clinical course:* Most acute cases are asymptomatic; symptoms in the noncompromised host usually self-limiting (within weeks) but infection persists for life; ocular infection is progressive and illness in immunocompromised host is rapidly fatal - both require combination drug therapy ●*Co-morbidities:* AIDS, immunosuppression

●*Procedure results:* Single or multiple ring-enhancing lesions on brain CT or MRI; positive toxoplasma IgM (for acute infection) or IgG (in the immunocompromised host), detection of toxoplasma DNA (by PCR) in CSF ●*Test findings:* Sightly elevated protein in CSF

Transient ischemic attack ●*Onset:* Usually middle age and older ●*Male:female ratio:* M=F ●*Ethnicity:* All ●*Character:* Focal, brief and reversible episodes of nonconvulsive neurologic disturbance, usually last less than 15 min, but by definition have to be less than 24h; no permanent sequelae; manifest in a variety of ways from memory lapse to localized weakness, dysarthria ●*Location:* Can occur in any vessel and manifest with symptoms consistent with ischemia of area supplied by the respective vessel ●*Pattern:* Single episodes can cause concern for both embolic or transient thrombotic event; repeat episodes more concerning for stroke; however, many attacks over a long period of time seem to pose less of a risk for stroke ●*Precipitating factors:* Mainly due to focal transient ischemia; hypotension, or cerebral vasospasm are hypothesized to contribute to the attacks; have been associated with outbursts of anger, coughing and exercise; hyperviscosity states must be ruled out; other causes include emboli from various sources such as a mural thrombus or carotid artery stenosis ●*Relieving factors:* Laying supine, rest from emotional outburst or exercise; usually reversible if a transient ischemic attack, and need supportive care and close observation ●*Clinical course:* Repeat episodes warrant a systemic workup; if attacks occur in the same pattern, atherosclerosis and embolism are considered culprits; of strokes that occur after transient ischemic attacks, 20% occur in one month after the first transient ischemic attack, and 50% in first year ●*Co-morbidities:* Polycythemia, hypertension, diabetes, older age, hyperviscosity due to malignancy, hyperlipidemia; macroglobulinemia ●*Procedure results:* Rarely any procedure required as the episodes are reversible ●*Test findings:* If sufficient time available, an MRI scan can help delineate area of ischemia before reversal occurs

Transient neonatal pustular melanosis ●*Onset:* Acute ●*Male:female ratio:* M=F ●*Ethnicity:* African American>Caucasian infant ●*Character:* Evanescent superficial pustules, ruptured pustules with fine scaled collarette, hyperpigmented macules ●*Location:* Anterior neck, forehead, lower back, scalp, trunk, limbs, palms, soles ●*Pattern:* Present at birth, one or all lesions may be found but pustules are earlier and macules are a later phase, pustules last 2-3 days and hyperpigmentation may last 3 months ●*Precipitating factors:* None relevant ●*Relieving factors:* Self-limited ●*Clinical course:* Self-limited ●*Co-morbidities:* None relevant ●*Procedure results:* Cultures negative, smears without eosinophils (as in erythema toxicum) ●*Test findings:* Biopsies in active phase show intra/subcorneal pustule with PMNs, debris, occasional eosinophils; maculae show increased melanization of epidermal cells

Traumatic ruptured diaphragm ●*Onset:* Acute ●*Male:female ratio:* M=F ●*Ethnicity:* All ●*Character:* Tachypnea, hypotension, absent breath sounds, abdominal distension, bowel sounds in chest. Chronic symptoms include vague upper abdominal or chest pain, nausea, or dyspnea. ●*Location:* Most commonly involves the left hemidiaphragm ●*Pattern:* Nonspecific ●*Precipitating factors:* Penetrating trauma to diaphragm or blunt trauma to chest or abdomen ●*Relieving factors:* ABCs, airway management, nasogastric tube, surgical repair ●*Clinical course:* If not recognized and repaired early, may develop chronic symptoms from intermittent herniation months or years later ●*Co-morbidities:* None relevant ●*Procedure results:* Laparoscopy or laparotomy may be required to visualize injury; diagnostic peritoneal lavage may reveal blood; radiographs may show abdominal contents in chest; CT scan, MRI may show rupture ●*Test findings:* No relevant tests

Traumatic tympanic membrane rupture ●*Onset:* Acute ●*Male:female ratio:* M=F ●*Ethnicity:* All ●*Character:* Pain and possibly bleeding at the time of trauma, followed by hearing loss ●*Location:* Affected ear ●*Pattern:* Nonspecific ●*Precipitating factors:* Use of Q-tip or other foreign object in the canal; slap injury to the ear ●*Relieving factors:* Cotton ball stuffed into ear ●*Clinical course:* Small perforations may repair themselves ●*Co-morbidities:* None relevant ●*Procedure results:* Perforated tympanic membrane seen on otoscopy ●*Test findings:* Audiogram may reveal hearing loss and tympanometry shows very large canal volume

Trench fever ● *Onset:* Acute ● *Male:female ratio:* M=F ● *Ethnicity:* All ● *Character:* Abrupt onset of fever, headache, photophobia, myalgia, progressive weight loss ● *Location:* Systemic illness involving bloodstream (bacteremia), meninges, muscles; localized symptoms are rare ● *Pattern:* Fever may be very high, paroxysmal; skeletal muscle pain is severe ● *Precipitating factors:* Homelessness, poor personal hygiene, crowding, body lice ● *Relieving factors:* None relevant ● *Clinical course:* Illness may persist for days to weeks, is relapsing, and requires prolonged antimicrobial therapy ● *Co-morbidities:* Body lice infestation ● *Procedure results:* No relevant procedures ● *Test findings:* Isolation of Bartonella henselae or quintana from blood culture after prolonged incubation (weeks)

Trichomoniasis ● *Onset:* Insidious ● *Male:female ratio:* M=F ● *Ethnicity:* All ● *Character:* Malodorous, yellow or green, vaginal discharge, with vulvar burning and erythema, and occasional dysuria or dyspareunia ● *Location:* Vagina, vulva, urethra, cervix, epididymis, prostate; gingiva (periodontal disease), GI tract ● *Pattern:* In men, the infection is usually asymptomatic. In women, vaginal discharge is purulent, malodorous, and associated with vulvar pruritus and erythema; dysuria and dyspareunia are common ● *Precipitating factors:* Unprotected sexual intercourse ● *Relieving factors:* Metronidazole - avoid in pregnancy ● *Clinical course:* Resolves with treatment ● *Co-morbidities:* None relevant ● *Procedure results:* No relevant procedures ● *Test findings:* Detection of the motile flagellates on microscopic examination of vaginal wet mounts or urethral secretions; specific direct immunofluorescent antibody (DFA) staining

Trichotillomania ● *Onset:* Subacute ● *Male:female ratio:* M=F ● *Ethnicity:* All ● *Character:* Compulsive pulling out of own hair ● *Location:* Scalp ● *Pattern:* Single non-inflamed balding patch with broken hairs of varying lengths ● *Precipitating factors:* Stress ● *Relieving factors:* Sedatives, psychotherapy ● *Clinical course:* Can resolve slowly ● *Co-morbidities:* Mental illness ● *Procedure results:* Skin biopsy helpful ● *Test findings:* No relevant tests

Tricuspid regurgitation ● *Onset:* Typically insidious ● *Male:female ratio:* M=F ● *Ethnicity:* All ● *Character:* TR murmur over right lower sternal border, augments with inspiration, leg-raise, liver compression ● *Location:* If heart failure present, edema typically in dependent places (lower extremities), RUQ abdominal fullness/pain ● *Pattern:* If leg/ankle edema, worse in day when patient is upright ● *Precipitating factors:* Walking; dangling legs makes edema worse ● *Relieving factors:* Leg elevation can reduce leg/ankle edema; treatment with diuretics, salt restriction improves symptoms ● *Clinical course:* Stable or gradually progressive over months-years ● *Co-morbidities:* Seen with RV and LV dysfunction, pulmonary hypertension, pulmonary embolism, tricuspid endocarditis, carcinoid syndrome, congenital RV or tricuspid valve disease, rheumatic heart disease ● *Procedure results:* No relevant procedures ● *Test findings:* Echo reveals tricuspid regurgitation, possibly enlarged right atrium, dilated IVC; right-heart cath reveals elevated RA pressure with CV waves

Tricuspid stenosis ● *Onset:* Insidious ● *Male:female ratio:* M=F ● *Ethnicity:* Increased in cultures with more frequent rheumatic fever ● *Character:* Prominent IJ a-wave, presystolic and diastolic murmurs over left lower sternal border vary with respiration/Valsalva maneuver ● *Location:* Edema typically in dependent places (lower extremities), RUQ abdominal pain. Right-sided heart failure (peripheral edema, liver tenderness, ascites, anorexia), neck fluttering, fatigue ● *Pattern:* Very gradual progression over months-years ● *Precipitating factors:* Rheumatic fever ● *Relieving factors:* Treatment with diuretics, salt-restricted diet improves symptoms ● *Clinical course:* Gradually progressive over months-years, either starting from birth or many years after rheumatic fever ● *Co-morbidities:* History of rheumatic fever, always associated with mitral valve involvement as well; congenital cardiac abnormalities ● *Procedure results:* EKG shows right atrial enlargement out of proportion to RVH ● *Test findings:* Echo reveals tricuspid valve thickening/stenosis with leaflet tip fusion, large right atrium, usually mitral valve thickening/stenosis; right-heart cath reveals elevated RA pressure with large a-wave and blunted y-descent, diastolic pressure gradient across tricuspid valve

Trigeminal neuralgia ●*Onset:* Subacute ●*Male:female ratio:* M<F ●*Ethnicity:* All ●*Character:* Characterized by paroxysms of pain in the distribution of the trigeminal nerve, with no symptoms between attacks; pain is searing or burning and comes on suddenly; each episode may last 15 min and the patient keeps their facial muscles still during the episode as talking can exacerbate the pain; there is no loss of sensation and there may be increased lacrimation ipsilateral to the pain ●*Location:* Distribution of the sensory fibers trigeminal nerve; the second division is involved more frequently than the third division ●*Pattern:* The pain starts from a 'trigger zone' that is a small area on the lip, cheek or nose; pain is rarely bilateral, in which case it can be associated with multiple sclerosis ●*Precipitating factors:* 'Trigger zone' trauma, talking, wind blowing on the trigger zone, stress; dental problems can also be precipitants ●*Relieving factors:* Evaluation of dentition and oral cavity to rule out precipitating factors; carbamazepine or other anticonvulsants may be helpful; surgical procedures may help if there is nerve compression ●*Clinical course:* Course varies, although once neuralgia develops, it needs a workup and therapy, rarely remits spontaneously ●*Co-morbidities:* Multiple sclerosis ●*Procedure results:* Decompression of trigeminal nerve, both for fibrosis and vascular loops, exploration of posterior fossa for patients who are difficult to control ●*Test findings:* CT or MRI scans may demonstrate spaceoccupying lesions in the posterior fossa or along the path of the trigeminal nerve

Tuberculosis ●*Onset:* Acute, subacute, or chronic, persistent for life ●*Male:female ratio:* M>F ●*Ethnicity:* All ●*Character:* Progressive fever, chills, night sweats, anorexia, and weight loss with productive cough, hemoptysis, and chest pain (in pulmonary infection) or any other localized symptom (based on site of infection) ●*Location:* Middle and lower lung zones (primary infection), apical and posterior segment of lungs (reactivation), pleurae, hilar lymph nodes, unilateral cervical lymph nodes, any other or generalized lymph nodes, upper airway and larynx, pericardium, genitourinary tract, spine (thoracic > lumbar > cervical), weightbearing joint (hip, knee > ankle, elbow, wrist); meninges (more at base of brain), GI (ileocecal > any site from mouth to anus), peritoneum, spleen, skin, choroid, any organ ●*Pattern:* Cough is productive; hemoptysis, progressive weight loss, and night sweats are common; paraspinal cold abscesses are common with spinal disease, may imitate any inflammatory disease ●*Precipitating factors:* Residence in/travel to/immigration from areas of high prevalence; HIV or AIDS; substance abuse; diabetes; silicosis; head or neck cancer; lymphoproliferative disease; renal failure; corticosteroid therapy; organ transplantation; known exposure to a case of respiratory tuberculosis ●*Relieving factors:* None relevant ●*Clinical course:* Primary tuberculosis (illness directly following infection) is most common in children; reactivation (postprimary tuberculosis) is most common within the first 1-2 years after infection; infection persists for life with an overall 10% lifetime risk of reactivation illness; reactivation risk is higher with immunosuppression, HIV, and chronic illness; reinfection is possible; mortality is high in the absence of prolonged combination therapy ●*Co-morbidities:* HIV and AIDS, substance abuse, diabetes, silicosis, head or neck cancer, lymphoproliferative disease, renal failure, corticosteroid therapy, organ transplantation, malnutrition, kyphosis, infertility ●*Procedure results:* Positive tuberculin skin test; detection of acid-fast organisms on smears from sputum, biopsy material; detection of Mycobacterium pneumonia (MTB) DNA (by PCR/other amplification technique) in clinical specimen, isolation of MTB from culture; upper lobe, posterior segment of lower lobe, or other lung zone infiltrate, calcified nodule(s), cavity (ies), and/or pleural effusion on chest imaging; pericardial thickening or effusion on echocardiogram; basilar meningeal enhancement or enhancing lesions on head CT/MRI; spinal osteomyelitis with spondylitis and adjacent cold abscess on spinal CT/MRI; caseating granulomata with giant cell reaction ●*Test findings:* Anemia, elevated ESR, thrombocytosis, monocytosis, pancytopenia (in miliary disease), pyuria, proteinuria, hematuria, lymphocytic (occasionally neutrophilic) CSF pleocytosis, low CSF glucose, elevated CSF protein, elevated alkaline phosphatase (in miliary disease), hypercalcemia

Tuberous sclerosis complex ● *Onset:* Subacute ● *Male:female ratio:* M=F ● *Ethnicity:* All ● *Character:* Infantile spasms, seizures, sebaceous adenomas, shagreen patch = orange peel-like raised lesion in lumbosacral area, sub/periungual fibromas, retinal lesions, hypopigmented skin lesions ● *Location:* Skin, brain, heart, eyes, kidneys, bone ● *Pattern:* Nonspecific ● *Precipitating factors:* Autosomal dominant TS gene chromosome 9q34 (TSC1) and 16p13 (TSC2) ● *Relieving factors:* None relevant ● *Clinical course:* Progressive, lifelong ● *Co-morbidities:* Cardiac rhabdomyomas, kidney hamartomas/polycystic disease, pulmonary angiomyolipomas ● *Procedure results:* Tubers/calcification on head MRI, abnormal EEG, ash-leaf lesion enhanced with Wood's lamp, abnormal retinal exam ● *Test findings:* No relevant tests

Tularemia ● *Onset:* Acute ● *Male:female ratio:* M>F ● *Ethnicity:* All ● *Character:* Abrupt onset of fever, chills, headache, and myalgia followed by tender localized lymphadenopathy and a skin ulcer, conjunctivitis, sore throat, atypical pneumonitis with pleural effusions, or nonspecific systemic illness ● *Location:* Systemic illness involving bloodstream, lymph nodes (head and neck > other), exposed skin (focal papule, ulcer, eschar), pharynx, conjunctiva, lungs, pleura, muscles, liver, spleen, (peritoneum, pericardium, endocardium, bones - less common) ● *Pattern:* Fever and chills begin abruptly, then subside, followed by localized symptoms; skin ulcer is indurated and persists, not healing, for weeks; adenopathy is tender; exudative or membranous pharyngitis ● *Precipitating factors:* Tick bite or tabanid flies contact in endemic areas, inhalation of aerosol from soil contaminated by infected domestic or wild animals, direct contact with infected animals occupational exposure (laboratory workers, hunters, veterinarians) ● *Relieving factors:* None relevant ● *Clinical course:* Fever occurs 2-5 days after inoculation; symptoms last 1-4 weeks but may continue for months or relapse; severe illness may be fatal; symptoms respond rapidly to antimicrobial therapy ● *Co-morbidities:* Tick bite ● *Procedure results:* Isolation of Francisella tularensis from lymph node aspirate, blood, other; fourfold rise in specific antibody, or a single value >=1:160, detection of F. tularensis DNA by PCR; bilateral patchy infiltrated, lobar consolidation, cavities, or pleural effusion on CXR ● *Test findings:* Normal or elevated WBC, mildly elevated hepatic transaminases

Turner's syndrome ● *Onset:* Subacute ● *Male:female ratio:* F ● *Ethnicity:* All ● *Character:* Infants: edema of dorsum of hands/feet/loose skin at nape of neck; neck webbing, low posterior hairline, broad chest/wide-spaced nipples, short stature, mental deficiency ● *Location:* Entire body ● *Pattern:* Nonspecific ● *Precipitating factors:* XO - major locus involved is on region of X chromosome (PAR 1) ● *Relieving factors:* Recombinant growth hormone, estrogen replacement therapy ● *Clinical course:* Lifelong ● *Co-morbidities:* Cardiac: aortic coarctation/stenosis, mitral valve prolapse; renal: pelvic/horseshoe kidney, double collecting system; hypertension, primary hypogonadism, thyroid disorders, inflammatory bowel disease (IBD), otitis media, sensorineural hearing loss, gonadoblastoma associated with mosaicism of Y chromosome ● *Procedure results:* U/S of heart, kidneys, ovaries, X-ray shows shortened 4 metatarsal/metacarpal/scoliosis, epiphyseal dysgenesis ● *Test findings:* Chromosomal analysis: XO, mosaic: XX/XO, XY/XO; elevated follicle-stimulating hormone (FSH)/luteinizing hormone (LH)

Typhoid fever ● *Onset:* Acute, insidious ● *Male:female ratio:* M=F ● *Ethnicity:* Seen in developing nations ● *Character:* Nonspecific illness with fever and abdominal pain; fever in travelers ● *Location:* Systemic (bacteremia), GI tract (ileocecal area>other), spleen, liver, CNS (delirium), skin (faint rash) ● *Pattern:* GI symptoms may resolve before the onset of fever. Salmon-colored rash on trunk only (30%, rose spots). Pulse-temperature dissociation (relative bradycardia) is common ● *Precipitating factors:* Worldwide distribution, more common in residents of/travelers to tropical areas; fecal-oral transmission ● *Relieving factors:* None relevant ● *Clinical course:* Incubation: 5-21 days, untreated clinical illness lasts 2-4 weeks with long convalescence; symptoms resolve within 3-5 days of appropriate antibiotic therapy ● *Co-morbidities:* Intestinal perforation or hemorrhage, immune complex glomerulonephritis, schistosomiasis ● *Procedure results:* Gram-negative rods on blood culture or punch biopsy of skin rash; isolation of Salmonella typhi from blood ● *Test findings:* Anemia, leukopenia (more often than leukocytosis), left shift, elevated hepatic transaminases, elevated CPK, GNRs in blood culture, isolation of S. typhi from blood

Ulcerative colitis ●*Onset:* Insidious ●*Male:female ratio:* M=F ●*Ethnicity:* More common in Jewish population ●*Character:* Diarrhea with blood, mucus; urgency and tenesmus are common; abdominal pain is variable, but can be severe; may have fever, malaise. Proctitis alone may cause constipation rather than diarrhea. Abdomen may be tender over affected regions of bowel; extraintestinal signs include episcleritis, uveitis, aphthous ulcers, erythema nodosum, pyoderma gangrenosum, ankylosing spondylitis ●*Location:* Abdomen ●*Pattern:* Diarrhea may be stimulated by food intake; nocturnal diarrhea is common ●*Precipitating factors:* Food intake ●*Relieving factors:* Proctitis or left colon disease may respond to hydrocortisone or mesalamine enemas; oral mesalamine and steroids are effective - in refractory cases, immunosuppressives such as 6-mercaptopurine may be effective; colectomy is curative ●*Clinical course:* Intermittent flares of disease activity of varying severity ●*Co-morbidities:* Primary sclerosing cholangitis; colon cancer (risk increases after 8-10 years of colitis); ankylosing spondylitis ●*Procedure results:* Colonoscopy reveals active inflammation and ulceration; biopsies show acute and chronic inflammation ●*Test findings:* WBC usually elevated during flares; ESR elevated; anemia may be present

Unstable angina ●*Onset:* Acute ●*Male:female ratio:* M>F ●*Ethnicity:* All groups ●*Character:* Usually substernal chest pain, pressure or heaviness with radiation to the jaw or left arm. Can present atypically with SOB, diaphoresis, nausea ●*Location:* Nonspecific ●*Pattern:* Chest pain which may get better with rest or sublingual nitroglycerin; can last as short as a few minutes to much longer, depending on acuity of presentation ●*Precipitating factors:* Unclear as to exact precipitating factors. Proposed factors that may lead to coronary plaque rupture include stress, physical exertion, vasoconstriction ●*Relieving factors:* Often, therapy is with nitrates, heparin, beta-blockers, morphine; also Gp IIb/IIIa inhibitors. May need coronary intervention with PTCA/stenting for pain relief ●*Clinical course:* Treated medically or may require more invasive evaluation and therapy ●*Co-morbidities:* Diabetes mellitus, hypertension, hyperlipidemia, smoking, cocaine use, positive family history of CAD ●*Procedure results:* May include ST/T wave changes on EKG, positive cardiac enzymes such as CK or troponins, positive cardiac stress test, coronary angiography revealing CAD ●*Test findings:* May include ST depressions or T wave inversions on EKG, positive cardiac enzymes such as CPK or troponins, positive cardiac stress test, coronary angiography revealing CAD

Upper GI bleeding ●*Onset:* Subacute to acute but if bleeding is slow can be insidious ●*Male:female ratio:* M=F ●*Ethnicity:* All ●*Character:* Melena, hematemesis, abdominal pain, lightheadedness, syncope, fatigue ●*Location:* Nonspecific ●*Pattern:* Nonspecific ●*Precipitating factors:* Nonsteroidal anti-inflammatory drugs, aspirin, Helicobacter pylori ●*Relieving factors:* Proton pump inhibitors, endoscopic therapy, removal of causal agent, treatment of Helicobacter pylori, for severe, refractory cases surgery is required ●*Clinical course:* Usually self-limited and treatable but has significant morbidity and mortality especially if in an elderly patient or associated with liver disease ●*Co-morbidities:* Liver disease ●*Procedure results:* Upper endoscopy: bleeding source; nasogastric lavage: blood ●*Test findings:* Anemia, elevated urea and creatinine

Upper respiratory tract infections ●*Onset:* Acute ●*Male:female ratio:* M=F ●*Ethnicity:* All ●*Character:* Clear nasal discharge, 'scratchy' throat - viral infections. Erythematous tonsils, exudates, tender adenopathy - bacterial and EBV pharyngitis ●*Location:* Nasal mucosa (rhinitis), throat (pharyngitis, tonsillitis), upper airways (croup, laryngotracheobronchitis bronchitis) ●*Pattern:* Contagious, clusters of patients ●*Precipitating factors:* Ill contacts ●*Relieving factors:* Decongestants, NSAIDs, antihistamines, lozenges ●*Clinical course:* Acute, self-limited; antibiotics shorten course of bacterial infections; untreated streptococcal pharyngitis may lead to rheumatic fever; epiglottitis may cause abrupt airway obstruction ●*Co-morbidities:* None relevant ●*Procedure results:* No relevant procedures ●*Test findings:* Streptococcal pharyngitis; throat culture grows strep

Urate nephropathy ●*Onset:* Acute to subacute ●*Male:female ratio:* M=F ●*Ethnicity:* All ●*Character:* May be asymptomatic; symptoms/signs of renal failure if rapid rising creatinine (i.e. nausea, fluid overload, poor urine output); may have flank pain if ureteral obstruction ●*Location:* Flank ●*Pattern:* Colicky pain, when present, may radiate to groin ●*Precipitating factors:* Gout; lymphoma, leukemia, or myeloproliferative disorders, especially right after chemotherapy (tumor lysis syndrome); other causes of hyperuricemia ●*Relieving factors:* Pre-treatment of chemo patients with allopurinol; alkalinization of the urine (uric acid crystals precipitate in acidic environment); IV fluids, diuretics to maintain urine output (flushing through kidney) ●*Clinical course:* Can cause acute renal failure ●*Co-morbidities:* Gout ●*Procedure results:* Urinalysis: protein; serum electrolytes: raised urea creatinine; urine chemistries: decreased creatinine clearance ●*Test findings:* Uric acid crystals; serum uric acid elevated; ratio of urinary uric acid to creatinine often >1:1; associated electrolyte abnormalities (tumor lysis syndrome) include hyperkalemia, hyperuricemia, hyperphosphatemia, and hypocalcemia

Uremic encephalopathy ●*Onset:* Acute to subacute ●*Male:female ratio:* M=F ●*Ethnicity:* All ●*Character:* Mental status changes; form of metabolic encephalopathy (confusion, usually nonfocal neurologic findings) ●*Location:* CNS ●*Pattern:* Confusion; decreased level of consciousness; difficulty with orientation ●*Precipitating factors:* Renal failure ●*Relieving factors:* Dialysis ●*Clinical course:* Usually continues as long as renal failure persists; no direct association with absolute blood urea nitrogen (BUN), but increasing incidence with BUN >100 ●*Co-morbidities:* Other manifestations of uremia: nausea/vomiting, dysfunctional platelets (bleeding), pericarditis ●*Procedure results:* No relevant procedures ●*Test findings:* Asterixis may be seen; abnormal mental status exam; elevated BUN, creatinine

Ureterocele ●*Onset:* Chronic or insidious ●*Male:female ratio:* M(1):F(4) ●*Ethnicity:* Almost exclusively in Caucasians ●*Character:* Mostly identified on prenatal ultrasound; UTI symptoms or pain from a mass effect occasionally seen ●*Location:* Abdomen, pelvis ●*Pattern:* Bilateral in 10% of patients; 80% arising from the upper pole of a duplicated renal system ●*Precipitating factors:* None relevant ●*Relieving factors:* Surgical correction ●*Clinical course:* Potential for infection, sepsis, calculus formation, urine retention, urinary incontinence and even obstruction of contralateral kidney if untreated ●*Co-morbidities:* Dysplastic kidney; vesicoureteral reflux ●*Procedure results:* No relevant procedures ●*Test findings:* Cystic mass in bladder on ultrasound; filling defect on IVP or cystogram

Urethral prolapse ●*Onset:* Subacute ●*Male:female ratio:* F ●*Ethnicity:* Almost exclusively in young African-American girls ●*Character:* Bloody spotting on underwear ●*Location:* Urethral meatus ●*Pattern:* Erythematous, inflamed protruding mucosa surrounding the urethral meatus ●*Precipitating factors:* Menopause in older women ●*Relieving factors:* Estrogen cream to meatus 2-3 times daily; sitz bath; surgical excision ●*Clinical course:* May not respond to clinical treatment and require surgical excision ●*Co-morbidities:* None relevant ●*Procedure results:* No relevant procedures ●*Test findings:* No relevant tests

Urethral stricture ●*Onset:* Chronic ●*Male:female ratio:* M ●*Ethnicity:* All ●*Character:* Difficulty in urination with obstructive and irritative voiding symptoms ●*Location:* Penis, urethra ●*Pattern:* Mild voiding symptoms initially, slowly progressing to urinary retention ●*Precipitating factors:* Urethral catheterization; prior urological surgeries; urethritis; balanitis xerotica obliterans; trauma ●*Relieving factors:* Dilation; internal urethrotomy; open reconstruction ●*Clinical course:* Progressive if untreated ●*Co-morbidities:* Urethral catheterization; urethritis; balanitis xerotica obliterans; UTI; prostatitis; epididymitis; trauma ●*Procedure results:* No relevant procedures ●*Test findings:* Urethroscopy and dynamic urethrogram to define location, length, depth, and density of stricture

Urethritis ●*Onset:* Subacute ●*Male:female ratio:* M=F ●*Ethnicity:* More prevalent in urban non Caucasians ●*Character:* Painful urination and discharge; suprapubic pain in women; men more often symptomatic ●*Location:* Pelvis, suprapubic area, genitalia/perineal area

●*Pattern:* Waxing and waning of symptoms ●*Precipitating factors:* Sexual intercourse; multiple sexual partners; poor hygiene; urinary tract instrumentation ●*Relieving factors:* Antibiotics, urinary tract analgesic agents ●*Clinical course:* Progressing to urethral strictures or PID if untreated ●*Co-morbidities:* None relevant ●*Procedure results:* Strictures, warts, or foreign body on urethroscopy or urethrography ●*Test findings:* Gram stain: PMN with intracellular Gram -ve diplococci = gonococcal urethritis; sheets of leukocytes without organism = nongonococcal urethritis; special cultures for chlamydia

Urinary tract infection ●*Onset:* Acute, subacute ●*Male:female ratio:* M<F ●*Ethnicity:* All ●*Character:* Any or all of the following: dysuria, urgency, frequency, pain, fever, hematuria ●*Location:* Pelvis, suprapubic area, flank ●*Pattern:* Recurrent or persistent in some cases ●*Precipitating factors:* Sexual intercourse; poor hygiene; urinary tract instrumentation; urinary outlet obstruction ●*Relieving factors:* Antibiotics; urinary tract analgesic agents ●*Clinical course:* Progressive if untreated; with treatment: symptoms improve within 24h for simple cystitis, 4-5 days before symptoms improve in pyelonephritis ●*Co-morbidities:* Urethral stricture, urine incontinence, pregnancy, urolithiasis, prostatitis, benign prostatic hyperplasia (BPH), diabetes, urethritis ●*Procedure results:* Any of the following on cystourethroscopy: strictures, outlet obstruction, stones; X-ray imaging (kidneys, ureter, bladder [KUB], intravenous pyelogram [IVP], CT, or U/S) to rule out stones and other abnormalities ●*Test findings:* Any of the following on urinalysis: pyuria, hematuria, bacteuria, positive nitrate, positive leukocyte esterase; urine culture and sensitivity: 100,000 bacteria/mL or lower counts in presence of pyuria are diagnostic

Urticaria ●*Onset:* Acute ●*Male:female ratio:* M=F ●*Ethnicity:* All ●*Character:* Itching ●*Location:* Any skin location ●*Pattern:* Circumscribed red edematous plaques ●*Precipitating factors:* Medicines, foods, cold temperature ●*Relieving factors:* Antihistamines, steroids ●*Clinical course:* Lesion gone in 24-48 hours, episode may last few weeks ●*Co-morbidities:* None relevant ●*Procedure results:* No relevant procedures ●*Test findings:* No relevant tests

Uterine myomas ●*Onset:* Insidious ●*Male:female ratio:* F ●*Ethnicity:* All ●*Character:* Irregular vaginal bleeding, infertility, pelvic pain/pressure, dysmenorrhea ●*Location:* Uterus/pelvis ●*Pattern:* Heavy/painful menstruation ●*Precipitating factors:* None relevant ●*Relieving factors:* Myomectomy ●*Clinical course:* Resolution after menopause ●*Co-morbidities:* Uterine sarcomas, infertility ●*Procedure results:* Homogeneous uterine lesions on ultrasound ●*Test findings:* No relevant tests

Uterine prolapse ●*Onset:* Gradual, insidious ●*Male:female ratio:* F ●*Ethnicity:* Most common in Caucasians ●*Character:* Heaviness or fullness in the pelvis associated with sensation of uterus descending into vagina ●*Location:* Descent of uterus into vagina either remaining within the vagina (primary); cervix protruding beyond introitus (secondary); entire uterus outside of vulva (third degree) ●*Pattern:* First degree prolapse may be intermittently symptomatic ●*Precipitating factors:* Pelvic relaxation following delivery; associated with chronic cough, ascites, weightlifting, habitual straining due to constipation ●*Relieving factors:* Perineal exercises (Kegel exercises) to strengthen pelvic floor, use of pessary or definitive surgery ●*Clinical course:* First degree prolapse may progress if untreated ●*Co-morbidities:* Urinary incontinence ●*Procedure results:* No relevant procedures ●*Test findings:* Diagnosed on pelvic examination; may require attempts to elicit prolapse with maneuvers/tenaculum

Uveitis ●*Onset:* Acute, subacute, insidious ●*Male:female ratio:* M=F ●*Ethnicity:* All ❶ *Character:* Achey eye pain; photophobia; cillary flush on examination ●*Location:* Uveal tract ❸ *Pattern:* Can affect one or both eyes simultaneously ●*Precipitating factors:* None relevant ●*Relieving factors:* Topical steroids or NSAIDs relieves symptoms ●*Clinical course:* Course variable depending on cause ●*Co-morbidities:* Can be associated with many conditions including sarcoidosis, connective tissue disorders, infectious conditions such as TB ●*Procedure results:* Workup tailored for each individual case which may include chest X-ray, ACE, PPD, fluorescent treponemal antibodoy test (FTA-ABs), HLA typing, Lyme titers, C-ANCA, others ●*Test findings:* Chest X-ray abnormal in TB or sarcoid; ACE elevated in sarcoidosis; certain HLA haplotypes typically associated with certain forms of uveitis; C-ANCA positive in Wegner's disease

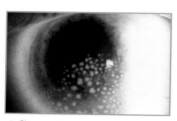

❶ *Character* Large, 'mutton-fat' keratic precipitates on the posterior corneal surface

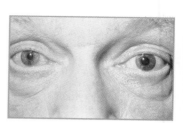

❸ *Pattern* Note the constricted pupil and ciliary injection in the right eye

Vaginal bleeding during pregnancy ● *Onset:* Acute ● *Male:female ratio:* F ● *Ethnicity:* All ● *Character:* Blood per vagina with or without pain ● *Location:* Vaginal ● *Pattern:* Bleeding ● *Precipitating factors:* Spontaneous; may be associated with trauma, intercourse ● *Relieving factors:* Variable ● *Clinical course:* Ranges from progression to delivery to self-limited ● *Co-morbidities:* Abruptio placentae, placenta previa, preterm labor, ectopic pregnancy ● *Procedure results:* U/S to eliminate placenta previa and ectopic pregnancy, determine fetal viability, and detect placental abruption ● *Test findings:* No relevant tests

Vaginal malignancy ● *Onset:* Insidious ● *Male:female ratio:* F ● *Ethnicity:* All ● *Character:* Irregular vaginal spotting/bleeding ● *Location:* Vagina ● *Pattern:* Irregular bleeding, vaginal ulcer, abnormal Pap test ● *Precipitating factors:* Exposure to intrauterine diethylstilbestrol (DES), prior chemotherapy, chronic vaginal irritation ● *Relieving factors:* Surgery; chemotherapy; radiotherapy ● *Clinical course:* Progression to invasion and distant metastasis ● *Co-morbidities:* DES exposure ● *Procedure results:* Abnormal Pap test ● *Test findings:* Pathologic suggestion of cellular dysplasia

Varicocele ● *Onset:* Subacute (most common); acute (least common) ● *Male:female ratio:* M ● *Ethnicity:* All ● *Character:* Three different presentations: asymptomatic (most common); infertility; or soft mass with dull ache ● *Location:* Upper scrotum ● *Pattern:* Majority on left side. Bilateral in 5-20% of cases. <2% unilateral right side ● *Precipitating factors:* Standing for long period of time; straining ● *Relieving factors:* Supine position; surgical correction; balloon embolization ● *Clinical course:* Slowly progressive; may indefinitely remain asymptomatic; surgical correction improving semen quality in up to 70% and pregnancy in 50% of couples; resolution of pain to be expected; recurrence of pain in 25% of patients ● *Co-morbidities:* None relevant ● *Procedure results:* Doppler ultrasound confirming diagnosis in subtle cases ● *Test findings:* Semen analysis: stressed pattern (decrease in number, motility, and morphology of sperms)

Varicose veins ● *Onset:* Insidious ● *Male:female ratio:* M(1):F(5) ● *Ethnicity:* All ● *Character:* Visible dilation and tortuosity of superficial veins; dull ache; may see edema; skin ulcerations ● *Location:* Varicosities seen in lower extremities, dull ache in legs, mild edema in ankles, skin ulcerations near ankles ● *Pattern:* Leg ache and edema worse during day, improved overnight ● *Precipitating factors:* Aching and edema worse with standing ● *Relieving factors:* Aching and edema improve with leg elevation; elastic compression stockings improve symptoms ● *Clinical course:* Symptoms may wax and wane, varicosities may gradually progress over years, elastic support hose can treat symptoms and slow progression ● *Co-morbidities:* DVT or venous insufficiency ● *Procedure results:* No relevant procedures ● *Test findings:* No relevant tests

Vascular aneurysm ● *Onset:* Acute, subacute, or insidious depending on cause ● *Male:female ratio:* M=F ● *Ethnicity:* All ● *Character:* Localized dilatation of a blood vessel wall with symptoms dependent on cause and location ● *Location:* Central, visceral, peripheral, cerebral arteries ● *Pattern:* Central and cerebral aneurysms may rupture. Peripheral aneurysms cause symptoms by thrombosis or embolization. Mass effect possible in all types ● *Precipitating factors:* Genetic predisposition ● *Relieving factors:* Surgery, stenting, risk modification (e.g. manage hypertension and hypercholesterolemia, discontinue smoking) ● *Clinical course:* Rate of progression depends on cause: with atherosclerosis, slow over years; with trauma or infection, subacute over days to months ● *Co-morbidities:* Atherosclerotic disease, genetic predisposition (e.g. in polycystic kidney disease, connective tissue disease), trauma, infection, vasculitis ● *Procedure results:* Angiography/CT/MRI/ultrasound/transesophageal echocardiography demonstrate vessel dilatation. Lumbar puncture demonstrates blood from leaking/ruptured intracerebral vessel ● *Test findings:* No relevant tests

Vasculitis ●*Onset:* Acute ●*Male:female ratio:* M=F ●*Ethnicity:* All ●*Character:* Constitutional complaints ●*Location:* Rash on trunk and lower extremities ●*Pattern:* No specific pattern ●*Precipitating factors:* None relevant ●*Relieving factors:* Corticosteroids or cytotoxic agents ●*Clinical course:* Acute onset, usually progressive ●*Co-morbidities:* None relevant ●*Procedure results:* Biopsy of involved organ reveals inflammatory infiltrate within affected vessel wall ●*Test findings:* Elevated acute phase reactants; some forms have increased levels of ANCA antibodies

Vasomotor rhinitis ●*Onset:* Chronic, insidious ●*Male:female ratio:* M=F ●*Ethnicity:* All ●*Character:* Diffuse bilateral clear rhinorrhea ●*Location:* Nasal cavity ●*Pattern:* Almost constant nasal drainage, often worse in the morning ●*Precipitating factors:* Emotional stress, solvent exposure ●*Relieving factors:* Over-the-counter antihistamines ●*Clinical course:* Usually chronic and persistent ●*Co-morbidities:* Allergic rhinitis ●*Procedure results:* No relevant procedures ●*Test findings:* Relatively normal examination on nasal endoscopy

Vasovagal response ●*Onset:* Acute ●*Male:female ratio:* M=F ●*Ethnicity:* All ●*Character:* Lightheadedness, warmth, yawning, nausea/vomiting, vision 'blacking out', sweating, pallor, possible fainting (loss of consciousness) ●*Location:* Systemic symptoms, mainly concerning sensation of feeling faint and losing consciousness ●*Pattern:* Relatively acute onset of symptoms, generally with progression over 1-5 minutes ●*Precipitating factors:* Commonly seen in setting of heat, fright, sight of blood or needles, fatigue, urination, severe coughing; can be associated with alcohol intake, dehydration; generally occurs when patient is upright (standing or seated) ●*Relieving factors:* Lying down and elevating legs helps relieve lightheadedness; symptoms abate spontaneously within minutes; caffeine can help relieve symptoms; atropine will reverse the bradycardia and hypotension ●*Clinical course:* Vasovagal episode typically resolves spontaneously over several minutes with no sequelae (unless syncope with fall and injury has occurred); patient may be prone to future episodes, especially in setting of similar predisposing factors ●*Co-morbidities:* Not necessarily related to other diagnoses or conditions; it is an independent, excessive reflex mediated by vagal fibers ●*Procedure results:* No relevant procedures ●*Test findings:* Tilt-table test may demonstrate sudden abnormal drop in heart rate and BP, although this test lacks sensitivity and specificity; during vasovagal episode, BP is low and heart rate is inappropriately slow

Venous insufficiency ●*Onset:* Insidious ●*Male:female ratio:* M<F ●*Ethnicity:* All ●*Character:* Dull ache and swelling in leg(s); possible erythema; hyperpigmentation and skin ulceration; may lead to cellulitis ●*Location:* One or both legs, edema seen distally, ulceration of medial and lateral malleoli ●*Pattern:* Symptoms worsen through day, are relieved overnight ●*Precipitating factors:* Prolonged standing or sitting can precipitate aching and swelling ●*Relieving factors:* Leg elevation improves symptoms; graduated compression stockings worn during day can palliate ●*Clinical course:* Symptoms may be stable or gradually progressive over years; compression stockings help; recurrent ulceration, edema, cellulitis may result ●*Co-morbidities:* DVT can lead to venous swelling and valve incompetence, but also see primary deep venous valve incompetence; varicose veins may result ●*Procedure results:* No relevant procedures ●*Test findings:* Venous ultrasound may show old DVT

Ventricular septal defect ●*Onset:* Acute ●*Male:female ratio:* M=F; M>F if due to myocardial infarction ●*Ethnicity:* All ●*Character:* Holosystolic murmur at left lower scapular/sternal border, short systolic ejection murmur at apex, mid-diastolic murmur if large ventricular septal defect (VSD); dyspnea, poor feeding, diaphoresis ●*Location:* Chest/cardiac ●*Pattern:* If large VSD, worsening symptoms ●*Precipitating factors:* Abnormal embryological development ●*Relieving factors:* Small VSD: spontaneous closure; large/persistent VSD: digoxin/diuretics surgical closure ●*Clinical course:* Progressive cardiac/congestive heart failure (CHF) symptoms ●*Co-morbidities:* Eisenmenger's complex, pulmonary stenosis, tetralogy of Fallot, chromosomal anomalies, prematurity ●*Procedure results:* Chest X-ray: normal or cardiomegaly, increased pulmonary vasculature if large VSD; ECG: normal or left ventricular hypertrophy (LVH)/right ventricular hypertrophy (RVH) if large VSD; abnormal echocardiogram ●*Test findings:* No relevant tests

Ventricular tachycardia ● *Onset:* Acute ● *Male:female ratio:* M=F ● *Ethnicity:* All ● *Character:* May be asymptomatic, fluttering in chest, possible presyncope or loss of consciousness ● *Location:* Nonspecific ● *Pattern:* Sudden paroxysmal onset of symptoms ● *Precipitating factors:* Spontaneous, can be provoked by acute or old MI, electrolyte imbalance (K+, Mg++, Ca++), medications with proarrhythmic properties ● *Relieving factors:* Spontaneous resolution, treatment with antiarrhythmic medication (lidocaine, amiodarone), electrical cardioversion ● *Clinical course:* Depending on VT rate and underlying cardiac function, fatal hemodynamic instability may result; depending on underlying cause and treatment, may recur ● *Co-morbidities:* Prior or acute MI, structural heart disease, prolonged QT interval (congenital or drug-related), metabolic disorders, RV dysplasia ● *Procedure results:* No relevant procedures ● *Test findings:* ECG reveals wide complex tachycardia (monomorphic or polymorphic), using Brugada criteria to distinguish SVT with aberrancy

Viral conjunctivitis ● *Onset:* Acute ● *Male:female ratio:* M=F ● *Ethnicity:* All ❶ *Character:* Painless red eye with mucoid, watery discharge and irritation; lids stick together.; normal vision, normal pupils, normal intraocular pressure ❷ *Location:* Conjunctivae - unilateral or bilateral ● *Pattern:* Worsens over the first week then improves over the next week or so ● *Precipitating factors:* Prior upper respiratory tract infection or exposure to someone with viral conjunctivitis ● *Relieving factors:* Cool compresses and artificial tears can relieve the associated itching and discomfort ● *Clinical course:* Self-limited ● *Co-morbidities:* Fever and pharyngitis are seen in the pharyngoconjunctival variant ● *Procedure results:* No relevant procedures ● *Test findings:* Mononuclear WBCs are seen on a conjunctival smear; palpebral conjunctival follicle formation and preauricular lymphadenopathy

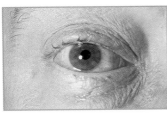

❶ *Character* Red eye, serous discharge, and normal pupil are characteristic

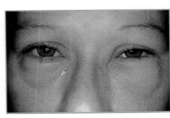

❷ *Location* Red eyes, serous discharge, and even lid edema can occur with acute viral conjunctivitis

Viral hepatitis ● *Onset:* Subacute ● *Male:female ratio:* M(2):F(1) for hepatitis B ● *Ethnicity:* All ● *Character:* Jaundice, fever, malaise, arthralgias, myalgias, right upper quadrant pain. Hepatitis B: prodrome of malaise, arthritis, or urticarial rash may precede onset of jaundice ● *Location:* Pain is in the right upper quadrant ● *Pattern:* Nonspecific ● *Precipitating factors:* Hepatitis A: contaminated food (shellfish, fruits, vegetables). Hepatitis B: unprotected sex or blood exposure. Hepatitis C: blood exposure. Hepatitis E: waterborne in endemic areas ● *Relieving factors:* Disease resolves over 3-6 weeks without treatment ● *Clinical course:* Symptoms persist for 3-6 weeks, then resolve; risk of liver failure is 0.3% in hepatitis A, 1% in hepatitis B; hepatitis C rarely causes hepatic failure; hepatitis E causes liver failure primarily in pregnant women ● *Co-morbidities:* None relevant ● *Procedure results:* Liver biopsy is not usually necessary for diagnosis ● *Test findings:* Serologic testing is usually diagnostic, but PCR (polymerase chain reaction) testing can be used to diagnose hepatitis B or C

Viral meningitis ●*Onset:* Acute ●*Male:female ratio:* M=F ●*Ethnicity:* All ●*Character:* Acute onset of severe headache, fever, meningismus, with lymphocytic pleocytosis of CSF ●*Location:* Meninges, CSF ●*Pattern:* Severe frontal/retro-orbital headache with meningismus, fever, malaise, mild drowsiness, pain with eye movement ●*Precipitating factors:* Causative organisms have seasonal variation ●*Relieving factors:* Acetaminophen, rest ●*Clinical course:* Self-limiting with full recovery within 1 week in most cases ●*Co-morbidities:* None relevant ●*Procedure results:* CSF: lymphocytic pleocytosis (usually <1000, may be neutrophilic very early in course), mildly elevated protein, normal glucose, no organisms on Gram stain. Positive specific viral serology ●*Test findings:* Blood: low, normal, mildly elevated WBC

Viral pneumonia ●*Onset:* Acute ●*Male:female ratio:* M=F ●*Ethnicity:* All ●*Character:* Fever, dry cough, headache, myalgias, malaise, fatigue, dyspnea ●*Location:* Chest ●*Pattern:* Bronchial breath sounds, inspiratory rales, egophony ●*Precipitating factors:* Exposure to ill contacts ●*Relieving factors:* Supportive care with hydration, supplemental oxygen as needed and antitussives. If influenza or varicella pneumonia, consider antiviral therapy ●*Clinical course:* Illness lasts days-weeks. Low mortality, unless influenza or varicella (esp. complicating pregnancy) ●*Co-morbidities:* Bacterial superinfection ●*Procedure results:* Some centers offer rapid viral isolation ●*Test findings:* Leukocytosis, focal or diffuse infiltrate(s) on chest X-ray, sputum with neutrophils with or without viral cytopathic changes

Vitamin B12 deficiency ●*Onset:* Insidious (years) ●*Male:female ratio:* M<F ●*Ethnicity:* Most common in Northern European Caucasians; incidence in African Americans approximately equal to non-Northern European Caucasians ●*Character:* Pallor, shortness of breath (manifestations of anemia); neurologic manifestations ranging from subacute combined degeneration of dorsal and lateral spinal columns to mental status or memory changes; hypercoaguable state may result from elevated homocysteine, which may be seen with B12 deficiency; glossitis possible; associated autoimmune disease may coexist (thyroiditis); increased risk of gastric cancer or gastric carcinoid ●*Location:* Anemia: bone marrow, peripheral blood; neurologic: CNS ●*Pattern:* Megaloblastic anemia; smear may also show hypersegmented polymorphs. Neurologic symptoms often involve symmetric neuropathy, affected legs>arms. Paresthesias and/or ataxia may develop. Loss of vibration and joint position sense. May develop clonus, paraplegia, fecal/urinary incontinence ●*Precipitating factors:* Gastric resection, achlorhydria, ileal resection or disease (parasites, Crohn's, blind loop, etc); autoimmune (pernicious anemia) accounts for majority of cases; dietary: lack of animal products (strict vegans, or vegetarians during pregnancy (increased requirements); other causes: pancreatic insufficiency, rare hereditary conditions (transcobalamin II deficiency or abnormal intrinsic factor) ●*Relieving factors:* Replenish stores - usually monthly IM injections until underlying disorder no longer exists; dietary modification ●*Clinical course:* Body stores (2-5mg) generally take years to deplete (typical diet has 5-20mcg/day); may coexist with folate deficiency; neurologic deficits can worsen over time; may not be reversible with long-standing duration; approx 10% of patients with B12 deficiency do not have anemia or neurologic findings ●*Co-morbidities:* Other autoimmune disease (i.e. thyroiditis) ●*Procedure results:* No relevant prcoedures ●*Test findings:* Blood smear with macro-ovalocytes, hypersegmented polymorphs. CBC with low hematocrit, elevated MCV. Abnormal Schilling test. Intrinsic factor Ab has 60% sensitivity, but high specificity. Antiparietal cell Ab has higher sensitivity but lower specificity. Serum homocysteine level may be elevated. Elevated methylmalonic acid seen in B12 deficiency, but not folate deficiency (can help distinguish these entities). Characteristic symmetric polyneuropathy can be suggestive. TSH should be screened every 1-2 years

Vitamin D excess ●*Onset:* Subacute to acute ●*Male:female ratio:* M=F ●*Ethnicity:* All ●*Character:* Hypercalcemia, metabolic bone disease ●*Location:* Increased absorption of calcium and phosphate from intestine, bone resorption, increased reabsorption of calcium and phosphate by kidney ●*Pattern:* Manifestations of hypercalcemia: nausea/vomiting, constipation, weakness, mental status changes, polyuria, polydipsia, muscle aches, pruritus, metastatic calcifications/nephrocalcinosis ●*Precipitating factors:* Increased ingestion of (dietary) vitamin D, excessively fortified milk, abnormal intestinal regulation/absorption, excessive exogenous vitamin D administration (i.e. for renal failure, hypoparathyroidism, osteoporosis), chronic granulomatous disease (granulomas produce 1,25 -(OH)2-D3) ●*Relieving factors:* IV fluids, stopping administration of vitamin D-containing substance sufficient in mild cases; lasix may be used after hydration; pamidronate if more severe hypercalcemia ●*Clinical course:* Persists as long as underlying cause exists (i.e. continued ingestion etc); ongoing effects at kidney, intestine, bone; feedback down-regulation of PTH often seen ●*Co-morbidities:* Bone disease; secondary effects of hypercalcemia (confusion, constipation, stones) ●*Procedure results:* No relevant procedures ●*Test findings:* High serum calcium; elevated 25-OH-D3. 1,25-(OH)2-D3 may also be elevated; PTH may be suppressed

Vitamin K deficiency ●*Onset:* Subacute to insidious ●*Male:female ratio:* M>F due to association with alcoholism ●*Ethnicity:* All ●*Character:* Poor clotting; bleeding diathesis, easy bruisability ●*Location:* Deep tissue (ecchymosis), bloody urine, stool, internal hemorrhage ●*Pattern:* Nonspecific ●*Precipitating factors:* Alcoholism, liver disease, poor nutrition (especially leafy greens), steatorrhea (inadequate absorption of fat-soluble vitamins), pancreatic insufficiency ●*Relieving factors:* Vitamin K supplementation; correction of underlying disorder ●*Clinical course:* Ongoing coagulopathy until deficiency corrected ●*Co-morbidities:* Bleeding diathesis (i.e. factor deficiency, thrombocytopenia) ●*Procedure results:* Serology ●*Test findings:* High INR in high risk patient

Vitiligo ●*Onset:* Subacute, insidious ●*Male:female ratio:* M=F ●*Ethnicity:* All ❶ *Character:* Skin lesions ❷ *Location:* Extensor bony surface, wrists, periorificial, lumbar ❸ *Pattern:* White macules ●*Precipitating factors:* None relevant ●*Relieving factors:* PUVA, steroids ●*Clinical course:* Persistent, progressive ●*Co-morbidities:* Thyroid, alopecia areata ●*Procedure results:* No relevant procedures ●*Test findings:* No relevant tests

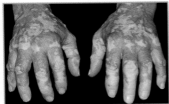

❶ *Character* Symmetric, sharply demarcated, loss of pigment on back of hands

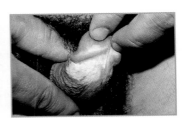

❷ *Location* The penis is a typical location

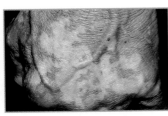

❸ *Pattern* Complete absence of pigment, sharp demarcation and scalloped borders

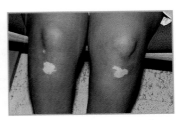

❸ *Pattern* Symmetric lesions on the legs

Vitreous opacities ●*Onset:* Acute, subacute, or insidious ●*Male:female ratio:* M=F ●*Ethnicity:* All ●*Character:* Can be asymptomatic; associated with blurred vision, floaters, or ocular redness, depending on the cause ●*Location:* One or both eyes ●*Pattern:* When symptomatic, there is generally no relation to time ●*Precipitating factors:* When secondary to endophthalmitis, there is often a history of recent cataract removal ●*Relieving factors:* Depends on the cause; only treatments directed to the underlying causes relieve symptoms ●*Clinical course:* Depends on the cause ●*Co-morbidities:* Vitreous opacities can be a sign of the benign condition asteroid hyalosis or a sign of many serious conditions such as pars planitis, endophthalmitis, leukemia ●*Procedure results:* Dilated fundus exam to ascertain the cause of vitreous opacities ●*Test findings:* RBCs, WBCs, tumor cells, pigment cells, or calcium deposits in the vitreous cavity

Vocal cord dysfunction ●*Onset:* Subacute to acute ●*Male:female ratio:* M:F ●*Ethnicity:* All ●*Character:* Inspiratory stridor; often normal voice; respiratory embarrassment ●*Location:* Vocal cord ●*Pattern:* Stridor often gradually progresses with time, diminishing exertional capacity ●*Precipitating factors:* Possibly antecedent viral illness ●*Relieving factors:* None relevant ●*Clinical course:* Slow progression of airway narrowing, often over the course of weeks to months ●*Co-morbidities:* Mediastinal malignancy; intracranial brain stem abnormality ●*Procedure results:* Flexible fiberoptic laryngoscopy reveals bilateral true vocal cord immobility, and narrow glottic airway ●*Test findings:* No relevant tests

Vocal cord nodules ●*Onset:* Subacute, insidious ●*Male:female ratio:* M=F ●*Ethnicity:* All ●*Character:* Hoarseness ●*Location:* Throat ●*Pattern:* Usually long-term history of hoarseness, often worse with additional voice use ●*Precipitating factors:* Excessive screaming, yelling, teaching, public speaking ●*Relieving factors:* Voice rest ●*Clinical course:* Poor-quality voice usually plateaus and persists for the long term ●*Co-morbidities:* None relevant ●*Procedure results:* Flexible fiberoptic laryngoscopy reveals bilateral true vocal cord nodules; laryngeal videostroboscopy confirms nodular nature of lesions ●*Test findings:* No relevant tests

Vocal cord polyp ●*Onset:* Variable ●*Male:female ratio:* M=F ●*Ethnicity:* All ●*Character:* Hoarseness ●*Location:* Throat ●*Pattern:* Persistent hoarseness, usually worse later in the day ●*Precipitating factors:* Excessive voice use; sudden screaming episode ●*Relieving factors:* Voice rest ●*Clinical course:* Usually persistent, requiring voice therapy or surgical therapy ●*Co-morbidities:* None relevant ●*Procedure results:* Flexible fiberoptic laryngoscopy reveals unilateral vocal cord polyp ●*Test findings:* No relevant tests

Volvulus ●*Onset:* Acute in infants, can be chronic in older children ●*Male:female ratio:* M=F ●*Ethnicity:* All ●*Character:* Gastric: severe epigastric pain/intractable nonbilious vomiting; midgut volvulus associated with malrotation: bilious emesis, abdominal pain, abdominal distension, diarrhea possibly asymptomatic ●*Location:* Abdomen ●*Pattern:* Acute can advance to perforation/chronic, can have usual symptoms and early satiety ●*Precipitating factors:* Gastric: absence/stretching of gastrohepatic/splenic/colic/phrenic ligaments; midgut volvulus associated with malrotation: incomplete rotation of intestine during fetal development; Ladd's bands ●*Relieving factors:* Surgery ●*Clinical course:* Acute or recurrent if chronic ●*Co-morbidities:* Gastric: intestinal malrotation, diaphragmatic defects, asplenia; midgut: malrotation, abdominal heterotaxia, asplenia-polysplenia, congenital heart syndrome ●*Procedure results:* KUB shows dilated stomach, upright films: double fluid level/beak near lower esophageal junction if mesenteroaxial volvulus (not seen in organoaxial volvulus); midgut: double bubble sign, UGI series shows abnormal ligament of Trietz position ●*Test findings:* No relevant tests

von Willebrand's disease ●*Onset:* Acute, insidious ●*Male:female ratio:* M=F ●*Ethnicity:* Scandinavia, Israel, Iran ●*Character:* Easy bleeding, bruising ●*Location:* Mucosal (epistaxis, gingival, menorrhagia), occasionally GI ●*Pattern:* Nonspecific ●*Precipitating factors:* Antiplatelet medications ●*Relieving factors:* Estrogen (pregnancy), presurgical - desmopressin acetate (for mild cases), factor VIII concentrates, cryoprecipitate, tranexamic acid (for dental procedures) ●*Clinical course:* Lifelong, mild, and often undiagnosed in mild cases ●*Co-morbidities:* None relevant ●*Procedure results:* No relevant procedures ●*Test findings:* Prolonged bleeding time (usually), reduced plasma vWF levels, reduced ristocetin cofactor activity

Vulval lichen sclerosis ●*Onset:* Insidious ●*Male:female ratio:* F ●*Ethnicity:* All ●*Character:* Soreness ●*Location:* Vulva ●*Pattern:* Shiny ivory white plaques ●*Precipitating factors:* None relevant ●*Relieving factors:* Topical steroids ●*Clinical course:* Persistent, progressive ●*Co-morbidities:* Morphea, vitiligo, squamous cell carcinoma ●*Procedure results:* No relevant procedures ●*Test findings:* Positive skin biopsy

Vulvar malignancy ●*Onset:* Insidious ●*Male:female ratio:* F ●*Ethnicity:* All ●*Character:* Long-standing vulvar pruritus, vulvar mass ●*Location:* Labia minora and majora ●*Pattern:* Raised, ulcerated, leukoplakic, wartlike ●*Precipitating factors:* Exposure to human papillomavirus ●*Relieving factors:* None relevant ●*Clinical course:* Progresses to invasion with distant metastases ●*Co-morbidities:* None relevant ●*Procedure results:* Dermal biopsy ●*Test findings:* Pathologic suggestion of cellular dysplasia

Wax in ear ●*Onset:* Insidious ●*Male:female ratio:* M=F ●*Ethnicity:* None ●*Character:* Ear pain, hearing loss, tinnitus ●*Location:* Affected ear ●*Pattern:* Persistent blockage ●*Precipitating factors:* Instrumentation of the ear by the patient ●*Relieving factors:* None relevant ●*Clinical course:* Chronic ●*Co-morbidities:* Dermatitis/eczema ●*Procedure results:* Otoscopy reveals wax plug in canal ●*Test findings:* No relevant tests

Weakness of pelvic floor muscles ●*Onset:* Insidious ●*Male:female ratio:* F ●*Ethnicity:* All ●*Character:* Incontinence, pelvic pressure ●*Location:* Vagina ●*Pattern:* Nonspecific ●*Precipitating factors:* Vaginal childbirth ●*Relieving factors:* Surgery, biofeedback, exercise ●*Clinical course:* Gradually worsens over years ●*Co-morbidities:* Multiple sclerosis ●*Procedure results:* Urodynamic testing to distinguish stress incontinence from detrusor instability ●*Test findings:* No relevant tests

Wegener's granulomatosis ●*Onset:* Subacute, insidious ●*Male:female ratio:* M(3):F(2) ●*Ethnicity:* All ●*Character:* Persistent rhinorrhea with purulent or bloody nasal discharge, oral and/or nasal ulcers, polyarthralgias, myalgias, sinus pain, cough, dyspnea, hemoptysis ●*Location:* Chest, upper airways, kidneys, joints, nervous system, skin, eyes, heart ●*Pattern:* Chest - focal or diffuse inspiratory rales, expiratory rhonchi, pleural rub. Upper airway - oral ulcers or purulent or bloody nasal discharge. Skin - vesicular, purpuric, or hemorrhagic lesions. Eyes - conjunctivitis or episcleritis. Nervous system - mononeuritis multiplex, cranial nerve abnormalities. Heart - pericardial rub, arrhythmia ●*Precipitating factors:* None relevant ●*Relieving factors:* Cyclophosphamide (1-2mg/kg/day orally) for 12-24 months (i.e. 6 months after remission) plus prednisone (0.5-1mg/kg/day orally for 7-14 days, then taper to 10-15mg/day until remission). Add trimethoprim/sulfamethoxazole three times weekly for Pneumocystis carinii pneumonia prophylaxis. Role of plasmapheresis is controversial. Renal replacement therapy as needed ●*Clinical course:* Progressive without treatment (90% mortality within 2 years), yet remission achieved in c.75% with 12-24 months of cyclophosphamide ●*Co-morbidities:* Other connective tissue diseases and antiglomerular basement membrane disease ●*Procedure results:* Biopsy of nasal mucosa or lung may reveal granulomatous inflammation with vasculitis; renal biopsy reveals segmental necrotizing glomerulonephritis with little Ig deposition ●*Test findings:* Positive serum antineutrophil cytoplasmic antibody (ANCA), chest X-ray may show nodules (some cavitate), interstitial, alveolar or pleural infiltrates; urinalysis reveals blood with RBC casts, peripheral blood - leukocytosis, thrombocytosis, normochromic, normocytic anemia, elevated sedimentation rate

Wernicke's encephalopathy ●*Onset:* Subacute, acute, insidious ●*Male:female ratio:* M=F ●*Ethnicity:* All ●*Character:* Ophthalmoplegia/nystagmus, mental status change/dementia, and ataxia/gait abnormality. Presence of all components not necessary for diagnosis ●*Location:* Nonspecific ●*Pattern:* Nonspecific ●*Precipitating factors:* Long term alcohol abuse ●*Relieving factors:* Administration of thiamine IV ●*Clinical course:* Usually improves slowly ●*Co-morbidities:* Korsakoff's psychosis presents with confabulation; loss of recent memory; loss of retention and recall ●*Procedure results:* No relevant procedures ●*Test findings:* No relevant tests

Whipple's disease ●*Onset:* Insidious ●*Male:female ratio:* M>F ●*Ethnicity:* All ●*Character:* Progressive arthralgia, abdominal pain, malabsorptive diarrhea, weight loss, wasting, skin pigmentation; occasional CNS, heart, or eye involvement ●*Location:* Small intestines, large joints, skin, myocardium, endocardium, CNS, cranial nerves, uvea, other ●*Pattern:* Low grade fever; steatorrhea, nystagmus, ophthalmoplegia, and memory loss are common with CNS involvement ●*Precipitating factors:* None relevant ●*Relieving factors:* None relevant ●*Clinical course:* Illness can progress to death within months without antimicrobial administration; remission common with prolonged antimicrobial therapy; relapse is common (40%) ●*Co-morbidities:* Malabsorption, vitamin deficiency, anemia ●*Procedure results:* Dilated lymphatics on jejunal biopsies; rod-shaped bacteria (Tropheryma whippelii) seen on electron microscopic evaluation of biopsy material; detection of T. whippelii DNA by PCR in blood or CSF ●*Test findings:* Anemia, hypoalbuminemia, impaired xylose absorption, periodic acid schiff staining granules in bowel macrophages

Williams syndrome ●*Onset:* Subacute ●*Male:female ratio:* M=F ●*Ethnicity:* All ●*Character:* Growth and mental deficiency, rounded facial features, medial eyebrow flare, stellate iris, strabismus, short palpebral fissures, depressed nasal bridge, prominent lips, hoarse voice, hypertension ●*Location:* Facies/cardiovascular ●*Pattern:* Nonspecific ●*Precipitating factors:* Microdeletion of 7q23- ●*Relieving factors:* Treat cardiovascular anomalies ●*Clinical course:* Lifelong ●*Co-morbidities:* Supravalvular aortic stenosis, peripheral pulmonary artery stenosis, pulmonic valvular stenosis, VSD/ASD, renal artery stenosis ●*Procedure results:* Abnormal Echo, cardiac catheterization ●*Test findings:* No relevant tests

Wilson's disease ●*Onset:* Autosomal recessive ●*Male:female ratio:* M=F ●*Ethnicity:* All ●*Character:* Hepatic dysfunction: malaise, anorexia, fluctuating jaundice, neurologic dysfunction: dystonic facies, dystonic upper extremity posturing, 'wing beating' tremor, loss of coordination, intellectual deterioration, Kayser-Fleischer ring ●*Location:* Liver ●*Pattern:* Nonspecific ●*Precipitating factors:* Autosomal recessive ●*Relieving factors:* Copper chelation with penicillamine, trientine, oral zinc, but normal function may not return; liver transplantation ●*Clinical course:* Progressive ●*Co-morbidities:* None relevant ●*Procedure results:* Slit lamp exam may reveal Kayser-Fleischer ring; liver biopsy shows increased copper ●*Test findings:* Low serum ceruloplasmin, increased urinary copper, hemolytic anemia

Wolff-Parkinson-White syndrome ●*Onset:* Congenital ●*Male:female ratio:* M>F ●*Ethnicity:* All ●*Character:* Usually asymptomatic, but may present with palpitations ●*Location:* Nonspecific ●*Pattern:* Palpitations are episodic ●*Precipitating factors:* Palpitations usually spontaneous, but may be precipitated by exercise, caffeine ●*Relieving factors:* Palpitations/arrhythmia may break with vagal maneuvers/AV-nodal medications. Avoid these therapies in WPW with atrial fibrillation ●*Clinical course:* Congenital condition that remains asymptomatic or results in episodic arrhythmia; electrophysiology study and radiofrequency ablation is curative ●*Co-morbidities:* Ebstein's anomaly ●*Procedure results:* No relevant procedures ●*Test findings:* Short PR interval on EKG (<0.12s), slurred QRS upstroke (delta wave)

Wrist injury ●*Onset:* Acute ●*Male:female ratio:* M=F ●*Ethnicity:* All ●*Character:* Pain, swelling, tenderness of wrist ●*Location:* Wrist ●*Pattern:* Nonspecific ●*Precipitating factors:* Fall on outstretched arm or direct blow to wrist ●*Relieving factors:* Splinting of sprains and nondisplaced fractures. Reduction of displaced fractures. Ice, anti-inflammatories ●*Clinical course:* Variable ●*Co-morbidities:* None relevant ●*Procedure results:* No relevant procedures ●*Test findings:* Radiographs required to rule out fractures or dislocations; scaphoid bone fracture may not be evident on initial radiographs

Yellow fever ●*Onset:* Acute ●*Male:female ratio:* M>F ●*Ethnicity:* All ●*Character:* Hemorrhagic fever - abrupt onset, followed by remission. Remittence with jaundice, hemorrhages, black vomit, anuria, delirium ●*Location:* Systemic - viremia, liver, GI tract, prerenal, brain (toxic-metabolic) injury ●*Pattern:* Biphasic - abrupt onset of fever, chills, myalgia and relative bradycardia. Remission follows - then recurrent fever with jaundice, hemorrhages, multi-organ involvement ●*Precipitating factors:* Mosquito bite in endemic areas - residence in/travel to tropical Africa and South America. Agricultural and forest work ●*Relieving factors:* Preventive vaccine ●*Clinical course:* More than 80% of cases subclinical; symptomatic illness incubates for 3-6 days, then 3-4 days viremia/early fever followed by short remission; 'intoxication', with 20-50% mortality on day 7-10 ●*Co-morbidities:* GI bleeding ●*Procedure results:* No relevant procedures ●*Test findings:* Early leukopenia, late leukocytosis; thrombocytopenia, albuminuria, elevated direct bilirubin, elevated hepatic transaminases, azotemia; late hypoglycemia and lactic acidosis

Yersinia ●*Onset:* Acute ●*Male:female ratio:* M=F ●*Ethnicity:* All ●*Character:* Abdominal cramps, low-grade fever and vomiting, diarrhea lasting around 14 days ●*Location:* Intestines and mesenteric lymph nodes; mesenteric veins, peritoneum, bile ducts and gall bladder, liver, pharynx; rarely bloodstream ●*Pattern:* Prolonged diarrhea, mesenteric adenitis may be confused with appendicitis; rarely generalized maculopapular rash ●*Precipitating factors:* Consumption of contaminated food (raw milk, meat, vegetables, fresh water), contact with contaminated soil, person-to-person fecal-oral transmission ●*Relieving factors:* None relevant ●*Clinical course:* Prolonged diarrhea, fecal bacteria excretions for 4-79 days; most cases self-limiting, but symptoms prolonged; persistent bacteremia may occur - severe complications possible ●*Co-morbidities:* Reactive arthritis, Reiter's syndrome, mesenteric vein thrombosis, bowel perforation, peritonitis, erythema nodosum ●*Procedure results:* No relevant procedures ●*Test findings:* Isolation of Y. enterocolitica from stool or other site (blood, lymph node aspirate, CSF, other), positive serologic tests; leukocytosis with a slight left shift

Zollinger-Ellison syndrome ● *Onset:* Insidious, subacute ● *Male:female ratio:* M(3):F(2) ● *Ethnicity:* All ● *Character:* Peptic ulcer disease - epigastric pain not responsive to standard antacid therapy; watery diarrhea, often predating ulcer; dyspepsia in 30-60%; gastrinoma ● *Location:* Epigastrium ● *Pattern:* Nonspecific ● *Precipitating factors:* None relevant ● *Relieving factors:* Therapy for pain and diarrhea; resection of gastrinoma ● *Clinical course:* No remission, 60% are malignant and slowly progress to metastatic disease ● *Co-morbidities:* Multiple endocrine neoplasia type I (MEN1) ● *Procedure results:* EGD: multiple duodenal ulcers. Octreotide scan: often shows duodenal/pancreatic gastrinoma ● *Test findings:* Fasting serum gastrin is markedly elevated